PHYSICAL DIAGNOSIS

SECRETS

Second Edition

Salvatore Mangione, MD

Associate Professor of Medicine
Director, Physical Diagnosis Course
Jefferson Medical College of Thomas Jefferson University
Philadelphia, Pennsylvania

MOSBY

ELSEVIER

MOSBY
ELSEVIER

1600 John F. Kennedy Boulevard, Suite 1800
Philadelphia, PA 19103-2899

Physical Diagnosis Secrets   ISBN-978-0-323-03467-8
Second Edition

NOTICE

Knowledge and best practice in this field are constantly changing. As new research and
experience broaden our knowledge, changes in practice, treatment and drug therapy
may become necessary or appropriate. Readers are advised to check the most current
information provided (i) on procedures featured or (ii) by the manufacturer of each
product to be administered, to verify the recommended dose or formula, the method and
duration of administration, and contraindications. It is the responsibility of the
practitioner, relying on his or her own experience and knowledge of the patient, to make
diagnoses, to determine dosages and the best treatment for each individual patient, and
to take all appropriate safety precautions. To the fullest extent of the law, neither the
Publisher nor the Editor assumes any liability for any injury and/or damage to persons or
property arising out or related to any use of the material contained in this book.

Library of Congress Cataloging-in-Publication Data

Mangione, Salvatore, 1954-
   Physical Diagnosis Secrets / Salvatore Mangione. – 2nd ed.
      p.; cm.
   Includes bibliographical references and index.
   ISBN 978-0-323-03467-8
   1. Physical Diagnosis–Miscellanea.   I. Title. [DNLM: 1. Physical Examination–
   Examination Questions.   2. Diagnostic Techniques and Procedures–Examination
   Questions.   3. Signs and Symptoms–Examination Questions.   WB 18.2 M277p 2008]
RC76.P524 2008
616.07'54076–dc22   2007003812

Senior Acquisitions Editor: James Merritt
Developmental Editor: Stan Ward
Project Manager: Mary B. Stermel
Marketing Manager: Alyson Sherby

Printed in China

Working together to grow
libraries in developing countries

www.elsevier.com | www.bookaid.org | www.sabre.org

ELSEVIER   BOOK AID International   Sabre Foundation

Last digit is the print number: 9   8   7   6   5   4   3   2   1

DEDICATION

To my dog Springy, who speaks softly but carries a big stick;

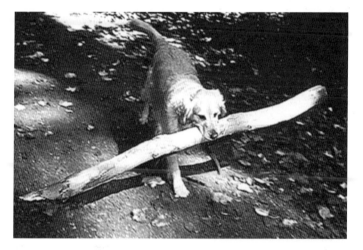

and to my daughter Gemma, who does the opposite.

Seek, and ye shall find.
Matthew 7:7

To be able to explore is, in my opinion, a large part of the Art.
Hippocrates, *Epidemics III*

It was six men of Indostan, to learning much inclined,
who went to see the elephant (though all of them were blind),
that each by observation might satisfy his mind.

The first approached the elephant and happening to fall,
against his broad and sturdy side, at once began to bawl:
"God bless me! But the elephant is nothing but a wall!"

The second, feeling of the tusk, cried, "Ho! what have we here,
so very round and smooth and sharp? To me 'tis mighty clear,
this wonder of an elephant is very like a spear!"

The third approached the animal, and happening to take
the squirming trunk within his hands, "I see," quoth he,
"the elephant is very like a snake!"

The fourth reached out his eager hand and feels about the knee:
"What most this wondrous beast is like, is mighty plain," quoth he,
"'Tis clear enough the elephant is very like a tree."

The fifth, who chanced to touch the ear, said: "E'en the blindest man
can tell what this resembles most: Deny the fact who can,
This marvel of an elephant is very like a fan!"

The sixth no sooner had begun about the beast to grope,
than, seizing the swinging tail, that fell within his scope,
"I see," quoth he, "the elephant is very like a rope!"

So, oft in theologic wars, the disputants, I ween,
tread in utter ignorance of what each other mean,
and prate about the elephant, not one of them has seen!

John Godfrey Saxe (1816–1887)

CONTENTS

CONTRIBUTORS

Enrica Arnaudo, MD
Clinical Assistant Professor of Neurology, Thomas Jefferson University, Philadelphia, Pennsylvania; Director, Neuromuscular Disease Program, Neuroscience and Surgery Institute of Delaware, Wilmington, Delaware

Michael D. Kim, MD
Neurology Fellow, Thomas Jefferson University, Philadelphia, Pennsylvania

PREFACE

Preface to the First Edition

Physical diagnosis occupies an uncertain position at the turn of the millennium. There has been recent interest in validating, refining, and sometimes discarding traditional methods and signs. A physical diagnosis interest group has arisen within the general internal medicine community. The *American College of Physicians* has sponsored an update course and bibliography on physical diagnosis, and The *Journal of the American Medical Association* has initiated a series of articles on the "rational clinical examination." Perhaps most importantly, physicians in practice rate history-taking and physical examination as their most valuable skills. On the other hand, a distressing literature documents the lack of competence in physical diagnosis among primary care residents and even physicians-in-practice. Few training programs provide structured teaching in these skills, and attending "rounds" too often avoid the bedside.

Still, there are plenty of reasons to promote the teaching of physical examination. Among these are cost-effectiveness, the possibility of making inexpensive serial observations, the early detection of critical findings, the intelligent and well-guided selection of costly diagnostic technology, and the therapeutic value of the physical contact between physician and patient. In times when the "fun" seems to have abandoned the practice of medicine, physical diagnosis and other bedside skills can even restore the satisfaction and intellectual pleasure of making a diagnosis using only our own wits and senses.

In reviewing the various maneuvers and findings which, over the centuries, created physical examination, we made a deliberate attempt at presenting some information about the men and women behind the eponyms (and for this we relied on that great little book by B.G. Firkin and J.A. Whitworth, *The Dictionary of Medical Eponyms*). We believe that learning about the character and personality of these physicians might shed some light on why physical diagnosis enjoyed so many contributions in the last century and so few in our own. The great bedside diagnosticians of the last century were passionately interested in everything human. Most, if not all of them, were humanists, lovers of the arts and literature, travelers and historians, poets and painters, curious of any field that could enrich the human spirit. William Osler, the pinnacle of 19th century bedside medicine, believed so strongly in the value of a liberal education that he provided his medical students with a list of ten books (ranging from Plutarch and Montaigne to Marcus Aurelius and Shakespeare) to read for half an hour before going to sleep.

As Bernard Lown puts it, today's physicians "seem at times more interested in laying on tools than laying on hands." Rejuvenating physical diagnosis might, therefore, require a revival of the time-honored link between the art and the science of medicine. We agree with William Osler that Medicine is "an art of probabilities and a science of uncertainties" and that these two aspects are inseparable, very much like Siamese twins: trying to separate one from the other would only kill both. Rekindling interest in the bedside and in the humanistic aspect of medicine, therefore, may represent two facets of the same challenge. We also agree with Socrates that one of the most effective ways to teach is to question. We hope that *Physical Diagnosis Secrets*, in following this tradition and that of the proven and time-tested *Secrets Series*, will serve as a valuable and engaging resource for learning and truly appreciating the art and science of physical diagnosis.

Salvatore Mangione, MD
Philadelphia, 2000

Preface to the Second Edition

It is amazing how quickly time flies. When I was preparing the first edition of *Physical Diagnosis Secrets*, my daughter was still sleeping in 101-Dalmatians bed sheets. Now that the first edition has been through four (and soon *five*) translations into foreign languages, she is about to graduate from college. And a new edition is ready to print.

Books we write have been compared to children, insofar as they teach us through the mistakes we make. Not that in my case (child or otherwise) there were many mistakes to learn from, but still it was good to have an opportunity for revisiting and expanding most of the chapters. Indeed, some were almost completely rewritten. In addition, we decided to make available to book buyers the online access to the highly successful *Heart and Lung Sounds Secrets* Cardio-Pulmonary Auscultation Workshop, which comes free once you activate the PIN found on the inside front cover by going to www.studentconsult.com. Since 40% of all errors in physical diagnosis are related to the cardiopulmonary exam, this simple but helpful tool will increase tremendously the educational value provided by the new edition. As for all other Elsevier books, buyers will also have complete free access to the Internet-based *Student Consult*, which not only provides an electronic version of *Physical Diagnosis Secrets* but also offers pictures and audiovisual adjuncts, plus algorithms that can help the user find a way through the various questions of each chapter.

Although these changes have surely made the new edition stronger, they have not altered the proven and time-tested Socratic approach of questions and answers that has made the *Secrets Series* so successful. This edition also continues to emphasize the evidence behind the signs and maneuvers so that readers can best sort the wheat from chaff in their daily practice. Finally, it has maintained the *whodunnit* approach to eponyms, rediscovering the men and women behind the signs, with all their quirks and rich humanity. We owe it to them and their ingenuity if medicine remains a science *and* an art. In this regard, we hope that the final product will continue to foster a lifelong interest in the time-honored art of bedside examination, one highly rewarding to its users, but also highly endangered—especially in our new millennium of high technology and low skills.

As one of the masters of physical exam (John Brereton Barlow) used to put it, we dedicate this book to *all students of medicine who listen, look, touch, and reflect. May they hear, see, feel, and comprehend.*

Salvatore Mangione, MD

TOP 100 SECRETS

These secrets are 100 of the top board alerts. They summarize the basic concepts, principles, and most salient details of physical diagnosis.

1. A postural *dizziness* (severe enough to stop the test) or an increase in heart rate of at least 30 beats/minute has sensitivity of 97% and specificity of 96% for blood loss >630 mL. *Unless associated with dizziness,* postural hypotension of any degree has little value.

2. Body fat "distributions" by *waist circumference* (WC) and *waist-to-hip ratio* (WHR) *are* much better markers for cardiovascular risk than the body mass index (BMI) alone. In fact, a WC <100 cm practically excludes insulin resistance.

3. An *acute* difference in systolic pressure >20 mmHg between the two arms usually indicates *aortic dissection* (complicated by aortic regurgitation in cases of more proximal dissection). If chronic, it indicates instead a subclavian artery occlusion or a *subclavian steal syndrome.*

4. An ankle-to-arm systolic pressure index (AAI) <0.97 identifies patients with angiographically proven occlusions/stenoses of lower extremities arteries with 96% sensitivity and 94–100% specificity. Most patients with claudication will have AAI values between 0.5 and 0.8, whereas those with pain at rest will have values <0.5. Indexes <0.2 are associated with ischemic or gangrenous extremities.

5. Paired, transverse, white nail bands in the second, third, and fourth fingers (Muehrcke's lines) suggest chronic hypoalbuminemia, occurring in more than three quarters of patients with nephrotic syndrome (<2.3 gm/100 mL) but also in liver disease and malnutrition.

6. In a study of 118 subjects with acrochordons (skin tags), 41% had either impaired glucose tolerance or overt type 2 diabetes.

7. Ten percent of patients with vitiligo have serologic or clinical evidence of autoimmune disorders; the most common are thyroid diseases, especially hypothyroidism of the Hashimoto variety. Diabetes, Addison's, pernicious anemia, alopecia areata, and uveitis (Vogt-Koyanagi syndrome) also are frequent.

8. Twenty percent of patients with acanthosis nigricans (AN) have an aggressive underlying neoplasm—a gastrointestinal (GI) adenocarcinoma in 90% of cases, and a gastric in 60%. Still, most patients with AN have just obesity and insulin resistance.

9. To separate icterus from the brownish color normally present in the bulbar conjunctiva of dark-skinned individuals, ask the patient to look upward. Then inspect the inferior conjunctival recess. This should be entirely white in nonicteric subjects, since the brownish discoloration of these individuals is the result of sunlight exposure.

10. *Earliest signs* of nonproliferative diabetic retinopathy include *microaneurysms* and *dot* intraretinal hemorrhages, with progression of disease characterized by an increase in number and size of microaneurysms and intraretinal hemorrhages (both *dot* and *blot*). Soft exudates are not as predictive, and hard exudates even less.

11. Diagonal earlobe creases in adults are an acquired phenomenon and a significant independent variable for coronary artery disease. *Hair in the external ear canal* also seems to be associated with coronary artery disease.

12. Findings that can best separate patients *with* and *without* strep throat are (1) pharyngeal or tonsillar *exudates,* (2) *fever* by history, (3) tonsillar enlargement, (4) tenderness or enlargement of the anterior cervical and jugulodigastric lymph nodes, and (5) absence of cough.

13. Multiple white, warty, corrugated, and painless plaques on the lateral margins of the tongue (*hairy leukoplakia*) represent an Epstein-Barr–induced lesion typical of HIV infection, even though this can also occur In severely immunocompromised *organ transplant patients.* If present, it carries a worse prognosis for HIV progression.

14. Pemberton's maneuver (reversible superior vena cava obstruction caused by a substernal goiter being "lifted" into the thoracic inlet as a result of arm raising) is a nonspecific finding that may be encountered in patients with substernal thyroid masses, lymphomas, or upper mediastinal tumors.

15. The average size of a thyroid nodule detected on exam is 3 cm. In fact, the larger the nodule, the more likely its detection (with <1 cm nodules being missed 90% of the time; <2 cm nodules 50% of the time).

16. Findings most suggestive of hyperthyroidism include lid retraction (likelihood ratio [LR] = 31.5), lid lag (LR = 17.6), fine finger tremor (LR = 11.4), moist and warm skin (LR = 6.7), and tachycardia (LR = 4.4). Findings more likely to rule *out* hyperthyroidism are normal thyroid size (LR = 0.1), heart rate <90/minute (LR = 0.2), and no finger tremor (LR = 0.3). Older hyperthyroid patients exhibit more anorexia and atrial fibrillation; more frequent lack of goiter; and overall *fewer* signs, with tachycardia, fatigue, and weight loss in more than 50% of patients (and all three in 32%).

17. Findings more strongly suggestive of hypothyroidism are bradycardia (LR = 3.88), abnormal ankle reflex (LR = 3.41), and coarse skin (LR = 2.3). No single finding, when absent, can effectively rule *out* hypothyroidism.

18. Clinical breast exam (CBE) has low sensitivity for the detection of breast masses, high specificity, and accuracy that can be increased by (1) longer duration of exam (at least 3 minutes per breast); (2) higher number of correct steps (a systematic and vertical search pattern, thoroughness, varying palpation pressure, use of three fingers, finger pads, and circular motion); and (3) examiner experience (previous training with silicone models).

19. A brisk arterial upstroke with a *widened pulse pressure* indicates *aortic regurgitation (AR).* A brisk arterial upstroke with a *normal pulse pressure* instead indicates either the simultaneous emptying of the left ventricle into a high pressure bed (the aorta) *and* a lower pressure bed (like the right ventricle in patients with ventricular septal defect, or the left atrium in patients with mitral regurgitation) or *hypertrophic obstructive cardiomyopathy* (HOCM).

20. The alternation of strong and weak arterial pulses despite *regular rate* and *rhythm* (pulsus alternans) indicates severe left ventricular dysfunction, with worse ejection fraction and higher pulmonary capillary pressure. Hence, it is often associated with an S_3 gallop.

21. Visible neck veins in the upright position indicate a central venous pressure >7 cmH$_2$O and thus are pathologic.

22. In chronic heart failure, jugular venous distention represents an ominous *prognostic* variable, independently associated with adverse outcomes, including risk of death or hospitalization. The presence of S_3 is similarly (and independently) associated with increased risk.

23. Presence of either end-inspiratory crackles or distended neck veins has high specificity (90–100%) but low sensitivity (10–50%) for increased *left-sided* filling pressure due to either systolic or diastolic dysfunction.

24. Positive abdominojugular reflux has equally high specificity (but better sensitivity, 55–85%) for increased *left-sided* filling pressure. S_3 gallop, downward and lateral displacement of the apical impulse, and peripheral edema also have high specificity (>95%) but low sensitivity (10–40%). Of these, only the S_3 and the displaced apical impulse have a positive likelihood ratio (5.7 and 5.8, respectively).

25. In patients presenting with dyspnea, an abdominojugular reflux argues in favor of *bi*-ventricular failure and suggests a *pulmonary capillary wedge pressure* >15 mmHg. Conversely, a negative abdominojugular reflux in a patient with dyspnea argues strongly *against* increased left atrial pressure.

26. *Posturally induced crackles (PICs)* after myocardial infarction (MI) carry an ominous significance, reflecting higher pulmonary capillary wedge pressure, lower pulmonary venous compliance, and higher mortality. After the number of diseased coronary vessels and the patient's pulmonary capillary wedge pressure, PICs rank third as most important predictor of recovery after an acute MI.

27. Ischemic heart disease patients with S_3 have a 1-year mortality that is much higher than those *without* it (57% versus 14%). The same applies to a displaced apical impulse (39% versus 12%).

28. Leg swelling without increased central venous pressure (CVP) suggests bilateral venous insufficiency or noncardiac edema (hepatic or renal).

29. The Valsalva maneuver has excellent specificity and sensitivity (90–99% and 70–95%, respectively) for detecting left ventricular dysfunction, either systolic or diastolic.

30. The PPP (*proportional pulse pressure*—arterial pulse pressure divided by the systolic blood pressure) has excellent sensitivity (91%) and specificity (83%) for identifying low cardiac index (CI). A PPP <0.25 has a positive likelihood ratio of 5.4 for CI of 2.2 L/min/m^2.

31. Patients with distended neck veins, dyspnea/tachypnea, tachycardia, and clear lungs should be thought of as having tamponade; thus, their *pulsus paradoxus* must be measured.

32. A pulsus paradoxus >21 mmHg has good sensitivity and excellent specificity for tamponade. It also may be palpable.

33. A paradoxical increase in venous distention during *inspiration* (Kussmaul's sign) is *not* a feature of tamponade but does occur in 30–50% of patients with "pure" constrictive pericarditis; 90% of patients with *constrictive pericarditis* also have a retracting apical impulse.

34. A loud S_1 should always alert the clinician to the possibility of mitral stenosis and should thus prompt a search for its associated diastolic rumble.

35. An audible physiologic splitting of S_2 is age dependent, present in 60% of subjects younger than 30 and 30% of those older than 60.

36. Wide splitting of S_2 usually reflects a delayed closure of the pulmonic valve because of either a right bundle branch block or pulmonary hypertension.

37. S_2 that remains audibly split *throughout respiration,* both in the supine and upright positions, with a *consistent interval* between its two components, argues in favor of an atrial septal defect.

38. S_2 that becomes audibly split only in *exhalation,* while remaining single in *inspiration* (*paradoxical or reversed splitting*), means pathology until proven otherwise. This is usually an increased impedance to left ventricular emptying (aortic stenosis, coarctation, or hypertension), a left bundle branch block, or a transient, left ventricular ischemia.

39. A loud and ringing S_2, rich in overtones and *tambour like* ("drum" in French), indicates a dilation of the aortic root. When associated with an aortic regurgitation murmur, it suggests Marfan syndrome, syphilis (Potain's sign), or a dissecting aneurysm of the ascending aorta (Harvey's sign).

40. S_3 is such an accurate predictor of *systolic* dysfunction (and elevated atrial pressure) that its absence argues in favor of an ejection fraction >30%.

41. In patients with congestive heart failure, S_3 is the best predictor for response to digitalis and overall mortality. It correlates with high levels of B-type natriuretic peptide (BNP), and if associated with elevated jugular venous pressure, it predicts more frequent hospitalizations and worse outcome. S_3 is also the most significant predictor of cardiac risk during noncardiac surgery. If preoperative diuresis is not instituted, it can also predict mortality. Finally, the presence of S_3 in mitral regurgitation reflects worse disease (i.e., higher filling pressure, lower ejection fraction, and more severe regurgitation).

42. S_4 reflects an increase in *late* ventricular diastolic pressure (hence a *diastolic* dysfunction); but, in contrast to S_3, it reflects normal atrial pressure, normal cardiac output, and normal ventricular diameter.

43. S_4 can be heard in as many as 90% of patients with MI, but eventually resolves. Presence of S_4 at more than 1 month after MI does predict a higher 5-year mortality rate.

44. An early systolic (ejection) sound indicates *normal* ejection of blood through an *abnormal aortic valve (i.e., bicuspid), normal* ejection of blood into a *stiffened and dilated* aortic root (i.e., hypertension, atherosclerosis, aortic aneurysm, or aortic regurgitation), or *forceful* ejection of blood into a *normal* aortic root (high output states like aortic regurgitation).

45. An aortic ES in patients with aortic regurgitation (AR) argues in favor of *valvular* AR, possibly due to a *bicuspid* valve.

46. In mitral valve prolapse (MVP), clickers stay clickers and murmurers murmurers. This may have implication for prophylaxis.

47. One tenth of all rubs are associated with a pericardial effusion. In fact, rubs can occur in up to one fourth of *tamponade* cases. Hence, *measure pulsus paradoxus in all patients with a rub.*

48. All right-sided auscultatory findings (*except the pulmonic ejection sound*) get louder on *inspiration* (Rivero Carvallo maneuver).

49. A murmur that intensifies with Valsalva or squatting-to-standing is due to either HOCM or MVP.

50. A longer diastolic pause (such as that following a premature beat) intensifies the murmur of *aortic stenosis* but not that of mitral regurgitation.

51. A benign "functional" murmur should be *systolic, short, soft* (typically <3/6), early peaking (never passing midsystole), predominantly *circumscribed* to the base, and associated with a well-preserved and normally split second sound. It should have an otherwise normal cardiovascular exam (i.e., *no bad company*); and it often disappears with sitting, standing, or straining (as, for example, following a Valsalva maneuver).

52. A "bad" systolic murmur instead should be long, loud (in fact, pathologic by definition if loud enough to generate a *thrill*), late peaking, nonlocalized, and associated with a soft-to-absent S_2 that does not normally split. It also should be accompanied by other abnormal findings/symptoms ("bad" company).

53. The murmur of *aortic sclerosis* is the most common systolic ejection murmur of the elderly, affecting 21–26% of persons older than 65 and 55–75% of octogenarians and carrying a 40% increased risk of myocardial infarction.

54. Presence of an *early systolic (ejection) click* in aortic stenosis (AS) usually indicates a *valvular* AS, typically due to a congenitally bicuspid aortic valve.

55. Some patients with AS may exhibit a dissociation of the systolic murmur into two components, with medium frequencies transmitted to the base and high frequencies to the apex, almost mimicking MR (Gallavardin phenomenon).

56. Findings arguing most strongly in favor of AS are a reduced/delayed carotid upstroke, a mid-to-late peak of the murmur, a soft-to-absent A_2, a palpable precordial thrill, and an apical-carotid (or brachioradial) delay. Conversely, lack of radiation to the right carotid artery argues most strongly *against* AS. A normal rate of rise of the arterial pulse argues also against the presence of significant AS, but only in the young.

57. The best bedside predictors for severity/clinical outcome of AS are (1) murmur *intensity* and *timing* (the louder and later-peaking the murmur, the worse the disease); (2) a *single* S_2; and (3) *delayed upstroke/reduced amplitude of the carotid pulse* (pulsus parvus and tardus). Still, no single physical finding has both high sensitivity and specificity for detecting *severe* valvular obstruction.

58. Presence of an audible S_4 in AS reflects severe left ventricular hypertrophy (with a transvalvular pressure gradient >70 mmHg), but *only* in younger patients (older subjects may already have a "normal" S_4). Yet, a *palpable* S_4 always reflects severe disease.

59. In cardiac auscultation, the louder (and the longer) the murmur, the worse the underlying disease. The only exception is severe aortic stenosis with decreased cardiac output.

60. *Plateau* mitral regurgitation (MR) murmurs are more likely to be *rheumatic*, whereas murmurs that start in midsystole and "grow" into S_2 are more likely to be due to either *mitral valve prolapse* or *papillary muscle dysfunction.*

61. The *acute* MR murmur is often early systolic (exclusively so in 40% of cases) and is associated with S_4 in 80% of the patients.

62. *Valvular* aortic regurgitation (AR) tends to be loudest over the Erb's point (left parasternal area), whereas "root" AR is loudest over the aortic area (right parasternal area).

63. The Austin-Flint murmur may occur in more than 50% of moderate to severe AR cases, usually requiring a regurgitant volume of at least 50 mL.

64. A palpable pulsus bisferiens usually reflects *moderate to severe aortic regurgitation* (with or without aortic stenosis).

65. A difference in systolic pressure $\geq$60 mmHg between upper and lower extremities (Hill's sign) has high specificity and a very high positive likelihood ratio for *severe aortic regurgitation*, but a sensitivity of only 40%. So do a diastolic blood pressure $\leq$50 mmHg *and* a pulse pressure $\geq$80 mmHg.

66. *Traube pistol shot sound(s)* and *Duroziez double murmur* have sensitivity of 37–55% for AR and specificity of 63–98%. Neither predicts severity.

67. The alternate reddening and blanching of the fingernails, coinciding with each cardiac cycle and easily visualized by lightly compressing the nail bed with a glass slide (*Quincke's pulse*), *is* one of the many peripheral signs of AR, albeit a nonspecific and vastly discredited one.

68. You diagnose *aortic* regurgitation in diastole, but you assess its severity in systole (through the presence of a flow murmur and possibly an ejection click). Conversely, you diagnose mitral regurgitation in systole, but you assess its severity in diastole (through the presence of an S_3 and possibly a diastolic flow rumble).

69. Tachypnea is so frequent in pulmonary embolism (92% of patients) that a normal respiratory rate argues strongly against the diagnosis.

70. Unlike orthopnea, platypnea (an obligatory "*supine respiration*") is usually due to a right-to-left shunt. This can be either intracardiac or intrapulmonary (typically bibasilar and common in cirrhotic patients—*hepatopulmonary syndrome*).

71. Abdominal paradox has high sensitivity (95%) and good specificity (71%) for impending respiratory failure, usually preceding arterial blood gases' deterioration.

72. Upward inspiratory motion of the clavicle in excess of 5 mm is a valuable sign of severe obstructive disease, correlating with FEV_1 of 0.6 L.

73. The distance between the top of the thyroid cartilage and the suprasternal notch (laryngeal height) is a strong predictor of postoperative pulmonary risk if $\leq$4 cm.

74. The *forced expiratory time* (FET) is the best bedside predictor of the *severity* of airflow obstruction. FETo >6 seconds corresponds to an FEV_1/FVC <40%. Conversely, FETo <5 seconds indicates an FEV_1/FVC >60%.

75. Crackles (and rhonchi) that clear with coughing suggest airflow obstruction. Conversely, crackles that *appear* after coughing (post-tussive crackles) argue in favor of tuberculosis.

76. *Bronchial breath sounds* reflect patent airways in a setting of *absent alveolar air*, with replacement by media that better transmit higher frequencies, such as liquids or solids (consolidation). If unaccompanied by crackles, they argue in favor of a pleural effusion.

77. Late inspiratory crackles can be detected by careful auscultation in 63% of young and healthy nursing students (in 92% if using an electronic stethoscope with high-pass filtration).

78. Timing of crackles predicts the site of production, with early inspiratory crackles reflecting bronchitis, mid-inspiratory crackles reflecting bronchiectasis, and late inspiratory crackles reflecting interstitial fibrosis or edema.

79. In asbestosis and idiopathic pulmonary fibrosis, the number of late inspiratory crackles correlates with disease severity.

80. In patients with pneumonia, crackles and diminished breath sounds appear first; bronchial breath sounds and egophony develop 1–3 days after onset of symptoms (i.e., cough and fever), and dullness to percussion (plus increased tactile fremitus) occurs even later. This time lag usually allows for x-ray to preempt diagnosis, thus making exam often irrelevant.

81. Wheezing on maximal forced exhalation has such a low sensitivity and specificity for asthma (57% and 37%, respectively) to be completely unreliable for diagnosing subclinical airflow obstruction.

82. Wheezes are neither sensitive nor specific for airflow obstruction. Although *unforced* wheezing argues strongly for chronic airflow obstruction, it can be absent in 30% of patients with FEV_1 <1 L. It may also resolve in acute asthmatics whose FEV_1 remains at 63% of the predicted value. In fact, in status asthmaticus, wheezing is the least-discriminating factor in predicting hospital admission or relapse.

83. Wheezing *intensity* does *not* correlate with severity of obstruction. Only *pitch* and *length* of wheezes are useful predictors of airway narrowing. Higher-pitched and longer wheezes reflect worse obstruction.

84. Bowel sounds lack sensitivity and specificity for intestinal obstruction, being decreased or absent in only one quarter of cases. Hence, they are clinically useless.

85. Lateral expansion of an abdominal mass >3 cm with pulsation suggests an abdominal aortic aneurysm. In cases of *small* aneurysms (3–5 cm in diameter), the finding is very specific, with the few false positives usually reflecting a tortuous aorta (yet, the finding is also poorly *sensitive,* detecting only one of five cases). In patients with *large* aneurysms (>5 cm), sensitivity increases to four out of five patients. In fact, lack of expansile pulsation in a thin patient should strongly argue against the presence of a large aneurysm.

86. Palpation of the liver edge is an unreliable way to estimate *hepatic consistency.* In fact, half of all palpable livers are not enlarged, and half of truly enlarged livers are not palpable.

87. A pulsatile liver edge may represent transmission of aortic pulsations through an enlarged liver but usually indicates one of two conditions: (1) constrictive pericarditis or (2) tricuspid regurgitation (TR). An inspiratory increase in the magnitude of pulsations will be typical of TR (especially in held mid-inspiration/end-inspiration), but not of constrictive pericarditis. *Pulsatility in a setting of hepatomegaly* instead is such a good indicator of *constrictive pericarditis* (present in 65% of patients) that its absence argues strongly against the diagnosis.

88. A painful arrest in inspiration triggered by palpation of the edge of an inflamed gallbladder (Murphy's sign) is a good test for cholecystitis, with sensitivity and specificity of 50–80% (specificity usually a little higher than sensitivity).

89. A palpable and nontender gallbladder in icteric patients strongly suggests that the jaundice is *not* due to hepatocellular disease, but to an *extrahepatic* obstruction of the biliary tract, more likely neoplastic. Albeit not too sensitive, this finding is highly specific.

90. In patients with splenomegaly, (1) concomitant *hepatomegaly* suggests primary liver disease with portal hypertension; (2) concomitant *lymphadenopathy excludes* primary liver disease and makes instead hematologic or lymphoproliferative disorders more likely; (3) *massive splenomegaly* (or left upper quadrant tenderness) also argues in favor of a myeloproliferative etiology; and (4) *Kehr's sign* (referred pain or hyperesthesia to the left shoulder) suggests impending splenic rupture.

91. Half of all patients with renovascular disease have a systolic murmur, whose significance depends on location and characteristics. Overall, *posterior murmurs are specific but not sensitive; anterior murmurs are sensitive but not specific; anterior bruits (i.e., continuous murmurs) are both specific and sensitive.*

92. Combining *all* bedside maneuvers provides a good bedside tool for the diagnosis of ascites, with overall accuracy of 80%. Still, the amount of volume necessary for these maneuvers to become positive (500–1000 mL) is much larger than that detected by ultrasound alone (100 mL).

93. Generalized adenopathy suggests a *disseminated malignancy* (especially hematologic), a *collagen vascular disorder*, or an *infectious process*. Adenopathy presenting with fever usually suggests infection or lymphoma.

94. A palpable supraclavicular node carries a 90% risk of malignancy for patients older than 40 years, and a 25% risk for younger patients.

95. A cranial nerve (CN) III palsy that spares pupils (i.e., ptosis and external rotation of the globe, but symmetric and equally reactive pupils) suggests diabetes, but also vasculitides and multiple sclerosis.

96. In a meta-analysis of almost 2000 patients, the signs with highest likelihood ratios for predicting neurologic recovery after a cardiac arrest were, at 24 hours: *absent corneal reflexes* (LR 12.9); *absent pupillary reflexes* (LR 10.2); absent motor response (LR 4.9); and absent withdrawal to pain (LR 4.7). At 72 hours, absent motor response predicted death or poor neurologic outcome.

97. Many traditional findings in *carpal tunnel syndrome*, including *Phalen, Tinel*, and *flick sign* have low sensitivity and limited or no value.

98. A positive straight-leg-raising test indicates nerve root impingement, usually by a herniated disk. It has high sensitivity (91%) but low specificity (26%), thus limiting its diagnostic accuracy. The "crossed" straight-leg raising test instead has low sensitivity (29%) but high specificity (88%). Hence, use them together.

99. A *composite* examination for anterior cruciate ligament (ACL) injuries has sensitivity >82% and specificity >94%, with an LR of 25.0 for a positive examination and 0.04 for a negative one. Overall, a positive Lachman test argues strongly in favor of ACL tear, whereas a negative is fairly good evidence against it. The anterior drawer is the least accurate test.

100. A *composite* examination for posterior cruciate ligament (PCL) injuries has sensitivity of 91%, specificity of 98%, and LRs of 21.0 (for a positive exam) and 0.05 (for a negative one). The posterior drawer test is the most reliable indicator, with mean sensitivity of 55%.

CHAPTER 1

GENERAL APPEARANCE, FACIES, AND BODY HABITUS

Salvatore Mangione, MD

"I knew you came from Afghanistan. From long habit, the train of thought ran so swiftly through my mind that I arrived at the conclusion without being conscious of immediate steps. There were such steps, however. The train of reasoning ran: 'Here is a gentleman of a medical type, but with the air of a military man. Clearly, an army doctor then. He has just come from the tropics, for his face is dark, and that is not the natural tint of his skin, for his wrists are fair. He has undergone hardship and sickness, as his haggard face says clearly. His left arm has been injured. He holds it in a stiff and unnatural manner. Where in the tropics could an English army doctor have seen much hardship and got his arm wounded? Clearly in Afghanistan.' The whole train of thought did not occupy a second. I then remarked that you came from Afghanistan and you were astonished."

–Arthur Conan Doyle, *A Study in Scarlet*, 1887

"You can observe a lot by watching."

–Yogi Berra

GENERAL APPEARANCE

1. **What is the value of carefully examining the patient's general appearance?**
   It is the Sherlockian value of making a diagnosis at first sight, sometimes while walking down a street. Attentive and knowledgeable observation is a time-honored skill of poets, physicians, and serial killers, beautifully articulated by Sir Arthur Conan Doyle (himself a doctor and a former student of the charismatic bedside diagnostician, Prof. Joseph Bell) in describing the first encounter between Holmes and Watson. The *Sherlockian* process requires practice and knowledge and is quite challenging. But it is also the most valuable, rewarding, and fun aspect of bedside diagnosis. It is best learned by having the luck to work with a physician who is skilled at it.

2. **Which aspects of the patient should be assessed?**
   - Posture
   - State of nutrition
   - State of hydration
   - Body habitus and body proportions
   - Facies
   - Apparent age
   - Apparent race and sex
   - Alertness and state of consciousness
   - Degree of illness, whether acute or chronic
   - Degree of comfort
   - State of mind and mood
   - Gait

   Often, the untrained eye is able to detect whether a patient "looks weird." But this awareness remains subliminal and never leads to a more cogent insight. The trained eye, on the other hand, is able not only to detect *weirdness,* but also to recognize the *reasons* behind it. Then, a mental database search attaches a medical label. As Holmes says, the entire process takes only a few milliseconds, yet it requires a series of intermediate intuitive steps.

A. POSTURE

3. **What information can be obtained from observing the patient's *posture*?**
   In *abdominal pain* the posture is often so typical as to localize the disease:
   - Patients with *pancreatitis* usually lie in the fetal position: on one side, with knees and legs bent over.
   - Patients with *peritonitis* are very still and avoid any movement that might worsen the pain.
   - Patients with *intestinal obstruction* are instead quite restless.
   - Patients with *renal* or *perirenal abscesses* bend toward the side of the lesion.
   - Patients who lie supine, with one knee flexed and the hip externally rotated, are said to have the "psoas sign." This reflects either *a local abnormality around the iliopsoas muscle* (such as an inflamed appendix, diverticulum, or terminal ileum from Crohn's disease) or inflammation *of the muscle itself*. In the olden days, the latter was due to a tuberculous abscess, originating in the spine and spreading down along the muscle. Such processes were referred to as "cold abscesses" because they had neither warmth nor other signs of inflammation. Now, the most common cause of a "psoas sign" is intramuscular *bleeding* from anticoagulation.
   - Patients with *meningitis* lie like patients with *pancreatitis*: on the side, with neck extended, thighs flexed at the hips, and legs bent at the knees—juxtaposed like the two bores of a double-barreled rifle.
   - Patients with a *large pleural effusion* tend to lie on the affected side to maximize excursions of the unaffected side. This, however, worsens hypoxemia (*see* Chapter 13, questions 48–51).
   - Patients with a *small pleural effusion* lie instead on the *unaffected* side (because direct pressure would otherwise worsen the pleuritic pain).
   - Patients with a large *pericardial effusion* (especially tamponade) sit up in bed and lean forward, in a posture often referred to as "the praying Muslim position." Neck veins are greatly distended.
   - Patients with *tetralogy of Fallot* often assume a squatting position, especially when trying to resolve cyanotic spells—such as after exercise.

4. **What is the posture of patients with dyspnea?**
   An informative alphabet soup of *orthopnea, paroxysmal nocturnal dyspnea, platypnea and orthodeoxia, trepopnea, respiratory alternans,* and *abdominal paradox*. These can determine not only the severity of dyspnea, but also its etiology (*see* Chapter 13, questions 35–51).

B. STATE OF HYDRATION

5. **What is hypovolemia?**
   A condition characterized by volume depletion and dehydration:
   - **Volume depletion** is a loss in *extracellular salt*, through either kidneys (diuresis) or the gastrointestinal tract (hemorrhage, vomiting, diarrhea). This causes contraction of the *total intravascular pool of plasma*, which results in circulatory instability and thus an increase in the serum urea nitrogen-to-creatinine ratio—a valuable biochemical marker for volume depletion.
   - **Dehydration** is instead a loss of *intracellular water*. It eventually causes cellular desiccation and an increase in serum sodium and plasma osmolality, two useful biochemical markers. Volume depletion occurs with or without dehydration, and dehydration occurs with or without volume depletion.

6. **Which is more common—volume depletion or dehydration?**
   It depends on the patient's age. For example, in children (especially younger than 5) the most common cause of hypovolemia is *volume depletion* without dehydration. This is usually due to excessive extrinsic loss of fluids from vomiting, diarrhea, or increased insensible water losses. Intravascular sodium levels are within reference range (*isonatremic* volume depletion), indicating that the entire plasma pool is contracted, with solutes (mostly sodium) and solvents (mostly water) lost in proportionate amounts. This is because in children younger than 5, significant fluid losses may occur rapidly, since the turnover of fluids and solute can be three times that of adults. In fact, worldwide diarrheal illnesses with subsequent volume depletion account for nearly 1 million deaths per year in infants and children.

7. **Is there any reason why these two processes should be kept separated?**
   The major one is management. *Volume depletion* is hemodynamically unstable, requiring rapid saline infusion. *Dehydration* is less dramatic, usually responding to 5% dextrose infusion.

8. **What are the goals of physical examination in assessing hypovolemia?**
   - To determine whether hypovolemia is present
   - To confirm its degree

9. **How do you determine the presence of hypovolemia?**
   Through the "tilt test," which measures postural changes in heart rate and blood pressure (BP):
   1. Ask the patient to lie supine.
   2. Wait at least 2 minutes.
   3. Measure heart rate and blood pressure in this position.
   4. Ask the patient to stand.
   5. Wait 1 minute.
   6. Measure heart rate and then blood pressure while the patient is standing. Measure rate by counting over 30 seconds and multiplying by two, which is more accurate than counting over 15 seconds and multiplying by four.

10. **Why is important to have the patient supine for at least 2 minutes before (s)he stands?**
    Because 2 minutes in the supine position is necessary to cause maximal leg pooling of blood, and thus maximal drop in cardiac output and maximal increment in heart rate upon restanding. Hence, 2 minutes in the supine position increases the sensitivity of the tilt test.

11. **What physiologic changes occur on standing?**
    Within 1–2 minutes, 7–8 mL/kg of blood (350–600 mL) shifts to the lower body. This decreases intrathoracic volume, stroke volume, and cardiac output while at the same time increasing circulating catecholamines. This, in turn, speeds heart rate and increases systemic vascular resistance. It also shifts blood from the pulmonary to the systemic circulation—all compensatory changes aimed at normalizing blood pressure. When these measures are ineffective (because of autonomic disregulation) or overwhelmed (because of blood loss), orthostatic changes will ensue.

12. **Should the patient lie supine for more than 2 minutes before standing up?**
    No. A longer period does *not* increase the sensitivity of the test.

13. **Is sitting equivalent to standing?**
    No. In fact, sitting greatly reduces the degree of leg "pooling" and thus the sensitivity of the test.

14. **What is the normal response to the tilt test?**
    Going from supine to standing, a normal patient exhibits the following:
    - *Heart rate* increases by 10.9 ± 2 beats/minute and usually stabilizes after 45–60 seconds.
    - *Systolic blood pressure* decreases only slightly (by 3.5 ± 2 mmHg) and stabilizes in 1–2 minutes.
    - *Diastolic blood pressure* increases by 5.2 ± 2.4 mmHg. This, too, stabilizes within 1–2 minutes.
    Hence, you should count the heart rate after 1 minute of standing, and only afterwards measure the blood pressure. This will allow an additional minute for blood pressure to stabilize.

15. **Does the tilt test changes with age?**
    Yes. As patients get older, age-related autonomic dysfunction will cause the postural increase in heart rate to become *smaller* and the decrease in blood pressure to become *larger*.

16. **What is orthostatic hypotension?**
    It is a persistent drop in *systolic blood pressure* >20 mmHg going from supine to a standing position. When not associated with dizziness, *this finding has low specificity for hypovolemia*; it is encountered with equal frequency in hypovolemic and normovolemic subjects (see later).

17. **What is the heart rate response to a tilt test?**
    It depends on the degree of hypovolemia. Most patients with *severe* blood loss (600–1200 mL) exhibit clear-cut orthostatic changes, like feeling dizzy upon standing (which practically stops the test) or experiencing a postural increase in heart rate (>30/min). As opposed to an isolated change in blood pressure, these findings are quite specific for hypovolemia, but sensitive only for *large* blood losses (100%). For *moderate* losses (<600 mL), their sensitivity is lower (10–50%).

18. **So what are the findings of a positive tilt test for hypovolemia?**
    - The most helpful is a *postural increase in heart rate of at least 30 beats/minute* (which has a sensitivity of 97% and a specificity of 96% for blood loss >630 mL). This change (as well as severe postural dizziness, see later) may last 12–72 hours if IV fluids are not administered.
    - The second most helpful finding is *postural dizziness so severe to stop the test*. This has the same sensitivity and specificity as tachycardia. *Mild* postural dizziness, instead, has no value.
    - *Hypotension of any degree* while standing has little value *unless associated with dizziness*. In fact, an orthostatic drop in systolic BP >20 mmHg *unassociated with dizziness* can occur in one third of patients >65 years old and 10% of younger subjects, with or without hypovolemia.
    - *Supine hypotension* (systolic BP <95 mmHg) and *tachycardia* (>100/min) may be absent, even in patients with blood losses >1 L. Hence, although quite specific for hypovolemia when present, supine hypotension and tachycardia have low sensitivity; they are present in one tenth of patients with moderate blood loss and in one third with severe blood loss. Paradoxically, blood-loss patients may even present with *bradycardia* as a result of a vagal reflex.
    Note that bedside maneuvers have been primarily studied in patients with blood loss. They have not been as extensively evaluated for hypovolemia from *vomiting, diarrhea,* or *decreased oral intake*.

19. **What is the significance of an orthostatic drop in systolic blood pressure?**
    It reflects *intravascular depletion*, usually from blood loss. Yet, this may also occur in normovolemia. Moreover, it has a sensitivity of only 9% for blood loss of 450–630 mL. Hence, it is not particularly useful—and definitely much less useful than the postural heart rate response.

20. **In addition to volume loss, are there any other causes of an abnormal tilt test?**
    The most common is the inability of the heart to increase its *output* as a result of pump failure. Postural changes can also be due to cardiac inability to increase *rate* (a common phenomenon in

the elderly), various neurogenic disorders, autonomic neuropathies, certain antihypertensives, prolonged bed rest, and even the weightlessness of space travel.

21. How do you assess *skin turgor*?
By pinching the abdominal skin with thumb and forefinger, pulling it upward over the abdominal plane, and then suddenly releasing it. Normal skin quickly returns to its original position.

22. What is poor skin turgor?
It is a loss of elasticity, another bedside indicator of *hypovolemia*. The physiology behind this test is rooted in the extreme changes in elastin caused by a decrease in moisture. Impaired elasticity (which may result from loss of as little as 3.4% in wet weight) prolongs the cutaneous recoil time by 40 times, delaying the skin's ability to spring back into place, and thus resulting in *"tenting"*—the lingering of the skin as a crease above the abdominal plane. Since older patients have less elasticity, this test has no real diagnostic value in adults. In children, instead, it is useful. Yet, since skin turgor may reflect not only the level of hydration (including electrolyte status) but also the level of *nutrition* (i.e., the amount of subcutaneous fat), "tenting" can be absent in cases of obesity or hypernatremic dehydration. Hence, the standard assessment of hypovolemia in *all* patients remains a set of basic laboratory tests: serum electrolytes, urea nitrogen, and creatinine.

23. What is the capillary refill time?
Another bedside assessment of volume status. This can be carried out through the "nail blanch test." Place the patient's hand at the same level as the heart, and then compress the distal phalanx of the middle finger for 5 seconds until it blanches. Release pressure, and measure how long it takes for the nail bed to regain its normal color. At room temperature (21°C), the upper limits of this *capillary refill time* (CRT) are 2 seconds for children and adult men, 3 seconds for adult women, and 4.5 seconds for the elderly. At colder temperatures, the normal upper limit may even be higher, raising questions regarding the reliability of the test in the prehospital setting.

24. What is the significance of a prolonged CRT?
It suggests tissue hypoperfusion and thus dehydration with possible hypovolemic shock. In adults, a prolonged CRT can also suggest heart failure or peripheral vascular disease.

25. How useful is CRT prolongation in estimating dehydration of infantile diarrhea?
Probably useful. In a study of 32 infants, 2–24 months of age, who had diarrhea, a CRT of <1.5 seconds was found to be indicative of a <50 mL/kg deficit or of a normal infant; 1.5–3.0 seconds suggested a deficit between 50–100 mL/kg, and >3 seconds suggested a deficit of >100 mL/kg. Conversely, in 30 age-matched normal controls, CRT was 0.81–0.31 seconds. Yet, in another study of approximately 5000 children evaluated in an emergency ward, a CRT >3 seconds was a poor predictor of the need for either intravenous fluid bolus or hospital admission.

26. How valuable is CRT in adults?
Not valuable at all. Using the age- and sex-specific upper limits of normal that were previously described, a prolonged CRT does *not* accurately predict 450 mL of blood loss (6% sensitivity, 93% specificity, positive likelihood ratio [LR], 1.0). Diagnostic performance is not improved by using an arbitrary upper limit of 2 seconds (11% sensitivity, 89% specificity, positive LR, 1.0). Hence, although the test has good interobserver agreement, its clinical value in adults is limited.

27. What other bedside findings can estimate the patient's volume status?
- Dry mucous membranes
- Dry axillae

- Sunken eyes
- Longitudinal tongue furrows

Interobserver agreement for these findings is moderate (80%). In a study of 100 ill elderly patients, dry axillae had a 50% sensitivity for detecting dehydration (percentage of dehydrated subjects *without* sweating) and a specificity of 82% (percentage of nondehydrated subjects *with* sweating). They also had a positive predictive value of 45% (percentage without sweating who were dehydrated) and a negative predictive value of 84% (percentage with sweating who were not dehydrated). Using likelihood rations, dry axillae *do* increase the probability of hypovolemia (positive LR, 2.8), although their sensitivity is rather low (50%). Conversely, *moist* axillae slightly decrease the probability of volume depletion (negative LR, 0.6).

28. **How valuable are *dry mucous membranes* in adults?**
    Valuable. In a study of elderly patients admitted to the emergency department, indicators that correlated best with dehydration severity (but were unrelated to patient age) included dry tongue, dry oral mucosae, and longitudinal tongue furrows (all with $p < 0.001$). Other statistically significant indicators are upper body muscle weakness and confusion ($p < 0.001$) and speech difficulty/sunken eyes ($p < 0.01$).

29. **What is the significance of dry mucous membranes in children?**
    It also indicates volume depletion. Still, several other findings may suggest this diagnosis, with their number increasing in proportion to the severity of the condition:
    - *Mild depletion* corresponds to <5% intravascular contraction (i.e., <50 mL/kg loss of body weight). This is usually determined by history alone, since physical signs are minimal or absent. Mucosae are moist, skin turgor and capillary refill normal, and pulse slightly increased.
    - *Moderate depletion* corresponds instead to 100 mL/kg loss of body weight. Mucosae are dry, skin turgor reduced, pulses weak, and patients are tachycardic and hyperpneic.
    - *Severe depletion* corresponds to >100 mL/kg loss of body weight. All previous signs are present, plus cold, dry, and mottled skin; altered sensorium; prolonged refill time; weak central pulses; and, eventually, hypotension.

C. STATE OF NUTRITION

30. **What information should be obtained about the patient's state of nutrition?**
    First, you should determine whether the patient is *well nourished* or *malnourished*. Then, whether (s)he is *overweight*, and, if so, to what degree. *Distribution* of obesity also should be determined.

31. **What is the BMI?**
    It is the acronym for *body mass index,* the federal government's standard for body weight. This represents the proportion of height to weight, expressed as the ratio between a subject's weight and height (*normal range*, 18.5–24.9). The BMI provides a much better measurement of body fat than the traditional weight and height charts. For example, currently anyone with a BMI >25 is considered overweight; however, older standards classify men with a BMI >27.3 as overweight and women with a BMI >27.8 as overweight. In fact, those with a BMI of 25.0–29.9 are *overweight,* and those with a BMI >30.0 are *obese*. In younger subjects, a BMI >25 is a good predictor of cardiovascular risk. Yet, this may not apply to the elderly (see later).

32. **How common is obesity?**
    Epidemic. Given the revised guidelines, more than half of all Americans age 20 or older are *overweight*; more than one fifth are *obese*—a percentage that has dramatically risen since the 1960s.

33. **Why is the BMI important?**
    Because a high BMI is associated with increased risk for serious medical problems:
    - Hypertension
    - Cardiovascular disease
    - Dyslipidemia
    - Adult-onset diabetes (type 2)
    - Sleep apnea
    - Osteoarthritis
    - Female infertility
    - Various cancers (including endometrial, breast, prostate, and colon) are more common in obese subjects (in one study, 52% higher rates in men and 62% in women).
    - Miscellaneous conditions, such as lower extremity venous stasis, idiopathic intracranial hypertension, gastroesophageal reflux, urinary stress incontinence, gallbladder disease, osteoarthritis, sleep apnea, and respiratory problems
    - Note that body weight has a U-shaped relationship with mortality, causing an increase when either very low or very high.

34. **What are the cutoffs for BMI?**
    In a *New England Journal of Medicine* study, subjects with a BMI <19 had the lowest death rate. Risk of death was 20% higher if BMI was 19–24.9; 30% higher if 25–26.9; 60% higher if 27–28.9; and twice as high (100%) if >29. This may vary if there are comorbid conditions.

35. **What is a comorbid condition?**
    Any condition associated with obesity that worsens as the degree of obesity increases, and, conversely, improves as obesity is successfully treated. Risk of disease based only on BMI increases whenever the patient has one or more comorbid conditions.

36. **How do you measure the BMI?**
    The best way is a BMI chart, wherein you simply locate the height (inches) and weight (pounds) of a patient and then find the corresponding BMI at the intersection of the two. BMI can also be determined by dividing weight in kilograms by height in meters squared (BMI = kg/m^2). The following formula provides a shortcut: (1) multiply weight (in pounds) by 703; (2) multiply height (in inches) by height (in inches); (3) divide the answer in step 1 by the answer in step 2.

37. **Is the BMI foolproof?**
    No. Although a better predictor of disease risk than weight alone, it may be inaccurate in growing children or frail and sedentary elderly patients. It may also be spuriously increased in competitive athletes and body builders (because of larger muscle mass), or pregnant and lactating women. Overall, indices of distribution of body fat have recently gained favor as better risk predictors.

38. **How important is the distribution of body fat?**
    Very important, since it strongly determines the impact of obesity on health. Fat deposition may be *central* (mostly in the trunk) or *peripheral* (mostly in the extremities) (Fig. 1-1).
    - **Central obesity** has a bihumeral diameter greater than the bitrochanteric diameter; subcutaneous fat has a "descending" distribution, being mostly concentrated in the *upper* half of the body (neck, cheeks, shoulder, chest, and upper abdomen).
    - **Peripheral obesity** has instead a bitrochanteric diameter greater than the bihumeral diameter; subcutaneous fat has an "ascending" distribution, being mostly concentrated in the *lower* half of the body (lower abdomen, pelvic girdle, buttocks, and thighs).

    Men tend to have *central* obesity, whereas women have *peripheral* obesity. Upper and central body fat distribution (especially if intra-abdominal rather than subcutaneous) is a greater

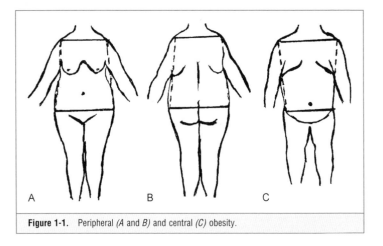

Figure 1-1. Peripheral *(A* and *B)* and central *(C)* obesity.

predictor of insulin resistance and cardiovascular risk than BMI alone. It also has higher association with hypertension, diabetes, atherosclerotic cardiovascular diseases, and other chronic metabolic conditions (*metabolic syndrome*). For example, a waist-to-hip ratio ≥ 1.0 is considered an "at risk" indicator for both men and women, confirming that an *apple* shape (extra weight around the stomach) is more dangerous than a *pear* shape (extra weight around hips or thighs). Subjects judged to be lean by BMI alone may be very insulin resistant if their body fat is centrally distributed.

39. **How do you assess body fat distribution?**
    By *waist circumference* (WC) and *waist-to-hip ratio* (WHR). Of these, WC is a better predictor of abdominal fat content, and both are much better markers for cardiovascular risk than BMI alone.

40. **How do you measure the WC?**
    By applying a measuring tape between the last rib and the iliac crest, at minimal inspiration and to the nearest 0.1 cm (0.04 in). This coincides with the narrowest waist level, just above the umbilicus.

41. **How do you measure the WHR?**
    As a *waist circumference* divided by *hip circumference*. To do so, tape-measure *hip* circumference at the widest part of the buttocks, and divide this by the previously measured *waist* circumference. The ratio is the WHR. This may be especially valuable in the elderly, since a recent British study by Fletcher et al. showed that in subjects older than 75 a high WHR (>0.99 in nonsmoking men and >0.90 in nonsmoking women) is associated with a 40% higher risk of cardiovascular disease/death than a lower WHR (≤ 0.8). The BMI was instead a less important predictor. In fact, older men and women with lower BMI (less than 23 and 22.3, respectively) were actually the ones most likely to die, suggesting that a low BMI in this population may indicate muscle loss or poor nutrition. Hence, in the elderly the WHR is a more accurate indicator of excess body fat.

42. **What is the WHR threshold for cardiovascular risk?**
    The cutoff seems to be a waist-to-hip ratio of 0.83 for women and 0.9 for men. Favoring WHR over BMI would result in a threefold increase in the population at risk for myocardial infarction. This would be especially valuable in Asia, where obesity by BMI is rare, but WHRs can be quite abnormal (Table 1-1).

TABLE 1-1. CARDIOVASCULAR RISK BASED ON WAIST-TO-HIP RATIO				
	Acceptable		Unacceptable	
	Excellent	Good	Average	High	Extreme
Male	<0.85	0.85–0.90	0.90–0.95	0.95–1.00	>1.00
Female	<0.75	0.75–0.80	0.80–0.85	0.85–0.90	>0.90

43. **What is the WC threshold for cardiovascular risk?**
It depends on age and sex. Overall, the cutoff for cardiovascular risk is 102 cm (40.2 in) in men and 88 cm (34.7 in) in women. Yet, a WC <100 cm practically excludes insulin resistance in *both* sexes (negative predictive value, 98%—*BMJ,* 2005.

44. **Why is abdominal obesity such a good marker of insulin resistance?**
Because hyperinsulinemia activates 11-Beta-hydroxysteroid dehydrogenase in omental adipose tissue, thus generating active cortisol and promoting a cushingoid fat distribution. Hence, WC is an excellent tool to either exclude insulin resistance or identify subjects at risk.

45. **Does WC correlate with BMI?**
Not necessarily. In fact, within the three BMI categories (normal, overweight, obese), subjects with higher WC values (men, >102 cm; women, >88 cm) are significantly more likely to have hypertension, diabetes, dyslipidemia, and the metabolic syndrome than those with *normal* WC (men, ≤102 cm; women, ≤88 cm). This is independent of other confounding variables, such as age, race, poverty–income ratio, physical activity, smoking, and alcohol intake.

46. **How do you define malnutrition on the basis of BMI?**
As *severe* (BMI <16), *moderate* (BMI 16–16.9), and *marginal* (BMI 17–18.4). Still, there are limitations to its use (see later).

47. **How else can you identify malnutrition?**
Through history and physical exam. Features of both can be combined in the subjective global assessment (SGA) of nutritional status, dividing patients into one of three groups:
- Class A (well-nourished)
- Class B (moderately malnourished)
- Class C (severely malnourished)

48. **What are the physical examination components of the SGA?**
Detecting loss of subcutaneous fat, loss of muscle, and shift of intravenous fluid. These are recorded as normal (0), mild (1+), moderate (2+), or severe (3+).
- The best locations for *assessing subcutaneous fat* are the triceps regions of the arms, the midaxillary line at the costal margin, the interosseous and palmar areas of the hand, and the deltoids of the shoulder. Loss of subcutaneous fat appears as lack of fullness, with skin loosely fitting over the deeper tissues.
- *Muscle wasting* is best assessed by *palpation* (although inspection may also help). Best locations for doing so are the quadriceps femoris and deltoids. Shoulders of malnourished patients appear "squared off" as a result of both muscle wasting and subcutaneous fat loss.
- *Loss of fluid from the intravascular to extravascular space* refers primarily to ankle/sacral edema and ascites. Edema is best assessed by *palpation*—that is, by pressing over the ankles or sacral area. Fluid displaced from subcutaneous tissues as a result of compression is its

hallmark. Such displacement is clinically manifested by a persistent depression of the compressed area (pitting), which lasts for more than 5 seconds.

Once gathered, these physical findings should be quantified (as normal, mild, moderate, or severe), combined subjectively with other clinical findings, and an SGA finally generated. There is no clear-cut weighting recommendation for combining these features, even though the following variables are usually important:

- Weight loss >10%
- Poor dietary intake
- Loss of subcutaneous tissue
- Muscle wasting

For example, patients with all three physical signs of malnutrition plus a weight loss >10% are usually classified as *severely malnourished* (class C). Note that the SGA technique is not highly sensitive for diagnosing malnutrition, but it is quite specific.

49. Why should one bother to evaluate for malnutrition?

Because it is a risk factor for major complications, such as *infection* or *poor wound healing*. In this regard, the SGA has been used successfully (both diagnostically and prognostically) in patients undergoing surgery, dialysis, and liver transplant. Conversely, a low BMI is *not* necessarily associated with adverse postoperative outcomes. In fact, it can easily overestimate severe malnutrition.

D. FACIES

50. What is facies?

It is the Latin word for *face*, and the term used to indicate the peculiar and often pathognomonic facial features of a particular disease. Physicians with a trained eye can quickly recognize a "facies" and often make a diagnosis by simply walking into the waiting room.

51. Which disease processes are associated with a typical facies?

Quite a few. The following list is not necessarily exhaustive (Table 1-2):

- **Facies bovina:** The cowlike face of Greig's syndrome: large cranial vault, huge forehead, high bregma, and occasional hypertelorism (widely spaced eyes)—all due to an enlarged sphenoid bone. It is often associated with other congenital deformities, such as osteogenesis imperfecta, syndactyly and polydactyly, Sprengel's deformity (scapular elevation), and mental retardation.
- **Elfin face:** An unusually flat face, with broad forehead, hypertelorism, short and upturned nose, low-set ears that are posteriorly rotated, puffy cheeks, wide mouth, patulous lips, hypoplastic teeth, and a deep husky voice. Patients are mentally retarded, but with a sweet and friendly personality. They are also typically short, and with congenital supravalvar aortic stenosis. Hypercalcemia may be present. First described by Williams in 1961.
- **Cherubic face:** The child-like face of *cherubism*, a familial fibrous dysplasia of the jaws, with enlargement in childhood and regression in adulthood. Also seen in forms of glycogenosis.
- **Hound-dog face:** The face of *cutis laxa* (*dermatochalasis*), a degenerative disease of elastic fibers, with skin progressively loose and hanging in folds—like that of a hound dog. Premature aging is common, and so are vascular abnormalities, gastrointestinal/bladder diverticula, and pulmonary emphysema. The face has an antimongoloid slant, slightly everted nostrils, prominent ears, and epicanthic folds. In contrast to Ehlers-Danlos syndrome, there is no joint laxity.
- **Hurloid face:** The coarse and gargoyle-like face of Hurler's syndrome (mucopolysaccharidosis type I, described in 1919 by the German pediatrician Gertrud Hurler). Because of lack of L-iduronidase, these patients accumulate intracellular deposits, with abnormal skeletal cartilage and bone, dwarfism, kyphosis, deformed limbs, limited joint

TABLE 1-2.	DISEASE PROCESSES ASSOCIATED WITH A TYPICAL FACIES	
Etiology	**Facies**	**Disease**
Congenital	Facies bovina	Greig's syndrome
	Elfin face	Williams' syndrome
	Cherubic face	Cherubism
	Hound-dog face	*Cutis laxa*
	Hurloid face	Hurler's syndrome
	Morquio's face	Morquio's syndrome
	Potter's face	Potter's syndrome
Infectious	Facies leonina	Leprosy
	Facies antonina	Leprosy
	Scaphoid face	Leprosy
	Tetanus face	Tetanus
Endocrine-metabolic	Renal face	Chronic renal failure
	Myxedematous face	Myxedema
	Graves' face	Graves' disease
	Acromegalic face	Acromegaly
	Cushing's face	Cushing's syndrome
Rheumatologic	Scleroderma face	Progressive systemic sclerosis
	Lupus face	Systemic lupus erythematosus
Cardiovascular	Aortic face	Aortic regurgitation
	Corvisart's face	Aortic regurgitation
	De Musset's face	Aortic regurgitation
	Mitral face	Mitral stenosis
Neurologic	Parkinson's face	Parkinson's disease
	Steinert's face	Myotonic dystrophy
	Myasthenic face	Myasthenia gravis
	Myopathic face	Various
Traumatic	Battle's sign	Basilar skull fracture
	Raccoon eyes	
Miscellaneous	Hippocratic face	Terminal illness
	Facies adenoid	Adenoids/chronic allergic rhinitis
	Rhinophyma	Various
	Saddle nose	Congenital syphilis/Wegener's/polychondritis
	Smoker's face	Tobacco

motion, spade-like hands, corneal clouding, hepatosplenomegaly, mental retardation, and, of course, a gargoyle-like face.

■ **Morquio's face:** The bizarre face of *Morquio syndrome* (mucopolysaccharidosis type IV). Like Hurler's, this is also associated with short stature, but intelligence is normal. The face is coarse, with corneal clouding, large mouth, anteverted nose, and short neck. In addition, there may be chest and limb deformities (short and kyphotic trunk, pectus carinatum, protruded abdomen, and genu valgum), hepatosplenomegaly, urinary excretion of mucopolysaccharides, and neutrophils with intracytoplasmic metachromatic granules (Alder-Reilly bodies). Severe spinal defects may eventually lead to fatal cord compression and respiratory failure.

- **Potter's face:** The characteristic facies of bilateral renal agenesis (Potter's *syndrome*) and other kidney malformations: hypertelorism, prominent epicanthal folds, low-set ears, receding chin, and flattened nose. There may also be pulmonary hypoplasia and cardiac malformations (ventricular septal defect, endocardial cushion defect, tetralogy of Fallot, and patent ductus arteriosus).
- **Facies leonina:** Also referred to as *leontiasis*, from the lion-like appearance. It is the face of advanced lepromatous leprosy, with prominent ridges and furrows of forehead and cheeks.
- **Facies antonina:** Another face of leprosy, with alterations in the eyelids and the anterior eye.
- **Scaphoid face:** From the Greek *scaphos* (boat-shaped, hollowed), this is the *dish-like* facial malformation of leprosy: protuberant forehead, prominent chin, depressed nose and maxilla.
- **Tetanus face:** The *risus sardonicus* of tetanus (sardonic grin in Latin): open mouth with transversally tightened lips, resembling the smirk of Batman's menace—the Joker.
- **Renal face:** The face of *chronic renal failure*. Very similar to that of myxedema, except that the swelling is *not* due to accumulation of connective tissue but of water (hypoproteinemia).
- **Myxedematous face:** Puffy and sallow facies from carotene accumulation, with coarse hair, boggy eyes, and dry, rough skin. The lateral third of the eyebrows is often missing.
- **Graves' face:** A typical and anxious-looking face, with exophthalmos and lid lag.
- **Acromegalic face:** Coarse facial features, thick bones, prominent mandible, protruding supraciliary areas, large nose and lips. From the Greek *akron* (extremity) and *megalos* (large), it is characterized by enlargement of the body's peripheral parts: head, face, hands, and feet.
- **Cushing's face:** A typical *moon face*: round, plethoric, oily, and ruddy. Acne, alopecia, and an increase in facial hair may also occur, as well as buffalo hump, buccal fat pads, striae, and central obesity.
- **Scleroderma face:** The facies of progressive systemic sclerosis—sharp nose and skin so tightly drawn that wrinkles disappear. Most patients also have hyperpigmentation, with patches of vitiligo and a few telangiectasias. Mouth opening is often quite narrow.
- **Facies of lupus erythematosus:** Malar and butterfly-like rash across the bridge of the nose.
- **Aortic face:** The pale and sallow face of early aortic regurgitation (AR).
- **Corvisart's face:** The characteristic facies of advanced AR or full-blown congestive heart failure—puffy, cyanotic, with swollen eyelids, and shiny eyes. First described by Jean Nicolas Corvisart, physician to Napoleon, Laënnec's teacher, and percussion zealot.
- **De Musset's face (or sign):** Bobbing motion of the head, synchronous with each heartbeat, and "diagnostic" of AR. First described in the French poet Alfred De Musset, it is neither sensitive nor specific, since it can also occur in patients with very large stroke volume (i.e., hyperkinetic heart syndrome) and even a massive left pleural effusion. A variant of De Musset's can occur in tricuspid regurgitation, even though in this case the systolic bobbing tends to be more lateral because of regurgitation along the superior vena cava.
- **Mitral face:** The acrocyanotic face of mitral stenosis (MS). Due to peripheral desaturation from low and fixed cardiac output, it typically affects the *distal parts of the body* (*akros,* distal in Greek): nose tip, earlobes, cheeks, hands, and feet. When MS evolves into right-sided heart failure and tricuspid regurgitation (from longstanding pulmonary hypertension), the skin turns sallow and often overtly icteric. This contrasts markedly with the cyanotic hue of the cheeks.
- **Parkinson's face:** The mask-like facies of Parkinson's. It has a fixed and apathetic look.
- **Steinert's face:** The expressionless facies of myotonic dystrophy (Steinert's disease)—frontal balding, cataracts, bilateral temporal muscle wasting, thin and beak-like nose, and tenting of the upper lip with tendency of the mouth to hang over.
- **Myasthenic face:** The facies of myasthenia gravis, with sagging mouth corners and drooping eyelids (ptosis). Weak facial muscles result in paucity of expression (apathetic look).

- **Myopathic face:** Seen in congenital myopathies. Similar to the myasthenic face—protruding lips, drooping eyelids, ophthalmoplegia, and a relaxation of facial muscles (Hutchinson's face).
- **Battle's sign:** The classic traumatic bruise over/behind the mastoid process. Due to basilar skull fracture with bleeding into the middle fossa. Can present at times as blood behind the eardrum. Battle's sign may occur on the ipsilateral or contralateral side of the skull fracture and can take as long as 3–12 days to appear. It has low sensitivity (2–8%) but 100% predictive value.
- **Raccoon eyes:** Periorbital bruises from external trauma to the eyes, skull fracture, and intracranial bleeding. Raccoon eyes may also occur in amyloidosis as a result of capillary fragility. In this case, the leak is often precipitated by a Valsalva-mediated increase in central venous pressure. This can be involuntary, as the one induced by proctoscopy.
- **Hippocratic face:** A tense and dramatic expression, with sunken eyes, sharp nose, hollow cheeks, fallen-in temples, open mouth, dry and cracked lips, cold and drawn ears, and a leaden complexion. First described by Hippocrates in protracted and terminal illnesses.
- **Facies adenoid:** The long, open-mouthed, and dumb-looking face of children with adenoidal hypertrophy. The mouth is open (because upper airway congestion renders them obligatory mouth-breathers); the nares are narrow, and the nose is pinched. Although typically adenoidal, this *facies* can also occur in recurrent *upper respiratory tract allergies*. Features include (1) *Dennie's lines* (horizontal creases under both lower lids, named after the American Charles Dennie); (2) *nasal pleat* (the horizontal crease above the tip of the nose, due to the recurrent upward wiping of nasal secretions by either palm or dorsum of hand—"the allergic salute"); and (3) *allergic shiners* (bilateral infraorbital shadows due to chronic venous congestion).
- **Rhinophyma:** A typical facial feature, immortalized by Ghirlandaio in his 1480 Louvre painting of an old man with grandson and then involuntarily popularized by W.C. Fields' potato nose.
- **Saddle nose:** The congenital (or acquired) erosive *indentation* of the nasal bone and cartilage. Due to congenital syphilis, Wegener's granulomatosis, and relapsing polychondritis.
- **Smoker's face:** A facies that is becoming increasingly familiar as a result of the tobacco epidemic. It is characterized by coarse features and a wrinkled, grayish, and atrophic skin that makes smokers look older. In fact, comparing smokers to nonsmokers may provide a much more effective prevention for teens (especially girls) than quoting the latest cancer statistics.

52. **Who was Greig?**

David Greig (1864–1936) was a Scottish surgeon and quite an interesting character. A graduate of Edinburgh University, he served in the army first in India and then in South Africa, where he participated in the Boer war. After returning to Scotland, he became supervisor at the Baldovan Institute for Imbecile Children and also curator of the Museum of the Royal College of Surgeons. Both these appointments fostered a peculiar fascination with *skulls* (either normal or abnormal) that lasted a lifetime and eventually gave him a shot at fame. He was so fascinated by them that he hoarded as many as 300 in his private collection. He wrote extensively about their deformities and even published a paper describing the skull characteristics of Sir Walter Scott. An avid reader, Greig also was interested in music and literature, eventually publishing a collection of his own poetry.

53. **What is Lincoln's sign?**

One of the varieties of De Musset's sign. The term refers to a picture of Abe Lincoln during the Civil War, showing the president quietly sitting with legs crossed and the tip of the raised foot fuzzy and indistinct. Since 19th-century photography required long exposure times, this clue suggested that Lincoln might have had aortic regurgitation, probably from Marfan's syndrome, and that the fuzziness of the foot could have been due to its bobbing with each heartbeat.

54. **Who was De Musset?**

Alfred De Musset was a Frenchman, he was a poet, and he lived in the 19th century. Hence, he had all the major risk factors for acquiring syphilis, which he compliantly did. The eponymous sign was first noticed by De Musset's brother (Paul) during a breakfast the two had in 1842 with their mother. When informed of his peculiar head motion, Alfred simply put forefinger and thumb to the chin, and calmly stopped the bobbing. Paul subsequently reported the event in a biography of his famous brother, and the rest is (medical) history. Incidentally, more than for this sign, De Musset is best known for his *lover* (George Sand) and for being eventually dumped by her for Frédéric Chopin—showing that Ms. Sand preferred tuberculous pneumonia to syphilitic aortitis.

E. APPARENT AGE

55. **Which conditions make you look *older* than your stated age?**

Other than a job in academic medicine, the most common reason is cigarette smoking. The next is chronic exposure to sunlight (especially its UV band), since this accelerates skin aging and wrinkling (*actinic face*). Progeria (Hutchinson-Gilford syndrome) is an exotic and much more ominous reason. It affects 1 in 8 million newborns, accelerating the aging process by 6–8 times. Symptoms begin around 18–24 months of age, with stunted growth, alopecia, and a small/bizarre face with receding jaw and pinched nose. Atherosclerosis and cardiovascular disease eventually follow, killing patients by their late teens. Cancer and dementia, however, are typically absent.

56. **What is Werner's syndrome?**

A rare and autosomal recessive disease of DNA replication, resulting in premature aging and death by the late 40s/early 50s. Patients grow and develop normally until puberty; then they start aging rapidly, with loss of hair, wrinkling of skin, and early cataracts. Extremities are thin, trunk is thick, and the face has a characteristic "bird-like" look. Age-associated disorders (such as diabetes, heart disease, and cancer) are common and a frequent cause of death.

57. **Which conditions make you look *younger* than your stated age?**

Not many, unfortunately. Good genes, of course, always help. Yet, there *are* a few conditions that can provide a youthful look:

- Hypogonadism and other endocrine disorders of developmental arrest or retardation
- Panhypopituitarism is also associated with a youthful look, but a sallow complexion and many fine wrinkles.
- Anorexia nervosa and some mental illnesses
- Immunosuppressive agents for organ-transplant protection can do it, too.
- Being mildly underweight also conveys an impression of youth and health, but this is probably more cultural and based on our ever-increasing obsession with thinness. In fact, when "consumption" from TB was still a major killer, being *overweight* was actually considered a sign of *health*. This is still the case in many parts of the world, where people's main concern is not to lose weight, but to put food on the table at least once a day.

58. **What is a toxic-looking patient?**

One who is anxious, flushed, sweaty, febrile, and tachycardic with rapid, shallow respirations. Such patients need immediate attention, since they are often septic. Poisoning (such as salicylate intoxication), thyroid storm, psychotic crisis, or heat stroke can also present in this fashion.

F. GAIT

59. Why is gait important?
Because gait *disturbances* are common, especially in the elderly, in whom they affect 15% of subjects older than 60, 25% of those older than 80, and half of all nursing home residents. Gait disturbances are also a risk factor for *falls*, and thus may contribute to *hip fractures*—the sixth leading cause of death in older patients. Moreover, by compromising independent ambulation they are often a reason for nursing home admission. Finally, they provide an *augenblick diagnose* (instant diagnosis).

60. What is the difference between stance and gait?
Stance is the position assumed by a *standing* person (from the French derivative of the Italian *stanza*). It is also one of the phases of ambulation. **Gait** is instead the individual's *ambulating style* (from the Old Norse *gata*, path), which is often so unique to be recognizable from a distance. In fact, gaits say a lot not only about neuromuscular (patho)physiology, but also about *mood* (like depression), *occupation,* and even *character*. Contrast, for example, the graceful and elegant walk of Henry Fonda with John Wayne's flamboyant and macho gait and Mae West's sexy waddle.

61. What are the two principal forms of human gaits?
Walking and *running*. Although a person who is running may at times be fully airborne, a person who is *walking* always maintains at least one foot on the ground. When referring to "gait" in this chapter, we will refer to *walking*.

62. What are the phases of a normal gait cycle?
Stance and *swing*. *Stance* begins when one heel strikes the ground, and it lasts for the entire period during which that foot stays grounded. Hence, it is a weight-bearing phase. *Swing* is instead the interval between the lifting of that foot's toes off the floor and the time the heel of the same foot strikes the ground again. Since during this period the foot is airborne, "swing" is a *non*–weight-bearing phase. *Stance* and *swing* make up a *stride*, which corresponds to the interval between the time one heel hits the floor until it strikes it again. Note that for 20–25% of the gait cycle the stance of the two legs overlaps, insofar as *both* feet are on the ground (double-limb support).

63. Which muscles contract during gait?
It depends. During *stance*, mostly the *extensors* contract: gluteus maximus early on, quadriceps in the middle, and plantar flexors (soleus and gastrocnemius) toward the end; during *swing,* instead, the *flexors* contract: iliopsoas (for hip), hamstrings (for knee), and tibialis anterior/toe extensors (for ankle).

64. What is the position of head, body, legs, and feet during gait?
The *body* is erect, the *head* straight, and the *arms* loose on each side; the *feet* are slightly everted, almost in line with each other; the *internal malleoli* come close to touching during walking; and steps are usually small and equal. During ambulation, the thorax rotates in a clock/counterclockwise direction (opposite the pelvic rotations), and the arms swing opposite to the leg movements.

65. How are stance and gait coordinated?
Through a highly sophisticated interplay of various structures, resulting in (1) *sensory input* (visual, proprioceptive, vestibular); (2) *motor output* (to muscles and joints); and (3) *good integration* (by various CNS centers). Hence, imbalance (and falls) usually results from failure of more than one of the following components:
- **Basal ganglia:** For automatic movements, including the automatic swinging of the arms

- **Locomotor region of the midbrain:** For initiating walking
- **Cerebellum:** For maintaining proper posture and balance; also controls the major characteristics of movement, such as trajectory, velocity, and acceleration.
- **Spinal cord:** For coordinating movements and relaying proprioceptive/sensory input from joints and muscles to the higher centers for feedback and autoregulation. Muscular tone must be high enough to resist gravity but low enough to allow movement.
- **Vision:** For feedback on head and body movement in relation to the surroundings, which allows for automatic balance adjustments whenever surface conditions change. Vision is *crucial* in case of reduced input from other sensory systems (e.g., proprioceptive, vestibular, and auditory).

66. **What are the two physiologic requirements of walking?**
    - **Equilibrium** (the ability to assume an upright posture and maintain balance)
    Antigravity support is provided by antigravity and postural reflexes in the spinal cord and brain stem that are responsible for maintaining full extension of hips, knees, and neck.
    - **Locomotion** (the ability to *initiate* and *maintain* rhythmic stepping—through propulsion and stepping)
    Propulsion involves leaning forward and slightly to one side. This permits the body to fall at a certain distance before being checked by the leg support.
    Stepping is a basic pattern of movement based on sensory input from the soles and body that is then integrated in the midbrain and diencephalus.
    Both *equilibrium* and *locomotion* require proper and coordinated function of the musculoskeletal and nervous systems. Equilibrium maintains center of gravity and balance during the shifting of weight from one foot to the other. This is very important, since during walking the *center of gravity* remains outside the base of support 80% of the time. To compensate, the body uses reactive and proactive adjustments. The *reactive* ones deal with unpredictable upsets of balance and thus depend on sensory input (proprioceptive, vestibular, auditory, and visual). *Proactive* adjustments counteract instead perturbations caused by gait movements per se and thus rely on vision to predict potential causes of disequilibrium and implement appropriate avoidance strategies.

67. **What is the impact of aging on gait?**
    It causes a greater sway while standing, slower postural support responses, a shorter and broader-based stride, reduced pelvic rotation and joint excursions, and a 10–20% reduction in velocity.

68. **What are the four most common reasons for gait disturbance?**
    - Pain
    - Immobile joint
    - Muscle weakness
    - Abnormal neurologic control
    To separate them, always notice whether the disturbance is *symmetric* (suggesting faulty neurologic control, except for the spasticity of hemiplegia) or *asymmetric* (suggesting instead pain, a fixed joint, or muscle weakness) (Fig. 1-2 and Table 1-3).

69. **What *historic information* should be gathered to adequately evaluate an abnormal gait?**
    In addition to symmetry versus asymmetry (previously discussed), one should inquire about:
    - Acute onset (usually suggesting vascular disease versus drugs: alcohol, benzodiazepines, neuroleptics, and agents causing orthostatic hypotension)
    - Presence of muscle weakness

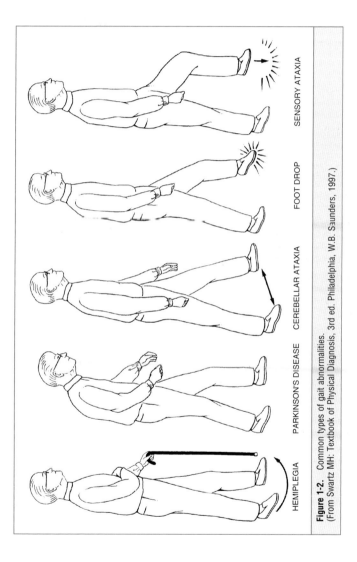

Figure 1-2. Common types of gait abnormalities. (From Swartz MH: Textbook of Physical Diagnosis, 3rd ed. Philadelphia, W.B. Saunders, 1997.)

TABLE 1-3. MAJOR CAUSES AND TYPES OF GAIT DISTURBANCE

Mechanism	Gait Disturbance	Disease
Pain	Antalgic gait	Osteoarthritis hip, knee, ankle
Immobile joint	Fixed joint gait	Osteoarthritis; prolonged periods of plaster immobilization
Muscle weakness	Trendelenburg gait	Unilateral weakness of hip abductors
	Anserine gait	Bilateral weakness of hip abductors
	High steppage gait	Weakness of hip abductors
		Charcot-Marie-Tooth disease
		Foot drop (peroneal paralysis)
Abnormal neurologic control	Gait of spinal stenosis	Myelopathy (cervical spondylosis)
	Gait of spastic paraplegia	Scissor gait
	Ataxic gait/cerebellar gait	Ataxia (sensory or cerebellar)
	Apraxic gait	Apraxia (frontal lobe disease)
	Hemiplegic gait	Hemispheric stroke
	Parkinsonian gait	Parkinson's disease

- Presence of stiffness in the limbs
- Difficulty in initiating or terminating walking
- Presence of bladder or bowel dysfunction
- Association with vertigo or light-headedness
- Association with pain, numbness, or tingling in the limbs
- Worsening of disturbance at night (because of darkness)

70. **How much information can be obtained through the assessment of a patient's gait?**
   It depends on the disease. Still, inspecting how a patient walks into your office (or climbs onto the examination table) can often unlock important neurologic or musculoskeletal diagnoses. At a minimum, it can sort out disorders due to *arthritis* (the most common reason for gait disturbance in primary care) from those resulting from *neurologic diseases* (stroke, Parkinson's, frontal gait disorders, myelopathy from spondylosis) or *other conditions* (claudication, orthostatic hypotension).

71. **How should one observe a patient with a gait abnormality?**
   By closely evaluating (from front, back, and side):
   - How the patient gets up from a chair (useful in Parkinson's or limb girdle dystrophy)
   - How the patient *initiates* walking (also useful in Parkinson's)
   - How the patient walks at a slow pace
   - How the patient walks at a fast pace
   - How the patient turns

- How the patient walks on *toes* (this cannot be mustered by patients with Parkinson's disease, sensory ataxia, spastic hemiplegia, or paresis of the soleus/gastrocnemius)
- How the patient walks on *heels* (diagnostic in motor ataxia, spastic paraplegia, or foot drop)
- How the patient walks a straight line in tandem (i.e., heel to toe) (useful in all gait disorders)
- How the patient *walks* with eyes first opened and then closed (a patient with sensory ataxia does much worse with closed eyes, whereas a patient with *motor* ataxia or *cerebellar* ataxia does poorly either way)
- How the patient *stands* erect with eyes first open and then closed (Romberg's)
- How the patient copes with sudden postural challenges, such as a modest pull from behind after adequate warning; inadequate postural reflexes (as often seen in nursing home residents) will cause a few steps of retropulsion, and even a tendency to fall backward.

Most gaits share nonspecific characteristics, such as a widened base while standing, short steps while walking, and greater proportion of the gait cycle spent in double-limb support (in some cases as much as 50%). A few gaits (cerebellar ataxia, coxarthritis, and Parkinson's) have unique features. Still, observation alone is limited and never as informative as a thorough physical exam.

72. What should be the focus of physical examination?
Detecting musculoskeletal, visual, and neurologic deficits. Hence, it should divide gait disorders into three groups:
- *Joint and skeletal abnormalities* (antalgic and fixed joint gait)
- *Motor abnormalities* (causing muscle weakness and thus interfering with initiation of walking: apraxic, spastic, rigid, and paralytic/paretic gait)
- *Impaired balance* (ataxic gait—sensory or cerebellar)

(1) GAIT DISTURBANCES DUE TO PAIN

73. What is an antalgic gait?
From the Greek "against the pain," this is a "limp" caused by discomfort on weight bearing. It is an *antalgic* strategy used by patients with either *hyperesthesia* (from neurologic disease) or pain in one of the weight-bearing joints (hips, knees, ankles, or just the bottom of the feet). The latter is very common, since by age 75, 85% of the population exhibit osteoarthritic changes of the large joints. These can all present in a unique (and diagnostic) fashion:
- **Gonarthrosis** is associated with knee stiffness and inability to flex or extend the leg during gait.
- **Coxarthrosis** causes instead a *coxalgic gait*, characterized by a limited range of *hip* extension and a "lateral (or adductor) lurch." This is an excessive lateral shift of the patient's upper body toward the affected side when standing on the painful limb, which effectively relocates the center of gravity, thus reducing the weight load.
- Finally, if the pain originates in the **foot**, there will be an incomplete (and very gentle) contact with the ground.

Whatever the source of pain, antalgic gaits are all characterized by *very short stance on the affected leg,* which is placed gingerly on the floor and lifted almost immediately, with weight rapidly redistributed to the normal leg.

(2) GAIT DISTURBANCES DUE TO IMMOBILE JOINTS

74. What are examples of abnormal gait due to a fixed joint?
In addition to loss of mobility from osteoarthritis, the most common example is the *plantar flexion contracture* of patients who have undergone prolonged periods of plaster immobilization. This may cause an inability of the foot to clear the ground, with compensatory foot-dragging or shifts in the center of gravity while walking. Immobile joints can be easily spotted by testing range of motion of hips, knees, and ankles.

(3) GAIT DISTURBANCES DUE TO MUSCLE WEAKNESS

75. **What is the most common gait abnormality due to muscle weakness?**
The one resulting from weak hip abductors (gluteus *medius* and *minimus*).

76. **What is the anatomy of gluteus *medius* and *minimus*?**
Both muscles originate on the *ilium*: between anterior and posterior gluteal lines (gluteus medius) and middle and inferior lines (gluteus minimus); both insert on the *greater trochanter* (lateral surface for gluteus medius, anterior surface for gluteus minimus); and both are innervated by the superior gluteal nerve ($L_{4,5}$–S_1). When contracting, both muscles pull the greater trochanter toward the lateral surface of the ilium, thus resulting in:
- Elevation of the *contralateral* pelvis
- *Ipsilateral* hip abduction and internal rotation

77. **What is a Trendelenburg gait?**
A gait produced by weakness of the hip abductors, causing the pelvis to *fall toward the unsupported side*. Normally, with each step the pelvis drops a few degrees to the side of the non–weight-bearing (or swinging) leg, but contractions of the hip abductors of the *opposite* (and weight-bearing) side usually minimize the extent of this fall. Yet, if these muscles are weak, they cannot hold up the *contralateral* pelvis, thus letting it sag toward the unsupported side. Hence, the "swinging" limb becomes too low to clear the ground. In an effort to raise the leg, patients learn to lean away from the unsupported side, with a compensatory "lateral lurch" toward the side of the weakened abductors. When both sides are weak, this "lateral lurch" becomes *bilateral*, producing a typical "waddling (or anserine) gait." Note that patients may also compensate by *stepping very high on the unsupported side*, thus allowing the "swinging" leg to clear the ground. This is known as "(high) steppage gait."

78. **What is an anserine gait?**
It is the duck-like waddle (from the Latin *anserinus*, goose) of girdle muscular dystrophy and progressive muscular dystrophy (or Duchenne's disease). Since these patients have *bilateral* hip adductors weakness, they walk with very short steps, *tilting their body from side to side in a characteristic sway*. They also keep their legs spread wide apart, with shoulders sloped slightly forward. On standing, they exhibit an exaggerated lumbar lordosis and a protuberant abdomen. They also have a very typical (not to mention difficult) way of getting up from a chair: first they bend forward (placing both hands on the knees); then they push themselves up by sliding their hands up the thighs. This *Gowers' maneuver* allows them to stand up from either a sitting or kneeling position, and it is so typical that it often allows an immediate diagnosis of muscular dystrophy. Note that if the arms are kept outstretched, standing becomes impossible.

79. **What are the causes of a Trendelenburg gait?**
The two most common are:
- **Neuromuscular weakness of the hip abductors** (nowadays resulting primarily from hip arthroplasty, but also from muscular atrophy/dystrophy—previously discussed)
- **Hip disease** (especially congenital dislocation)

80. **Describe the gait of "foot drop."**
It is a (high) steppage gait. "Foot drop" (i.e., the inability to dorsiflex the ankle while walking because of weak tibialis anterior and toe extensors) presents with two unique features:
- **High steppage:** This consists of knees raised unusually high to allow the drooping foot to clear the ground. And yet, since the toes of the lifted foot remain pointed *downward*, they may still scrape the floor, thus resulting in frequent stumbles and falls. A foot drop can often be

diagnosed by simply looking at the patient's shoes, since wears and tears will be typically asymmetric, *especially affecting the toes*.

- **"Foot slap":** After the heel touches the ground, the forefoot is brought down suddenly and in a slapping manner. This creates a typical *double loud sound of contact* (first the heel and then the forefront).

81. **What are the causes of foot drop?**

The most common are lower motor neuron disease, peripheral neuropathy, peroneal injury, and muscular atrophies. If the proximal (girdle) muscles are affected, then the patient acquires a waddling (anserine) gait.

82. **What is a *Charcot-Marie-Tooth* (CMT) gait?**

It is another (high) steppage gait. In earlier forms, this can be easily identified by having the patient run and by noticing how high the knees are raised in order for the drooping toes to clear the ground.

83. **What is CMT?**

A progressive and hereditary degeneration of peripheral nerves and roots that leads to wasting of the distal muscles of the extremities. CMT involves feet and legs initially (*peroneal nerve paralysis*), and hands and arms later. It rarely involves muscles more central than the elbows, or above the mid-third of the thighs. The first sign of the disease is often *pes cavus* (an exaggeration of the normal foot arch due to involvement of the extensor and everter muscles of the foot). The foot becomes plantarflexed, inverted, and adducted, producing a typical equinovarus deformity. Calluses and perforating ulcers are also common. Later, all muscles below the middle third of the thighs may atrophy, causing the patient's lower extremities to resemble a "stork leg." Deficits may involve touch and pain (usually in feet earlier than hands), as well as proprioception. Deep tendon reflexes of the involved limbs are usually absent.

84. **Who were Charcot, Marie, and Tooth?**

Jean M. Charcot (1825–1893) was a legend of French medicine. Axel Munthe described him as "short, with the chest of an athlete, the neck of a bull and an impressive appearance: pale, smoothly shaved face, low forehead, cold, piercing eyes, aquiline nose and sensitive lips: the mask of a Roman Caesar." This Roman Caesar almost single-handedly created neurology, with 15 medical eponyms to his credit—including the first description of amyotrophic lateral sclerosis, the characterization of multiple sclerosis as a separate entity (while observing the disease in his housemaid), and several studies in hysteria and hypnotism. He also was an interesting man, albeit cold and a bit aloof. For one, he was an animal lover (who detested the Brits because of fox hunting and researchers because of vivisection). He also was a talented artist, especially in drawing and painting, two skills that helped him become an astute bedside observer. Finally, he was a Beethoven fanatic, who spent Thursday evenings on music, strictly forbidding any medical talk. Yet Charcot was primarily a *charismatic teacher*, who inspired the likes of Pierre Marie, Joseph Babinski, Vladimir Bekhterev, Desiré Bourneville, Gilles de la Tourette, and 29-year-old Sigmund Freud. He was especially famous for his theatrical and flamboyant teaching style, which replaced traditional hospital rounds with patient interviews in the amphitheater of the Salpêtrière. This had been the arsenal and gunpowder store of Louis XIII, but under Charcot it became a hospice for more than 5000 indigent patients—many with *hysteria*. In fact, "hysteria shows" were Charcot's unique specialty, eventually making him a household name. This did not prevent him from developing angina and dying at 68 of pulmonary edema. Still, his contributions as diagnostician were staggering and aptly summarized in his own words: "We tend to see only what we are *ready* to see, what we have been taught to see. We eliminate and ignore everything that is not part of our prejudices. Hence, if the clinician wishes to see things as they really are, he must make a *tabula rasa* of his mind and proceed without any preconceived notion." Words still valid today.

Pierre Marie (1853–1940) was a student of Charcot, whom he eventually succeeded at the Salpêtrière. He had actually started in law, but soon switched to medicine, and eventually to neurology, where he contributed the first description of acromegaly and three aphasia papers.

Henry Tooth (1856–1925) was a British army surgeon during the Boer war and World War I, where he distinguished himself at Malta and on the Italian front. Well liked by students and peers, Dr. Tooth was also an excellent spare-time carpenter and musician. He described CMT disease in his Cambridge doctorate of medicine thesis, the same year (1886) as Charcot and Marie.

(4) GAIT DISTURBANCES DUE TO ABNORMAL NEUROLOGIC CONTROL

85. **What are the most common causes of *neurologic* gait disturbance?**
    Myelopathy (16% of all neurologic cases), followed by *ataxia* (cerebellar 8%; sensory 17%), *apraxia* (upper motor neuron and frontal lobe disease in 20% of cases), and *Parkinson's disease* (10%).

86. **What is the most common cause of *myelopathy*?**
    Cervical spondylosis, with B_{12} deficiency a distant second. Osteophytic protrusions are epidemic in the elderly, causing cervical cord impressions in one tenth of patients older than 70, often with no neck discomfort or radicular pain. Eventually, chronic cord compression (*spinal stenosis*) may lead to spasticity and hyperreflexia in the lower extremities, urinary urgency, and posterior column signs.

87. **Describe the gait of spinal stenosis.**
    The early gait is stiff-legged, with circumduction and reduced toe clearance. Later it becomes wide-based, unsteady, shuffling, and spastic. This is because *lumbar* encroachment may result in both abnormal proprioception (with sensory ataxia) *and* spasticity. Hence, the slow, unsteady, and yet stiff gait of spinal stenosis. The diagnosis should be suspected in older patients with severe lower-extremity pains that resolve on sitting. Thigh pain after 30 seconds of lumbar extension is also a good predictor. Neurologically, there is usually an abnormal Romberg's sign (inability to stand with feet together and eyes closed for more than 60 seconds), abnormal Achilles reflex, decreased strength (of knee flexors and extensors, ankle dorsiflexors and plantar flexors, and extensor hallucis longus muscle), and dorsal column signs (vibration and weakened pinprick). Difficulties with sphincter control can also be present, but only in 20% of the cases.

88. **Describe the gait of spastic *paraplegia*.**
    With hips adducted and internally rotated (so that thighs rub together), and legs slightly flexed at the hips and knees. Overall, patients appear to be crouching. Because of their excessive adduction, legs are unable to move straight forward. Instead, they swing across each other in a typical criss-cross motion at the knees ("scissor gait"). Since ankles are plantarflexed, patients walk on tiptoe, with feet scraping the floor (and soles becoming typically worn along the toes). To compensate for the stiff movement of the legs, patients may move the trunk from side to side. For an illustration of the gait of spastic paraplegia, go to *http://web. macam98.ac.il/~shayke/hebrew/ppt/adaptask/adaptation/walk.htm*.

89. **What are the causes of a spastic paraplegic gait?**
    The most common is *spinal cord disease,* causing lower motor neuron involvement with spasticity and weakness in both lower extremities. In contrast to Parkinson's, toes of spastic paraplegia always stay on the ground.

90. What is an *ataxic* gait?

The unsteady and uncoordinated walk of *sensory/cerebellar ataxia*. The base is wide, and the feet are thrown outward.

91. What is the gait of *sensory* ataxia?

It is the gait of patients who have lost sensory and proprioceptive sensation in the lower extremities. In the golden days of syphilis, this used to be pathognomonic of *tabes dorsalis*, but now it is mostly due to neuropathy of large afferent fibers. Patients with sensory ataxia are unaware of their limbs' position in space; hence, they walk by taking steps that are higher than necessary, while at the same time carefully monitoring the ground. Although their gait is as wide as that of *cerebellar ataxia*, only patients with *sensory* ataxia typically *slap* the foot onto the ground (to increase peripheral input). And although their stance is as wide based as that of cerebellar ataxia, only sensory ataxia patients have positive a Romberg's sign (swaying and falling after loss of compensatory visual input). This is also why they have difficulty walking at night.

92. What is Drachman-Hart syndrome?

A form of sensory ataxia due to multiple sensory deficits, including vision, vestibularis, and proprioception. Described by Drachman and Hart in dizzy diabetics.

93. What is a *cerebellar* gait?

It is the unsteady, staggering, and cautious gait of *cerebellar ataxia*: totally irregular in rate, range, and direction. This is accompanied by swaying to one side or the other, so that patients often look for something to lean on, whether a cane, bed rail, or even the wall. Balance typically fails when attempting to walk heel to toe. *Stance* is widened, but not enough to prevent staggering. Titubation while standing worsens considerably when patients are asked to close their feet together, causing wobbling and even falling. Still, in contrast to *sensory* ataxia, opening (or closing) of the eyes neither improves nor destabilizes stance. Since the cerebellum is responsible for proper balance and posture, a cerebellar gait results from either cerebellar disease or alcohol intoxication. Hence, it differs from sensory ataxia since it is associated with other signs of cerebellar deficit, like dysmetria, dysarthria, nystagmus, hypotonia, and intention tremor.

94. Describe the gait of a toxic-metabolic encephalopathy.

It is a gait associated with motor disturbance, altered sensorium, wide base, asterixis, and tendency to fall backward. Although typical of *uremia* or *hepatic* failure, it can also occur with neuroleptics and benzodiazepines, since these impair postural reflexes and thus predispose to falls.

95. What is a gait of spastic *hemiplegia* (circumduction gait)?

It is the stiff and foot-dragging walk of patients who have suffered a hemispheric stroke (*hemiplegic gait*), although some simply have a history of vascular disease. On the affected side, there are (1) upper extremity adduction and *flexion* at all levels (elbow, wrist, and fingers); and (2) lower extremity *extension* at all levels (hip, knee, and ankle). The foot is internally rotated. Spastic hemiplegic patients have great difficulty in flexing the involved hip and knee and in dorsiflexing the ankle (which remains flexed downward and inward—equinovarus deformity). As a result, they do not drag the foot limply behind them, but swing it on the affected side in a half-circle (*circumduction*), with the foot scraping the ground on its lateral edge, in a typical wear-and-tear of the shoes. The upper body tilts to the opposite side (compensating for the semicircular movement of the leg), and the walk is overall difficult and slow. Asymmetric arm-swinging is another typical feature, even though this may also occur in 70% of normal subjects.

96. What is *apraxic* (frontal) gait?

A wide-based gait characterized by hesitation in starting and short, shuffling steps that rarely leave the floor. Hence, the term "magnetic gait," as if the feet were glued to the ground. Some patients also have difficulty in maintaining an upright posture, due to the forward flexion of the upper trunk, arms, and knees. They also lack reflexes against sudden perturbation. This not only causes them to fall, but also makes turns difficult, often leading to a misdiagnosis of Parkinson's (even though apraxic patients typically maintain arm swinging). Mild cognitive deficits are also common, such as constructional dyspraxia (inability to draw a five-pointed star) and memory impairments (of the retrieval type). Apraxic gait is *not* due to muscle weakness, paralysis, or other motor/sensory impairments, but to the inability to carry out familiar purposeful movements. Hence, sensory response and deep tendon reflexes are usually normal (although the plantar reflex may be of the Babinski type). The neuroanatomic basis is a disconnection of prefrontal and frontal regions from the other parts of the motor control system.

97. **What are the causes of apraxic gait?**
The most common are small subcortical strokes of the white matter of the frontal regions (Binswanger's disease). This is usually the result of smoking, hypertension, diabetes, or aging. Other causes include *frontal lobe tumors* and *normal pressure hydrocephalus,* where the apraxic gait is associated with bladder urgency, urinary incontinence, dementia, and a cerebrospinal fluid pressure <180 mmHg. Response to removal of 40–50 mL of cerebrospinal fluid is often diagnostic.

98. **What is a *Parkinsonian* gait?**
The frozen gait of Parkinson's disease. This is so typical that in the absence of tremor it provides the most reliable sign of the disease. Its main feature is axial *rigidity*—resulting in a rather *slow* walk, characterized by a series of small and narrow-based steps that barely clear the ground. It is especially difficult to *initiate* the gait, not only when trying to rise from a chair, but also when starting to walk after long standing. Very characteristic are also the *freezing episodes,* which typically occur when crossing a threshold, facing a door, turning a corner, or simply transitioning from hardwood to carpet floor. Turns are also rather slow (*en bloc*) due to bradykinesia and postural instability. Overall, patients walk with trunk bent forward, arms immobile at the side (or flexed ahead of the body—*but never swinging*), and legs bent at the hips, knees, and ankles. Other typical features include:

- *Festination* (progressively shorter and accelerated steps after the walk has finally begun, from the Latin *festino*, accelerate)
- *Propulsion* (a tendency to fall forward, and the reason for festination)
- *Retropulsion* (a tendency to involuntarily walk *backward*)
- *Rigidity*, causing not only a forward stoop, but also small shuffling steps, with dragged feet that scrape the ground

Festination is usually a late phenomenon, resulting from all the manifestations of the disease: flexion of hips and knees, forward stoop, and shuffling steps. Especially crucial is the forward leaning (and advancing center of gravity), since patients have to keep moving in order to regain it. This is eventually inadequate, thus causing them to fall. As for *stance,* Parkinson's is characterized by a stooped, rigid, and primarily flexed posture: in the head (bent downward), thoracic spine (bent forward), arms (moderately flexed at the elbows), and legs (slightly flexed at both hips and knees). This may resemble the "simian stance" of spinal stenosis (which is an antalgic posture, since it reduces the pull on the compressed lumbosacral nerves), but in contrast to spinal stenosis, the stance of Parkinson's is completely painless. It is also associated with the typical Parkinsonian gait.

99. **What is a *malingering* gait?**
The gait of either hysterical or malingering patients seeking medico-legal compensation. It is characterized by (1) no objective signs of neurologic deficit; and (2) all kinds of arm and leg movements that follow no physiologic pattern. Despite the theatrics, patients are usually quite capable of maintaining their balance and never allow themselves to fall.

SELECTED BIBLIOGRAPHY

1. Baraff LJ, Schriger DL: Orthostatic vital signs: Variation with age, specificity, and sensitivity in detecting a 450-mL blood loss. Ann Emerg Med 10:99–103, 1992.

2. Bergenwald L, Freyschuss U, Sjostrand T: The mechanism of orthostatic and haemorrhage fainting. Scand Clin Lab Invest 37:209–216, 1977.

3. Detsky AS, Smalley PS, Chang J: The rational clinical examination. Is this patient malnourished? JAMA 271: 54–58, 1994.

4. Eaton D, Bannister P, Mulley GP, Conolly MJ: Axillary sweating in clinical assessment of dehydration in ill elderly patients. BMJ 308:1271, 1994.

5. Ebert RV, Stead EA, Gibson JG: Response of normal subjects to acute blood loss. Arch Intern Med 68:578–590, 1941.

6. Eisner LS: Diagnosing Gait Disorders (videotape). Secaucus, NJ: Continuing Medical Education, 1987.

7. Green DM, Metheny D: The estimation of acute blood loss by the tilt test. Surg Gynecol Obstet 84:1045–1050, 1947.

8. Gross CR, Lindquist RD, Woolley AC, et al: Clinical indicators of dehydration severity in elderly patients. J Emerg Med 10:267–274, 1992.

9. Janssen I, Katzmarzyk PT, Ross R: Body mass index, waist circumference, and health risk. Arch Intern Med 162:2074–2079, 2002.

10. Knepp R, Claypool R, Leonardi D: Use of the tilt test in measuring acute blood loss. Ann Emerg Med 9:72–75, 1980.

11. McGee S, Abernathy WB 3rd, Simel DL: Is this patient hypovolemic? JAMA 281:1022–1029, 1999.

12. McGee S: Evidence-Based Physical Diagnosis. Philadelphia, W.B. Saunders, 2001.

13. Ralston LA, Cobb LA, Bruce RA: Acute circulatory effects of arterial bleeding as determined by indicator-dilution curves in normal human subjects. Am Heart J 61:770–776, 1961.

14. Sapira JD: The Art and Science of Bedside Diagnosis. Baltimore, Urban & Shwarzenberg, 1990.

15. Shenkin HA, Cheney RH, Govons SR, et al: On the diagnosis of hemorrhage in man. Am J Med Sci 208:421–436, 1944.

16. Skillman JJ, Olson JE, Lyons JH, et al: The hemodynamic effect of acute blood loss in normal man, with observations on the effect of the Valsalva maneuver and breath holding. Ann Surg 166:713–738, 1967.

17. Wahrenberg H, Hertel K, Leijonhufvud BM, et al: Use of waist circumference to predict insulin resistance: Retrospective study. BMJ 330:1363–1364, 2005.

18. Wallace J, Sharpey-Schafer EP: Blood changes following controlled haemorrhage in man. Lancet 241:393–395, 1941.

19. Warren JV, Brannon ES, Stead EA Jr, et al: The effect of venesection and the pooling of blood in the extremities on the atrial pressure and cardiac output in normal subjects with observations on acute circulatory collapse in three instances. J Clin Invest 24:337–344, 1945.

20. Willis JL, Schneiderman H, Algranati PS: Physical Diagnosis. Williams and Wilkins, Baltimore, 1994.

21. Witting MD, Wears RL, Li S: Defining the positive tilt test. Ann Emerg Med 23:1320–1323, 1994.

CHAPTER 2

VITAL SIGNS

Salvatore Mangione, MD

> "Immediately below a completely compressed artery (with obliteration of the lumen) no sounds are heard. As soon as the first drop of blood escapes from under the site of pressure, we hear a clapping sound very distinctly. This sound is heard when the compressed artery is released and even before the appearance of pulsation in the peripheral branches."
>
> —N.S. Korotkoff, on methods of studying blood pressure. Bull Imperial Acad Med St. Petersburg 11:365, 1905.

> "Humanity has but three great enemies: Fever, Famine and War. Of these by far the greatest, by far the most terrible, is fever."
>
> —Sir William Osler, JAMA 26:999, 1896.

> "A quartan fever kills old men and heals young." —Italian proverb

GENERALITIES

Measuring vital signs is the initial but still essential part of bedside examination. Unfortunately, this task is often relegated to nonphysicians, sometimes even technicians. Yet, as the word implies, *vital* signs can provide a wealth of crucial information, some requiring special skills and knowledge.

A. VITAL STATISTICS

1. **What are the vital statistics?**
   They are *weight* and *height*, both important measurements (*see* Chapter 1, General Appearance, questions 30–49). In contrast to vital *signs*, vital *statistics* are usually stable and thus less clinically helpful.

B. VITAL SIGNS

2. **What are the vital signs?**
   They are crucial (and thus *vital*) measurements that should be obtained in every meaningful patient interaction. They include *heart rate* and *rhythm*, *respiratory rate*, *temperature*, and *blood pressure*. To these, hemoglobin oxygen saturation (O_2 sat) has been recently added.

C. TEMPERATURE

3. **What is a fever?**
   A bodily temperature >98.6°F (37°C). This is the value traditionally considered "normal," based on 19th-century data by Wunderlich, who took 1 million axillary temperatures in 25,000 subjects. Yet, many normal people can get higher than 98.6 simply because of exercise or exposure. Moreover, gender differences (temperatures are usually higher in women than men) and

swings over time (lowest values between 1–8 AM and highest between 4–9 PM) make "normal" a bit more flexible. A more recent study by Mackowiak et al. indicates that the upper limit of *normal* should be considered an oral temperature of 99.9°F (37.7°C). Fever, therefore, is anything above it.

4. **Which is higher, rectal or oral temperature?**
   Rectal temperature. The difference is around 1°F (0.55°C) but can be even greater in mouth-breathing or tachypneic patients, whose rectal values may average 1.67°F (0.93°C) more than oral values.

5. **Are there any other conditions that can alter oral temperature?**
   Beside tachypnea (which decreases oral temperature by 0.5°C for every 10 breaths/minute increase in respiratory rate), recent ingestion of cold or hot substances (including smoking a cigarette) may also change it—something well known to anyone who ever tried to play hooky from school (*see factitious fever* in question 17).

6. **What about tympanic membrane temperatures?**
   They are lower than oral temperatures and better suited to reflect *core* temperatures. Yet, they can be lowered by cerumen (hence, always check for it) and, depending on time of recording, may exhibit greater swings than other modalities of measurement.

7. **What about axillary temperatures?**
   To Wunderlich's chagrin, they are very inaccurate and should be avoided. Especially in patients with hemiparesis, where the affected site always exhibits a significantly lower temperature.

8. **How long does it take for a thermometer to equilibrate when placed under the tongue?**
   Three minutes with the old mercury thermometers, and around one with the newest models.

9. **What is the clinical significance of a fever?**
   It usually indicates the presence of an *infection*. Fever, however, can also be present in *inflammatory processes* (like autoimmune diseases), *cancers*, *drug reactions*, or even *environmental exposure* (heat stroke). They may also occur in *dysmetabolic and endocrine disorders*, such as Graves' disease and Addisonian crisis.

10. **What are the most commonly encountered fever patterns?**
    There are four classic ones:
    - **Sustained or continued** (little variability from day to day): This used to be the pattern of *lobar pneumonia*, steady until abruptly resolving by either *crisis* or death. Nowadays, a sustained pattern is mostly seen in *gram-negative sepsis*, but also in central nervous system (CNS) diseases.
    - **Intermittent:** With complete resolution between episodes (see later)
    - **Remittent:** Abating every day, but still not completely resolving. This used to be the pattern of *typhoid fever*.
    - **Relapsing:** With a series of febrile attacks, each lasting several days, and all separated by afebrile intervals of about the same length. A relapsing fever is usually *infectious* (brucellosis, borreliosis, or relapsing typhoid, but also tuberculosis [TB]), but can occur in Hodgkin's, too, or familial Mediterranean fever.

11. **What are the most common fever types?**
    Intermittent or *remittent*. In fact, since the introduction of antibiotics, all the aforementioned associations have become more historic than diagnostic. Yet, a *continued* pattern in the face of antibiotics should still suggest four primary explanations:
    - Resistant organism
    - Closed space infection

- Superinfection
- Allergic reaction

It might also suggest a noninfectious etiology, such as an occult neoplasm or autoimmune disease.

12. **What are the main types of "intermittent" fever?**

The classic ones are those of *malaria*, one of the three great *medical* killers of mankind (the others being TB and HIV, plus, of course, war and organized religion). Intermittent malarial fevers vary considerably, based on organism involved:

- **Quotidian fever:** From the Latin *quotidianus*, daily. This is a fever whose paroxysm (and resolution) occurs every day. It is usually caused by a *double tertian malaria*, due to infection by two distinct groups of *Plasmodium vivax*, alternately sporulating every 48 hours. It may also be caused by the most pernicious malarial parasite (*P. falciparum*), combined with vivax, or by two distinct falciparum generations that mature on different days, thus resulting in a fever that occurs twice a day. Note that a *double quotidian fever* is a daily two-spikes fever that is *not* malarial, but gonococcal. It used to be present in 50% of endocarditis cases, but today is mostly extinct.
- **Tertian fever:** From the Latin *tertianus*, third. This is a *P. vivax* fever that recurs every third day, counting the day of an episode as the first. Hence, it occurs every 48 hours (every other day).
- **Quartan fever:** From the Latin *quartanus*, fourth. This is a *P. malariae* fever that recurs every fourth day, counting the day of an episode as the first. Hence, it occurs every 72 hours. Note that a *double quartan* is instead an infection with two independent groups of quartan parasites, so that the febrile paroxysms occur on two successive days, followed by one without fever.
- **Malignant tertian fever:** This is the fever of *P. falciparum* (*falciparum fever*, or *aestivo-autumnal fever*, or *Roman fever* because it was a common ailment in the countryside of Rome up to World War II). It is characterized by 48-hour paroxysms of a severe form of malaria, occurring with acute cerebral, renal, or gastrointestinal manifestations. These are usually due to clumping of the infected red blood cells, causing secondary capillary obstruction and ischemia.

13. **What are the other most common types of *intermittent* fever?**

They are Charcot's intermittent fever and "hectic" fever.

14. **What is *Charcot's intermittent fever*?**

It is a special *intermittent* fever that is usually accompanied by chills, right upper-quadrant pain, and jaundice. It is due to stones transiently obstructing the common duct.

15. **What is a "hectic" fever?**

From the Greek *hektikos* (habitual), this is a form of *intermittent fever* characterized by wide swings, usually greater than 2.5°F (1.4°C). It has a typical daily afternoon spike, often accompanied by facial flushing, and is traditionally linked to active tuberculosis.

16. **What is Pel-Ebstein fever?**

It is the fever of 16% of Hodgkin's cases. It is characterized by episodes lasting for hours or days, followed by afebrile periods of days and even weeks. It is, therefore, a typical *relapsing* fever. It was first described in the 19th century by the Dutch Pieter Pel and the German Wilhelm Ebstein. The latter is probably better remembered for his extracurricular interests, ranging from arts and literature to history. He even wrote a couple of books on the diseases of famous Germans (including Luther and Schopenhauer) and a medical reinterpretation of the Bible.

17. **What is factitious fever?**

A self-induced and artificial fever (from the Latin *factitius*, made by art). This can occur in many ways, the most common being the ingestion (and mouth holding) of hot liquids prior to a temperature check. Factitious fever can often (but not always) be counteracted by measuring rectal temperature (which may even serve as a punitive deterrent) or urinary temperature on voiding. If doing so, remember that urinary temperature is a little lower than oral temperature.

18. **Are there any other terms in this alphabet soup of "fevers"?**
    Quite a few, once again primarily of historic value. For a smorgasbord:
    - **Ephemeral fever:** A febrile episode lasting only a day or two
    - **Epimastical fever:** From the Greek *epakmastikos*, coming to a height. A fever that increases steadily until reaching an acme, and then declines by crisis or lysis (*crisis* indicates a sudden drop, whereas *lysis* indicates a more gradual defervescence).
    - **Exanthematous fever:** A fever associated with an exanthem, i.e., a skin rash
    - **Fatigue (exhaustion) fever:** An elevation of body temperature that follows excessive and continued muscular exertion. It may last sometimes for up to several days.
    - **Miliary fever:** An infectious fever characterized by profuse sweating and the production of *sudamina* (i.e., minute vesicles of fluid retention in sweat follicles, a.k.a. "milia"). Typical of past epidemics.
    - **Monoleptic fever:** A *continued* fever that has only one paroxysm
    - **Polyleptic fever:** From the Greek *poly* (multiple) and *lepsis* (paroxysm). A fever that occurs in two or more paroxysms, as typically seen in malaria.
    - **Undulant fever:** The long and wavy temperature curve of brucellosis

19. **What is an "essential" fever?**
    One with an unknown etiology, whether ultimately due to infection or other processes. It is defined as a temperature of at least 100.4°F (or 38°C), lasting 3 weeks or longer, and with no identifiable cause—often referred to as FUO (*fever of unknown origin*).

20. **What are the causes of an essential fever?**
    FUO in adults is most commonly due to *infection*, either closed space (abscess) or disseminated (malaria, tuberculosis, HIV, endocarditis, fungemia). Other less common causes include *cancer* (particularly lymphomas, hypernephromas, hepatomas, and hepatic metastasis of extrahepatic tumors); *autoimmune diseases* (collagen vascular diseases and vasculitis); and *drug reactions*. Patients with iatrogenic fever often have temperature/pulse dissociation, appear well in spite of high fever, and have other allergic signs, like skin rash or eosinophilia.

21. **What is a temperature/pulse dissociation?**
    A rise in temperature that is not matched by an equivalent rise in heart rate. Normally, for each degree of temperature increase there is a 10 beats/minute increase in heart rate. This, however, may not always occur. Fever with *relative bradycardia* has a narrow differential diagnosis, usually *infectious* (including, among others, salmonellosis and typhoid fever, brucellosis, legionellosis, mycoplasma pneumonia, and meningitis with increased intracranial pressure), but possibly *iatrogenic* (like a drug fever) or simply the use of digitalis or beta blockers.

22. **What are the causes of *extreme pyrexia*?**
    Very high temperatures (>105°F, or 40.6°C) are usually due to neurologic thermodysregulations (i.e., *central* fever). These include heat stroke, cerebrovascular accidents, or major anoxic brain injury following a cardiac arrest. *Malignant hyperthermia* and *neuroleptic malignant syndrome* are other important causes of very high fevers of central origin, often raising temperature >106°F (or 41.2°C). Fevers of this degree *can* be due (but often *not*) to an infectious process like gram-negative sepsis. The exception is a CNS infection, such as meningitis or encephalitis.

23. **What are the causes of an inappropriately *low* fever?**
    Fever lower than expected is typical of patients with *chronic renal failure* (especially if uremic), but also of those receiving antipyretics (such as acetaminophen) and nonsteroidal anti-inflammatory agents. Inappropriately low temperature may also be caused by *shock*.

24. **What other physical findings may help identify the cause of a fever?**
    - *Anhidrosis* argues in favor of either heat stroke or drugs interfering with diaphoresis.
    - *Muscle rigidity* suggests neuroleptic malignant syndrome or malignant hyperthermia.

- *Jaundice* may be seen in bacterial infections, independent of their direct involvement of the hepatobiliary system (such as cholangitis or hepatitis, *see* question 14).
- *Shaking chills* argue only modestly in favor of bacteremia. Conversely:
- *Historic predictors* (such as *diabetes mellitus* and *old age*) plus the degree of *leukocytosis* and the presence of *hypotension* argue very strongly in favor of bacteremia.

25. **What is *hypothermia*?**
    It is a core temperature below 98.6°F (37°C). Yet, given the normal fluctuations, true hypothermia is considered anything below 95°F (35°C). At this low level of temperature, the body usually becomes unable to generate heat, and thus core temperature continues to fall. In fact, at 86°F (30°C), body temperature equilibrates with the environment. Based on this premise:
    - *Mild hypothermia* is a core temperature of 89.6–95°F (32–35°C).
    - *Moderate hypothermia* is one of 82.4–89.6°F (28–32°C).
    - *Profound hypothermia* is one less than 82.4°F (<28°C). Temperatures of this degree are missed by routine thermometers and thus require thermistors.

26. **What are the causes of hypothermia?**
    Various. Based on its mechanism, hypothermia is usually classified as:
    - *Primary* (typically due to accidental exposure)
    - *Secondary* (due instead to failure of thermoregulation)
    Depending on its setting, the most common cause of hypothermia is *overwhelming sepsis* or *environmental exposure*. Other major causes include *cerebrovascular accidents* (anorexia nervosa, multiple sclerosis, stroke, coma of any cause, spinal cord injury), *low cardiac output* following acute myocardial infarction, *endocrine disorders* (hypoglycemia, hypothyroidism, panhypopituitarism, adrenal insufficiency), and *intoxication* (drugs and alcohol). Note that patients who appear hypothermic to touch are often simply peripherally vasoconstricted.

27. **What are the signs and symptoms of hypothermia?**
    They vary, depending on the degree of hypothermia and the type of underlying disorder (a *stroke*, for example, may obscure the signs of hypothermia). Moreover, symptoms and signs are often a continuum, and there is major variability among patients (Table 2-1).

TABLE 2-1. SIGNS AND SYMPTOMS OF HYPOTHERMIA

Mild Hypothermia	Moderate Hypothermia	Severe Hypothermia
Confusion	Level of consciousness diminishes	Unresponsiveness or coma
Tachypnea	Delirium	May appear dead*
Tachycardia	Bradycardia	Loss of reflexes
Vasoconstriction	Bradypnea	Very cold skin
Lethargy	Shivering stops	Hypotension
Shivering	Reflexes slowed	Pulmonary edema
Ataxia	Cold diuresis	Respiratory failure
Dysarthria		Profound acidemia and ventricular fibrillation
Loss of fine motor coordination		

*Hence, you are never dead until you are *warm* and dead (*see* Chapter 20, Coma).

D. HEART RATE AND RHYTHM

28. **What is the history behind the measurement of heart rate through the arterial pulse?**
Interpretation of a *weak pulse* as a bad prognostic indicator goes all the way back to third-millennium Egypt, but only in Ptolemaic and Hellenistic Alexandria (third and second century BC) did such knowledge eventually get applied to the *heart rate*. The two leading figures of the time were *Herophilus of Chalcedon* and his rival *Erasistratus of Cos*, both Hippocratic Greeks who had moved to Egypt to perform dissections, practice medicine, and conduct research. Erasistratus gave heart valves the names they still carry today and eventually committed suicide because of incurable cancer. Herophilus described not only the duodenum (which he named after the Greek word for 12 fingers, the measurement of its length), but also the liver, spleen, circulatory system, eye, brain, and genital organs. He gave great importance to drugs ("the hands of God") and was the first to suggest that physicians could be guided diagnostically by the *arterial pulse*, which he counted by using a portable water clock. Influenced by musical theories, he even developed a classification of pulse *characteristics*, based on rate, rhythm, strength, and amplitude.

Five hundred years later, the Romans perfected this knowledge through the work of Galen, who defined the diagnostic significance of the pulse in terms of force, length, and speed. Half a millennium later, the Chinese developed an even more complicated classification, requiring analysis of the pulse at various sites and simultaneous timing with the physician's own respiration. Four pulsations to each respiratory cycle constituted the normal adult rate. To avoid possible distractions, practitioners were asked to banish all extraneous thoughts prior to an exam and to conduct their assessments in the morning (and on an empty stomach).

Things got a little easier in the 18th century, when the British physician John Floyer (1649–1734) asked a local watchmaker to build him a portable clock with a special second hand that ran exactly for 1 minute. This allowed him to accurately determine the speed of the pulse and to publish in 1707 "The Physician's Pulse Watch," a little treatise that suggested the use of the watch for a more objective determination of the pulse. Floyer also had other and more eccentric interests. One, for example, involved Dr. Samuel Johnson, whom he examined as a 5-year-old child, eventually recommending a healthy dose of "Royal Touch" as remedy against various evils (Dr. Johnson's mother complied, and so did Queen Anne, who touched and reportedly "healed" the child). Other eccentricities concerned a lifelong fascination with minerals, vegetables, and animals (he wrote a book about discovering their virtues through taste and smell) and a similarly lifelong fascination with cold bathing (he wrote a book on that, too). Maybe because of all this baggage, Floyer's recommendations on the pulse went mostly unheard, so that for decades practitioners continued to rely more on their "feel" of the pulse, than on an objective assessment of rate and rhythm.

It was only during the mid-19th century that measurement through a watch became the standard of medical care. That was also the time when Adams and Stokes made the connection between an inappropriate slowing of the pulse and some episodes of syncope and seizure, thus shifting attention from the brain to the heart (and to physical exam).

29. **How should the pulse be examined?**
It depends. If you are simply assessing *rate* and *rhythm*, the best (and most accurate) technique is to count the pulse at the wrist for 30 seconds, and then double the figure. Alternatively, you could count the *apical* rate, which is more accurate in situations of pronounced tachycardia, especially atrial fibrillation (where *pulse deficit* commonly occurs). In this case, counting 60 seconds may further improve accuracy. Finally, if you want to assess the *characteristics of the waveform*, then you should assess the pulse of a *central* artery (*see* Chapter 10, questions 3–56).

30. **What is a pulse deficit?**
It is the absence of a palpable arterial pulse despite a precordial heartbeat. This is expressed as apical rate minus pulse rate per minute. A pulse deficit is very common in atrial fibrillation, since some ventricular contractions may be too weak to empty into the aorta and cause a

waveform. Missed pulses also can be encountered after premature beats, or in other tachycardic states. Hence, always measure heart rate over both precordium and wrist, especially in tachycardia.

31. So what is a normal heart rate?
The traditionally reported range is 60–100/minute, even though 50 is probably a more accurate lower boundary. Hence, anything <50 is *bradycardia,* whereas anything >100 is *tachycardia.*

32. In addition to rate, which other characteristics should be assessed in a pulse?
Its *regularity*—and if the pulse is irregular, whether the irregularity itself is *regular* or *irregular*. This is especially important in the evaluation of tachycardia.

33. What is the clinical significance of tachycardia?
Usually ominous. Common in infection and ischemia, a *sinus* tachycardia predicts poor outcome in pneumonia, sepsis, pontine hemorrhage, myocardial infarction, gallstone pancreatitis, and congestive heart failure.

34. What bedside information can help to evaluate an arrhythmia?
In times of electrocardiograms (ECGs), it seems almost anachronistic to discuss the physical examination of arrhythmias. Yet a thorough and astute exam, comprising an assessment of arterial pulse (especially when coordinated with apical impulse—*see pulse deficit* in question 30), venous waveform, and characteristics of heart sounds, can often deliver a diagnosis.

35. What are the features of the pulse one should consider when evaluating arrhythmias?
Its *regularity* (or lack thereof) and its *response to vagal maneuvers*. In this regard:

- A *regularly irregular tachycardia* is a sign of bigeminy or trigeminy. But it can also indicate atrial flutter with variable atrioventricular block (in this case, look for *flutter waves* in the neck veins) or a second-degree heart block in which skipped beats occur at regular intervals.
- An *irregularly irregular tachycardia* is most commonly seen in atrial fibrillation. This is differentiated from frequent premature contractions because the latter may present with occasional cannon "A" waves (*see* Chapter 10, questions 78–88).
- A *regularly regular tachycardia* can be due to atrial flutter (with constant A-V block), paroxysmal atrial tachycardia, ventricular tachycardia, and, of course, sinus tachycardia. Response to vagal maneuvers might be helpful in separating these entities.
- A tachycardia that resolves abruptly after either Valsalva's maneuver or carotid artery massage is a *paroxysmal atrial tachycardia* (typically associated with a unique feeling of "pounding in the neck" due to the simultaneous occurrence of carotid pulsations and cannon "A" waves).
- One that only slows down is usually *sinus tachycardia.*
- One that halves in rate is typically *atrial flutter.*
- *Ventricular tachycardia* is usually unchanged by vagal maneuvers. Ventricular tachycardia, however, typically presents with findings of atrioventricular dissociation, such as cannon "A" waves, and variable intensity of S_1.

36. What other findings might help to recognize an arrhythmia?
- The presence and characteristics of a *pause between heartbeats*. A pause preceded by a premature beat, for example, usually indicates an atrial (or a ventricular) premature contraction, whereas one *not* preceded by a premature beat usually indicates a heart block.
- A premature beat associated with a *cannon "A" wave* on venous exam (*see* Chapter 10, questions 86 and 87) usually indicates an atrial contraction against a closed tricuspid valve and, therefore, a *ventricular* rather than an atrial premature contraction. Cannon "A" waves might also consistently occur in *paroxysmal atrial tachycardia* due to the almost

simultaneous contraction of atria and ventricles in this condition. Conversely, they might occur randomly in *complete heart block*.

- A very loud, almost "cannon-like," S_1 occurring at times in patients with regular rhythm usually suggests the coincidental contraction of atria *just before ventricles*. This argues in favor of an escape ventricular rhythm from complete heart block.
- A "regular" *pulse deficit* (for example, a rate at the wrist that is exactly half of that at the apex) argues in favor of bigeminy, with the premature beats being always unable to achieve ejection. This needs to be differentiated from *pulsus alternans* (*see* Chapter 10, question 23).

E. BLOOD PRESSURE

37. How is blood pressure measured?

It depends. In clinical practice, the standard of measurement is the *indirect* method, which relies on a blood pressure cuff (sphygmomanometer) and can be either *palpatory* or *auscultatory*. The gold standard, however, remains *direct* determination, based on intra-arterial rigid-walled catheter.

38. Why is it important to measure blood pressure accurately?

Because unrecognized hypertension may lead to cardiovascular disease and thus reduce life expectancy. Hypertension is a common medical problem, affecting as many as 1 of 5 North American adults. It is easily treatable but often clinically silent, at least in its initial phases. Only regular and accurate blood pressure measurements can detect it early enough to initiate therapy. In addition, erroneous pressure overestimates may label a normal person as hypertensive, with significant economic, medical, and psychologic repercussions. Hence, correct and frequent ambulatory measurements are key in every physician's armamentarium.

39. What does sphygmomanometer mean?

It is Greek for "measure of a weak pulse" (*sphygmos,* pulse; *manos,* scanty; *metron,* measure).

40. Who invented it?

In contrast to failures (that are almost always orphans), the *sphygmomanometer* has many proud fathers: the French Pierre Potain, the Italian Scipione Riva-Rocci, the Russian Nicolai Korotkoff, and the American Harvey Cushing. Cushing did not really participate in the ideation of the device but was instrumental (no pun intended) in its diffusion to North America. Incidentally, the mercury sphygmomanometer just celebrated his 111th anniversary (it was invented in 1896).

41. Who made the first *direct* measurement of blood pressure?

Stephen Hales, an English botanist and part-time chemist, who in 1733 decided to sacrifice his mare to see whether indeed a "blood pressure" existed. He cannulated the left carotid of the poor animal and then measured the height of the column of blood extending from her artery into a brass pipe until she finally died. Since the blood rose 8 feet and 3 inches above the level of the left ventricle, Hales concluded that there was indeed something he called "blood pressure," and suggested that this varied between arteries and veins, cardiac dilations and contractions, and larger and small animals. He published it under the title "Haemasticks," and then went on to bigger and better things, like telling housewives that putting an inverted teacup in their pies would prevent the crust from getting soggy.

42. Who was Potain? How did he contribute to the measurement of blood pressure?

Pierre Potain was one of the several well-rounded giants produced by 19th-century French medicine. A true humanist who never went to sleep without reading a few pages of his beloved Pascal, he was also an interesting man. As an intern, he survived a rendezvous with cholera (which he contracted during the 1849 epidemic) and then an even more dangerous rendezvous with the Prussians (whom he faced during the 1870 war, fighting as a simple foot soldier). Unscathed by these experiences, Potain went on to become one of Trousseau's protégés, a great promoter of cardiac auscultation, and a very compassionate teacher (he was famous for answering his own question if an examinee failed to provide the answer in time). Before dying peacefully in his sleep at age 76, he made many landmark contributions: he was the first to describe (and name) the gallop rhythms, the opening snap of mitral stenosis, the *tambour* S_2 of syphilitic aortitis ("Potain's sign"), the hepatic pulsatility of tricuspid regurgitation, and the waveform analysis of the internal jugular vein. He even inspired the figure of the great Parisian diagnostician in Proust's *Remembrance of Things Past*. His unique contribution to blood pressure measurement consisted of a contraption made of a compressible bulb filled with air and attached by a rubber tube to an aneroid manometer. To measure the blood pressure, the bulb was pressed on the peripheral artery of the patient until the pulse disappeared. The manometric recording at time of pulse disappearance reflected the patient's systolic blood pressure. Potain also taught Riva-Rocci, the next link in this blood pressure saga.

43. **Who first thought of the mercury sphygmomanometer?**
The Italian Scipione Riva-Rocci, who became interested in noninvasive blood pressure measurement while studying air-filling of the pleural cavity at controlled pressures, a technique pioneered by Forlanini for the control of tuberculosis. In 1896, at age 33, Riva-Rocci came up with the idea of "Un nuovo sfigmomanometro" (*a new sphigmomanometer*), which he reported in the *Gazzetta Medica di Torino*. His device was attached to a manometer in which the varying pressures were shown by differences of elevation in a column of mercury rather than by a revolving pointer, as in Potain's *aneroid (or dial) manometer*. The idea was quite good for medicine, but may have been fatal for Riva-Rocci, who years later died of a chronic neurologic condition he probably contracted in the laboratory. Still, he had good insights and made several improvements on Potain's instrument:
- He used the *brachial rather than the radial artery*, making measurements easier and more accurate.
- He used a *wraparound inflatable rubber cuff* that greatly reduced the frequency of Potain's over-readings (later Von Recklinghausen increased the cuff width from 5 to 13cm).
- He suggested *guidelines* for the correct use of the instrument, aimed at minimizing errors.
- He proposed an instrument so *simple and easy to carry* that it made blood pressure measurement feasible even at the bedside. Indeed, with only minor modifications, his original sphygmomanometer is still very much in use 100 years later.
- Finally, Riva-Rocci was also the first to describe the "white-coat" effect of blood pressure measurement (*see* question 61).

44. **How did Riva-Rocci's device reach the United States?**
Serendipity. Despite its achievements, Riva-Rocci's *sfigmomanometro* might have remained a little Italian secret were it not for Harvey Cushing's visit to Pavia in 1901. Cushing spent several days with Riva-Rocci at the Ospedale di San Matteo, made a drawing of the instrument, received one as a gift, and brought everything back to Johns Hopkins. The rest is history.

45. **What were the problems of Riva-Rocci's tool? Who perfected the "indirect" method?**
Both Riva-Rocci's and Potain's devices only provided a *systolic* reading (by releasing the arterial pulse, after its obliteration). Thirty-year-old Nicolai Sergeievich Korotkoff came to the rescue. As often happens in medical breakthroughs, he actually stumbled onto his discovery of *auscultatory recording of blood pressure*. A surgeon in the Czar's army, he had completed a tour of duty in the Russian–Japanese war and was working in St. Petersburg on an animal model of post-surgical arteriovenous fistulae. One day, while listening over a dog's artery before releasing a tourniquet, he suddenly heard loud sounds. Intrigued, he noticed that these

correlated with systole and diastole, and in 1905 reported his observation in the "Izvestie Imp Voiennomedicinskoi Akademii" of St Petersburg. It was a brief report (only 281 words) that suggested that listening for the appearance and disappearance of *pulse sounds* might serve as a signal for maximal and minimal blood pressure. Written in Russian, the paper did not create much noise in Europe, but stirred quite a ruckus at home, winning Korotkoff an enviable reputation as a madman. It was only after the article finally reached Germany (and from there England) that his auscultatory method replaced the pulse obliteration technique of Riva-Rocci and Potain. Modern measurement of systolic and diastolic blood pressure was finally born. Korotkoff did not enjoy the rewards, though. Arrested during the Russian revolution of 1917, he soon died of TB.

46. **What is the systolic pressure?**
    It is the *highest* intra-arterial pressure that can be produced during ventricular systole.

47. **What is the diastolic pressure?**
    It is the *lowest* intra-arterial pressure prior to the next systolic event.

48. **What are the various Korotkoff phases?**
    They are acoustic marks that take place after gradual deflation of the cuff. Validated by intra-arterial recordings, they were first suggested by Goodman and Howell in 1911. They include:
    - **Phase 1:** First appearance of low-frequency tapping sounds
    - **Phase 2:** Softer and longer sounds
    - **Phase 3:** Crisper and louder sounds
    - **Phase 4** (often absent): Initial muffling of sounds
    - **Phase 5:** Complete disappearance of sounds

    Use phase 1 to determine systolic pressure and *phase 5* for diastolic (using phase 4 would overestimate it by close to 20 mmHg).

49. **Where (and how) are Korotkoff sounds produced?**
    They are produced under the distal portion of the cuff, by the systolic reopening of a completely collapsed artery. Note that the sudden tensing of the arterial wall (and its resulting sound) can only occur *between systolic and diastolic pressure* because values above systolic will keep the artery collapsed, whereas values below diastolic will keep it totally open (and, thus, silent).

50. **What is the proper technique for indirect measurement of blood pressure?**
    The American Heart Association has published guidelines for indirect (auscultatory) measurement (Table 2-2). Italicized parts ought to be paid special attention. Note that you should use the stethoscope's *bell* and not the diaphragm (because Korotkoff sounds are low in frequency).

51. **When should blood pressure be measured?**
    In every significant patient interaction, whether ambulatory or hospital based. Always obtain two or more readings from the same arm, with patient supine or seated. Then record the average value. If diastolic readings differ by more than 5 mmHg, take additional measurements until a stable pressure is reached. Measure blood pressure in both arms at the first visit, and then use the arm with the higher pressure thereafter (the arm with the lower pressure is abnormal). When indicated, also measure the pressure in the lower extremities and/or in different positions (supine versus *standing*).

52. **How about comparison of upper extremities' pressure?**
    Blood pressure should be measured at least once in *both* upper extremities. This requires two independent observers, working simultaneously on the two arms and then switching sides.

TABLE 2-2. TECHNIQUE FOR MEASURING BLOOD PRESSURE

The intent and purpose of the measurement should be explained to the patient in a reassuring manner, and every effort should be made to put the patient at ease. (*Include a 5-minute rest before the first measurement.*) The sequential steps for measuring the blood pressure in the upper extremity, as for routine screening and monitoring purposes, should include the following:

1. Have paper and pen at hand for immediate recording of the pressure.

2. *Seat the patient* in a quiet, calm environment [*with feet flat on the floor, and back supported against the chair*] with his or her bared arm resting on a standard table or other support *so that the midpoint of the upper arm is at the level of the heart.*

3. Estimate by inspection, or measure with a tape, the circumference of the bare upper arm at midpoint between acromium and olecranon, and select an appropriately sized cuff. *The bladder inside the cuff should encircle 80% of the arm in adults* and 100% in children less than 13 years old. If in doubt, use a larger cuff. If the available cuff is too small, this should be noted.

4. Palpate the brachial artery and place the cuff so that the midline of the bladder is over the arterial pulsation; then wrap and secure the cuff snugly around the patient's bare arm. Avoid rolling up the sleeve in such a manner that it forms a tight tourniquet around the upper arm. Loose application of the cuff results in overestimation of the pressure. The lower edge of the cuff should be 1 in (2 cm) above the antecubital fossa where the head of the stethoscope is to be placed.

5. Place the manometer so that the center of the mercury column (or aneroid dial) is at eye level (except for tilted-column floor models) and easily visible, and tubing from cuff is unobstructed.

6. Inflate the cuff rapidly to 70 mmHg, and increase by 10 mmHg increments while palpating the radial pulse. Note the level of pressure at which the pulse disappears and subsequently reappears during deflation. This palpatory method provides a necessary preliminary approximation of the systolic BP, and ensures an adequate level of inflation for the actual, auscultatory measurement. The palpatory method is particularly useful to avoid underinflation of the cuff in patients with an auscultatory gap and overinflation in those with very low BP.

7. Place the earpieces of the stethoscope into the ear canals, angled forward to fit snugly. *Switch the stethoscope head to the low-frequency position (bell).* The setting can be confirmed by listening as the stethoscope head (i.e., the bell orifice) is tapped gently.

8. Place the head of the stethoscope over the brachial artery pulsation, just above and medial to the antecubital fossa but below the edge of the cuff, and hold it firmly (but not too tightly) in place, making sure that the head makes contact with the skin around its entire circumference. Wedging the head of the stethoscope under the edge of the cuff may free one hand but results in considerable extraneous noise (and is nearly impossible with the bell in any event).

9. *Inflate the bladder rapidly and steadily to a pressure 20–30 mmHg above the level previously determined by palpation;* then partially unscrew (open) the valve and deflate the bladder at 2 mm[Hg]/sec while listening for the appearance of the Korotkoff sounds.

10. As pressure in the bladder falls, note the level of pressure on the manometer at the first appearance of repetitive sounds (Phase I), at the muffling of these sounds (Phase IV), and when they disappear (Phase V). While Korotkoff sounds are audible, *rate of deflation should be no more than 2 mm per pulse beat,* thus compensating for both rapid and slow heart rates.

Continued

TABLE 2-2. TECHNIQUE FOR MEASURING BLOOD PRESSURE—CONT'D

11. After the Korotkoff sound is heard, the cuff should be deflated slowly for at least another 10 mmHg to ensure that no further sounds are audible and then rapidly and completely deflated. The patient should be allowed to rest for at least 30 seconds.

12. The systolic (Phase I) and diastolic (Phase V) pressures should be recorded immediately, *rounded off (upward) to the nearest 2 mmHg*. In children, and when sounds are heard nearly to a level of 0 mmHg, Phase IV pressure also should be recorded (example: 108/65/56 mmHg). All values should be recorded together with the name of the patient, the date and time of the measurement, the arm on which the measurement was made, the patient's position, and the cuff size (when a nonstandard size is used).

13. *Measurement should be repeated after at least 30 seconds, and the two readings averaged*. Additional measurements can be made in the same or opposite arm, same or alternative position.

53. **What is a significant difference between the two arms?**
A difference in systolic pressure >10–15 mmHg. If >20, this usually indicates a subclavian artery occlusion, whose etiology varies based on setting. In an acute situation, it usually suggests *aortic dissection* (with aortic regurgitation in cases of more proximal dissection). In more chronic settings, it would instead indicate a *subclavian steal syndrome*, wherein blood is "stolen" from the vertebral circulation to feed a hypoperfused arm. Patients with this condition usually present with vertebrobasilar symptoms, such as vertigo, hemiparesis, ataxia, and visual changes. They can also have a diminished arterial pulse and an ipsilateral bruit over the subclavian artery.

54. **Which factors can affect the accuracy of blood pressure measurement?**
Several, and these can be related to patient, equipment, or examiner (Table 2-3). Conversely, some factors have no effect on blood pressure: menstrual phase, chronic caffeine ingestion, phenylephrine nasal spray, cuff self-inflation, discordance in gender or race of examinee and examiner, thin shirt sleeve under cuff, bell versus diaphragm, cuff inflation per se, hour of day (during work hours), and room temperature.

55. **How variable can pressure be?**
Quite variable. With >2 measurements at each visit, the standard deviation between visits is 5–12 mmHg systolic and 6–8 diastolic. Between-visits variability is greater than *within-visit* fluctuation. Hence, more visits are needed to ensure diagnostic precision. That is why the Joint National Committee on Prevention, Detection, Evaluation, and Treatment of High Blood Pressure recommends repeat measurements within 1 month for initial values in the range of 160–179 mmHg systolic or 100–109 mmHg diastolic (stage 2 hypertension), within 2 months for stage 1, within 1 week for stage 3, and immediate evaluation for stage 4. Arrhythmias (especially atrial fibrillation) also may cause beat-to-beat variations in cardiac output and thus increase interobserver variation in blood pressure measurements. Averaging several readings may help.

56. **And how about the physician's expertise?**
Although interobserver agreement is usually high for blood pressure measurement, examiners may also be responsible for errors. In fact inter examiners differences of 10/8 mmHg are quite common. A common physician's error is excessive pressure with the stethoscope (which can

TABLE 2-3. FACTORS AFFECTING THE IMMEDIATE ACCURACY OF OFFICE BLOOD PRESSURE

Examinee		Examiner		Examination	
Increase	Decrease	Increase	Decrease	Increase	Decrease
Soft Korotkoff sound	Soft Korotkoff sounds	Expectation bias	Reading to next lowest 5 or 10 mmHg or expectation bias	Cuff too narrow	Left versus right arm
Missed auscultatory gap	Recent meal	Impaired hearing	Impaired hearing	Cuff not centered	Resting for too long (25 min)
DBP (rare, huge)	Missed auscultatory gap			Cuff over clothing	Elbow too high
Pseudohypertension	High stroke volume			Elbow too low	Too rapid deflation
"White coat" reaction	Habituation			Cuff too loose	Excessive bell pressure
To physician	Shock (additional pseudohypotension)			Too short rest period	Parallax error (aneroid)
To nonphysician				Back unsupported	Noisy environment
Paretic arm (due to stroke)				Arm unsupported	Faulty aneroid device
Pain, anxiety					Low mercury level
Acute smoking					Leaky bulb
Acute caffeine					
Acute ethanol ingestion					

Distended bladder	Too slow deflation
Talking, signing	Too fast deflation
Setting, equipment	Parallax error
Environmental noise	Using phase IV (adult)
Leaky bulb valve	
Blocked manometer vents	Too rapid remeasure
Cold hands or stethoscope	Cold season (versus arm)

SBP = systolic blood pressure, DBP = diastolic blood pressure. (Modified from Reeves RA: Does this patient have hypertension? How to measure blood pressure. JAMA 273:1211–1217, 1995.)

lower the diastolic reading). Another error is placing the patient's arm either higher than the level of the heart (which lowers both systolic and diastolic readings) or *lower* (which increases them).

57. What is the most common "equipment" error?

The wrong cuff size (shorter cuffs overestimate blood pressure, whereas larger ones underestimate it). Also, aneroid instruments (used by 34% of practices) often go out of calibration, usually *downward*. In surveys, one third of office devices were off by >10 mm. Hence, the need for periodical recalibration.

58. How do you calibrate an aneroid sphygmomanometer?

Against a mercury unit, and by using a Y connector to link the cuff to both devices.

59. What is the silent or auscultatory gap?

A finding present in one fifth of elderly patients with hypertension. It consists of a temporary disappearance of Korotkoff sounds after the systolic reading (and during phase II Korotkoff), with sudden reappearance of sounds just above diastolic values. This may *underestimate* the systolic pressure, *unless one simultaneously palpates the radial pulse* (which persists throughout the "gap"). The phenomenon was first described by Krylov in 1906, just a year after Korotkoff's initial report. Its potential clinical relevance was then suggested by Cook and Taussig in 1917.

60. How common is the auscultatory gap? What are its causes?

In a recent study by Cavallini et al., classic gaps were present in 21% of 168 hypertensive patients, otherwise healthy and not on medications. Gaps were associated with female gender, increased arterial stiffness, prevalence of carotid atherosclerotic plaques—all independent variables—and also with *older age*—not an independent variable. These findings suggest that auscultatory gaps are related to the atherosclerosis and increased arterial stiffness of hypertensive patients. Hence, they may have *prognostic relevance*, making hypertensive patients with gaps more likely to develop cardiovascular disease, independent of age, blood pressure, and other risk factors.

61. How accurate is blood pressure measurement by sphygmomanometer?

Accurate, but with some limitations:
- Values recorded *indirectly* (auscultatory method) correlate quite well with simultaneous *direct* intra-arterial recordings (r = 0.94 to 0.98). Still, Korotkoff phase I sounds do not appear until 4–15 mmHg *below* direct systolic blood pressure, whereas Korotkoff phase V sounds disappear *above* the direct diastolic value (by 3–6 mmHg). Hence, there is some minor underestimation and overestimation.
- Physicians may also cause inaccuracies. For example, despite previously agreeing to use *three* readings for diagnosis, a group of British general practitioners diagnosed hypertension after only one measurement in half of the cases. Similarly, 37% of German ambulatory physicians determined diastolic pressure using Korotkoff phase IV (muffling), rather than the more accurate phase V. Still, the most common physician's error is failure to use sufficiently large cuffs. In one survey, only 25% of primary care offices had them available. Of interest, auscultatory automatic monitors have fewer discrepancies than experienced clinicians.
- Finally, in some patients the blood pressure measured in the physician's office is considerably and consistently higher than the daytime ambulatory value. This phenomenon is called the "white coat" effect and is seen in as many as 10–40% of untreated and borderline hypertensive patients. Even treated patients often show blood pressure differences that are >20/10 mmHg. The phenomenon is more pronounced in female than male patients and results more often in responses to the white coat of doctors than to that of nurses.

62. What is the palpatory systolic blood pressure?

The value that coincides with arterial reopening (i.e., the reappearance of peripheral pulse). It can be obtained by palpating either the brachial artery below the cuff or the radial artery at the wrist.

63. **Can the palpatory method be used to determine diastolic pressure?**
   Yes, but with some expertise. The most-used technique consists in feeling the brachial pulse just below the deflating cuff. The point where a sudden decrease in volume (and peak) makes the pulse less bounding coincides with the diastolic blood pressure.

64. **Are there differences in systolic pressure determined by palpation versus auscultation?**
   Yes, but not a lot. *Palpatory* values are about 7mmHg lower than *auscultatory* values. Hence, physicians with hearing impairment may still rely on it to get accurate systolic *and* diastolic values.

65. **How common is hypertension?**
   Very common. It affects nearly one fourth of the adult U.S. population, in whom it is also the most common outpatient diagnosis. The lifetime risk for hypertension is also quite high: 90% percent of those who, at age 55, do not yet have it will eventually develop it. Still, 30% of affected patients are unaware that they have it, which is sad, since effective blood pressure control is indeed achievable and can substantially reduce the risk of stroke, myocardial infarction, and heart failure.

66. **How is hypertension defined?**
   With great difficulty. Overall, the risk of cardiovascular disease begins at 115/75 mmHg and doubles with each increment of 20mmHg systolic blood pressure and 10mmHg diastolic. This means that if a patient's blood pressure were to increase from 115/75 mmHg to 135/85 mmHg, the risk of stroke and heart attack would double. Hence, even "mild" hypertension should receive serious consideration. And *systolic* hypertension should not be disregarded either. In fact, in patients older than 50, a systolic pressure >140 mmHg is a more important cardiovascular risk factor than its diastolic counterpart. Overall, general consensus defines hypertension as the *blood pressure level* above which the risk for stroke and heart disease increases significantly. This threshold is set by the World Health Organization (WHO) at a systolic blood pressure >139 mmHg and/or a diastolic blood pressure >89 mmHg in an adult patient who is not receiving antihypertensive medication and is not acutely ill. Recent evidence, however, shows that this threshold should be lowered to 130/80 mmHg for patients with diabetes, heart failure, or chronic kidney disease.

67. **What are the key aspects of the latest guidelines?**
   The Seventh Report of the Joint National Committee on Prevention, Detection, Evaluation, and Treatment of High Blood Pressure (released in 2003) is an update of the 1997 guidelines (Table 2-4). It combines stages 2 and 3 hypertension, and it also contains a new

TABLE 2-4. COMPARISON OF 2003 AND 1997 JNC GUIDELINES			
New Classification (2003)		**Previous Classification (1997)**	
140/90 or above	High	High	140/90 or above
120–139/80–89	Prehypertension	Borderline	130–139/85–89
		Normal	129/84 or below
119/79 or below	Normal	Optimal	120/80 or below

Joint National Committee on Prevention, Detection, Evaluation, and Treatment of High Blood Pressure 2003: The Seventh Report of the Joint National Committee on Prevention, Detection, Evaluation, and Treatment of High Blood Pressure. Bethesda, MD: U.S. Department of Health and Human Services, 2003. NIH Publication No. 03–5233.

category of *prehypertension* (120/80–139/89 mmHg). Prehypertensive patients are at increased risk of progressing to hypertension (those in the 130/80–139/89 mm Hg range have twice the risk of developing hypertension as those with lower values) and thus should initiate lifestyle modifications. These include weight reduction, a DASH diet (Dietary Approaches to Stop Hypertension), lowering of sodium intake, increased physical activity, moderate consumption of alcohol, and no tobacco.

68. **What is *pseudo*hypertension?**
An elevated *indirect* recording of blood pressure in patients with normal intra-arterial measurements. It is uncommon, seen in fewer than 2% of otherwise healthy elderly people.

69. **What is the cause of *pseudo*hypertension?**
A stiffening of the arterial wall. This leaves the vessel *patent* (and thus able to produce Korotkoff sounds), even when the cuff pressure has exceeded the systolic blood pressure.

70. **What is Osler's maneuver?**
A bedside test for the detection of *pseudohypertension*. It is carried out by first inflating the cuff until it obliterates the radial *pulse,* and then by feeling the radial artery. If the cuff is unavailable, the radial pulse can be obliterated by compressing the brachial artery with the other thumb. The maneuver is positive when the artery remains palpable as a firm "tube" (positive Osler's *sign*).

71. **What is the significance of a positive Osler's sign?**
Palpability of an artery in the absence of its pulse is a sign of *arteriosclerosis*. It suggests that both systolic and diastolic pressures might be overestimated (pseudohypertension).

72. **How useful is Osler's sign?**
Probably not as much as traditionally taught. It has moderate to modest intraobserver and interobserver agreement, and occurs frequently in the elderly, hypertensive or not. Also, many Osler's cases do not really have pseudohypertension, since both indirect and intra-arterial recordings actually show *lower* blood pressure.

73. **What is malignant hypertension?**
A form of hypertension associated with one or more of the following end-organ damages: rapid deterioration of renal function, retinal hemorrhages or optic nerve involvement, left ventricular failure, myocardial ischemia, or cerebrovascular accidents. This may occur independently of the level of hypertension. Hence, patients with very high pressure may not develop malignant hypertension, whereas those with pressures as low as 180/120 mmHg may present with it.

74. **What is pseudo*hypo*tension?**
A condition seen in shock, where the high peripheral vascular resistance tightens arteries to the point of impairing the generation of Korotkoff sounds. This prevents effective measurement of systolic and diastolic pressures, and may lead to gross *underestimation*. Both pseudohypertension and pseudo*hypo*tension can be counteracted by a direct intra-arterial recording.

75. **What is the clinical significance of hypotension?**
In acute settings, it always carries a bad prognosis. Data confirm this ominous significance in cases of acute myocardial infarction, pneumonia, and intensive care unit hospitalization in general.

76. **What is a mean arterial pressure?**
Not a wicked pressure, but instead the sum of systolic plus twice the diastolic pressure, divided by three. This is in recognition of the different durations of systole and diastole (with the latter being usually twice as long as systole), thus contributing unequally to average blood

pressure values. Hence, in a patient with a blood pressure of 120/80 mmHg, the mean arterial pressure would be $(120 + [2 \times 80]) \div 3 = 280 \div 3 = 93.33$.

77. **What is a *pulse pressure*?**
It is the difference between systolic and diastolic pressure. Thus, in a patient with a systolic value of 120mmHg and a diastolic value of 80, the normal pulse pressure is 40.

78. **What is a *wide* pulse pressure? What are its causes?**
An abnormally large ("wide") pulse pressure is one that is greater than 50% of the systolic blood pressure. Hence, in a patient with a systolic of 140mmHg and a diastolic of 60, the *pulse pressure* is 80. The most common cause is a *hyperkinetic heart syndrome,* a high output state characterized by increased stroke volume and low peripheral vascular resistance. This is seen in various conditions, including:
- Aortic regurgitation
- Patent ductus arteriosus (PDA)
- Exercise
- Anxiety
- Fever
- Anemia
- Arteriovenous fistulas
- Beriberi
- Paget's disease
- Cirrhosis
- Pregnancy
- Thyrotoxicosis
- Severe exfoliative dermatitis

Many of these are characterized by arteriovenous (A-V) fistula(s) that may be large and single (as in PDA), or small and multiple. The latter are seen in Paget's disease (the fistulas are in the *bone*); exfoliative dermatitis (the fistulas are in the *skin*); cirrhosis (the fistulas are both hepatic and extrahepatic); and pregnancy (the entire *placenta* functions as a big A-V fistula). Shunt from fistulas is then responsible for the high output and hyperdynamic state.

79. **What is the significance of a wide pulse pressure in aortic regurgitation (AR)?**
If >80 mmHg, it reflects moderate to severe AR—a finding moderately sensitive but highly specific.

80. **What is the significance of a wide pulse pressure in only one extremity?**
It indicates the presence of an A-V fistula in that extremity. A Branham's sign would confirm it.

81. **What is Branham's sign?**
It is the typical bradycardia that occurs after compression (or excision) of a large A-V fistula. This is caused by inhibition of the Bainbridge reflex, which operates continuously in patients with large fistulas and is responsible for a compensatory *increase* in heart rate as a result of the higher right atrial pressure commonly induced by the large shunt. This right atrial stretching will then cause compensatory tachycardia through inhibition of vagal influence and activation of sympathetic acceleration. Note that the Bainbridge reflex is also responsible for the supraventricular tachyarrhythmias of patients with acute pulmonary embolism.

82. **How does one test for the Branham's sign?**
By inflating a blood pressure cuff over the suspected limb: the heart rate will slow down, only to reaccelerate upon deflation of the cuff (and secondary reopening of the A-V fistula).

83. **Who were Branham and Bainbridge?**
    Henry Branham was a 19th-century American surgeon. *Francis Bainbridge* (1874–1921) was an English physiologist and a small, quiet, and unimpressive lecturer with interest in exercise.

84. **When is a pulse pressure considered "narrow"? What are its causes?**
    A pulse pressure is abnormally *small* ("narrow") if <25% of the systolic value. Hence, a patient with a systolic of 100 mmHg and a diastolic of 90 has a narrow *pulse pressure* of 10. The most common cause is a drop in left ventricular stroke volume because of obstruction to left ventricular *filling* (tamponade, constrictive pericarditis) or *emptying* (aortic stenosis, even though this usually presents with normal pulse pressure). It may also occur in a tachycardia so severe to reduce ventricular filling time, and in *shock* (because of increased peripheral vascular resistance).

85. **What is *pulsus paradoxus*?**
    It is an exaggeration of the normal respiratory variation in *systolic* blood pressure (the diastolic changes little) characterized by a decrease with *inspiration* and an increase with *exhalation*. Although these swings are physiologic, in some disease states they may become large enough to be detectable at the bedside, *even on simple palpation of a peripheral artery*. In this case, the pulse will grow stronger on *expiration* and weaker on *inspiration*. It may even disappear.

86. **How wide does this swing in systolic pressure have to get to become palpable?**
    At least 20 mmHg. Of course, an easier and more sensitive way of detection is by blood pressure measurement. In this regard, an abnormal pulsus paradoxus is defined as an *inspiratory* drop in systolic pressure >12 ± 2 mmHg (some authors even quote lower values, such as 6 ± 3).

87. **Why is it called *paradoxical*?**
    Because changes in pulse *volume* are independent of changes in pulse *rate*. This paradox goes back to the original patients described by Kussmaul in 1873, who had such an inspiratory decrease in systolic pressure to completely lose their peripheral pulse, even though they still maintained consciousness and an apical beat. This was a paradox to Kussmaul; hence, his choice of the Latin term *pulsus respiratione intermittens* (i.e., "intermittent pulse as a result of respiration"). Pulsus paradoxus had actually already been described in 1669 by the Cornish physician Richard Lower, who reported a case of constrictive pericarditis in his treatise on the heart. Subsequently, the British physician Floyer (the same who recommended measuring the arterial pulse with a portable clock) made a similar observation in asthma, and so did William in 1850. Since none of these (Kussmaul included) had a sphygmomanometer (it had not been invented yet), they had to exclusively rely on the peripheral pulse; hence, Kussmaul's choice of the term "pulsus." This, however, has become outdated, not only because it describes an exaggerated *physiologic* (and not paradoxical) phenomenon, but also because nowadays these respiratory changes are *not* detected by arterial pulse, but by blood pressure.

88. **Describe the pathophysiology of pulsus paradoxus**
    It is an exaggeration of the *inspiratory drop* in systolic pressure, and thus in the fullness of the pulse.
    - *Inspiration* lowers intrathoracic pressure, which then increases venous return to the *"right"* ventricle. Conversely, it *reduces* venous return to the *left* ventricle (because of blood pooling in the inflated lungs and a leftward shift in the ventricular septum). In turn, the smaller end-diastolic left ventricular volume results in lower stroke volume and, thus, lower systolic pressure.
    - *Exhalation*, on the other hand, *increases* left ventricular filling (because of blood being "squeezed" by lung deflation, and also because of rightward shift in the ventricular septum). This increased ventricular filling results in higher left-ventricular stroke volume and systolic pressure.

All these respiratory variations are physiologic, but in certain pathologic states they become large enough to cause more profound (and detectable) changes in blood pressure and pulse volume.

89. **How does one measure pulsus paradoxus?**
   - Position yourself at the bedside in such a way to simultaneously monitor the respiratory movements of the patient and the column of the sphygmomanometer.
   - Don't ask the patient to breathe too vigorously, since this might generate an abnormal pulsus paradoxus even in the normal subject.
   - Fully inflate the blood pressure cuff until you achieve auscultatory silence.
   - Start deflating the cuff very slowly, while at the same time paying attention to both chest and abdominal wall expansions.
   - As soon as you hear the first Korotkoff sounds, stop deflating the cuff, and record the systolic pressure reading. You will notice that sounds are only heard in *exhalation*.
   - Restart deflating the cuff, very slowly, until you hear Korotkoff sounds both in inspiration *and* expiration. Record the second systolic blood pressure reading.
   - The difference between the two systolic recordings, in mmHg, is the pulsus paradoxus.

90. **Can pulsus paradoxus be identified on arterial tracing?**
   Yes, since it causes visible inspiratory *and* expiratory swings in systolic pressure.

91. **Which arteries are best suited for detecting pulsus paradoxus: peripheral or central?**
   Peripheral (i.e., better at the wrist than at the arm or at the neck) because peripheral arteries magnify elastic swings. Hence, they are very good for detecting *pulsus paradoxus* and *pulsus alternans*, but very bad for the *parvus* and *tardus* of aortic stenosis.

92. **What are the values to remember for pulsus paradoxus?**
   Age of puberty, age of drinking, and age of driving. In other words, the normal respiratory swing in systolic pressure is usually in the range of a magic number frequently encountered in clinical medicine: *age of puberty* (but also anion gap, osmolar gap, alveolar–arterial oxygen gradient, Hill's sign, and pulsus paradoxus)—all 12 ± 2. To stretch this analogy a bit further, we might even say that a pulsus paradoxus can be normal all the way up to 16 (i.e., the *age of driving*). For values between 16 and 21 (*age of drinking*), a "pulsus paradoxus" has been reported (albeit not consistently) in:
   - Pulmonary embolism
   - Right ventricular infarction
   - Right ventricular failure
   - Severe congestive heart failure

   Values in this range also occur in *tamponade*, and 30–45% of patients with *constrictive pericarditis*, but this must have an exudative component and not be completely "dry." Conversely, values *above* 21 are due to only two conditions: tamponade and status asthmaticus.

93. **What is cardiac tamponade?**
   It is a medical emergency characterized by a pericardial collection large enough to render intrapericardial pressure greater than intracardiac diastolic pressure. This not only prevents adequate filling of the heart (and thus ventricular ejection), but also creates a situation wherein the cardiac chambers start competing for the limited intrapericardial space. This leads to major respiratory swings in ventricular septa, ventricular filling, and systolic blood pressures.

94. **What are the characteristics of pulsus paradoxus in tamponade?**
   Almost 100% of patients will have a "pulsus" >12 mmHg. This percentage is lower (70%) in more chronic cases, but close to 100% for rapid fluid accumulation. A cut-off of 21 mmHg (age of drinking) will decrease sensitivity (only 78% of tamponade cases have it) but improve specificity.

95. **In addition to pulsus paradoxus, what are the other clinical features of tamponade?**
    They consist of a *tetrad*, present in close to 100% of patients:
    - Tachycardia
    - Dyspnea/tachypnea
    - Distended neck veins
    - Clear lungs

96. **What is Beck's triad?**
    It is a triad described by the American surgeon Claude Beck (who also pioneered open cardiac massage in patients "too good to die") and considered, until recently, typical of tamponade:
    - Hypotension
    - Distended neck veins
    - Small, quiet heart
    These findings are still seen in tamponade, but only in very advanced cases. Conversely, the tetrad just outlined (coupled with the presence of a *pulsus*) is probably a much better tool for early diagnosis.

97. **Can pulsus paradoxus be falsely negative in tamponade?**
    Yes. It may be absent in 2% of cases, usually because of compensatory mechanisms that prevent major septal shifts in inspiration. The most common are:
    - **Isolated right heart tamponade:** This has been described in patients with chronic renal failure who are on hemodialysis. Regional tamponade can also occur in loculated pericardial effusions. In both cases, the pericardial "water bag" is too asymmetric to cause a "real estate" competition between ventricles.
    - **Aortic regurgitation (AR):** In AR, the left ventricle can fill from the aorta during inspiration, which then prevents the development of a "pulsus." Hence, patients with aortic dissection (who have both AR and tamponade) may often present *without* pulsus paradoxus.
    - **Large atrial septal defect:** The normal inspiratory increase in systemic venous return is counterbalanced by a decrease in left-to-right shunt, resulting in minimal change in right ventricular volume.
    - **Elevated left ventricular diastolic pressures:** These occur in cases of severe left ventricular dysfunction. The left ventricular pressure is too high to allow any ipsilateral septal shift in inspiration.
    - **Severe rheumatoid spondylitis or disease of the bony thorax:** Wide changes in intrathoracic pressure are prevented by the relative immobility of the chest wall.
    - **Severe hypotension and shock**
    - **Coexistent conditions producing *"reversed pulsus paradoxus"*** (*see* question 101)

98. **What other conditions can cause pulsus paradoxus >10 mmHg?**
    See Table 2-5.

99. **What about pulsus paradoxus in airflow obstruction?**
    Obstructive lung disease (especially status asthmaticus) can indeed cause pulsus paradoxus. The mechanism is probably lung hyperinflation, causing excessive *inspiratory pooling of blood*, and thus a greater drop in systolic blood pressure. Since this form of pulsus paradoxus depends on respiratory rate and effort, it is not a very sensitive indicator of severe bronchospasm (in fact, only half of status asthmaticus patients have a pulsus >10). It is, however, quite specific, with values >20 usually indicating FEV_1 <0.5–0.7 L. Hence, it can serve as a "poor man's" spirometer (or peak flow meter) for situations in which these devices are not readily available.

TABLE 2-5. CONDITIONS RESPONSIBLE FOR PULSUS PARADOXUS >10 MMHG		
Cardiac causes	**Extracardiac pulmonary causes**	**Extracardiac nonpulmonary causes**
Cardiac tamponade	Bronchial asthma	Anaphylactic shock (during urokinase administration)
Pericardial effusion	Tension pneumothorax	
Constrictive pericarditis*		Hypovolemic shock
Restrictive cardiomyopathy		Volvulus of the stomach
Pulmonary embolism		Diaphragmatic hernia
Right ventricular infarction		Superior vena cava obstruction
Right ventricular failure		Extreme obesity
Cardiogenic shock		

Modified from Khasnis A, Lokhandwala Y: Clinical signs in medicine: pulsus paradoxus. J Postgrad Med 48:46–49, 2002.
*Seen in 30–45% of patients, but the condition must have an exudative component and not be completely "dry."

100. **How does pulsus paradoxus behave in intubated and mechanically ventilated patients?**
It may present as respiratory variations in the baseline tracing of pulse oximetry (with the height of oscillation correlating with the severity of *pulsus* and the degree of auto-PEEP [positive end-expiratory pressure]). Hence, pulse oximetry assessment of pulsus paradoxus can provide a useful noninvasive monitor of air trapping severity. Still, beware that positive pressure ventilation can reverse the respiratory changes in intrathoracic pressure, so that the lowest systolic blood pressure will be recorded during *expiration* (reversed pulsus paradoxus—*see* question 101), rather than inspiration. Although the correlation between pulsus paradoxus and pulse oximetry recordings might not be influenced by the state of respiration (spontaneous or mechanical ventilation), reversed pulsus paradoxus is not a good indicator of disease severity in patients receiving mechanical ventilation because the magnitude of the *pulsus* depends (at least in part) on the applied ventilatory pressures.

101. **What is "reversed" pulsus paradoxus?**
A drop in systolic pressure that coincides with *expiration* rather than inspiration. This is typical of HOCM (hypertrophic obstructive cardiomyopathy), where the ventricle is too stiff to adequately fill. It also can be seen in patients with left ventricular failure who are on *positive pressure ventilation* (PPV). In this case, PPV displaces the wall of the ventricle inward during systole, thus assisting ventricular emptying and causing a slight rise in systolic pressure during mechanical inspiration. Note that a reversed pulsus paradoxus in ventilated patients is a sensitive indicator of hypovolemia. Finally, a reversed pulsus paradoxus can also be seen in patients with isorhythmic dissociation. The atrial activity precedes the ventricular activity during inspiration, and *follows* it during expiration. The atrial contribution during inspiration increases stroke volume, while the lack of it during exhalation *decreases* it.

102. **What is *pseudo*-pulsus paradoxus?**
It is a term used by Salel et al. to describe a patient with isorhythmic dissociation from complete heart block who was misdiagnosed as having pulsus paradoxus. This was in reality due to increased sinus rate from inspiration, which temporarily positioned the P waves in front of the QRS, thus synchronizing (and maximizing) atrioventricular contraction. The misdiagnosis can be avoided by strictly adhering to the guidelines for pulsus paradoxus laid down by Gauchat and Katz:

- The pulse must be felt in *all* the accessible arteries.
- There is *no* need for deep inspiration.
- There must be *no irregularity of cardiac action.*

103. What is the usefulness of Kussmaul's sign in pulsus paradoxus?
Kussmaul's sign is a paradoxical increase in venous distention (and pressure) during *inspiration* (*see* Chapter 10, The Cardiovascular Exam). This should not be confused with the exaggeration of the normal *expiratory* increase in venous pressure that is often seen in patients with pulmonary disease. Instead, Kussmaul's sign reflects some sort of obstruction to right-sided venous return, like superior vena cava syndrome, tricuspid stenosis, right ventricular hypertrophy or infarction, constrictive pericarditis, pulmonary emboli, and severe pulmonary hypertension. Of interest, patients with *tamponade do not demonstrate Kussmaul's sign;* yet, they *do* demonstrate pulsus paradoxus. Conversely, "pulsus" (albeit one that is never >21 mmHg) *may* occur in some patients with Kussmaul's.

104. What is Trousseau's sign?
There are actually *two* Trousseau's signs:
- *Recurrent thrombophlebitis* associated with a visceral carcinoma (Trousseau's *syndrome*). The phlebitis may be superficial or deep, often with a *migratory* pattern (thrombophlebitis migrans). This presents with successive crops of tender nodules in the affected vessels, with different veins being involved either simultaneously or randomly. It reflects a prothrombotic state from an underlying visceral malignancy, usually an adenocarcinoma (pancreas or lung, but also stomach, breast, and prostate). First described in 1861 by Trousseau, who in 1867 recognized it on himself as part of the pancreatic cancer that eventually killed him.
- *Carpal spasm* in patients with overt tetany (Trousseau's *phenomenon*). This is associated with extension of the foot (carpo*pedal* spasm), extension of the body, and opisthotonos. The spasm of the hand involves wrist flexors and finger extensors, so that the fingers are flexed at the metacarpophalangeal joints and extended at the phalangeal joints; the thumb is flexed and adducted into the palm. Thus shaped, the hand so typically resembles that of a physician making a vaginal examination to often be referred to as the "obstetrician's hand" (*main d'accoucheur,* from the original Trousseau's description).

105. What are the causes of an "obstetrician's hand"?
Those predisposing to tetany: alkalemia, hypocalcemia, hypomagnesemia, or hypophosphatemia.

106. How can one trigger carpal spasm in patients with "latent" tetany?
- By occluding the arterial pulse for 5 minutes with a blood pressure cuff. This has sensitivity of 66% for hypocalcemia, with a false positive rate of 4%. Hence, it does not eliminate the need for blood testing.
- By *Chvostek's sign*. This test of muscular hyperexcitability is performed by tapping the bone anterior to the ear, which corresponds to the exit point of cranial nerve VII. The test is positive when it triggers facial twitching. Chvostek sign has low sensitivity for latent tetany (27%), and very high false positive rates (19–74% in children and 4–29% in adults).

107. Who was Trousseau?
Armand Trousseau (1801–1867) was one of the great leaders of 19th-century Parisian medicine. Among his "firsts" were the performance of tracheostomy (in France), the use of thoracentesis, and the creation of the term "aphasia." Trousseau was a superb clinician, a much beloved teacher, and a lecturer who could present cases with the elegance of a novelist. He popularized eponyms such as Addison's, Graves', and Hodgkin's disease and was a passionate advocate of bedside teaching through clinical demonstration. Totally adored by students and colleagues alike, he trained, among others, Potain, Lasegue, Brown-Sequard, and Da Costa. Trousseau was also active in politics, especially after the revolution of 1848, holding

important positions, including a membership in the legislative body. His advice to students still stands 150 years after his death: "Observe the practice of many physicians; do not implicitly believe the mere assertion of your master; be something better. Do not fear to confess your ignorance. In truth, it seems that the words 'I do not know' stick in every physician's throat. Take care not to fancy yourself as a physician as soon as you have mastered scientific facts; they only afford to your understanding an opportunity of bringing forth fruit, thus elevating you to the high position of *a man of art*."

108. Who was Chvostek?
Frantisek Chvostek (1835–1884) was a Moravian-born Austrian surgeon who described the homonymous sign in 1876. His field of interest, however, was the pathology and treatment of neurologic disease, where he even experimented with electrotherapy.

109. What is the Rumpel-Leede sign?
It is an old test of *capillary fragility*, carried out by raising the venous pressure in the forearm through either inflation of a blood pressure cuff or the closing of a tourniquet. The test is positive when it causes petechial eruptions (presumably because of fragile capillaries bursting open). It is named after the two physicians who first described it at the turn of the century: the German Theodore Rumpel and the American Carl Leede. Yet, it is often referred to as the Hess test, from Alfred Hess (1875–1933), the American who first noticed it while treating scorbutic children.

110. What is Hill's sign?
A sign of *severe aortic regurgitation*, first described in 1909 by the British physician Leonard Hill. It is characterized by an exaggerated difference in *systolic* pressure between upper and lower extremities. Note that there is already a *physiologic* difference of around 12 ± 2 mmHg (with legs having higher systolic pressure than arms). Conversely, a difference of >20 and <40 is considered pathologic, but with low specificity and sensitivity for AR. A difference of >60 mmHg has high specificity (and a very high positive likelihood ratio) for *severe* AR, but a sensitivity of only 40%.

111. Is Hill's sign real?
No. The "normal" difference in systolic pressure between foot and arm is only present on *indirect* recording. By *direct* intra-arterial measurement there is no discrepancy.

112. What is the mechanism of Hill's sign?
It's not entirely clear. According to one theory, a high stroke volume generates a summation between the regular *pulse wave* of the aortic pressure and a *rebound wave* from the periphery. Because of the rebound wave's characteristics, the summation only occurs in the legs.

113. So what about Hill's sign in AR?
It also is not real. There are no *intra-arterial* differences in systolic pressure between upper and lower extremities. Hence, the differences at the cuff are just a sphygmomanometric artifact, most likely due to enhanced transmission of pressure wave. Still, it can predict AR severity.

114. Is Hill's sign specific for AR?
No. It also can be encountered in other hyperdynamic states (previously discussed).

115. How do you perform Hill's test?
By measuring in the supine patient the *systolic* pressure at the foot, and then subtracting the one recorded at the arm. The pressure at the foot is obtained by wrapping the cuff around the calf and then *palpating* either the dorsalis pedis or the tibialis posterior (whichever value is higher).

116. **What causes the systolic pressure to be less in the *lower* than in the upper extremities?**
It depends on the age of the subject. In elderly individuals, the most common cause is aortic obstruction (atherosclerotic), or dissection. In younger patients, the predominant reason is instead aortic coarctation. In this case, the lower extremities also have *reduced* and *delayed* pulses, and a systolic blood pressure at least 6mmHg lower than that in the upper extremities.

117. **What is the standard bedside test for assessing chronic lower extremity ischemia?**
The *ankle–brachial pressure index* (ABPI), also known as the ankle-to-arm systolic pressure index (AAI).

118. **How is the ABPI measured?**
According to the guidelines of the Standards Division of the Society of Interventional Radiology:
1. With the patient supine, measure brachial and ankle systolic pressure by handheld Doppler.
2. To obtain an ABPI, divide the highest systolic pressure of the dorsalis pedis (or tibialis posterior) for each foot by the highest systolic pressure at the arm. For example:
- To obtain the left ABPI, first measure the systolic brachial pressure in both left and right arms. Select the higher value as your brachial artery pressure measurement. There should be a difference of less than 10 mmHg between each brachial pressure measurement.
- Next, measure the left dorsalis pedis (or tibialis posterior) arterial systolic pressures. Select the higher of these two values as the ankle pressure measurement.
- Then, divide the selected ankle pressure measurement by the previously selected brachial artery systolic pressure measurement.

Normal values range between 0.97 and 1.1; values <0.97 identify patients with angiographically proven occlusions or stenoses, with 96% sensitivity and 94–100% specificity. Most patients with claudication will have an ABPI between 0.5 and 0.8, whereas those with pain at rest will have values <0.5. Indexes <0.2 are associated with ischemic or gangrenous extremities.

119. **Can the ABPI be misleading?**
Yes, because it only measures pressure at the ankle and therefore does not account for possible distal occlusions, such as microemboli or small atherosclerotic plaques. Moreover, the ABPI may be falsely elevated in Mönckeberg's sclerosis, the medial wall calcification of many diabetic patients. In this condition, the ABPI reflects more the ability of the heavily calcified vessel to resist compression than the true blood flow (and pressure) within it. In these patients, toe pressure determinations may more accurately reflect lower extremity perfusion.

120. **Who was Hill?**
Sir Leonard Hill (1866–1952) was an English physiologist who modified the original Riva-Rocci mercury sphygmomanometer by using a pressure gauge. In 1923, he won the Nobel Prize in physiology for his studies of heat production and muscle metabolism.

121. **What is the Valsalva's maneuver? How does it modify blood pressure?**
Valsalva is a great little test for assessing the reflex autonomic control of the cardiovascular system, both sympathetic and vagal. It does so by modifying blood pressure, heart rate, and venous return—all as a result of respiratory swings in intrathoracic pressures. It can be difficult to perform, though, and thus should always be well explained to the patient, especially the need to keep on straining until told to stop, and to breathe as quietly as possible after stopping straining. Valsalva consists of two major *periods*, comprising a total of four *phases* (Fig. 2-1):
Period 1: a held (or strain) period. This is carried out by asking the patient to fully inspire and then forcefully exhale against closed glottis for at least 10 seconds. It can be easily

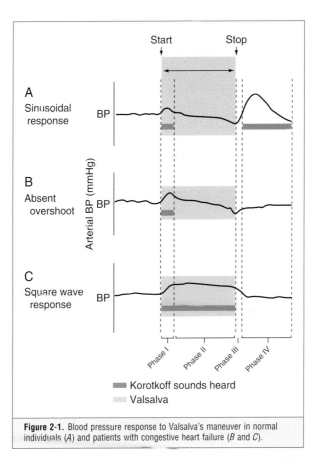

Figure 2-1. Blood pressure response to Valsalva's maneuver in normal individuals (*A*) and patients with congestive heart failure (*B* and *C*).

accomplished by having the patient "bear down as if having a bowel movement," or alternatively, by placing a fist onto the midabdomen of a supine patient and then having him or her strain against it (it could even be accomplished more formally by having the patient blow for 10 seconds against an aneroid manometer at a constant pressure of 40 mmHg). Whatever the technique, the resulting *strain* causes an increase in intrathoracic pressure, a drop in venous return, a reduction in left ventricular diameter, and a fall in cardiac output. These can be quite dramatic (in fact, when first experimenting with Valsalva's, Weber, in typical Teutonic fashion, managed to give himself a syncope and a seizure; then he recovered and wrote the paper). This "strain" comprises two phases:

- *Phase I:* After onset of straining, systolic pressure increases (due to aortic compression), and heart rate decreases (due to reflex bradycardia from baroreceptor activation).
- *Phase II:* Characterized instead by a drop in venous return because of straining-induced compression of the vena cava. This eventually leads to a fall in cardiac output, a secondary fall in aortic pressure (which therefore slowly returns to the baseline level), and a secondary increase in heart rate (still mediated by the baroreceptor reflex). During the rest of the straining period, the arterial mean and pulse pressures continue to slowly fall, and the heart rate continues to slowly increase.

Period 2: a release period. This is carried out by asking the patient to stop bearing down, or alternatively, by releasing the fist pressure on the abdomen. It also comprises two phases:

- *Phase III:* As soon as straining is released (and the subject starts breathing again), there is a small but transient drop in systolic pressure due to sudden loss of aortic compression. This, in turn, causes a further reflex acceleration of the heart rate.
- *Phase IV:* When the vena cava compression completely resolves, venous return suddenly increases. This causes a rapid rise in cardiac output, which, in turn, makes the systolic pressure overshoot above baseline values (due to increased systemic resistance from phase II sympathetic activation) and heart rate to drop (because of baroreceptor reflex).

This normal hemodynamic response to Valsalva can be quite altered in *congestive heart failure*.

122. **How good is Valsalva for detecting congestive heart failure?**
Very good. Valsalva has excellent specificity and sensitivity (90–99% and 70–95%, respectively) for detecting left ventricular dysfunction, either systolic or diastolic. It also has significant likelihood ratios (both negative and positive—the latter being 7.6). To perform the test, inflate the blood pressure cuff 15mmHg above the patient's resting systolic pressure, and then maintain this value throughout the 10 seconds of *strain* and the 30 seconds of *release*. While doing so, auscultate over the brachial artery, looking for Korotkoff's sounds. When the patient starts straining, a normal response consists of an initial increase in systolic pressure with clear-cut sounds (phase I); this is then followed by a drop in systolic pressure with disappearance of sounds (phase II) and then, after release of straining, by an overshooting in pressure with reappearance of sounds (phase IV). Note that Korotkoff's sounds should always be heard during phase I. If not, the patient has failed to adequately increase intrathoracic pressure. Patients with heart failure have instead a quite different response: they either maintain sounds throughout the *entire* 40 seconds of the maneuver (as a result of an increase in systolic pressure that matches the increase in intrathoracic pressure—*square wave response*), or they fail to gain them back after strain release (because of the failing ventricle's inability to produce a systolic pressure overshoot after the hypotension induced by straining—*absent overshoot*). In fact, the degree of overshoot is directly related to left ventricular ejection fraction, and thus provides a marker for systolic dysfunction. Note, however, that an abnormal Valsalva response may also reflect high filling pressures (and thus provide a marker for *diastolic dysfunction*).

123. **In addition to an abnormal Valsalva response, are there other findings that might diagnose congestive heart failure (CHF)?**
Yes, and they involve most of the five "fingers" of the cardiovascular exam (*see* Chapter 20, Cardiovascular Examination). On the venous side, for example, the presence of either end-inspiratory crackles or distended neck veins has high specificity (90–100%) but low sensitivity (10–50%) for increased *left-sided* filling pressure due to either systolic or diastolic dysfunction. Of these two signs, only an elevated jugular venous pressure has a significant positive likelihood ratio (3.9). Positive abdominojugular reflux has equally high specificity, but better sensitivity (55–85%), and an even stronger likelihood ratio (8.0). S_3 gallop, downward and lateral displacement of the apical impulse, and peripheral edema also have high specificity (>95%) but low sensitivity (1–40%) for elevated diastolic filling pressures; of them, only the S_3 and the displaced apical impulse have a positive likelihood ratio (5.7 and 5.8, respectively). Given their negative likelihood ratios, only an absent abdominojugular reflux and an abnormal Valsalva response argue against the presence of high filling pressures. Finally, S_4 has high sensitivity (71%), but low specificity (50%), and nonsignificant likelihood ratios.

124. **And what about patients with "systolic" dysfunction?**
They not only have high diastolic filling pressure (the hallmark of heart failure, whether systolic or diastolic), but also *low ejection fraction* (<50%). Hence, they present with both dyspnea *and*

fatigue. Of all bedside signs, only an abnormal Valsalva response has high sensitivity *and* specificity for their identification (>70% and >90%, respectively, with a positive likelihood ratio of 7.6). S_3 and displaced apical impulse have positive likelihood ratios (3.8 and 5.7, respectively) but specificities that are much higher than sensitivity (>90% and 10–50%, respectively). Hence, absence of these findings does *not* exclude an ejection fraction <50% (although absence of S_3 *does* exclude an ejection fraction <30%). All other signs (crackles, distended neck veins, peripheral edema, hepatomegaly, mitral regurgitation) have high specificity (>90%) but sensitivity too low for significant likelihood ratios. The PPP (*proportional pulse pressure*) is another finding with excellent sensitivity (91%) and specificity (83%) for identifying low cardiac index (CI). It is calculated by dividing the arterial pulse pressure by the systolic blood pressure. In dilated cardiomyopathy, a PPP <0.25 has a positive likelihood ratio of 5.4 for CI of 2.2 L/min/m^2.

125. **Can physical exam predict *outcome* in patients with CHF?**
Yes. CHF findings are valuable and independent predictors of worse clinical outcome. For example, ischemic heart disease patients with S_3 have a 1-year mortality that is much higher than those *without* it (57% versus 14%). The same applies to a displaced apical impulse (1-year mortality of 39% if present and 12% if absent).

126. **Who was Valsalva?**
Antonio Valsalva (1666–1723) was a professor of anatomy in Bologna, a student of Malpighi, and himself the teacher of Morgagni. He developed his maneuver as a bedside tool for cleaning and inflating the eustachian tube, and reported it in 1704 in a book on the ear. Weber rediscovered it 150 years later, mostly for its effects on cardiac physiology, and the rest is history.

127. **What are the diagnostic and therapeutic uses of Valsalva?**
Two major **diagnostic** applications:
- Identification of congestive heart failure (previously discussed)
- Enhancement of the murmurs of hypertrophic obstructive cardiomyopathy (HOCM) and mitral valve prolapse (MVP) (*see* Chapter 21, Cardiac Murmurs)

Valsalva also has four **therapeutic** applications:
- Interrupting supraventricular tachyarrhythmias (by increasing vagal tone)
- Helping patients with multiple sclerosis whose flaccid bladder cannot fully empty
- On rare occasions, diminishing chest pain in patients with mild coronary disease
- Last but not least, helping men avoid premature ejaculation (I am not making this up)

As for its use in angina, keep in mind that this has to be done with great care, since Valsalva profoundly affects venous return and cardiac output (remember the syncope and seizure of Weber while experimenting with it) and thus may have untoward effects not only in patients with severe coronary artery disease or recent myocardial infarction, but also in patients with moderate to severe hypovolemia and recent surgery/hemorrhage of the eye or central nervous system.

F. RESPIRATION

Respiratory Rate and Rhythm

128. **How useful is it to assess the patient's rate, rhythm, and depth of respiration?**
Very useful. In fact, an intelligent observation of these respiratory parameters may generate an entire alphabet soup of terminology, often conducive to specific diagnoses. For a more detailed description of these terms and disease processes, please refer to Chapter 13, Chest Inspection, Palpation, and Percussion; and Chapter 14, Lung Auscultation.

SELECTED BIBLIOGRAPHY

1. Bailey R, Bauer JH: A review of common errors in the indirect measurement of blood pressure (sphygmomanometry). Arch Intern Med 153:2741–2748, 1993.

2. Bor DH, Makadon HJ, Friedland G, et al: Fever in hospitalized medical patients: Characteristics and significance. J Gen Intern Med 3:119–125, 1988.

3. Cavallini MC, Roman MJ, Blank SG, et al: Association of the auscultatory gap with vascular disease in hypertensive patients. Ann Intern Med 124:883, 1996.

4. Dock W: Korotkoff's sounds. N Engl J Med 302:1264–1267, 1980.

5. Enselberg CD: Palpatory measurement of diastolic blood pressure. N Engl J Med 265:272–274, 1961.

6. Erickson RS, Kirklin SK: Comparison of ear-based, bladder, oral, and axillary methods for core temperature measurement. Crit Care Med 21:1528–1534, 1993.

7. Hla KM, Samsa GP, Stoneking HT, Feussner JR: Observer variability of Osler's maneuver in detection of pseudohypertension. J Clin Epidemiol 44:513–518, 1991.

8. Joint National Committee on Prevention, Detection, Evaluation, and Treatment of High Blood Pressure 2003: The Seventh Report of the Joint National Committee on Prevention, Detection, Evaluation, and Treatment of High Blood Pressure. Bethesda, MD, U.S. Department of Health and Human Services, 2003.NIH Publication No. 03–5233.

9. Kishan CV, Talley JD: Hill's sign: A non-invasive clue of the severity of chronic aortic regurgitation. J Ark Med Soc 95:501–502, 1999.

10. Kuwajima I, Hoh E, Suzuki Y, et al: Pseudohypertension in the elderly. J Hypertens 8:429–432, 1990.

11. Mackowiak PA, Wasserman SS, Levine MM: A critical appraisal of 98.6 degrees F, the upper limit of the normal body temperature, and other legacies of Carl Reinhold August Wunderlich. JAMA 268:1578–1580, 1992.

12. McGee S: Evidence-Based Physical Diagnosis. Philadelphia, W.B. Saunders, 2001.

13. Musher DM, Fainstein V, Young EJ, et al: Fever patterns: Lack of clinical significance. Arch Intern Med 139:1225–1228, 1979.

14. Neufeld PD, Johnson DL: Observer error in blood pressure measurement. Can Med Assoc J 135:633–637, 1986.

15. Pickering TG, Hall JE, Appel LJ, et al: Recommendations for blood pressure measurement in humans and experimental animals: Part 1: Blood pressure measurement in humans: A statement for professionals from the Subcommittee of Professional and Public Education of the American Heart Association Council on High Blood Pressure Research. Circulation 111:697–716, 2005.

16. Reeves RA: Does this patient have hypertension? How to measure blood pressure. JAMA 273:1211–1218, 1995.

17. Sacks D, Bakal CW, Beatty PT, et al: Position statement on the use of the ankle brachial index in the evaluation of patients with peripheral vascular disease. J Vasc Interv Radiol 14:S389, 2003.

18. Tsapatsaris NP, Napolitana GT, Rothchild J: Osler's maneuver in an outpatient clinic setting. Arch Intern Med 151:2209–2211, 1991.

CHAPTER 3

THE SKIN

Salvatore Mangione, MD

"The power of making a correct diagnosis is the key to all success in the treatment of skin diseases; without this faculty, the physician can never be a thorough dermatologist, and therapeutics at once cease to hold their proper position, and become empirical."

–Louis A. Duhring (1845–1913)

"Beauty's but skin deep."

–John Davies of Hereford (1565–1618)

BASIC TERMINOLOGY AND DIAGNOSTIC TECHNIQUES

1. **How many skin *diseases* exist? What are the two main categories of skin *lesions*?**
   There are more than 1400 skin diseases. Yet, only 30 are important, common, and worth knowing. The first step toward their recognition is the separation of *primary* from *secondary* lesions (Table 3-1).
   - **Primary lesions** result only from disease and have not been changed by additional events (such as trauma, scratching, or medical treatment; *see* Table 3-1). To better identify primary lesions, pay attention to their colors, shape, arrangement, and distribution.
   - **Secondary lesions** instead have been altered by outside manipulation, medical treatment, or their own natural course.

2. **What are the major *primary* lesions?**
   - **Macules:** *Flat,* nonpalpable, circumscribed areas of discoloration ≤0.5 cm in diameter. Typical macules are the familiar freckles.

   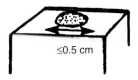

   ≤0.5 cm

   - **Patches:** *Flat,* nonpalpable areas of skin discoloration >0.5 cm in diameter (i.e., a large macule). A typical patch is the one of vitiligo.

   >0.5 cm

   - **Papules**: *Raised* and *palpable* lesions ≤0.5 cm in diameter. They may or may not have a different color from the surrounding skin. A typical papule is a raised nevus.

   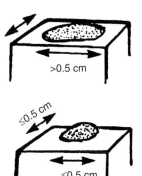

   ≤0.5 cm

   ≤0.5 cm

TABLE 3-1. DERMATOLOGIC LESIONS

Skin Lesions		
Primary	**Secondary**	**Special**
Solid (Nonpalpable)	Crusts	Purpurae
• Macules (≤0.5 cm)	Scales	Petechiae
• Patches (>0.5 cm)	Ulcers	Ecchymoses
	Fissures	Teleangiectasias
Solid (Palpable)	Excorations	Comedones
• Papules (≤0.5 cm)	Scars	Burrows
• Plaques (>0.5 cm)	Erosions	Target lesions
• Nodules (*deeper* plaques)	Lichenification	
• Wheals (*pruritic* plaques)	Atrophy	
• Tumors (*larger* nodules)	Scars	
	Sinuses	
Fluid-Lesions		
• Vesicles (fluid-filled *papules*)		
• Pustules (*pus*-filled *papules*)		
• Bullae (fluid-filled *plaques*)		
• Cysts (fluid-filled *nodules*)		

- **Plaques:** *Raised* and *palpable* lesions >0.5 cm in diameter (i.e., a large papule). Usually confined to the superficial dermis, they may result from the *confluence of papules*. A typical plaque is that of psoriasis.

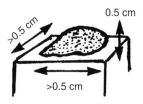

- **Nodules:** *Raised, palpable*, and *elevated* lesions >0.5 cm in diameter, which, unlike plaques, go *deeper* into the dermis. Since they are *below* the surface of the skin, the overlying cutis is usually mobile. Typical nodules are those of erythema nodosum.

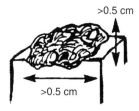

- **Tumors:** *Nodules* that are either >2 cm in diameter or poorly demarcated. Usually neoplastic.

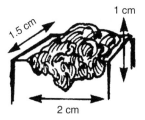

- **Wheals (hives):** *Raised,* circumscribed, edematous, and typically pruritic plaques that are pink or pale but typically transient. Classic wheals are the lesions of urticaria, or of a mosquito bite.

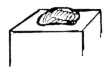

- **Vesicles (blisters):** Fluid-filled, circumscribed, and raised lesions that contain *clear serous fluid* and are ≤0.5 cm in diameter. Typical vesicles are those of herpes simplex.

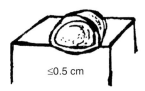

≤0.5 cm

- **Bullae:** Vesicles >0.5 cm in diameter. Commonly seen in patients with second-degree burns. Presence of a *bulla* is so important that it usually trumps all other concomitant primary lesions.

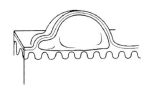

- **Cysts:** Raised and *encapsulated* lesions that contain fluid or semi-solid material. Typical are the cysts of acne.

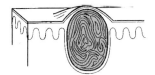

- **Pustules:** Pus-filled papules. Typically seen in patients with impetigo or acne.

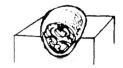

- **Purpura:** Skin extravasation of red cells, which, based on size, may present as petechiae or ecchymoses. *Palpable* purpura is never normal and argues for an antigen-antibody complex (vasculitis). Often localized to the lower extremities, the lesions of Henoch-Schönlein are typical examples of a palpable purpura. Internal organs (kidneys, GI tract) are often involved too.

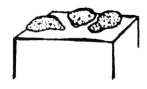

- **Petechiae:** Reddish-to-purple discolorations, caused by a microscopic hemorrhage. These are <0.5 cm in diameter and usually in clusters. With the exception of color, they resemble *papules* or *macules* (depending on whether they are palpable or not). Typical petechiae are those of typhus. The lesions of thrombocytopenic thrombotic purpura (TTP) are typical petechiae too.

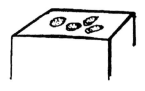

- **Ecchymoses (bruises):** Reddish-to-purple discolorations larger than petechiae. Except for color, they resemble *plaques* and *patches* (depending on whether they are palpable or not). Typically located below an intact epithelial surface.

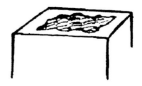

- **Spider angiomas:** These are *arterial* teleangiectasias, i.e., vascular arterial lesions that resemble the legs of a spider. They fill from the center and blanch whenever this is compressed.

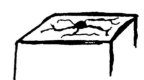

- **Venous spiders:** These are *venous* teleangiectasias, i.e., vascular venous lesions that also resemble the legs of a spider. Hence, they fill from the periphery, *not* the center. They empty with pressure.

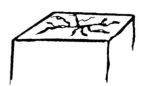

(Figures adapted from Willms JL, Schneiderman H, Algranati PS: Physical Diagnosis. Baltimore, Williams & Wilkins, 1994, with permission.)

3. **What are the major secondary lesions?**
   - **Excoriations:** Linear *erosions* produced by scratching. Often raised, *scratch marks* may also present as crust on top of a primary lesion that has been partially scratched off. They are almost exclusively confined to the *eczematous diseases*.

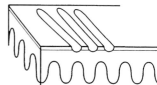
Excoriation

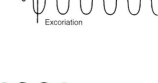

   - **Lichenification:** A typical skin thickening seen in chronic pruritus with recurrent scratching. Resembles the callus formation of palms and soles after recurrent trauma. Lichenified skin is hardened, leather-like, with prominent markings and some scaling. Like excoriation, lichenification is typical of *eczematous diseases*. In fact, it is considered pathognomonic of *atopic dermatitis*.

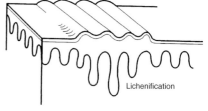
Lichenification

- **Scales:** *Raised* lesions presenting as flaking of the upper skin surface. In fact, they represent thickening of the stratum corneum, the uppermost layer of the epidermis. Scales may be white, gray, or tan. They may also be small or rather large. They provide the

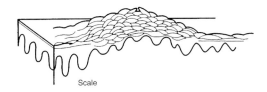

Scale

squamous component to papulosquamous diseases. They are extremely common in the scalp, where they suggest either banal processes (dandruff) or more serious conditions (seborrheic dermatitis, psoriasis, and tinea capitis).

- **Crusts:** *Raised* lesions produced by dried serum and blood cell remnants. Usually preceded by fluid-filled primary lesions (i.e., vesicles, pustules, or bullae). The most familiar crust is the "scab" of impetigo.

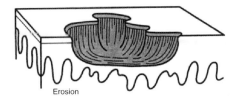

Crust

- **Erosions:** *Depressed* lesions produced whenever the epidermis is either removed or sloughed. They are moist, usually red, and well circumscribed. Classic erosions are those of chickenpox following rupture of a vesicle.

Erosion

- **Ulcers:** *Depressed* lesions produced whenever not only the epidermis but also part (or all) of the dermis is gone. Ulcers are *concave*, often moist, and at times inflamed or even hemorrhagic. They heal with scarring. A classic ulcer is that of the syphilitic chancre.

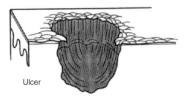

Ulcer

■ **Fissures:** *Depressed* lesions presenting as narrow, linear, and vertical cracks that penetrate through the epidermis, reaching at least part of the dermis. Classic fissures are those of the athlete's foot.

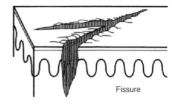

■ **Atrophy:** Usually the nonspecific end-product of various skin disorders. It is characterized by a pale and shiny area, with loss of cutaneous markings and full skin thickness.

■ **Sinuses:** Connective channels between the surface of the skin and deeper components.

(Figures from Fitzpatrick JE, Aeling JL: Dermatology Secrets. Philadelphia, Hanley & Belfus, 1996, with permission.)

4. **Are there other ways to classify skin lesions?**
Many ways. One divides lesions into four groups based on the *relationship with the surrounding skin*:
   ■ **Flat, nonpalpable:** Macule, patch, purpura, ecchymosis, spider angioma, venous spider
   ■ **Raised, solid, palpable:** Papule, plaque, nodule, tumor, wheal, scale, crust
   ■ **Raised, cystic, palpable:** Vesicle, pustule, bulla, cyst
   ■ **Depressed:** Atrophy, erosion, ulcer, fissure

5. **What is the *pattern* of distribution?**
Beside the distribution in the body (i.e., generalized versus localized), this descriptor refers to the relationship of lesions to one another:
   ■ **Clustered (grouped, herpetiform)** lesions are in close proximity, occurring in a group or series of groups.
   ■ **Confluent (coalescent)** lesions are multiple and blending together.
   ■ **Dermatomal** lesions are typically distributed along neurocutaneous dermatomes. Like herpes zoster (shingles).

6. **What is the *configuration* of a skin lesion?**
It is the *outline* of the lesion as observed from above. The most common configurations are:
   ■ **Annular:** Doughnut-shaped lesions. Fungal infections present as red rings with the scaly surface.
   ■ **Linear:** Lesions arranged in a line. For example, streaks of small vesicles on an erythematous base. The most common linear lesion is the rash of poison ivy, also called rhus dermatitis (*rhus* is the Greek word for sumac, which describes various shrubs or small trees). Some species of sumac, or rhus, include poison ivy and poison oak—both cause an acute itching rash on contact.
   ■ **Reticular:** Lesions organized in a net-like cluster
   ■ **Gyrate:** Lesions with a serpiginous (or polycyclic) configuration—as in gyrate erythema

7. **How should an initial cutaneous exam be done?**
From head to toe. Patients should fully disrobe, so that the entire body can be inspected—including palms, soles, scalp, and mouth. If a total skin exam is not feasible, a *targeted* exam of lesions, as guided by history, is also appropriate. Either way, always attempt to complete at least an upper body exam, since the trunk represents a large but easily examinable surface area.

8. **How should a specific lesion be examined in order to better classify it?**
   Not only by looking at it, but also by *touching* it, which is key for determining its characteristics and relationship to the surrounding skin: papular, sclerotic, soft, mobile, rough, or smooth. Note that, in contrast to other fields of medicine, a thorough physical examination is key for dermatologic diagnoses. In fact, it is much more key than history.

9. **And so, what are the required components of a dermatologic diagnosis?**
   Based on the aforementioned criteria, a dermatologic diagnosis requires first of all the recognition of both the *primary* and the *secondary* lesions. Once that is done, lesions must be assessed based on:
   - **Morphology:** Color, shape, dimensions (width and height, if necessary), elevation/depression, and palpable features (smoothness, induration, tenderness, scaling, and crusting)
   - **Distribution (body location):** Generalized versus localized
   - **Distribution (arrangement to one another):** Clustered, confluent, dermatomal
   - **Configuration:** Annular, reticular, linear, gyrate

10. **What are the *tools* necessary for a dermatologic diagnosis?**
    Primarily three:
    - **Magnifying glass**
    - **Wood's lamp:** A fluorescent and long-wave ultraviolet light that has been narrowed to 360 nm. Developed by Robert Wood (1868–1955), it is commonly relied on for detecting fungal lesions, areas of hypopigmentation, and porphyrin compounds. In a darkened room, it reveals fungal infections (like tinca capitis) as sharply marginated patches of bright blue-green. Since melanin absorption is at 360 nm, it also identifies areas of vitiligo or tinea versicolor (*hypopigmented* patches as pale-white, and *depigmented* areas as bright-white). Finally, it makes porphyrin compounds stand out as coral red fluorescence, like in erythrasma, a bacterial infection of intertriginous areas (axillae).
    - **Scalpel:** To get scrapings for fungi or arthropods (scabies)

11. **How does one prepare a potassium hydroxide (KOH) stain for fungi?**
    Scrape a few scales off the skin, and place them onto a glass slide. Then, pour potassium hydroxide (10%) onto the slide, and apply a coverslip. After gently warming up the slide (usually over a match), examine the preparation under a microscope for hyphae and spores.

12. **What is a *Tzanck* test?**
    A test commonly used for herpes virus infection. Pioneered by the Russian dermatologist Arnault Tzanck (1886–1954), it is carried out by unroofing a vesicle with a scalpel, scraping its base, applying the material to a microscope slide, fixing it with 95% alcohol, and preparing it with a standard Wright or Giemsa stain. If positive, the test reveals *multinucleated giants cells*, confirming that the cause of the lesion is either herpes simplex or varicella zoster.

13. **What skin appendages should be part of a thorough dermatologic exam?**
    Definitely *hair* (including eyebrows, eyelashes, and scalp), but also *fingernails* and *toenails*. As opposed to hair, these are rarely of concern to the patient, yet they may narrow the differential diagnosis, guide work-up, and provide important clues for the identification of systemic illnesses. Hence, it is the physician's responsibility to examine them thoroughly.

14. **How should *fingernails* and *toenails* be assessed?**
    If covered by polish, clean them first with a solvent like acetone. Then pay attention to color and shape but also to anatomic details (Fig. 3-25):
    - **Lunula:** The white half-moon at the proximal edge of the nail bed
    - **Cuticle:** The thin skin adherent to the nail at its proximal portion
    - **Perionychium:** The epidermis forming the ungual wall at the sides and back of the nail

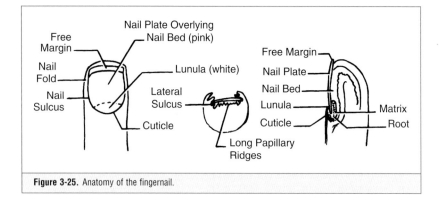

Figure 3-25. Anatomy of the fingernail.

Although fingernails tend to be more informative than toenails (since they grow more rapidly and suffer fewer traumas), always examine them *both*. Inspect them first without applying any pressure. Then, blanch the fingertip to see if a pigmented lesion changes color (which would argue for discoloration of the vascular bed rather than the nail plate). Finally, place a penlight against the finger pulp and shine it through the nail. If upon illumination a discoloration disappears, it is also more likely to be in the vascular bed than in the soft tissue or matrix. When indicated, scrape the nail plate surface, and do a potassium hydroxide preparation to rule out fungal disease. Note that nail changes due to systemic disease (as opposed to trauma) often occur in the *matrix*, so that the leading edge of the abnormality (for example, a pigmentation change) is usually shaped like the distal portion of the matrix. To estimate the time of initial insult, measure the distance from the proximal nail fold (cuticle) to the leading edge of the pigmentation change, remembering that nails grow 0.1–0.15 mm/day.

15. **What systemic conditions are associated with changes in nail *shape* or *growth*?**
    - **Clubbing:** Inflammatory bowel disease, pulmonary malignancy, asbestosis, chronic bronchitis, chronic obstructive pulmonary disease, cirrhosis, congenital heart disease, endocarditis, atrioventricular malformation and fistulas (*see* also question 19)
    - **Koilonychia (spoon nails)** (Fig. 3-26): Iron deficiency anemia, hemochromatosis, Raynaud's disease, systemic lupus disease, trauma, nail-patella syndrome
    - **Onycholysis:** Psoriasis, infection, hyperthyroidism, sarcoidosis, trauma, amyloidosis, connective tissue disorders
    - **Pitting:** Psoriasis, Reiter's syndrome, incontinentia pigmenti, alopecia areata
    - **Beau's lines** (*see* Fig. 3-26): Any severe systemic illness that disrupts nail growth, Raynaud's disease, pemphigus, trauma
    - **Yellow nail:** Lymphedema, pleural effusion, immunodeficiency, bronchiectasis, sinusitis, rheumatoid arthritis, nephrotic syndrome, thyroiditis, tuberculosis, Raynaud's disease

16. **What systemic conditions are associated with changes in nail *color*?**
    - **Terry's nails** (*see* Fig. 3-26): Hepatic failure, cirrhosis, diabetes, congestive heart failure, hyperthyroidism, malnutrition
    - **Azure lunula:** Wilson's disease, silver poisoning, quinacrine
    - **Lindsay's nails (half-and-half nails)** (*see* Fig. 3-26): Specific for renal failure
    - **Muehrcke's lines:** Specific for hypoalbuminemia
    - **Lines of Mees'** (*see* Fig. 3-26): Arsenic poisoning, Hodgkin's disease, congestive heart failure, leprosy, malaria, chemotherapy, carbon monoxide poisoning, other systemic insults
    - **Dark longitudinal streaks:** Melanoma, benign nevus, chemical staining, normal variant in darkly pigmented people

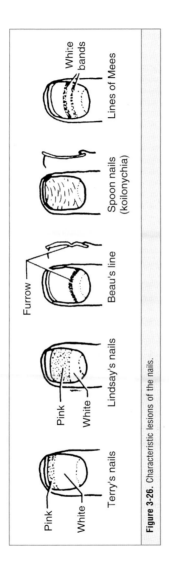

Figure 3-26. Characteristic lesions of the nails.

- **Longitudinal striations:** Alopecia areata, vitiligo, atopic dermatitis, psoriasis
- **Splinter hemorrhage:** Subacute bacterial endocarditis, systemic lupus erythematosus, rheumatoid arthritis, antiphospholipid syndrome, peptic ulcer disease, malignancies, oral contraceptive use, pregnancy, psoriasis, trauma
- **Telangiectasia:** Rheumatoid arthritis, systemic lupus erythematosus, dermatomyositis, scleroderma

17. **How are nail findings classified?**
    - Disturbances of growth
    - Transverse linear lesions
    - Longitudinal linear lesions
    - Vascular and nail bed changes
    - Infections

NAILS

Growth Disturbances

18. **What are the main growth disturbances of the nail?**
    They are clubbing, onycholysis, nail pitting, koilonychia, yellow nail, beading, onycogryphosis, onychorrhexis, and Reedy nails.

19. **What is *clubbing*?**
    A condition that can be (1) idiopathic; (2) congenital (dominant trait); or (3) a clue to serious underlying pathology, including cardiovascular, hepatobiliary, mediastinal, endocrine, gastrointestinal, neoplastic, infectious, and, especially, pulmonary (*see* Chapter 13, questions 101–116).

20. **What is *onycholysis*?**
    "Loosening of the nail" in Greek, it consists of separation of the nail plate from the nail bed. This begins at the free edge and progresses proximally, causing a traumatic uplifting of the distal plate. Usually incomplete, it results in white discoloration of the affected area, often complicated by secondary microbial colonization. Typically traumatic, it may also result from any local problem that separates the plate from the nail bed, such as periungual warts or onychomycosis. It also may originate from eczematous or drug disorders, reactions to acrylic nails or nail-hardeners, and *psoriasis*. The latter may at times occur with *complete separation of the nail*, which is either mechanically lifted off the bed or separated by traumatic bleeding. Absent local explanations, thyrotoxicosis must be ruled out ("Plummer's nails"). This may also cause brown nail discoloration.

21. **What is *nail pitting*?**
    An early but nonspecific sign of psoriasis that can also occur in alopecia areata and chronic dermatitis. Nails are pocked by multiple tiny depressions, which may eventually cause the nail to crumble. Pitting is due to loss of parakeratotic cells from the surface of the plate, starting in *the proximal nail matrix* and migrating distally.

22. **What are the nail findings of psoriasis?**
    Many, affecting 10–55% of patients and <5% of those with no other cutaneous manifestation. If untreated, they can lead to functional and social impairment. They are especially common in psoriatic *arthritis* (53–86% of patients), even though only 10–20% of all psoriatic patients have the arthritis.
    - **Pitting** (previously discussed)
    - **Oil spot or salmon patch/nail bed:** The most diagnostic nail sign; it consists of a translucent, yellow-red discolored patch in the nail bed, resembling a drop of oil beneath the plate.

- **Beau's lines in the proximal nail matrix** (see later)
- **Leukonychia:** Areas of white nail plate; due to parakeratotic foci in the mid-matrix
- **Subungual hyperkeratosis:** Excessive proliferation of the nail bed that can lead to onycholysis
- **Onycholysis**
- **Nail plate crumbling:** Weakened nail plate, bed, and matrix from diseased underlying structures
- **Splinter hemorrhages:** Longitudinal black lines due to tiny capillary hemorrhages between the nail bed and plate; analogous to *Auspitz sign* (pinpoint bleeding under the psoriatic plaque)
- **Dilated tortuous capillaries in the dermal papillae**
- **Spotted lunula:** Distal matrix involvement characterized by erythema of the lunula

23. **What is *koilonychia* (spooning)?**
    A "spoon-shaped" deformity of the nail, usually large enough to hold a drop of liquid. Normal in *infants* (but resolving after the first few years of life), it also may result from trauma, recurrent exposure to petroleum-based solvents, or *nail-patella syndrome*. It is also seen in Raynaud's disease or lupus erythematosus, but rarely in isolation. Finally, it can occur with iron deficiency (with or without anemia) or, paradoxically, hemochromatosis (check iron, hemoglobin).

24. **What is *yellow nail syndrome*?**
    An autosomal-dominant disease characterized by absent/hypoplastic and easily dislocated patellae, skeletal abnormalities, nephropathy, glaucoma, and fingernail dysplasia. This consists of slow nail growth, with a "heaped-up" or thickened appearance, excessive transverse curvature, loss of the lunula, and a *yellowish/greenish discoloration*. Eventually, the nail thickens and may even detach. Yellow/green nails may result from *any* condition that slows nail growth (such as infection, like *Pseudomonas*) or impedes lymphatic circulation. Hence, they have been associated with lymphedema of the extremities or face. They also have been linked to respiratory involvement (including chronic bronchiectasis or sinusitis), pleural effusions, internal malignancies, immunodeficiency syndromes, and rheumatoid arthritis (usually as a result of *thiol drugs*, such as bucillamine and gold sodium thiomalate). Microvascular hyperpermeability with protein leakage would explain the link of yellow nail syndrome with infection, hypoalbuminemia, pleural effusion, and lymphedema.

25. **What are brittle nails (*onychorrhexis*)?**
    Nails whose distal plate *splits* into layers, with irregular, frayed, and torn borders—almost resembling the scaling of dry skin. Present in 20% of adults (and even more in older subjects), brittle nails may be hereditary or simply aging-related. They also may be due to strong solvents or repeated immersion in water (e.g., dishwashers). Dysmetabolic states (such as hyperthyroidism, malnutrition, and iron or calcium deficiency) must always be ruled out.

26. **What is longitudinal ridging (*Reedy nails*)?**
    A normal variant of patients older than 50, but one that also can occur in younger subjects. It may even represent a *brittle nail* variation. Ridges typically extend from the proximal nail fold to the distal plate, with some being very prominent, especially in older women. They are usually multiple, but at times may be single—like in patients with lichen planus (*see* questions 38 and 210–216).

27. **What is nail *beading*?**
    A condition due to faster matrix turnover. It is quite common in rheumatoid arthritis (RA). In a study of 119 RA patients and an equal number of controls, "global" beading (i.e., involving >50% of the nail) on at least six fingernails (or four toenails) was highly suggestive of underlying disease, with

a positive predictive value of 95%. Beading, however, is uncommon in *early* RA, thus limiting its diagnostic value. Beading can occur with itraconazole too, since this also increases nail growth.

28. What is *onychogryphosis*?
A thickened nail plate, often due to trauma plus mycotic infection. Eventually, the nail curves *inward*, resembling a claw (*gryphon* is dragon in Greek) and "pinching" the nail bed (pincer nail).

Transverse Linear Lesions

29. What are the main transverse linear lesions of the nail?
They are leukonychia, trauma, Beau's lines, bitten nail lesions, Muehrcke's lines, and Mees' lines.

30. What is *leukonychia*?
A condition characterized by white spots, patches, or streaks between the nail and nail bed. It is due to tiny bubbles of subungual air trapped in the plate layers after trauma. Leukonychia (white nail in Greek) may involve the entire nail (*total*), or present instead as lines (*striate*) or dots (*punctate*). Total leukonychia is a congenital dominant disorder, whereas striate or punctate forms are instead traumatic. The latter resolve with time, since spots eventually grow out with the nail plate

31. What are *Beau's lines*?
Transverse grooves on the fingernails of patients recovering from a serious illness (like a myocardial infarction). This produces a transient intermittent inflammation of the matrix, resulting in arrested growth. Grooves will progress distally with the nail, eventually coming into view and finally moving out as the nail elongates. First described by the French Joseph H.S. Beau (1806–1865).

32. What are *bitten nails lesions*?
Lesions that may resemble Beau's lines, insofar as they, too, are transversal indentations (no pun intended), although, more commonly, they present as absence of the free nail edge, produced by nervous biting and chewing. They are an important clue to underlying psychosocial pathology.

33. What are *Muehrcke's lines* (ML)?
Two arcuate, narrow, and transverse white lines—parallel to the lunula and separated by an otherwise normal nail. Named after the American nephrologist who first described them in 1956, ML usually involve the second, third, and fourth fingers. They reflect a vascular abnormality in the nail *bed* (typically, subungual edema), and *not* in the nail plate. Hence, they do *not* progress distally with nail growth. Common in hypoalbuminemia (<2.2 gm/100 mL), they disappear with its resolution. In his original study, Muehrcke found paired, transverse, white bands in 23/31 (74%) patients with nephrotic syndrome and 8/9 with hypoalbuminemia (<2.3 gm/100 mL) from other causes. Lines were instead absent in all healthy subjects, and in those with albumin >2.2 gm/100 mL. Bands were more prominent after albumin had been <1.8 gm/100 mL for at least 4 months. In another study by Conn and Smith, Muehrcke lines were seen in 10/44 (23%) patients with hypoalbuminemia from various debilitating illnesses, but absent in those with normal serum levels. Hence, ML occurs in hypoalbuminemia from *many* reasons, including nephrotic syndrome, but also liver disease and malnutrition. Additionally, they can occur in pellagra, Hodgkin's disease, sickle cell anemia, or nail damage from paraquat and chemotherapeutic agents. Although transverse white bands in the nail plate are often due to *trauma* to the matrix at the proximal nail fold (leukonychia), Muehrcke's (and Mees') lines are instead associated with a *systemic* disease. They typically span the entire breadth of the nail bed/plate, tend to be more homogenous, have a contour similar to the distal lunula (with a rounded distal edge and smoother borders), occur on several nails at once, and typically follow a generalized insult. Trauma-induced transverse white bands tend to be more linear, do not spread across the entire breadth of the nail plate, resemble the contour of the proximal nail fold (where trauma occurred), and have a history of localized trauma to the cuticle.

34. What are Mees' lines?
They are transverse white lines distal to the cuticle, and typically laid down during a generalized illness or after a poisoning. In contrast to Muehrcke's lines, Mees' lines (also called Reynolds' or Aldrich's) are in the *nail plate*. Hence, they move distally with it. Differential diagnosis includes arsenic or thallium (2–3 weeks after an acute poisoning, or following chronic exposure), cancer chemotherapy, Hodgkin's lymphoma, and other systemic disorders, such as severe cardiac or renal disease. They were first described by the Dutch physician R.A. Mees.

35. What are the traumatic changes of the nail?
Subungual hematomas are posttraumatic hematogenous extravasation in the nail bed. When partially digested and oxidized, a subungual hematoma may turn into a brownish and transversal dark band, often associated with indentation or damage of the nail plate.

Longitudinal Linear Lesions

36. What are the main longitudinal linear lesions of the nail?
They are longitudinal melanonychia and lichen planus.

37. What is *longitudinal melanonychia*?
A condition characterized by brownish/blackish longitudinal streaks or bands. Very common in dark-skinned individuals, it reflects melanin deposition from a normal increase of melanocytes in the nail bed. Yet, it also may indicate a much more ominous *subungual* melanoma. Hence, it presents a clinical challenge. When in doubt, always biopsy the nail matrix and bed.

38. What is *lichen planus* of the nail?
A condition present in 10% of patients with lichen planus. The most common finding is thinning of the nail plate, leading to longitudinal grooving and *ridging* (*see* also question 26). Hyperpigmentation, subungual hyperkeratosis, onycholysis, and longitudinal melanonychia can also be present.

Vascular and Nail Bed Changes

39. What are the main vascular and nail bed changes of the nail?
Splinter hemorrhages, azure half-moons in nail beds, Lindsay's and Terry's nails, red half-moons in nail beds, and vasculitic changes.

40. What are *splinter hemorrhages*?
Tiny and linear red hemorrhages, extending from the free margin of the nail bed toward the proximal end. Traditionally linked to subacute bacterial endocarditis or trichinosis, they are more commonly due to trauma. According to conventional teaching, *traumatic* "splinters" extend all the way *into the edge of the nail*, whereas *embolic* splinters (like those of endocarditis) are fully contained within the nail bed. There is, however, little evidence to support this differentiation.

41. What are *azure half-moons in nail beds*?
The nails of Wilson's disease (hepatolenticular degeneration). Lunulae are not white, but bluish.

42. What are *Lindsay's nails*?
Half-and-half nails, with a white proximal half, and a dark distal half (usually brownish, but also reddish or pink). Named after the American physician who first described them in 1967, Lindsay's nails have a sharp linear demarcation between the two halves, parallel to the nail edge. Of the 25 patients first described by Dr. Lindsay, 21 had chronic renal failure and two had minor nephropathy.

43. **What are *Terry's nails*?**

Nails characterized by whitening of the *proximal 80%* of the nail, leaving a small rim of peripheral reddening, usually as sharply demarcated as in Lindsay' nails. Named after the British physician who described them in 1954, Terry's nails are seen in older subjects and patients with heart failure, cirrhosis, or non–insulin-dependent diabetes. They probably are due to subungual edema.

44. **What are *red* half-moons in nail beds?**

A variety of Terry's nails, also described by him in the same 1954 *Lancet* paper. They are characterized by a lunula that is not white, but *red*. They also are called the nails of cardiac failure. In fact, all these half-and-half nails (Lindsay's, Terry's, and the red half-moons in nail beds) reflect conditions causing subungual edema, such as cardiac, hepatic, and renal disease.

45. **How does *vasculitis of the nail* present?**

With typical nail fold changes, like cuticular hypertrophy (with small, hemorrhagic infarcts) and periungual telangiectasias. These are common in scleroderma or dermatomyositis.

Infections

46. **What are the main infections of the nail?**

They are tinea (also called *onychomycosis*), paronychia, and *Pseudomonas* infections.

47. **What is *tinea unguium*?**

A dermatophytic infection of the nail, characterized by *onychauxis* (hypertrophy of the nail plate caused by keratin pileup); *onycholysis* (nail plate separation from the nail bed); and *dystrophic*, thickened, broken, and discolored nails (white, yellow, brown, black). Browning of the plate (with peeling and splitting of the edge) also occurs, together with ridging and white spots. Note that, although *dystrophic nails* are often onychomycotic, half of them are not (and instead due to trauma, psoriasis, or lichen planus). Hence, always do scraping and KOH staining to rule out fungal infection.

48. **What is *paronychia*?**

An acute or chronic inflammation of the *perionychium*, with redness, swelling, and tenderness.

49. **How does *pseudomonal infection of the nail* present?**

With a *greenish* nail, due to iron compounds produced by pseudomonas organisms invading the nail between the nail plate and nail bed. The darker the discoloration, the deeper the bacterial progression into the plate layers. This eventually causes it to lift altogether from the nail bed.

50. **What are *blue lines*?**

The result of minocycline therapy.

HAIR

51. **How is the hair assessed?**

Region by region, first the scalp and then the body—including axillae, extremities, and pubic region. Evaluate *quantity* and *distribution* of hair, plus *thickness* and *texture*. Since alopecia is often caused by inflammation of the scalp, look for scaling, redness, crusts, and papules. Note that of the three scaling scalp lesions (seborrheic dermatitis, psoriasis, and tinea capitis), only tinea is associated with *alopecia*.

52. **What is folliculitis?**
An infection of hair follicles, most commonly due to staphylococci, but also gram-negative organisms and even fungi. In fact, *Pityrosporum*, the organism responsible for tinea versicolor, can overgrow in the follicles of patients with HIV and cause folliculitis.

53. **What is *eosinophilic folliculitis*?**
A disorder of unknown etiology, characterized by recurrent crops of sterile pustules and papules, often intensely pruritic, and presenting in multiple cycles of remissions and exacerbations. Although labeled as a *folliculitis*, it is actually a "sterile eosinophilic pustulosis" since lesions are not restricted to the hair follicle. It is probably an autoimmune response against sebocytes or some other components of sebum that usually occurs in the third to fifth decade of life. It can affect all races, but predominates in Asians. It presents as an area of erythematous papules and pustules, facial in 85% of patients, but also on the back and extensor surface of upper extremities. Papules eventually become confluent, creating indurate plaques with a healing center and a spreading periphery. These ultimately fade away, leaving residual hyperpigmentation and scaling. In HIV-infected patients, eosinophilic folliculitis (EF) presents with widespread urticarial lesions or large erythematous plaques with excoriations, often severe and persistent. Also seen in lymphoma, leukemia, myelodysplastic syndrome, atopy, and bone marrow transplantation.

> **Pearl:**
> In the immunocompromised patient, common things look uncommon.

FLUID-FILLED LESIONS: PUS (PUSTULES)—TABLE 3-2

Acne

54. **What does acne look like?**
The hallmark of acne (from the Greek *acme*, blooming) is the *variety* of its lesions, both inflammatory and noninflammatory, blossoming on the face and trunk of patients. Noninflammatory lesions include *closed comedones* (whiteheads) and open comedones (blackheads). *Comedo* is the Latin word for glutton, since this is indeed a juicy clump of sebum and keratin around a hair follicle. Closed comedones are dome-shaped papules 1–2 mm in size. When open, their content is exposed to air and thus blackened through oxidation. Hence, open comedones are 1–2-mm papules with a black keratinous plug closing the orifice of a sebaceous follicle. Inflammatory lesions are instead *papules* and *pustules*, as well as *cysts* (suppurative nodular lesions). Cystic lesions are more likely to scar if left untreated. Scarring may be pitted, hypertrophic, or papular.

55. **Who develops acne?**
Usually puberal teens, although girls may develop it one or more years before menarche. Men tend to have more severe acne, but this usually resolves by the second decade. In women, it often lingers well into the 40s and 50s, often with perimenstrual flares.

56. **What are the other clinical presentations of acne?**
The two most common are *steroid acne* and *acne rosacea*, although the latter is more than a variant of acne, and probably a completely different process of middle-aged and older people.

57. **What is *acne rosacea*?**
An acne-like rash that affects the central and flush/blush areas of the face (forehead, nose, cheeks, chin). Vascular lability is so typical that many patients have a history of *facial flushing*

TABLE 3-2. FLUID-FILLED LESIONS		
Fluid-Filled Lesions		
Pus-Filled	Clear Fluid	
Pustular	Vesiculo-Bullous	Bullous
Acne vulgaris	H. simplex	Pemphygus vulgaris
Acne rosacea	H. zoster/varicella	Pemphygoid
Steroid acne	Dermatophytoses	Drug reactions • Erythema multiforme • Stevens-Johnson • TEN
Folliculitis (bacterial/fungal)	Insect bites	Poison ivy/contact dermatitis
Intertriginous candidiasis	Dermatitis herpetiformis	Bullous impetigo
		Porphyria cutanea tarda
		Lupus erythematosus

in childhood or early teens, often triggered by dietary and environmental factors (like hot drinks, alcohol, spicy foods, but also temperature changes and even emotions). Ocular rosacea may be accompanied by conjunctival injection, and rarely, chalazion and episcleritis. Although rare, there may be extrafacial involvement of the neck and upper part of the chest. Overall, symptoms of rosacea are intermittent, but can progressively lead to permanent flushing of the skin, with telangiectasias of cheeks and nose, lymphedema, and, ultimately, skin coarseness with acne-like papulopustular eruption. Yet, unlike acne, there is neither seborrhea (i.e., greasiness of the skin) nor comedones. In fact, rosacea may present with *drying* and *peeling*. Hyperplasia of sebaceous glands may eventually lead to a thickened and disfigured nose (*rhinophyma*). Still, this can be an isolated finding, and in fact, some authors even consider it a separate entity. Note that although rosacea is much more frequent in subjects of Celtic ancestry, it has also been described in dark-skinned individuals, such as African-Americans.

58. **What is *steroid acne*?**
An acne-like rash that may begin as early as 2 weeks after administration of systemic corticosteroids. In contrast to plain acne, lesions are *monomorphous* (generally pustules and dome-shaped papules) and covering the trunk, shoulders, and upper arms. A rosacea-like syndrome (including perioral dermatitis) also can result from the indiscriminate use of potent corticosteroids on the face.

59. **How is acne diagnosed?**
Clinically, based on a mixture of lesion types in the appropriate location.

FLUID-FILLED LESIONS: CLEAR FLUID (VESICULOBULLOUS DISEASES)

Herpes Simplex

60. **How does herpes simplex present?**
With pain or tingling. This precedes the onset of small erythematous papules/plaques of uniform size and shape, which eventually develop into grouped umbilicated vesicles on an erythematous

basis, progress to *pustules*, and finally ulcerate, erode (especially in the genital areas), and crust. The most common locations are *labial* (vermilion border of the lip) and *genital*, although other areas may be affected, including the eye and presacrum.

61. **Who develops herpes simplex?**
Any age group, even though certain involvements are age-specific, such as stomatitis in children, labialis in adults, genitalis in sexually active subjects, and lumbosacral in patients older than 40.

62. **What is the typical clinical course of herpes simplex?**
- **Primary (initial) outbreaks:** Usually more severe, with pain, edema, and a prolonged course. Still, the majority of primary infections go unnoticed because symptoms are either absent or so minimal that only the recurrent episodes are recognized.
- **Secondary (recurrent) disease:** Less severe and shorter in duration. In fact, the hallmark of mucocutaneous herpes simplex is its ability to remain dormant in ganglia, eventually recurring in areas of primary infection. Frequency of recurrences varies, but for genital and labial herpes, the average is four episodes per year. Approximately 50% of patients with genital herpes have one or more episodes, often from local trauma, menses, and even stress.

63. **What are the other clinical presentations of herpes simplex?**
- **Herpetic gingivostomatitis:** Presents in children and young adults with fever, malaise, sore throat, painful vesicles, and erosions of tongue, palate, gingiva, buccal mucosa, and lips
- **Herpetic whitlow** (middle English for *white flaw*; also referred to as a *felon*): This is an occupational hazard of medical and dental professionals caused by exposure to the virus in a patient's mouth. It is characterized by vesicles and edema of a digit, sometimes associated with erythema, lymphangitis, and lymphadenopathy of the arm. It may last for several weeks.
- **Herpes simplex in immunosuppressed patients:** Frequently produces more severe and persistent ulceration, as well as disseminated cutaneous and systemic lesions

64. **How is herpes simplex diagnosed?**
Usually by clinical appearance (grouped umbilicated vesicles on an erythematous base). Still, a Tzanck preparation is diagnostic. Direct immunofluorescent antibody staining of infected cells is also an effective and rapid method of diagnosis. Viral cultures grow herpes simplex virus in several days. Biopsy of lesions demonstrates reticular and ballooning degeneration of the epidermis, multinucleated giant cells, and intranuclear inclusions.

Varicella

65. **What are the features of varicella?**
The classic lesion is a 2–3-mm elliptical *vesicle* surrounded by erythema, commonly described as a "dew drop on a rose petal." This quickly converts into a *pustule*, then umbilicates and crusts. The crust falls off in 1–3 weeks, leaving a shallow pink depression that may result in scarring. New vesicles appear in successive crops, resulting in nonclustered lesions in *all* stages of development. These first appear on the face and scalp, then the trunk, and 2–3 days later on the arms and legs in a centrifugal fashion. Mucous membranes are also involved, especially the mouth.

66. **Who develops varicella?**
Mostly children younger than 10 years. Only 5% of cases occur in subjects older than 15.

67. **What is the typical clinical course of varicella?**
Incubation is 2 weeks, with patients being highly contagious for 2–4 weeks (from 1–2 days before exanthema until crusting of all lesions).

68. **How are the other clinical presentations of varicella?**
More severe in adults than in children, with higher fever, constitutional symptoms, and pneumonia (4% of cases). During pregnancy, varicella can be transmitted to the fetus, producing serious developmental abnormalities. In immunocompromised patients, it causes a more extensive and persistent rash, with higher morbidity and mortality, and even hemorrhagic complications.

69. **How is varicella diagnosed?**
By the classic appearance of the rash, often supported by a history of recent exposure. Conversely, to distinguish disseminated herpes simplex from varicella, a culture is often needed.

Herpes Zoster

70. **What are the clinical features of herpes zoster?**
The hallmark of zoster (*girdle* in Greek) is its *clustered* pattern, as opposed to the nonclustered pattern of varicella. The rash is usually preceded by paresthesia and *pain* in the involved dermatome (*Saint Anthony's fire*). This is often mistaken as musculoskeletal, due to its intensity and deep location. Hence, zoster should always be considered in patients with deep dermatomal pain with no historical or physical explanations. The prodromal discomfort is then followed by the appearance of erythematous plaques, which, in sequence, develop into (1) grouped vesicles, (2) pustules, (3) umbilicated pustules, and (4) crusts. The rash is unilateral, does not cross the midline, and generally appears in only one dermatome, with trigeminal and T3 to L2 being the most common. It is not unusual to see a few vesicles just outside the involved dermatome.

71. **Who develops herpes zoster?**
Older subjects, with more than two thirds of cases occurring in patients older than 50 and less than 10% of cases in those younger than 20. It is also more common in immunosuppressed patients. Zoster in infants is usually associated with a history of maternal varicella infection during gestation.

72. **What is the typical clinical course?**
The rash erupts and progresses to complete crusting over 1 week, then resolves over several weeks. *Postherpetic neuralgia* (pain persisting after all crusts have fallen off) occurs in 15% of patients and is more common in the older population.

73. **What are the other presentations of herpes zoster?**
- **Involvement of the eye (ophthalmic branch):** Heraldic lesions appear on the tip of the nose, due to infection of the nasociliary nerve. Get immediate ophthalmologic consultation.
- **Ramsay Hunt syndrome:** Due to involvement of the geniculate ganglion with facial paralysis. Lesions occur over the external auditory canal or tympanic membrane, with or without vertigo, tinnitus, deafness/hyperacusis, unilateral loss of taste, and decrease in tear formation and salivation. Described by the Philadelphia neurologist James Ramsay Hunt (1874–1937).
- **Zoster in immunocompromised patients:** Seen in patients with AIDS and malignancies (especially lymphocytic leukemia or Hodgkin's) and those undergoing immunosuppressive therapies. Usually more severe and often disseminated. Chronic eruptions can be the first sign of HIV infection.

Scabies (*see* questions 255–257)

Dermatitis herpetiformis

74. **What is dermatitis herpetiformis (DH)?**
An immune-mediated blistering disease. First described by Duhring in 1884, DH is uniformly linked to gluten-sensitive enteropathy—usually asymptomatic. Hence, it can be controlled by a gluten-free diet. Typical of 20- to 40-year-old Northern Europeans. May degenerate into cancer.

75. **What are the skin lesions of DH?**
They are clusters of flesh-colored to erythematous herpetiform papules and vesicles. These are inflammatory, pruritic, and mostly located on the extensor surfaces (elbows, knees, buttocks, shoulders, and the posterior/nuchal scalp). Lesions may often present *not as vesicles*, but as *erosions* and *crusts*. Palms and soles usually are spared, and so is the buccal mucosa.

76. **What is the course of DH?**
A lifelong one, with remissions and exacerbations. Symptoms can be controlled with dapsone in 24–48 hours. A gluten-free diet can also provide control without medications.

Pemphigus and Pemphigoid

77. **What is Pemphigus?**
A group of autoimmune and potentially life-threatening mucocutaneous diseases characterized by intradermal blisters and circulating IgG against keratinocytes. Binding of autoantibodies results in *acantholysis* (i.e., loss of cell–cell adhesion), and antibody titers correlate with disease activity. Pemphigus (from the Greek *pemphix*, blister) comprises three subsets: pemphigus vulgaris (70% of all cases), pemphigus foliaceus, and paraneoplastic pemphigus.

78. **What are the clinical features of *pemphigus vulgaris* (PV)?**
It can affect all races, although more commonly Jewish and other Mediterranean groups. Its peak of onset is during the fifth and sixth decades. The primary lesion is a flaccid *blister* filled with clear fluid, and originating from a normal or erythematous skin base. Since blisters are fragile, they rupture easily, producing large, shallow, and painful *erosions* that heal slowly. Hence, erosions are the most common skin manifestation of the disease. Still, *mucosal* lesions (usually oral) are the most common *presenting* manifestation, affecting 50–70% of patients and often preceding cutaneous involvement by several months. Since intact bullae are rare in the mouth, most patients have irregularly shaped erosions of gingival, buccal, or palatine mucosa. These are painful, slow to heal, and interfere with eating, drinking, or swallowing. Other involved mucosae include conjunctiva, esophagus, larynx, labia, vagina, cervix, penis, urethra, and anus.

79. **Are there any other causes of PV?**
A form of PV (but also BP, see question 80) can be drug induced, resulting from penicillamine, captopril, thiol-containing compounds, and rifampin. Emotional stress can also trigger it. Finally, PV may occur in other autoimmune diseases, including myasthenia gravis and thymoma.

80. **What is *bullous pemphigoid* (BP)?**
Another autoimmune and blistering skin disease, except that in contrast to PV it rarely involves mucous membranes, it rarely erodes (lesions are subepidermal and thus the bullae have thicker roofs), and it is typically pruritic. Caused by the binding of circulating IgG autoantibodies to the skin basement membrane, BP is more common than PV, affects older patients (average age 65), and runs a chronic course marked by remissions and exacerbations. Onset may be subacute or acute, with widespread, tense, and often pruritic blisters. These may at times arise from persistent urticarial lesions, but also from chronic nonbullous inflammatory diseases, such as lichen planus and psoriasis. Rupture of the blisters leaves painful and disabling erosions, especially when involving palms and soles. Still, the primary lesion of BP is the *bulla*: tense, arising from normal-appearing as well as erythematous skin, and affecting any part of the body (even though flexural areas are usually a preferential site). Involvement of ocular and oral mucosae is rare (only 10–25% of patients), but when it occurs, oral intake may be limited because of dysphagia.

81. **What is *Nikolsky's sign*? What is its significance?**
It is a sign described in 1896 by Pyotr W. Nikolsky, a Russian dermatologist who taught at Warsaw and Rostov. It consists in the superficial separation of normal-appearing epidermis into

an *erosion*, as a result of the shearing stress produced by sliding a finger on it. It is due to poor adhesion of the epidermal cells (acantholysis). Hence, it occurs in bullous diseases like pemphigus, but *not* pemphigoid, where the epidermal split is much deeper. Still, it is not entirely specific for PV, since it can occur in other active blistering diseases, such as scalded skin syndrome.

82. **What is *Asboe-Hansen* sign?**
Another sign of PV; lateral pressure on the edge of a blister may spread it into unaffected skin.

Drug Reactions

83. **What are the most important cutaneous manifestations of drug reactions?**
Erythema multiforme (EM), toxic epidermal necrolysis (TEN), and *Stevens-Johnson syndrome (SJS)*. Even though EM may be entirely distinct, SJS and TEN probably represent different manifestations of a single disease. A recent classification based on percentage of *epidermal detachment* defines SJS as denuding <10% of body surface area (BSA), overlapping SJS/TEN as denuding 10–30%, and classic TEN >30%. *Bullous* EM, previously grouped with SJS, causes epidermal detachment in <10% of BSA, but has *acral target lesions* or raised atypical targets.

84. **What is *erythema multiforme* (EM)?**
A relatively benign process characterized by target or targetoid lesions, with or without blisters, *in a symmetric and acral distribution*. In fact, the rash favors palms and soles, dorsum of hands, face, and extensor surfaces of extremities (Fig. 3-27). It is often associated with oral lesions, but rarely involves more than one mucosal surface. Although it can be caused by drugs, it is most commonly a sequela of herpes virus infection. It has low morbidity, no mortality, but frequent recurrences. It may be associated with epidermal detachment, yet *denudation always involves <10% of BSA*.

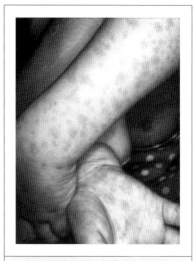

Figure 3-27. Erythema multiforme. The eruption consists of annular and papular erythema over the acral areas. (From Fitzpatrick JE, Aeling JE: Dermatology Secrets. Philadelphia, Hanley & Belfus, 1996.)

85. **What is *Stevens-Johnson syndrome* (SJS)?**
A potential dermatologic emergency. First described in 1922 by the American pediatricians Albert Stevens and Frank Johnson, SJS is characterized by *widespread* purpuric macules and targetoid lesions, usually more common on face and torso, and with concomitant *mucosal involvement* of *more than one site* (usually the eyes, mouth, and genitalia; Fig. 3-28). Lesions may undergo full-thickness epidermal necrosis, although this is limited by definition to <10% of cutaneous surface. Hence, mortality is much less than in TEN (only 5%).

86. **What is *toxic epidermal necrolysis* (TEN)?**
Also known as Lyell's syndrome, this is a true dermatologic emergency characterized by widespread skin *and* mucosal *denudation*. Skin lesions are erythematous and target-like macules associated with full-thickness epidermal necrosis and detachment of >30% BSA (Fig. 3-29). It is fatal in 50% of the cases, usually because of sepsis and respiratory distress.

Mortality is related to BSA involvement: 11% for BSA (which is actually more of a SJS-TEN *transitional* form), and 35% for BSA >30%.

87. **Describe the presentation of SJS/TEN**
    Constitutional symptoms (fever, cough, or sore throat) precede the cutaneous lesions by 1–3 days. Then photophobia appears, followed by a diffuse "cayenne pepper" eruption that is extremely tender to touch and symmetrically distributed on the face and upper torso. This consists of poorly defined erythematous macules with darker purpuric centers (targetoid lesions) that coalesce, blister, and ulcerate. Sheets of skin may then lift off as in a severe thermal burn, especially in TEN.

88. **What is the difference between "targetoid" lesions of SJS/TEN and "targets" of EM?**
    The SJS/TEN lesions have only two zones of color: a central dusky purpura (or central bulla), surrounded by a macular erythema. Conversely, a classic target lesion of EM has *three* zones of color: a central dusky purpura (or central bulla), a surrounding edematous pale zone, and a surrounding macular erythema. Except for the central bulla, the initial lesion of SJS/TEN is also typically flat. Conversely, lesions of EM are more likely palpable.

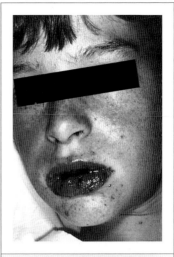

Figure 3-28. Stevens-Johnson syndrome. Typical mucosal inflammation of the mouth, lips, andf conjunctiva. (From Fitzpatrick JE, Aeling JE: Dermatology Secrets. Philadelphia, Hanley & Belfus, 1996.)

89. **What are the skin manifestations of SJS/TEN?**
    Lesions begin symmetrically on face and upper torso, and then extend rapidly. Maximal extension occurs in 2–3 days, but occasionally takes only a few hours. Individual macules are usually present around large areas of confluence. Lesions may predominate in sun-exposed areas, but may also affect the entire epidermis, including nail beds. The hairy scalp, however, usually remains intact. Palms and soles develop a painful edematous erythema. Flaccid blisters are typically present, together with full-thickness epidermal necrosis. Nondenuded areas have a wrinkled paper appearance. A Nikolsky sign is easily demonstrated by applying lateral pressure to the bullae. Full skin detachment usually occurs in areas subjected to pressure, such as shoulders, sacrum, or buttocks. Areas of denuded epidermis are dark red with oozing surfaces.

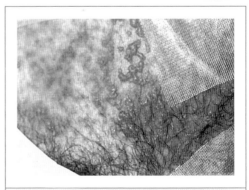

Figure 3-29. Toxic epidermal necrolysis. The patient demonstrates the typical "telangiectatic" blanching erythema and blistering that progress to denuding of the epidermis. (From Fitzpatrick JE, Aeling JE: Dermatology Secrets. Philadelphia, Hanley & Belfus, 1996.)

90. **Is there any _mucosal_ involvement in SJS/TEN?**

Yes. Mucosae are involved in almost _all_ patients with SJS/TEN—not only those with extensive cutaneous manifestations. In fact, mucosal lesions may precede _skin_ lesions. Preferential sites include the oropharynx and esophagus, tracheobronchial tree, GI tract, genitalia, and anus. Painful oral erosions cause severe crusting of the lips, increased salivation, and impaired alimentation. Intact expectorated cylindrical casts of bronchial epithelium may also occur, and involvement of genitalia can lead to painful micturition. Patients with GI manifestations often develop a profuse protein-rich diarrhea. Of all mucosal lesions, the most problematic are the _ocular_ ones, since they often leave sequelae. Initially, the conjunctivae are erythematous and painful, with lids often stuck together. Efforts to loosen them may result in tearing of the epidermis. Eventually, pseudomembranous conjunctival erosions form synechiae between the eyelids and conjunctivae, with inverted eyelashes, keratitis, corneal erosions, and corneal/conjunctival neovascularization.

91. **What are the sequelae of SJS/TEN?**

Variable. Some patients rapidly lose large areas of the skin in just a few days, whereas others begin re-epithelialization almost as quickly. Predicting the course at initial presentation is not possible. Overall, re-epithelialization is usually complete within 3 weeks, but pressure and mucosal areas may remain eroded and crusted for 2 weeks or longer. Long-term sequelae of SJS/TEN vary based on site:

- Disabling eye lesions may cause blindness in 40% of TEN survivors. Persistent watery eyes or a sicca-like syndrome can also occur.
- Cutaneous lesions may resolve with a mottling of hyperpigmentation and hypopigmentation.
- Genitourinary lesions may result in phimosis or vaginal synechiae.
- Fingernails and toenails may regrow abnormally.

92. **What is the cause of SJS/TEN?**

Almost exclusively a drug reaction, 1–3 weeks from administration. The most frequent offenders are _antibiotics_ (especially trimethoprim-sulfamethoxazole and other sulfonamides, but also aminopenicillins, quinolones, and cephalosporins); _anticonvulsants_ (including phenobarbital, phenytoin, valproic acid, and carbamazepine), and finally _nonsteroidal anti-inflammatory drugs, allopurinol,_ and even _corticosteroids_. HIV patients have greater risk of TEN, and often tend to be younger. This may be related to their increased use of sulfonamides. Finally, TEN has been reported in systemic lupus erythematosus or acute graft versus host disease. Infections with _herpesvirus, Mycoplasma pneumoniae,_ or _Yersinia_ may also occur in SJS, but even more in EM.

93. **What is the mechanism of TEN?**

Unclear. Early histology shows full-thickness epidermal necrosis, with little or no lymphocytic infiltrate, suggesting that TEN is _not_ induced by inflammation but by a _cellular toxin,_ which is why steroids and immunosuppressive therapy are _not_ effective and, in fact, possibly detrimental.

94. **How do you separate _staphylococcal scalded skin syndrome_ (SSSS) from TEN?**

TEN is characterized by a deeper split in the epidermis (i.e., at the dermoepidermal junction). The split in SSSS is instead higher, and just inferior to the stratum corneum (the uppermost layer of the epidermis). Hence, SSSS lesions are more superficial and heal more quickly, while TEN is usually treated in burn units (which is crucial for survival: referral in less than 7 days after onset has a mortality rate of 4%, whereas referral beyond 7 days has a mortality rate of 83%). SSSS, on the other hand, is commonly treated with antibiotics, since it is induced by a staphylococcal toxin. Note that TEN also is called _toxic epidermal necrolysis of the Lyell type_ (from the British dermatologist who first described it) to distinguish it from _toxic epidermal necrolysis of the Ritter type_ (from the Austrian dermatologist who described it in 1878)—another name for SSSS.

95. What are the other major cutaneous manifestations of drug reactions?
- Urticaria (hives)
- Morbilliform rash
- Phototoxic reaction (doxycycline)
- Erythema nodosum (panniculitis, often pretibial)
- Pigmentary changes
- Fixed eruptions
- Vasculitis
- Bullous eruptions
- Lichenoid eruptions
- Nail changes, such as onycholysis

96. What is a drug-induced *photosensitivity reaction*?
A cutaneous disease resulting from the *combined* effects of light *and* a chemical substance—administered either systemically (medication) or topically (cream). A drug-induced photosensitivity is more likely to be triggered by UV-A (320–400 nm) than UV-*B* wavelengths (290–320 nm). Conversely, UV-B wavelengths are more likely to cause sunburn and nonmelanoma skin cancer.

97. What are the most common photosensitizing medications?
The usual suspects:
- Antibiotics (especially tetracyclines, fluoroquinolones, sulfonamides)
- Nonsteroidal anti-inflammatory drugs
- Diuretics
- Retinoids
- Miscellaneous agents (amiodarone, diltiazem, enalapril)

These are mostly responsible for *phototoxic* reactions. Topical substances are instead photosensitizing through a *photoallergic* reaction. Among these are *fragrances* (musk ambrette) and *sunscreens* (especially if containing salicylates, cinnamates, benzophenones, and para-aminobenzoic acid). Some drugs are photoallergic, too, including dapsone, hydrochlorothiazide, quinidine, and hypoglycemic agents (sulfonylureas, such as glipizide and glyburide). As for all drug reactions, consider timing, rates of reactions, response to withdrawal, and re-challenge.

Urticaria

98. What is *urticaria* (hives)?
A flat-topped and vascular reaction consisting of blanching, raised and palpable wheals, typically migratory and transient. It is quite common, affecting one fifth of the U.S. population. Causes are many, but not identifiable in >50% of the cases. Management is straightforward and generally successful.

99. What are the skin manifestations of urticaria?
The primary lesion is the *wheal*, a whitish-to-reddish, well-demarcated, edematous papule or plaque with a pale center. This is usually surrounded by a halo and quite pruritic. Wheals may be linear, round, oval, annular, arcuate, serpiginous, or generalized. They vary from several millimeters to 10 cm, affecting mostly the trunk, buttocks, and chest, although they also can occur anywhere. They last from minutes to hours, always resolving with no postinflammatory pigmentary changes or scaling. If *individual* lesions last longer than a day (and are associated with pigmentary changes or symptoms other than pruritus—such as pain or burning), consider performing a biopsy to exclude *urticarial vasculitis*, a forme fruste of leukocytoclastic vasculitis that may be associated with internal organ involvement.

100. What is angioedema?
An urticarial variant characterized by subcutaneous swelling in the distensible tissues of eyelids, lips, and oral mucosal membranes (including tongue). May result in respiratory distress.

101. **What is the clinical course of urticaria?**
   - **Acute urticaria** resolves in 4–6 weeks. It is usually associated with drugs (penicillin, sulfonamides, aspirin); food allergens (e.g., chocolate, shellfish, eggs, cheese, nuts, peanut butter, berries, tomatoes, strawberries); new pets; or infections (upper respiratory infection, especially streptococcal in children). Pregnancy may aggravate it into *pruritic and urticarial papules and plaques of pregnancy* (PUPPP syndrome).
   - **Chronic urticaria** is instead longer than 6 weeks and may last for years. One half of patients are free of symptoms at 12 months, but 20% have lesions that persist for decades. In 80% of cases, the etiology remains unknown, with possibilities including the same causes of acute urticaria, as well as cryoglobulins, autoimmune diseases, food additives, inhalants, viruses (hepatitis B), parasites, arthropods (scabies and fleas), neoplasms, and even *stress* (often responding to hypnosis). Still, physical factors are the most commonly identifiable etiologies of chronic urticaria, being responsible for one out of five cases. Among them are cold, water, sun, pressure, vibration, and even stroking (demographism), often coexisting in the individual patient. Physical urticarias are easily recognized by challenge testing.

102. **What are the other clinical presentations of urticaria?**
   1. **Hereditary angioedema:** Autosomal dominant, it presents in the second to fourth decade of life with sudden attacks of angioedema that often last for days and can be life threatening. Due to low or nonfunctional C1 inhibitor, with diagnosis being suggested by a low C4 level.
   2. **Physical urticarias:** appear in response to a stimulus, such as cold, sunlight, trauma, water:
      - *Dermatographism* (wheals at site of skin-stroking)
      - *Pressure urticaria* (severe swelling with deep pain several hours after localized pressure is applied, most commonly on feet and buttocks)
      - *Aquagenic urticaria* (elicited by water, as in a cold or hot shower)
      - *Cold urticaria* (from rewarming of skin exposed to cold; most common on hands and feet)
      - *Solar urticaria* (urticaria on unshielded skin after exposure to sunlight)
      - *Cholinergic urticaria* (on face and trunk, pruritic, induced by exercise and emotional stress)

103. **How is urticaria diagnosed?**
   By its classic and fleeting lesions. Always inquire about association with medicine intake, food exposure, recent illness, and physical stimuli, but delay work-up for underlying causes until the problem becomes chronic. Then, do a thorough physical exam, a complete blood count and differential, biochemistry screening, urinalysis, hepatitis B surface antigen, sinus films, oral examination, stool specimens for ova and parasites, and an elimination diet.

Miscellaneous

104. **Are there any other diseases that may cause *vesiculobullous* lesions?**
   Impetigo, insect bites, contact dermatitis, porphyria cutanea tarda, and lupus erythematosus.

SOLID LESIONS: TAN OR PINK—TABLE 3-3

Warts

105. **What are warts?**
   Benign, keratotic (rough-surfaced), mucocutaneous proliferations due to human papilloma viruses (HPV). There are more than 150 known types of HPV, whose manifestations include *common warts, genital warts, deep palmoplantar warts,* and *flat warts*. Ubiquitous, they affect 7–12% of the general population, 10–20% of school-aged children, and an even greater percentage of immunosuppressed patients and meat handlers ("butcher warts"). They are difficult to treat and may resolve spontaneously.

TABLE 3-3. SOLID LESIONS

Solid Lesions			
Tan/Pink	**White**	**Brown**	**Yellow**
Keratotic Papules/Nodules (Rough-Surfaced)	*Patches/Plaques*	*Macules*	*Smooth-Surfaced*
• Warts	• Vitiligo	• Tinea versicolor	• Xanthomas
• Actinic keratosis	• Tinea versicolor	• Acanthosis nigricans	• Xanthelasmas
• Squamous cell carc.		• Freckles	• Necrobiosis lipoidica
• Bowen's disease		• Lentigenes	
• Corns and calluses			
Nonkeratotic Papules/Nodules (Smooth-Surfaced)		*Papules/Nodules*	*Crusted*
• Basal cell carc.		• Melanocytic nevi	• Misc. infections
• Acrochordons		• Dysplastic nevi	
		• Seborrheic Keratoses	
		• Leser-Trélat sign	
		• Melanoma	
		• Actinic damage	
		• Café au lait spots	

106. **How are warts transmitted?**
By direct or indirect contact, especially when the normal epithelial barrier has been disrupted.

107. **What are the major types of warts?**
   - **Common wart:** Often referred to as *verruca vulgaris*, it presents as a rough-surfaced, scaly, and circumscribed papule, <1 mm to >0.5 cm in size. Most commonly located on hands and knees, although it can occur anywhere (Fig. 3-30). Often accompanied by "*black seeds*" (i.e., thrombosed capillaries). Usually asymptomatic, warts may cause cosmetic disfigurement or tenderness.

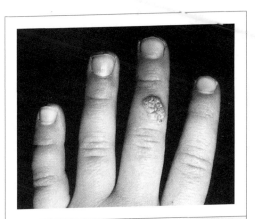

Figure 3-30. Common wart of the hand. (From Fitzpatrick JE, Aeling JE: Dermatology Secrets. Philadelphia, Hanley & Belfus, 1996.)

- **Filiform wart:** Long and slender growth, usually around lips, eyelids, or nares
- **Condyloma:** A genital wart, mostly of the anus, vulva, or glans. Presents as a flat-topped papule with an irregular surface. Condylomata may be pink at first, but turn tan or brown with time.
- **(Palmo)plantar wart:** Involving the soles or dorsi of feet, but also toes. Often callused, it presents as a white, irregularly surfaced area--with or without black dots. Plantar warts are usually painful, and when extensively involving the soles, they may impair ambulation. Deep palmoplantar warts are also termed *myrmecia* (from the Greek *murmekos*, ants). They begin as small shiny papules that progress into deep and sharply defined rounded lesions, with a rough keratotic surface and a smooth collar of thickened horn. Since they grow deep, they are more painful than common warts.
- **Flat wart:** Also called "plane warts" (or verruca plana). Flat and flesh-colored papules, >1–5 mm in size. Smooth or slightly hyperkeratotic, they may number just a few or in the hundreds, at times becoming grouped or confluent, and often acquiring linear distribution after scratching or trauma (Koebner's phenomenon). Although possible anywhere, they typically involve the face (Fig. 3-31), shins, and dorsum of hands. May regress spontaneously, often after an inflammatory flare.

Actinic Keratosis

108. What is actinic keratosis (AK)?

Actinic (or solar) keratosis (literally "sun-induced"; *aktis*, ray in Greek) is the most common premalignant lesion in humans. It is a sun-related growth that affects an estimated 60% of individuals older than 40, typically the fair-skinned and blue-eyed easy burners, who tan poorly and have occupations/hobbies that expose them to lots of sun. Most have at least one actinic keratosis per year. Many have several.

Histologically, AK represents a partial-thickness atypia of the epidermis and, if left untreated, may degenerate into squamous cell carcinoma (SCC). Lesions usually develop as a single, small erythematous plaque, 3–10 mm in diameter, typically located over exposed surfaces, such as nose, forehead, temples, cheeks, ears, bald scalp, forearms, and dorsum of the hands (but also the back, chest, and legs). The lesions have an erythematous base that is usually covered by a scale (hyperkeratosis), often on a background of solar-damaged skin, with telangiectasias, elastosis, pigmented lentigines, and multiple erythematous keratoses. They flare and become more visible during time of immune suppression, acute sun exposure, or chemotherapy. One in 20 eventually breaks through into the dermis, becoming invasive and possibly metastatic. These are typically the most elevated, erythematous, and indurated. Although more common in older individuals, AK may also affect people in their 20s and 30s, especially fair-skinned redheads and blonds who do not use sunscreen and live in the "sun belt" (Australia is the nation with the highest AK prevalence).

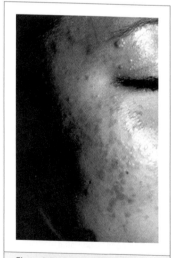

Figure 3-31. Flat warts of the face. (From Fitzpatrick JE, Aeling JE: Dermatology Secrets. Philadelphia, Hanley & Belfus, 1996.)

Squamous Cell Carcinoma (SCC)

109. **How does SCC present?**

In a myriad of morphologic variants, although typically as a scaly, erythematous, and hyperkeratotic *plaque*, often with superficial *ulceration* and no defined translucent border (Fig. 3-32).

110. **Where in the skin does SCC originate?**

From keratinocytes located in the epidermis, just above the basal layer.

111. **Describe the evolution of SCC. Why is it important?**

SCC starts as a group of atypical cells in sun-exposed areas, such as *head and neck* in 70% of the cases (mostly the lower lip, external ear, and periauricular region, but also forehead and scalp), and arms and hands in the remainder. At this early stage, the lesion presents as *actinic*

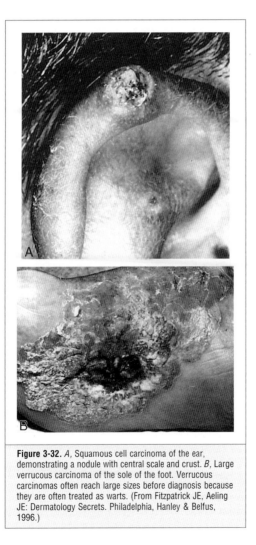

Figure 3-32. *A,* Squamous cell carcinoma of the ear, demonstrating a nodule with central scale and crust. *B,* Large verrucous carcinoma of the sole of the foot. Verrucous carcinomas often reach large sizes before diagnosis because they are often treated as warts. (From Fitzpatrick JE, Aeling JE: Dermatology Secrets. Philadelphia, Hanley & Belfus, 1996.)

keratosis (i.e., a flat, scaly, and pink macule). This is precancerous but may *not* evolve into SCC. As the atypical cells fill the entire epidermis but do not breach the basal layer, the lesion becomes *SCC in situ* (*Bowen's disease*). The next and final step is progression to *invasive SCC*, wherein the atypical cells penetrate below the basement membrane and into the dermis.

112. What is the course of SCC?
When it arises in actinically damaged skin, SCC rarely metastasizes. Risk factors for spread include depth of invasion, degree of cellular differentiation, and *origin in a mucous membrane*. Therefore, SCC of the lips has a much greater potential for systemic metastases.

Bowen's Disease

113. What is Bowen's disease (BD)?
A condition first described in 1912 by the Harvard dermatologist John T. Bowen—shy lecturer and reclusive bachelor. BD is a full-thickness, keratotic atypia of the epidermis, considered equivalent to SCC *in situ* with the potential for progression (although less than 5% of cases advance to invasive SCC). Lesions originate on both sun-exposed and covered skin, since BD is not only due to chronic solar damage, but also to inorganic arsenic ingestion and HPV. Early papers reported a 15–70% association with internal malignancies, but most recent studies have refuted it. BD occurs more commonly in older white subjects, where it presents as a single lesion in two thirds of cases, usually on the head and neck, but also the hands, limbs, and any other mucocutaneous surface. In fact, it may also affect the glans penis, where it is referred to as *erythroplasia of Queyrat*. The typical lesion is an asymptomatic and slowly enlarging erythematous patch or plaque that is scaly, relatively flat, and may eventually become hyperkeratotic, crusted, fissured, or even ulcerated. Lesions vary in size from a few millimeters to several centimeters, usually ending with a sharply demarcated and irregular border. They are rarely pigmented, and since they are often asymptomatic and benign looking (especially early on), they often go undiagnosed.

Basal Cell Carcinoma (BCC)

114. How does BCC present?
As a pink, pearly, and nonkeratotic (smooth-surfaced) *papule* with a rolled, translucent border and a few telangiectasias. Typical of sun-exposed areas of face and ears, it may occur anywhere. BCC may "outgrow" its blood supply and become necrotic in the center ("rodent ulcer").

115. What is the usual clinical course of BCC?
Usually so benign that it used to be called *basal cell epithelium*. If untouched, it grows locally, with the potential of becoming highly destructive, but rarely metastatic.

Acrochordons (Skin Tags)

116. What are acrochordons (skin tags)?
From the Greek *akros* (apical) and *khorde* (elongated structure), these are benign, flesh-colored, and usually pedunculated soft neoplasms 2–5 mm in diameter with a nonkeratotic (smooth) or variegated appearance. They arise most frequently in intertriginous areas (neck, axillae, groins, and eyelids), but also trunk, abdomen, and back. They occur more rarely in oral, anal, and vulvovaginal areas. They increase with age, so that by 70 they are found in 60% of the population. Usually asymptomatic, they may become painful when inflamed or irritated, usually as a result of friction from jewelry or clothing.

117. What are the causes of skin tags?
Unknown. Proposed etiologies include:
- **Frequent irritation:** Hence, the predilection for intertriginous areas, especially in obese patients

- **Human papilloma virus (HPV):** Frequently cultured in skin tag biopsies, suggesting at least a co-factor role
- **Paraneoplastic:** Acrochordons may coexist with various neoplasms, especially gastrointestinal and renal, suggesting a role for tumor-secreted growth hormones. Still, the association with colonic polyps is controversial at best.
- **Hormonal imbalances:** Hyperestrogenemia and hyperprogesteronemia of pregnancy, the high growth hormone levels of acromegaly, and the hyperinsulinemia of type 2 diabetes

118. **What is the evidence behind the association between skin tags and type 2 diabetes?**
Suggestive. In a study of 118 subjects with acrochordons, 41% had either impaired glucose tolerance or overt type 2 diabetes. There was, however, no correlation between glucose intolerance and location, size, color, or number of acrochordons.

SOLID LESIONS: WHITE

Vitiligo

119. **What is vitiligo?**
A common, acquired, and progressive destruction of some (or all) of the melanocytes in the interfollicular epidermis and follicles, resulting in skin and hair depigmentation. The disease has hereditary predisposition and age of onset between 10 and 30.

120. **How does vitiligo present?**
As milky white, nonscaly, and sharply demarcated macules and patches of variable size (Fig. 3-33). These are often symmetric, and commonly involving areas of repeated trauma, such as elbows, ventral wrists, knees, axillae, dorsal hands, and feet. Other targets include mucous membranes and periorificial sites (eyes, nose, ears, lips, gums, genitals, areolas, and nipples). Lesions eventually increase in number and become confluent, taking on bizarre shapes. They may also appear at sites of injury (*koebnerization*). *Localized vitiligo* (i.e., restricted to one area) is less common

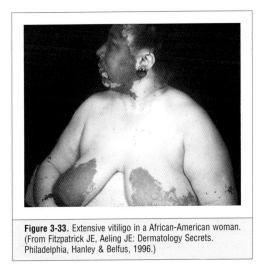

Figure 3-33. Extensive vitiligo in a African-American woman. (From Fitzpatrick JE, Aeling JE: Dermatology Secrets. Philadelphia, Hanley & Belfus, 1996.)

121. **What are the other associated cutaneous findings?**
Prematurely gray hair, piebaldism (*see* question 122), halo nevi, alopecia areata, and ocular abnormalities, such as chorioretinitis, retinal pigmentary abnormalities, and iritis. The scalp is the hair most frequently involved, followed by eyebrows, pubis, and axillae. Vitiligo of the scalp usually presents as a localized patch of white or gray hair, but total scalp depigmentation (*leukotrichia*) may also occur, usually indicating low likelihood of repigmentation.

122. **What is piebaldism?**
A rare autosomal dominant disease of melanocyte development, characterized by a focal lack of melanocytes resulting in a congenital white forelock and multiple symmetric hypopigmented or depigmented macules. From the old English *piebald*, spotted, this phenomenon was first described by Roman, Greek, and Egyptian writers. In time, the presence of a stable white forelock in families even led to the creation of telltale surnames, such as Whitlock, Horlick, and Blaylock.

123. **What are the characteristics of piebaldism?**
Eighty to ninety percent of individuals have a white forelock, typically from birth. The central frontal scalp can also be permanently white, as may be eyebrow and eyelash hair. Finally, white spots may occur on the face, trunk, and extremities. Piebaldism is one of the cutaneous signs of *Waardenburg's syndrome*, along with heterochromia of irides, lateral displacement of inner canthi, and deafness (*see* Chapter 4, questions 106 and 107).

124. **When does vitiligo appear?**
At any age, although most frequently in the first two decades of life. It affects 1–2% of the U.S. population and is considered autoimmune, a mechanism corroborated by its association with other autoimmune disorders. People of color are affected more frequently, but are also more apt to seek treatment because of the greater cosmetic impact. Male-to-female ratio is equal. One third of patients report another affected family member, suggesting a genetic component.

125. **What is the typical course of vitiligo?**
Unpredictable, but generally characterized by slow progression, which may be interrupted by periods of stability. Spontaneous repigmentation also may occur, but generally is incomplete.

126. **What are the other clinical presentations of vitiligo?**
   - **Segmental vitiligo:** Characterized by unilateral depigmented macules and patches in a dermatomal or quasi-dermatomal distribution. It generally has a stable course.
   - **Focal vitiligo:** One or more pale macules in an area that is single but not segmental
   - **Universal vitiligo:** It results in total or nearly total body involvement.

127. **How is vitiligo diagnosed?**
Clinically. In patients with fair skin, the lack of contrast between normal and diseased areas may make the identification of lesions more difficult, so that a Wood's lamp becomes necessary. A biopsy will demonstrate no melanocytes, but their presence does not exclude the diagnosis.

128. **What systemic diseases are associated with vitiligo?**
At least 10% of patients have serologic or clinical evidence of autoimmune disorders, the most common being thyroid diseases, especially hypothyroidism of the Hashimoto variety. Diabetes, Addison's, pernicious anemia, alopecia areata, and uveitis (Vogt-Koyanagi syndrome) are also frequent. A careful history and appropriate screening are therefore necessary. Still, treatment of concomitant diseases does not influence the course of vitiligo.

Tinea Versicolor

129. What is tinea versicolor (TV)?
A common, benign, and superficial fungal infection, characterized by hypo/hyperpigmented macules, patches, and thin plaques, widely covering chest and back. The cause is *Malassezia furfur,* part of the normal skin flora (present in 20% of infants and close to 100% of adults). In situations of predisposition (genetics, immunosuppression, malnutrition, Cushing's disease, and warm/humid environments—hence its predilection for Western Samoa and relative rarity in Scandinavia), the saprophytic yeast undergoes conversion to the parasitic and mycelial form, thus infecting the stratum corneum of the epidermis and thereby causing clinical disease. TV is not contagious, but in predisposed individuals may chronically recur. It is most common in the first and second decades, when the sebaceous glands are more active. Conversely, it is rare before puberty or after age 65.

130. How does TV look?
As the name implies (*versicolor* means multicolor), the condition is characterized by numerous, well-marginated, finely scaly, oval-to-round macules over the trunk and/or chest. These range in color from white to red to brown, and can be pruritic. They eventually coalesce, forming irregular patches of discoloration. The diagnosis is usually confirmed by potassium hydroxide (KOH) examination of scales. This demonstrates both the cigar-butt mycelial *hyphae* and the round thick-walled *spores*, in a pattern often referred to as "spaghetti and meatballs," or "bacon and eggs." Note that TV is more noticeable during the summer, since lesions cannot tan, thus making the discrepancy with surrounding skin even more apparent.

131. How does TV present in immunocompromised hosts?
As an inverse form, affecting not the trunk, but the face, extremities, and flexural regions. Cell-mediated immunity plays a pathogenetic role, since lymphocyte function is impaired in TV.

SOLID LESIONS: BROWN

Tinea Versicolor (previously discussed)

Acanthosis Nigricans

132. What is acanthosis nigricans (AN)?
A condition characterized by brown-to-black, poorly defined, velvety plaques that may occur anywhere, although typically on the intertriginous areas of axilla and groin. The umbilicus is also a preferred site, as are the posterior and lateral folds of the neck, especially in children. In hyperandrogenic and obese females, the vulva is the most commonly involved area. Lesions are often associated with skin tags (acrochordons) and may even occur on mucous membranes—such as the oral cavity, esophagus, and nasal/laryngeal mucosa. Nipple areolas are another common target.

133. What are the *causes* of AN?
The most common are factors that stimulate epidermal keratinocyte and dermal fibroblast proliferation. In benign AN, these may be either insulin or an insulin-like growth substance; in the *malignant* form, they are instead neoplastic products. Overall, AN can occur with:

- **Obesity and insulin resistance:** Lesions are weight dependent and may completely regress with slimming.
- **Congenital syndromes:** Typical of young women with type A or type B syndromes. The type A is also referred to as HAIR-AN syndrome (*H*yper*A*ndrogenemia, *I*nsulin *R*esistance, and AN syndrome). It affects primarily young African-American women, with polycystic

ovaries, high testosterone levels, and signs of virilization (hirsutism and clitoral hypertrophy). The type B syndrome occurs instead in women with uncontrolled diabetes, ovarian hyperandrogenism, or an autoimmune disease (such as systemic lupus erythematosus [SLE], scleroderma, Sjögren's syndrome, or Hashimoto thyroiditis). Anti-insulin receptor antibodies are often present.
- **Drug reaction:** Due to nicotinic acid, insulin, pituitary extract, systemic corticosteroids, and diethylstilbestrol
- **Internal malignancy**

134. **How common is acanthosis nigricans associated with malignancy? How does it present?**
It comprises one fifth of all cases, usually due to an aggressive underlying neoplasm—a GI adenocarcinoma in 90% of cases and a gastric in 60%. AN often develops concurrently with the tumor, although it may predate the tumor (by up to 15 years) or follow it. In 25–50% of patients, AN presents as *oral* lesions (mostly tongue and lips), which are seldom pigmented. Indistinguishable from the benign form, malignant AN is usually *not* associated with obesity. Instead, its skin lesions are more extensive, more rapidly spreading, atypical in location (palms, soles, and mucosae), and often symptomatic. Regression and progression follow the course of the underlying tumor.

Melanocytic Nevi (Common, Atypical, Dysplastic)

135. **What are melanocytic nevi?**
Benign neoplasms composed almost exclusively of melanocytes. These are so common to be considered a normal part of the skin, such as cherry angiomata or seborrheic keratoses. They typically form during early childhood, usually in response to sun exposure. In fact, early use of broad-spectrum sunscreens can effectively reduce their development. Nevi often appear after blistering events, such as sunburns or second-degree thermal burns, suggesting once again their actinic etiology. Incidence of acquired melanocytic nevi increases in number throughout childhood and early adulthood, peaking during the fourth to fifth decade of life, with significant reduction in later years. In fact, acquired melanocytic nevi have been said to be absent at birth and at *death*, reflecting their slow involution with age.

136. **What about *congenital* nevi?**
They are nevi that are present at birth or soon thereafter. They are probably hamartomas, since they contain many skin elements, but a predominance of melanocytes. Large congenital nevi have a low (5%) but real risk for malignant transformation into melanoma. Hence, the need for prophylactic excision. In a rare autosomal dominant condition, family members acquire with time many large nevi, sometimes more than 100 (*see* FAMMM, discussed in question 141).

137. **List and describe the different types of common nevi (moles).**
Melanocytic nevi are classified according to histology:
- **Junctional nevus:** Usually a macule or thinly raised papule with well-circumscribed borders and homogeneous brown to black pigment. Cells are located in the *dermoepidermal junction*.
- **Compound nevus:** A *raised* papule, brown or tan and often lighter than a junctional nevus. Pigmentation and border are even, and cells are at the *dermoepidermal junction/upper dermis*.
- **(Intra-) Dermal nevus:** Also a papule, usually dome-shaped, pedunculated or warty-surfaced. Cells are in the *dermis*. Color is brown or even flesh-like, since melanin is often lacking.

138. What are the features of a melanocytic nevus?
The most important is *stability*—in size, height, color, and outline. Also, lack of symptoms (i.e., not itchy, painful, irritated, or bleeding), even color (usually tan to brown), and small size (<1 cm).

139. What are *atypical or dysplastic nevi* (Clark nevi)?

They are acquired variants typical of families of northern European descent, with fair skin, light-colored hair, freckles, and other Celtic features. The United Kingdom, Netherlands, Germany, and occasionally Poland and Russia are the most affected countries. Patients present with hundreds of relatively broad lesions that are flat or thinly papular. The more numerous the nevi, the greater the likelihood of melanoma (*see* discussion on familial atypical multiple mole and melanoma in question 141). Still, dysplastic nevi are just a marker for risk, and not necessarily a precursor. Hence, removal of *all* dysplastic nevi may not really alter the risk.

140. Describe the characteristics of dysplastic nevi.
They are larger than common moles (5–15 mm in diameter) and often *variegated* (tan to dark brown to pink). They occur in both sun-exposed *and* sun-protected areas, more commonly the back, chest, buttocks, breasts, and scalp. Since they grow through lateral extension, they often assume the configuration of a fried egg, with a central papule and a surrounding macular area of differing pigmentation. Due to their lateral extension, they have notched and poorly defined rims.

141. What is FAMMM?
It is the *familial atypical multiple mole and melanoma* (FAMMM) syndrome (also known as dysplastic nevus syndrome), in which family members develop >100 melanocytic nevi, which is far more than the average number of common nevi (15–20). Lifetime risk for melanoma is high. In fact, close to 100% for individuals with >100 lesions and more than two family members with melanoma history.

Seborrheic Keratoses

142. What are seborrheic keratoses?

The most common benign tumors of old age, present in as many as 90% of people older than 65 and increasing in number with age. They have a variety of appearances and pigmentation and are due to proliferation of epidermal cells. Although entirely benign, they can be cosmetically unappealing and often provide a daily reminder of the annoying effects of aging. In fact, they are often referred to as *benign senile verrucae*, or *senile warts*. They also can grow, itch, become irritated, and even infected, especially from scratching or other mechanical irritation.

143. Describe the morphology of seborrheic keratoses (SK).
Lesions are round to oval, pigmented, initially flat, but subsequently raised and with a velvety to finely verrucous surface. Margins are sharp (as if stuck on normal skin) and have a soft and greasy look. Usually <1 cm at onset, they grow thicker and larger with time, while new lesions continue to appear. Often aligned in the direction of skin folds, they can have keratotic plugging on the surface. Although more common in sun-exposed areas (and often arising from *solar lentigines*), they may occur anywhere, except for the palms, soles, and mucous membranes.

144. What is *dermatosis papulosa nigra*?
An SK variant, with earlier onset than the ordinary form. It affects the upper cheeks and lateral orbits of dark-skinned individuals, with small, multiple, pedunculated, and heavily pigmented lesions.

Signs of Leser–Trélat

145. What is the sign of Leser-Trélat?
An important paraneoplastic syndrome characterized by the explosive blooming of hundreds and hundreds of seborrheic keratoses—on chest, back, and face. First described by the German Edmund Leser (1828–1916) and the French Ulysse Trélat (1828–1890), it is most commonly due to an *adenocarcinoma*, especially of the GI tract. Yet, an eruption of seborrheic keratoses may also develop after an inflammatory dermatosis, such as a severe sunburn or eczema.

Melanoma

146. Summarize the risk of developing melanoma.
Increasing, with Australia and New Zealand leading the way (37.7 cases/100,000 men and 29.4 in 100,000 women). In American whites, incidence has more than tripled in just two decades, with a prevalence of 6.4 cases/100,000 men and 11.7/100,000 women. In fact, the U.S. lifetime risk for melanoma has increased 2000% since 1930 (from 1/1500 to 1/65). If noninvasive melanoma *in situ* is included, the risk is now 1/37 Americans. Hence, the need for prompt diagnosis, since unlike basal and squamous cell carcinomas, melanomas are very aggressive. They cause six of seven skin cancer deaths. In fact, one American dies each hour from metastatic melanoma.

147. Who gets melanomas?
Light-skinned individuals with (1) excessive childhood sun exposure and blistering sunburns, (2) numerous or atypical nevi, and/or (3) a family history of the disease. Hence, do regular and thorough skin exams, since these may detect lesions at an earlier and thinner stage. Median age of onset for *superficial spreading melanoma* (by far the most common type) is 44, but melanomas are also the most common reported cancers in whites during the second and third decades.

148. What are the morphologic warning signs of melanoma?
As always, start with history. Since half of all melanomas are initially discovered by the patient, inquire about new moles or preexisting ones that have recently changed size, color, shape, or sensation. Note that melanomas often develop in melanocytic nevi, but half arise de novo. Tenderness, pain, itching, and bleeding suggest instead more invasive lesions. Ask about personal or family history of melanoma, tendency to burn, and prior sunburns. On physical exam, rely on (1) the ABCD(E) checklist, and (2) the revised Glasgow 7-point checklist.

149. What is *the ABCD(E) checklist*?
A commonly used acronym for identifying the warning signs of malignant melanoma. Developed in 1985, it considers a lesion suspicious when it has more than one of the five following features (*see* Fig. 3-34):
- **A** = **A**symmetry (if the lesion is bisected, one half is not identical to the other half)
- **B** = **B**order irregularity (a border that is uneven or ragged as opposed to smooth and straight)
- **C** = **C**olor variegation (more than one shade of pigment)
- **D** = **D**iameter increase (defined as a diameter greater than 6 mm)
- A suggested addition to this list is a final **E**, for **E**levation above the skin surface; however, since elevation is also a feature of many benign nevi, E is often excluded.

150. How good is the ABCD(E) checklist?
Two studies have assessed its accuracy. The first found a 92% sensitivity for lesions with >1/5 diagnostic features. The second evaluated instead the accuracy of only the BCD items, and found 100% sensitivity and 98% specificity for lesions with *all three features*. Still, the major

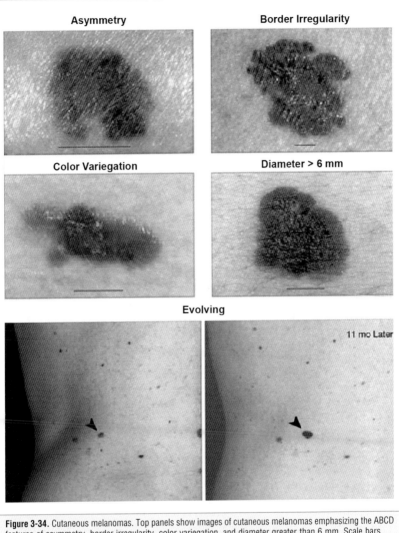

Figure 3-34. Cutaneous melanomas. Top panels show images of cutaneous melanomas emphasizing the ABCD features of asymmetry, border irregularity, color variegation, and diameter greater than 6 mm. Scale bars represent approximately 5 mm. Bottom panels show the back of a male patient with numerous moles, demonstrating evolution of one mole into melanoma over an 11-month period. Note the increased diameter and darkening of the lesion in the right panel compared with the left panel. (From Abbasi NR, Shaw HM, Rigel DS, et al: Early diagnosis of cutaneous melanoma: Revisiting the ABCD criteria. JAMA. 292[22]:2771—2776, 2004, with permission.).

problem is D, since some melanomas are <6 mm. Because D considerably lowers the checklist's sensitivity, some authors have suggested dropping it altogether. Yet, available data argue against this approach and propose instead changing the "E" from "Elevation" and "Enlargement" to "Evolving" because significant elevation is not apparent in most early melanomas, and thus not a good warning sign of early disease; enlargement can be inaccurate, too, since it focuses primarily on change in *size* and not, for example, in *color*, which can be very important in the progress of the disease. Evolving, on the other hand, would include not only evolution (i.e., change of any kind, color included), but also elevation and enlargement. It also supports the observation that 89–95% of 100 consecutively accrued melanomas demonstrate changes in these features, and 100% show changes in at least one feature. Hence, beware of evolving nevi that change size, shape, surface (especially bleeding), symptoms (itching, tenderness), or shades of color. Also, beware of new pigmented lesions.

151. **How capable are physicians of recognizing melanomas?**
It depends. Overall, ability to detect melanomas has a 50–97% sensitivity and 96–99% specificity. Dermatologists' examinations are more sensitive, both in real patients and images of lesions. Nondermatologists provide the correct diagnosis significantly less frequently than dermatologists (60% versus 74% of the time). Early detection through history and physical exam is crucial, since thickness of the tumor at excision is the primary prognostic determinant.

152. **What is the Revised Glasgow 7-Point Checklist?**
A British-developed diagnostic aid that relies on four major and three minor criteria. It also relies heavily on the concept of evolution (i.e., change). In fact, the three major criteria are historical (change in size, shape, and color), while the four minor are instead physical and often late-appearing: (1) inflammation, (2) crusting or bleeding, (3) sensory change, and (4) diameter >7 mm. A scoring system assigns two points for each major criterion and one for each minor. Patients with >1 major criterion should be referred to a dermatologist. Patients with scores >3 should be referred, too.

153. **How good is the 7-point checklist?**
Several studies have found sensitivity of 79–100% and specificity of 30–37%.

> **Pearl:**
> Both the ABCD checklist (especially when positivity does not require the presence of all four features) and the 7-point checklist are very sensitive tools that lack, however, specificity.

154. **How should the physical exam be conducted?**
As thoroughly as possible: head to toe in a well-lit room. Always include scalp, oral mucosa, genital area, nails, and interdigital skin of hands and feet. Complete cutaneous examinations are 6.4 times more likely to detect a melanoma than only partial examinations. In cases of multiple nevi, pay special attention to those with unusual features. Remember that melanomas may also arise from the skin, eyes, ears, GI tract, leptomeninges, and orogenital mucosae.

155. **What are the major clinical-histopathologic types of melanoma?**
They are five, and all first growing radially (often for months and years) before eventually going deep. Only nodular melanoma grows vertically right away. Hence, it lacks the typical ABCDE warning signs and presents instead with elevation and/or ulceration/bleeding.
- **Superficial spreading melanoma:** The most common subtype (>70% of cases) and the one most frequently found near existing nevi. Onset is during the third to fifth decade, usually over the back of men, legs of women, and trunk of both genders. Lesions are flat or slightly raised, brown, variegated (with black, blue, pink, or white discoloration), >6 mm in diameter, and with irregular borders.
- **Nodular melanoma:** 15–30% of all melanomas. It presents as a papule or dome-shaped nodule, on legs and trunk, and black or brown-to-bluish in color, even though it may also be amelanotic. It often grows rapidly over just a few months, often with ulceration and bleeding, especially after minor trauma. It originates at the dermoepidermal junction, growing vertically into the dermis with little radial extension.

- **Lentigo maligna:** An *in situ* (i.e., intraepithelial) precursor of *lentigo maligna melanoma*. This presents as a flat and relatively large (>3 cm) hyperpigmented area with variegated pigment and an irregular border, commonly located on sun-exposed areas, especially head, neck, and arms. Late occurring (fifth and sixth decades), it exists for 10–15 years before undergoing malignant transformation. This is nonetheless rare (estimated 5–8%) and usually heralded by new brown-to-black macular pigmentation or raised blue-black nodules. Growth is *radial*. Often called *Hutchinson's freckle* from the English surgeon who also described the Hutchinson's triad of congenital syphilis.
- **Lentigo maligna melanoma:** 4–15% of all melanomas. Almost exclusive of sun-damaged areas of the elderly. Large in size (>3 cm), it typically grows slowly over a period of many years. More variegated in color than lentigo maligna.
- **Acrolentiginous melanoma:** The rarest in whites (2–8%), but the most common in dark-skinned groups (African Americans, Asians, and Hispanics), in whom it accounts for 29–72% of all melanomas. Because of delayed diagnosis, it carries a worse outcome. It occurs on palms, soles, or beneath the nail plate, presenting as one or more dark papules against a pigmented and unevenly speckled background—often resembling *lentigo maligna melanoma*. The subungual variety may occur as diffuse nail discoloration, or a longitudinal pigmented band within the nail plate. A hallmark finding is pigment spreading to proximal or lateral nail folds (*Hutchinson's sign*).

156. **What is the major prognostic indicator of stage I melanoma?**
The histologic level of the lesion. The thinner and higher in the skin, the better. Patients with lesions <0.75 mm in thickness have 98% 5-year survival, whereas those with lesions >4 mm have survival rates <50%. Overall, lesions >1.0 mm have a more ominous outcome. Other factors associated with a worse prognosis are vertical growth phase, high mitotic rate, involvement of blood vessels, presence of microscopic satellites, and ulceration with decreased lymphoid infiltrates. The best outcome is in young women with lesions on the extremity rather than the trunk or head.

Signs of Sun Damage

157. **What are the characteristic signs of sun damage?**
- **Solar lentigo (lentigines):** From the Latin *lentigo* (*lentil*), these are sun-induced, well-circumscribed, light brown or tan macules that resemble a freckle, except for regular border, microscopic proliferation of the rete ridges, and persistence even after the tan or sunburn fades. Typically on sun-exposed areas of the face, hands, and shoulders, they range in size between 5–20 mm. They have no potential for neoplastic degeneration, and yet a lentigo with black, pinhead-sized speckles (*lentigo maligna*) may degenerate over years into *lentigo maligna melanoma*.
- **Freckles:** From the Old English *freken* (ephelis), these are yellowish/brownish sun-induced macules on exposed areas, typical of light-complexioned individuals with red or blond hair. Lesions increase in number after exposure to the sun. The epidermis is microscopically normal, except for increased melanin. A freckle resembles a solar lentigo, except that (1) it appears early in life (lentigines do not occur until mid-adulthood); (2) it is usually smaller (only 1–2 mm in diameter); and (3) it may disappear with time. It has no malignant potential. Still, clustered freckles (especially over lips and fingertips) should raise the possibility of Peutz-Jeghers (*see* Chapter 6, question 74).
- **Rhytides:** From the Greek for *wrinkles*, these are the familiar skin changes of sun-exposed individuals, such as farmers, fishermen, and ski instructors who do not believe in sunscreen.
- **Evidence of sun-induced cellular atypia:** This includes actinic keratosis and squamous or basal cell carcinoma. Of course, a melanoma is the deadliest of all sun-damage effects.

SOLID LESIONS: YELLOW

158. What are the most common yellow lesions of the skin?
Cutaneous xanthomas and necrobiosis lipoidica (*see* also questions 258 and 259).

159. What are xanthomas?
Lesions caused by accumulation of lipid-laden macrophages, usually because of primary (familial, congenital) or secondary dyslipidemia. Secondary *hypercholesterolemia*, for example, can occur in pregnancy, hypothyroidism, cholestasis, and acute intermittent porphyria. Secondary *hypertriglyceridemia* is instead associated with diabetes, alcoholism, pancreatitis, gout, and oral contraceptives. Combined disorders occur in nephrosis, chronic renal failure, and steroid therapy.

160. What is the significance of cutaeous xanthomas?
Other than being a cosmetic nuisance, they suggest *dysmetabolism*. They also may precede a diagnosis of hyperlipidemia, although this is often known through atherosclerosis or pancreatitis.

161. How do xanthomas present?
The hyperlipidemic xanthomas present as *xanthelasmas* or *true xanthomas* (tuberous, tendinous, eruptive, plane, and generalized plane). The normolipemic xanthomas are instead more *disseminated* or *verruciform*.

162. What is *xanthelasma palpebrarum*?
The most common cutaneous xanthoma, often presenting in the absence of xanthomas anywhere else, even though histologically identical. In contrast to true xanthomas (that can occur at any age), xanthelasmas usually affect older subjects (>40) and women twice as often as men. From the Greek *xanthos* (yellow) and *elasma* (beaten metal plate), they present as soft, yellow, velvety, and sharply marginated plaques that eventually grow into papules and may even coalesce into larger lesions. Typical of the inner canthus of the eyelids (*upper* more than lower), they are often bilateral and symmetric, flat-topped, and totally asymptomatic. They are associated with hyperlipidemia in 50% of cases, usually one of the primary types (II or IV mostly), but occasionally a secondary, too.

163. What are *tuberous* xanthomas?
They are firm, painless, and red-yellow *nodules* that classically develop in pressure areas, such as the buttocks and the extensor surfaces of knees and elbows. They also may occur in the eyelids and yet not be xanthelasmas since nodular in type. Lesions come in many sizes but often coalesce to form large and multilobated tumors. Tuberous xanthomas are associated with hypercholesterolemia and increased low-density lipoprotein (LDL) levels, either primary or secondary.

164. What are *tendinous* xanthomas?
Slowly enlarging subcutaneous *nodules* that are typically present over tendons (Achilles) and other extensor surfaces of feet and hands. Often related to trauma, they occur in patients with severe hypercholesterolemia and high LDL, either primary or secondary.

165. What are *eruptive* xanthomas?
Small and red-yellow papules on an erythematous base, typically erupting in crops over the buttocks, shoulders, and extensor surfaces of extremities (more rarely over the face or oral mucosa) (Fig. 3-35). Often pruritic and tender, they usually resolve spontaneously in a few weeks. Eruptive xanthomas are associated with hypertriglyceridemia, particularly types I, IV,

and V (high very low-density lipoprotein [VLDL] level and chylomicrons), yet they also may occur in *secondary* hyperlipidemias, especially if related to diabetes.

166. **What are plane xanthomas?**
Macular lesions, only rarely raised, and occurring anywhere in the skin, including the face, neck, thorax, and flexures. *Generalized* plane xanthomas can cover very large areas. They may occur in secondary hyperlipidemias (especially cholestasis), whereas in type III dysbetalipoproteinemia, they typically involve the palmar creases. They also can coexist with monoclonal gammopathy.

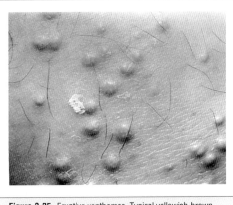

Figure 3-35. Eruptive xanthomas. Typical yellowish-brown papules. White material was applied by the patient to remove these "warts." (From Fitzpatrick JE, Aeling JE: Dermatology Secrets. Philadelphia, Hanley & Belfus, 1996.)

167. **What is *xanthoma disseminatum and verruciform*?**
Two forms of xanthomas that can occur in normolipemic adults, usually as a reaction to local stimuli. The course is benign, often with spontaneous resolution—especially the *disseminatum* form, which presents as red-yellow papules and nodules over flexures. The *verruciform* form instead involves the oral cavity, presenting as a single papillomatous yellow lesion, often requiring excision.

SOLID LESIONS· RED OR PURPLE—TABLE 3-4

Scaling Diseases *Without* Epithelial Disruption

Psoriasis

168. **What is psoriasis?**
A common, chronic, and genetically determined inflammatory disease of the skin, characterized by rounded and erythematous scaling patches. Probably due to accelerated epidermopoiesis.

169. **What is the cause of psoriasis? Who gets it?**
There is a strong but still undefined genetic influence, particularly in cases with earlier onset. Gender ratios are equal, and overall prevalence is 1–2% in the United States. Although it may appear at any time, the peak of onset is the third decade, with a much smaller group developing it in their 60s.

170. **What are the clinical features of psoriasis?**
Classic *psoriasis vulgaris* (from the Greek *psoriasis*, itchy—which indeed these lesions are) presents as sharply demarcated, circular to oval erythematous papules and plaques of varying size. These are often covered by a white *scale* due to epidermal hyperproliferation and dermal inflammation. Scales may be thick and "mica-like" (*micaceous*) because of a silvery white

TABLE 3-4. RED/PURPLE LESIONS (1)

Red-Purple Lesions

A. Scaling

Without Epithelial Disruption		With Epithelial Disruption	
Papulo-Squamous Diseases		*Eczematous Diseases*	
Prominent Plaque Formation	*Predominantly Papular*	*With Prominent Excoriation*	*Without Excoriation*
• Psoriasis	• Pityriasis rosea	• Atopic dermatitis	• Seborrheic dermatitis
• Dermatophytoses	• Secondary syphylis	• Stasis dermatitis	• Contact dermatitis
• Lupus erythematosus		• Lichen simplex chronicus	
		• Lichen simplex chronicus	

look. Their removal typically causes tiny bleeding droplets (*Auspitz sign*). Associated pitting and dystrophy of the nails are also quite common. Sites of predilection include the scalp, elbows, knees, genitalia, lumbosacral region, and extensor surfaces of the extremities. Degree of involvement is variable.

171. **What are other characteristics of psoriatic lesions?**
Newly developed lesions tend to be small (1–3 mm) but easily coalescing, resulting in large plaques with often a gyrate pattern. Note that psoriasis, lichen planus, vitiligo, and warts are the only skin diseases characterized by the Koebner's phenomenon, in which lesions appear 7–14 days after skin trauma (scratching, for example). Koebner's occurs in 40–80% of *plaque psoriasis* cases.

172. **Who was Koebner?**
Heinrich Koebner (1838–1904) was a German dermatologist with a penchant for melodrama. This included self-inoculation with various kinds of skin infections so that he could demonstrate typical lesions during lectures—all because PowerPoint had not been invented yet.

173. **What is the typical clinical course of psoriasis?**
One of variable extent and duration, even though usually as a lifelong disease. Spontaneous remissions occur with unpredictable frequency, and patients may move from one clinical form to another. Acute flares may evolve into more severe disease, such as pustular or erythrodermic (*see* question 174).

174. **What are the other clinical presentations of psoriasis?**
Psoriasis is a heterogeneous disorder with a spectrum of clinical variants:
- **Intertriginous** (axillary, inframammary, inguinal, perianal): Lack of maceration prevents scales.
- **Guttate:** Sudden explosion of hundreds of small, erythematous, and nonconfluent papules, widely distributed and not very scaly. Palms and soles are rarely affected, and nail changes like pits, ridges, and the oil-drop sign (typical of chronic psoriasis) may be absent. Guttate psoriasis often occurs in young adults and children and may be triggered by a streptococcal infection, as well as by a viral upper respiratory infection. In fact, all psoriatic

forms can be exacerbated by infections, especially upper respiratory infections (URIs) by *Streptococcus* and *Staphylococcus.*
- **Erythrodermic:** Total body erythema with scaling, possibly hypothermia and heart failure
- **Pustular:** The most serious form, presenting in a generalized and systemic fashion, with fever anemia, leukocytosis, erythema, and overlying pustules (Von Zumbusch type). A more localized form involves instead the palms and soles, with no systemic symptoms (Barber type).

175. How Is psoriasis diagnosed?
Appearance usually suffices. Distribution of lesions (scalp, elbows, knees, and gluteal folds), Koebner's phenomenon, and nail pitting are also classic clues. A skin biopsy may help in more perplexing cases and typically shows acanthosis, parakeratosis, neutrophils in the stratum corneum, and a lymphohistiocytic infiltrate in the papillary dermis.

176. What other disease is often associated with psoriasis?
Psoriatic *arthritis*, in one tenth of cases. When this precedes skin involvement, you must do a complete exam, especially of scalp, genitalia (looking for hidden plaques), and nails.

Dermatophytes

177. What are dermatophytoses?
From the Greek *dermato* (skin) and *phyton* (plant), they are cutaneous fungal infections caused by dermatophytes (ringworm). Their hallmark is invasion of dead keratin—in the skin, hair, or nails.

178. What is tinea?
Tinea (from medieval Latin, *a gnawing worm*) originally indicated larvae of insects that fed on clothes and books. Subsequently, it came to indicate parasitic infestation of the skin. By the mid-16th century, the term was used to describe diseases of the hairy scalp, with the term *ringworm* indicating instead those skin diseases that assumed a ring form, including tinea per se. Only in 1880, through the work of Sabouraud, was the agent of *tinea capitis* infection demonstrated, and it became clear that the disease was due to a class of fungi, the dermatophytes.

179. How are dermatophytoses classified?
By the body region involved (Table 3-5). Note that fungal involvement can affect multiple sites. Hence, if you see lesions on the buttocks, always ask, "Can I see your feet?" Almost invariably there will be typical fungal lesions in the fourth web space.

180. What are the clinical features of dermatophyte infections?
The main symptom is *pruritus*. On exam, areas affected tend to be those with humid or moist skin, which provides a favorable environment for fungal growth. Different types of tinea may present with different findings, especially based on area involved. Still, the primary lesions remain the same: pruritic, erythematous, and scaly plaques, with active border and central clearing. Papules, vesicles, and bullae may occur too.

181. What is the frequency of dermatophytoses?
It depends. *Tinea corporis* occurs in any age group. *Tinea cruris* and *pedis* predominantly affect the adult population, particularly individuals using communal showers or pools. *Tinea pedis* is the most common dermatophytosis worldwide (10% of the U.S. population). *Onychomycosis* is quite common, too, with prevalence in adult American males of approximately 3% and incidence that increases steadily with age. Conversely, *tinea capitis* is usually a disease of children.

TABLE 3-5. CLASSIFICATION OF DERMATOPHYTOSES BY BODY REGION		
Disease	Location	Clinical Presentation
Tinea capitis	Scalp	Infection of scalp hair. It causes erythematous patches of alopecia and scaling, with broken hair. *Kerion celsi*, an inflammatory variant, produces tender abscesses with purulent drainage that may result int scarring alopecia. *Favus* (also termed tinea favosa) is severe tinea capitis with yellow, cup-shaped crusts around infected hair follicles.
Tinea corporis	Body	Infection of exposed areas of trunk and extremities. Characterized by circular lesions with central clearing and erythematous/raised edges (ringworm) eventually evolving into annular scaly plaques. May also present with pustules and vesicles.
Tinea faciale	Face	Red scaly plaques sometimes lacking central clearing and elevated border.
Tinea barbae	Beard	Infection of beard and neck area, characterized by erythema, scaling, and pustules.
Tinea cruris (jock itch)	Groin	Infection of groin and pubic region. Causes plaques with central clearing and raised scaly border. On inguinal fold and adjacent skin, but not scrotum.
Tinea manus	Hand	Infection of palms and finger webs, usually in association with tinea pedis. Lesions consist of annular plaques on the dorsum of hand, with hyperkeratosis of palms. Scaling and erythema may also be present. Affects only one hand (but often *two* feet).
Tinea pedis	Feet	Infection of interdigital webs, usually third and fourth. Presents with erythema, scaling, fissuring, and maceration (athlete's foot). Hyperkeratosis and scaling may extend to the sole's instep. Variations include bilateral moccasin distribution (scaling of soles and lateral surfaces) or vesicopustules on the instep. Onychomycosis may also occur, and is often the portal of entry for other tinea lesions.
Tinea unguium (onychomycosis)	Nail	Yellow-brown discoloration of nail plate associated with subungual hyperkeratosis.

182. **How are dermatophytoses diagnosed?**

By microscopic examination. This relies on the presence of septate hyphae on potassium hydroxide (KOH) preparation of lesion scrapings or nail clippings (conversely, examination of hairs from scalp infection typically demonstrates spores involving the hair shaft). As a general rule, "if it scales, you should scrape it" (and then do a KOH on it). This rule applies to *all* scales, independent of location. If the KOH exam is negative, a culture should be obtained on Sabouraud's dextrose agar with antibiotics.

Lupus Erythematosus (*see* later)

Pityriasis Rosea (PR)

183. **What is pityriasis rosea?**
A benign and noncontagious papulosquamous disease that may resemble secondary syphilis. First described by Camille Melchior Gibert in 1860.

184. **Who gets it?**
Any age group, although usually 10- to 35-year-olds—women twice more frequently than men.

185. **What are the clinical features of pityriasis rosea?**
From the Greek *pityron* (bran, dandruff) and *rosea* (pink), PR presents half of the time with a solitary 2–3 cm macule that heralds the eruption (the *herald patch*). This is a round or oval lesion, salmon colored (rosea), and usually located on the trunk. Over a few days it enlarges into a larger patch (up to 10cm), with a collarette of fine scale (pityron) just inside a well-demarcated border. Because of its annular shape, the lesion may be mistaken for tinea corporis, hence, the frequent need for a KOH preparation. The herald patch is followed in 1–2 weeks by a *diffuse eruption* on the trunk, neck, and inner aspects of the proximal extremities. During this phase (which also lasts 2 weeks), 50–100 isolated, small (0.5–1.5 cm), bilateral, and symmetric *macules* may appear. Lesions are nonconfluent and similar in morphology to the herald patch (i.e., oval or football shaped), although with much less (if any) scaling. They typically have their long axis along the lines of cleavage of the skin, parallel to the rib lines, thus forming a *Christmas tree* pattern. Mild to moderate pruritus occurs in 75% of patients, and photosensitivity also may be present. Oral involvement is uncommon (<10% of cases), as it is lymphadenopathy. Hence, its difference with syphilis. The eruption eventually resolves completely over 6 weeks, but may range 2–10 weeks.

186. **What is the typical clinical course of pityriasis rosea?**
Benign. The rash generally resolves without sequelae or recurrence. Yet, in dark-skinned individuals there may be a residual postinflammatory hyperpigmentation.

187. **What are the causes of pityriasis rosea?**
Although no agent has been isolated, some data suggest it might be a viral exanthema, possibly due to an upper respiratory infection:
- It tends to cluster in families and close contacts.
- It is more common in stressed or immunocompromised patients.
- A single outbreak provides lifelong immunity.
- Increased amounts of cutaneous CD4 T cells suggest viral processing.

188. **How is pityriasis rosea diagnosed?**
By clinical observation of the rash characteristics:
- Herald patch
- Oval shape of lesions
- Typical distribution (trunk and upper but not lower extremities)
- Lesions parallel to rib lines (Christmas tree pattern)
Note that biopsy is nondiagnostic, while serology may become necessary to rule out secondary syphilis.

Secondary Syphilis (*see* later)

Scaling Diseases *With* Epithelial Disruption

Eczematous Diseases: Atopic Dermatitis

189. **What is atopic dermatitis?**

   A pruritic disease of unknown origin that starts in early infancy and is characterized by pruritus, eczematous lichenified lesions, and xerosis of the skin.

190. **What are the clinical features of atopic dermatitis?**

   The hallmark is uncontrolled scratching in response to itching, causing an itch-scratch cycle that eventually leads to the classic lesions. The *"primary"* lesion of atopic dermatitis (AD) has actually been debated, and indeed multiple skin findings may coexist:

   - Erythematous papules and plaques, which at times may be follicular
   - Vesicles, pustules, weeping, and crusting; usually due to superinfection with herpes or staphylococci
   - Chronic excoriations leading to secondary changes, such as linear erosions and lichenification (thickening and accentuation of skin markings)

   Other supporting features of AD include *involvement of skin creases* (such as fronts of ankles or neck, folds of elbows, and areas behind the knees); *history of generally dry skin* (xerosis); and *history of atopic diseases*. Visible *flexural* dermatitis (or dermatitis involving the cheeks, forehead, or outer limbs of children younger than 4 years) is also quite supportive.

191. **Describe the distribution of atopic dermatitis lesions.**

   Age-related:

   - **Infants:** Face (especially the cheeks) and extensor surfaces
   - **Children:** Hands, feet, antecubital and popliteal fossae
   - **Adults:** Flexures (including genitalia) but also the face (eyelids and forehead), neck, hands, and feet

   Generalized involvement may develop at any age (*see* Fig. 3-36).

192. **Who develops atopic dermatitis?**

   Usually children, with 85% of cases in the first year of life and 95% before age 5. Prevalence is high and rising, with 10–12% of American children and 0.9% of adults being affected. Patients often have a personal or family history of other atopic diseases, such as allergic rhinitis, asthma, hay fever, or urticaria. Associated findings include dry, lackluster skin, Hertoghe sign (lateral thinning of eyebrows), and Dennie-Morgan fold (an extra infraorbital eyelid fold).

193. **Describe the course of atopic dermatitis.**

   More severe and persistent in childhood, but eventually improving with age. Still, in 50% of patients the disease persists well into adulthood. Risk factors for persistence include a family history of atopy, early disease in childhood, and severe cutaneous lesions.

194. **What are the other clinical presentations of atopic dermatitis?**

   The most severe forms progress to *erythroderma*, which consists of generalized scaling and redness associated with fever, high-output cardiac failure, systemic infection, and heat loss. This represents a severe complication and may require hospitalization. Note that erythroderma can occur in other skin diseases, such as psoriasis, seborrheic dermatitis, and drug reactions.

195. **How is atopic dermatitis diagnosed?**

   Clinically. Major criteria include typical morphology and distribution, chronic or relapsing course, and personal or family history of atopy and pruritus. Elevated serum IgE levels and specific IgE-mediated sensitization (as measured by skin test or radioallergosorbent test

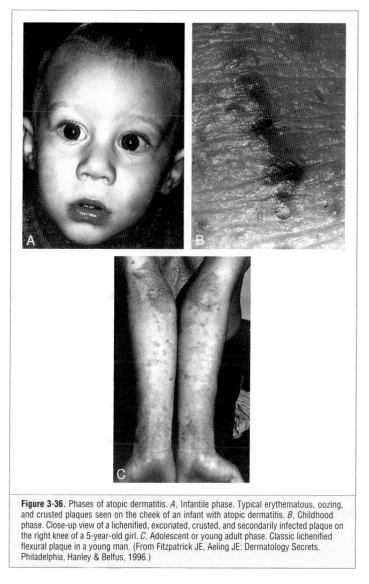

Figure 3-36. Phases of atopic dermatitis. *A,* Infantile phase. Typical erythematous, oozing, and crusted plaques seen on the cheek of an infant with atopic dermatitis. *B,* Childhood phase. Close-up view of a lichenified, excoriated, crusted, and secondarily infected plaque on the right knee of a 5-year-old girl. *C,* Adolescent or young adult phase. Classic lichenified flexural plaque in a young man. (From Fitzpatrick JE, Aeling JE: Dermatology Secrets. Philadelphia, Hanley & Belfus, 1996.)

[RAST]) also support the diagnosis. Biopsy is nondiagnostic, with varying degrees of acanthosis, spongiosis, and mixed dermal infiltrate. Note that pruritus unaccompanied by rash can occur not only in atopic dermatitis, but also in scabies, dermatitis herpetiform, pre-bullous pemphigoid, drug eruption, liver disease, renal disease, polycythemia fever, and malignancies (especially lymphoma).

196. **What other skin diseases can be associated with atopic dermatitis?**
Definitely superinfections, especially with *S. aureus* (hallmark being oozing and crusting), but also warts, molluscum contagiosum, dermatophytosis, and herpes simplex. The latter may progress to Kaposi's varicelliform eruption, a disseminated form of the disease.

Eczematous Diseases: Stasis Dermatitis

197. What is stasis dermatitis?
The earliest cutaneous sequela of venous insufficiency and a precursor of more serious manifestations, such as venous leg *ulceration*.

198. How does it present?
With erythematous, scaly, and eczematous plaques of the lower extremities, brown hyperpigmentation, and edema. An aching discomfort is often present (at times pruritic), but severe pain is rare. Diffuse red-brown discolorations representing intradermal deposits of hemosiderin (from degraded, extravasated erythrocytes) are also quite common. Lesions typically involve the medial ankle, but with time may progress to the foot and/or medial lower leg. In severe cases, an ulceration may develop. Superinfection with bacteria leads to honey-colored crusting, whereas superimposed cutaneous candidiasis causes monomorphous pustules.

199. Who develops stasis dermatitis and ulceration?
Adults older than 50 (with prevalence reaching 20% by age 70); women are more frequently affected than men. It is often preceded by a history of dependent leg edema, due to venous insufficiency or phlebitis.

200. What is the clinical course?
Chronic, with large and recalcitrant ulcers that heal with elevation and compression bandages. Dermatitis usually responds to mid-potency steroids and compression stockings.

201. How are stasis dermatitis and ulceration diagnosed?
Clinically. Still, a vascular evaluation is necessary to rule out arterial disease. Pulses are normal.

Eczematous Diseases: Seborrheic Dermatitis

202. What is seborrheic dermatitis (SD)?
A papulosquamous disorder of sebum-rich areas, such as the scalp, face, and trunk. It varies in severity from mild dandruff to exfoliative erythroderma.

203. What causes it?
Nobody knows. It has been linked to *Malassezia furfur,* immunologic abnormalities, and complement activation, with exacerbations related to stress, scratching, and changes in humidity or seasons. Very common in Parkinson's and in people with AIDS, among whom it is widespread and refractory.

204. What are the primary lesions of seborrheic dermatitis?
Erythematous papules and plaques, with greasy-appearing yellow scales and crusts (*inflammatory dandruff*). The yellow color is usually the result of serum exuding on the surface of the scale. Although lesions may occur in both hairy and nonhairy skin, the word *seborrhea* is Greek for overflow of sebum. Hence, oily and hairy areas of the head and neck are the most hit. These include the scalp, forehead, eyebrows, glabella, lash line, nasolabial folds, beard, and retroauricular skin, but also the ear canal and submentum. More severe disease may involve the central chest (midsternum), back, and intertriginous regions (umbilicus, axillae, inframammary and inguinal folds, perineum, or anogenital crease). Involvement of *intertrigines* is usually nonscaling. The scalp may be varyingly affected: from small and patchy scaling versus diffuse and adherent crusts. Blepharitis also may occur, and pruritus is common.

205. Who develops seborrheic dermatitis?
Mostly subjects with oily skin, males slightly more than females. Onset is after puberty, with peak in the fourth and seventh decades. Yet SD is also common in infants younger than 6 months old.

206. **How does SD present in babies?**
As erythematous plaques covered with greasy-appearing scales and crusts, typically involving the scalp (*cradle cap*) and intertriginous regions. Spontaneous resolution is the rule, usually by 6 months.

207. **What is the typical course of seborrheic dermatitis in adults?**
Chronic, with periods of exacerbation (winter/early spring) and remission (summer). Activity is heralded by burning, scaling, and itching, followed by lesions that present as greasy and brownish scalings over an inflamed skin. Superinfection with oozing and crusting is common.

208. **How is seborrheic dermatitis diagnosed?**
By the typical clinical appearance. Biopsy is nondiagnostic.

Nonscaling Lesions—Table 3-6

Cherry Angiomas

209. **What are cherry angiomas?**
The most common cutaneous vascular lesion. They consist of benign proliferations of dilated *venules*, presenting as tiny, dome-shaped, cherry-red papules or macules. These can be quite widespread, although they typically tend to be limited to the skin, sparing all mucous membranes. They appear during the third or fourth decade of life, increasing in frequency with age (*senile angiomas*). Lesions have a variable appearance, ranging from small red macules to large dome-topped or polypoid papules. They are bright cherry-red in color, but also may be violaceous, and, occasionally, dark brown to black. This darker hue usually indicates

TABLE 3-6. RED/PURPLE LESIONS (2)		
Red-Purple Lesions		
B. Nonscaling		
Dome-Shaped	**Flat-Topped**	**Drug Reactions**
Inflammatory Papules	*Vascular Reactions*	*Minor-to-Major*
• Cherry angiomas	A. *Nonpurpuric (Blanchable)*	• Morbilliform fine pink papules
• Pyogenic granuloma	• Toxic erythema	• Urticaria
• Insect bites	• Erythema multiforme	• Vasculitis
• Lichen planus	• Vascular reactions	• Erythema multiforme
	• Urticaria	• Stevens-Johnson
		• TEN
	• Erythema nodosum	
	B. *Purpuric (Nonblanchable)*	
	• Palpable purpura	
	• Miscellaneous petechiae and ecchymotic disease	

hemorrhage, and prompts a differential diagnosis with malignant melanoma. Most lesions occur in healthy individuals, although some reports have described unusual blooming of cherry angiomas in patients with malignancies.

Lichen Planus

210. What is lichen planus (LP)?
A flat-topped, pruritic, and papular eruption that is most likely autoimmune. In fact, it often coexists with various immune disturbances, such as ulcerative colitis, alopecia areata, dermatomyositis, vitiligo, myasthenia gravis, but also chronic active hepatitis, hepatitis C, and primary biliary cirrhosis.

211. Who gets lichen planus?
Men and women in their 40s; 10% have positive family history, suggesting genetic predisposition.

212. What is the primary lesion of lichen planus?
The *papule*. This is characterized by five Ps: *planar, purple, polygonal, pruritic,* and *papular*. LP lesions are shiny, 1–4 mm in size, flat-topped, violaceous, occasionally scaling, and invariably pruritic. Morphologically, however, they can be quite variable, and even bullous and verrucoid. LP papules typically affect the trunk (especially sacral areas) and extremities (tibial areas and flexor surfaces of the wrists). They can be discrete, but more often occur in clusters of lines or circles, usually coalescing into small 1–2 cm plaques. Wickham striae (white or gray streaks forming a reticular pattern on a violaceous background) are often present, especially on oral lesions. Indeed, lesions are called lichen planus because they are flat (*planus* in Latin) and often aggregate like lichens on a rock. LP is one of the few skin diseases with Koebner's phenomenon.

213. What other sites beside the skin may be involved?
LP can occur on mucous membranes, genitalia, nails (*see* question 38), and the scalp. The latter can progress to *atrophic cicatricial alopecia*.

214. How common are mucosal lesions?
Common. They can occur without skin involvement and may be asymptomatic or slightly burning. Usually localized on the tongue and buccal mucosa, they are often associated with Wickham striae. Ulcerated lesions tend to be *painful*, and in men may undergo malignant transformation. LP lesions also can occur on other mucosae, such as the tonsils, larynx, GI tract, and conjunctivae.

215. How about the genital lesions of LP?
In men they present as *papules on the glans*, with a typical annular configuration and associated cutaneous manifestations. Vulvar involvement ranges instead from reticulate papules to severe erosions, causing pruritus, dyspareunia, and even vulvar and urethral stenosis.

216. What is the course of lichen planus?
Characterized by an initial and localized eruption followed in a week or so by a generalized rash. This reaches maximal spread at 2–16 weeks. Lesions resolve within 6 months in 50% of patients and within 18 months in 85%. Oral LP lasts longer (5 years on average). Recurrences are rare.

VASCULAR REACTIONS

Purpura

217. What is purpura?
From the Latin *purpura* (a shellfish that yields purple dye), these are *violaceous* lesions.

218. **What are the two major types of purpura?**
Noninflammatory and inflammatory (vasculitis).

219. **What is *noninflammatory* purpura?**
It is blood extravasation into the skin or mucous membranes, nonindurated and nonpalpable. The most common is a *traumatic* bruise. Yet, noninflammatory purpuras usually reflect a *hemostatic* problem, such as (1) thrombocytopenia (most common cause of purpura) and platelet dysfunction, (2) thrombocythemia, and (3) vascular disorders (e.g., structural vessel malformation, disorders of connective tissue, small vessel vasculitis).

220. **How are noninflammatory purpuras classified?**
By size, shape, and depth. In this regard, blood extravasations can be divided into four groups:
- **Petechiae:** Superficial, pinpoint (<3 mm), red or purple, nonblanching macules. Mostly located on dependent areas, usually caused by platelet-related issues or vessel disease.
- **Ecchymoses:** Larger (>3 mm) and flat, usually due to more significant extravasation. Also known as bruises. They form an initial purple patch, eventually turning yellow and fading.
- **Vibices:** Linear purpuric lesions due to scratching
- **Hematomata:** Deeper collections of blood within the skin. They may be fluctuant.

221. **What about the "inflammatory" purpura?**
It is a lesion due to extravasation not only of red cells, but also *leukocytes*. Hence, inflammatory purpura is by definition indurated and *palpable*. It indicates small vessel vasculitis.

222. **What is leukocytoclastic vasculitis (LCV)?**
A histopathologic term for small-vessel vasculitis. LCV may be acute or chronic and usually carries a good prognosis unless internal involvement is present.

223. **How do LCV lesions present?**
They may be either *localized to the skin* or *extended to internal organs*, most commonly the GI tract, kidneys, and joints—but also the lungs, heart, and central nervous system.

224. **What are the characteristics of LCV lesions?**
- **Palpable purpura:** The most common cutaneous small-vessel vasculitis. Lesions are usually on the legs, even though any area can be involved; round; small (1–3 mm in size, but at times coalescing into plaques); palpable (if only barely); and rarely ulcerated (a more common feature of *large* vessels vasculitis). Subungual splinter hemorrhages also may occur.
- **Urticarial lesions:** Of longer duration (often >24 hours) than regular urticarial lesions. Usually resolving with residual pigmentation or ecchymosis. More burning than pruritic.

225. **What is *livedo reticularis*?**
A rare manifestation of cutaneous vasculitis, since it reflects involvement of medium-sized rather than small-sized vessels. It is characterized by a purplish, streak-like net.

226. **What are the causes of cutaneous vasculitis?**
It depends on the patient's age:
1. In **children** the most common cause is *Henoch-Schönlein purpura,* followed at a great distance by *leukocytoclastic hypersensitivity* (i.e., drug reaction).
2. In **adults**, cutaneous vasculitis is often due to immune complexes, although other autoantibodies can do it, too. Yet, 30–50% of all cases are idiopathic. The rest are caused by:
   - **Drugs**, especially antibiotics (particularly beta-lactams), diuretics, nonsteroidal anti-inflammatory drugs, but also foods or food additives.

- **Infections**, including upper respiratory tract infections (particularly beta-hemolytic streptococcal), viral hepatitis (especially C, probably through the presence of cryoglobulins), HIV, and endocarditis. Vasculitis usually postdates the infection.
- **Collagen vascular diseases**, especially rheumatoid arthritis, Sjögren syndrome, and lupus erythematosus. Vasculitis often denotes active disease and possibly poorer prognosis. Note that cutaneous vasculitis is rarely seen in patients with involvement of larger vessels, such as polyarteritis nodosa, Churg-Strauss syndrome, or Wegener's syndrome.
- **Inflammatory bowel disease** (such as ulcerative colitis or Crohn's disease).
- **Malignancy** (especially lymphoproliferative diseases, particularly hairy cell leukemia). Still, cancer is a rare cause, accounting for <1% of all cases of cutaneous vasculitis.

MISCELLANEOUS DISORDERS

Kaposi's Sarcoma

227. **What are the major types of Kaposi's sarcoma? Describe each.**
- **Classic** (traditional): Now relatively rare, this is the KS of shins or feet of older men of either Mediterranean or Eastern European descent (Ashkenazi Jews). It begins as purplish papules slowly progressing to plaques. Rarely fatal. In fact, most patients die *with* KS rather than *of* KS.
- **Epidemic** (AIDS-associated): Present in more than one third of AIDS patients. Lesions are more varied and widespread than in the classic form, ranging from macules to papules, to plaques or ulcers, all red-purple in color (Fig. 3-37). Mean survival is 15–24 months, although antiretroviral therapy has extended it. Visceral involvement is common, including genital, oral, GI, and pulmonary sites.
- **Endemic** (African): Cutaneous and/or lymphatic. Common (10% of all cancers), aggressive, 15:1 male-to-female ratio, and possible in children. Endemic in Uganda, Congo, and Zambia.
- **Iatrogenic:** From immunosuppression, may regress with its termination. Often with GI bleeding.

228. **What is the presentation of KS?**

- Usually begins as bilateral and symmetric discrete *skin patches*, red or purple in color but occasionally violaceous, typically involving the lower extremities. These eventually become elevated, evolving into spongy nodules and plaques (*localized nodular form*).
- May also present in a *locally aggressive form*, either as a large infiltrating mass or multiple cone-shaped friable tumors, firmly adhering to underlying anatomic structures, like bone.
- Finally, it may spare the skin and present with *visceral involvement* (including lymph nodes).
- Course ranges from indolent (if limited to skin) to fulminant (if affecting multiple internal organs).

229. **What is the cause of KS?**
There is definitely a KS-associated herpes virus (human herpesvirus [HHV] type 8), first identified in 1994, and subsequently linked to all four types. Yet, HHV-8 is probably necessary but *not* sufficient. Also, it is unclear whether KS is a hyperplasia or tumor and whether it is multicentric or metastatic.

230. **How is Kaposi's sarcoma (KS) diagnosed?**
It is suspected clinically and diagnosed histologically.

231. **Who was Kaposi?**
Moritz Kaposi (1837–1902) was a Viennese dermatologist. Born Moritz Kohn in Kaposvar, Hungary, he chose to rename himself after his native town when he converted to Catholicism.

A conceited chap famous for never saying, "I don't know," Kaposi linked his name not only to KS, but also to one of the earliest descriptions of lupus erythematosus and dermatitis herpetiform.

Lupus Erythematosus

232. What is lupus erythematosus (LE)?
A connective disease that is either limited to the skin or with devastating systemic involvement (systemic lupus erythematosus [SLE]).

233. What are the *cutaneous* manifestations of LE?
Primarily three:
- *Acute* cutaneous lupus erythematosus (ACLE)
- *Subacute* cutaneous lupus erythematosus (SCLE)
- *Chronic* cutaneous lupus erythematosus (CCLE), also called *discoid lupus* (DLE)

These are histopathologically similar but clinically very different.

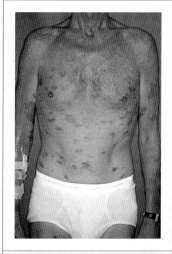

Figure 3-37. Kaposi's sarcoma. Multiple violaceous plaques following the lines of skin cleavage in a pityriasis rosea-like pattern are seen on the trunk of an HIV-positive patient. (From Fitzpatrick JE, Aeling JE: Dermatology Secrets. Philadelphia, Hanley & Belfus, 1996.)

234. What is the presentation of *acute cutaneous lupus erythematosus*?
The typical one is an acute and *focal* butterfly rash, involving the cheeks and bridge of the nose. This is often painful or pruritic and may even be photodistributed (forehead, periorbital area, chin, ears, and neck). In fact, a temporal association with sun exposure is very common. More rarely (and usually in older patients), ACLE presents with a *generalized* maculopapular rash that represents a photosensitive dermatitis. At times may even occur as a widespread blistering phototoxic reaction, resembling toxic epidermal necrolysis (TEN).

235. Is ACLE associated with SLE?
It is strongly associated with the *systemic* manifestations of LE (i.e., SLE) and its serology. In fact, malar rash occurs in 55–90% of all SLE patients; generalized maculopapular eruption in 35%.

236. What is the course of ACLE?
A waxing and waning, with sun-related exacerbations lasting for days to weeks. At times, it can become quite protracted, usually resolving with postinflammatory hyperpigmentation. It rarely scars, but at times ulcerates. Ulcerations of oral and nasal mucosae are also common, either painful or painless. ACLE may coexist with SCLE, but much more rarely with CCLE (i.e., discoid lupus).

237. What laboratory studies are positive in ACLE?
The same studies that are positive in SLE:
- **Antinuclear antibodies (ANA)** are invariably present (95% sensitivity). They have, however, low specificity, even though they are much less common in dermatomyositis, a condition that can otherwise mimic LE.

- **Anti–double-stranded DNA (anti-dsDNA)** antibodies are present in 60–80% of ACLE patients. More specific for SLE. They may also correlate with the degree of activity of lupus in general, and with the level of nephritis.
- **Anti-Sm antibodies** are very specific for SLE. Hence, if negative, they exclude underlying systemic involvement.
- **Complement levels** are uniformly depressed.

238. **What are the lesions of SCLE?**
Although at times generalized, these are primarily subacute lesions of sun-exposed areas in white subjects, predominantly women. They begin as erythematous papules or plaques, eventually evolving into annular lesions (mimicking erythema annulare) or papulosquamous and scaling ones resembling psoriasis or lichen planus. Usually asymptomatic (at times mildly pruritic), they wax and wane, *always healing with neither scarring nor atrophy*. They may, however, leave residual dyspigmentation. Sunscreens, topical steroids, and antimalarials can be effective.

239. **Is SCLE associated with SLE?**
Only with *very few* manifestations of SLE, except for musculoskeletal symptoms, which are present in one half of all SCLE patients (arthralgia, often symmetric, of the hands and wrists). Yet full-blown arthritis is less common (<2%). Laboratory abnormalities, like ANA and, especially, anti-Ro (SS-A) autoantibodies, are very common. One half of SCLE patients have four or more of the diagnostic criteria for SLE, but a less severe disease. Still, some SCLE patients may manifest SLE symptoms; hence, look for pleuritis, pericarditis, neurologic involvement, and renal impairment. They also may have nonspecific cutaneous manifestations of lupus erythematosus, such as livedo reticularis, palpable purpura, urticaria, ischemic changes of the distal fingertips (from Raynaud's phenomenon), or mucosal ulcerative lesions.

240. **Can any drugs elicit SCLE skin lesions?**
Mostly hydrochlorothiazide, but also calcium channel blockers, angiotensin-converting enzyme (ACE) inhibitors, and griseofulvin.

241. **What is the association with discoid lupus erythematosus (DLE)?**
Some SCLE patients can have lesions of DLE. Some may even develop small vessel vasculitis.

242. **What is discoid lupus?**
The chronic cutaneous form of lupus erythematosus. It is also the most common form, accounting for 50–85% of all cutaneous manifestations of LE.

243. **What is the difference between DLE and the discoid lesions of SLE?**
DLE occurs in the absence of other systemic involvement and in patients who rarely develop SLE. It affects middle-aged subjects with low ANA titers and *absence of* more SLE-specific antibodies, such as anti-native DNA and anti-Sm. DLE *may* also occur in 20% of patients with SLE, and indeed some DLE patients (<5%) may progress to SLE. Yet, the two are fundamentally separate. DLE patients rarely fulfill four or more of the criteria for SLE, and serologic abnormalities are uncommon. Still, some DLE patients may also have lesions of SCLE, and some may even have a malar rash.

244. **How does DLE present?**
As a chronic, scarring, and atrophy-producing photosensitive dermatosis. Discoid lesions begin as sharply demarcated erythematous papules and plaques, with slight to moderate scaling, usually arising over a sun-exposed area, such as the cheeks, nose, ears, face, and scalp. In severe disease, however, they may involve the upper chest, back, and arms, and, on rare occasions, even the legs and unexposed skin. DLE lesions are mostly asymptomatic, although at times they may be pruritic and occasionally painful. Eventually, they spread centrifugally and

may merge. As they do so, scales thicken and become adherent, causing hyperpigmentation at the active border and hypopigmentation in the central and inactive areas. As lesions age, dilation of follicular openings occurs with a keratinous plug, termed *follicular plugging*. There also may be telangiectasias. Resolution of the active lesion results typically in pink or white depressed scars and alopecia of the scalp. In fact, *atrophy* and disfiguring *scarring* are the hallmark of the disease. Hence, the term "lupus," since, like a wolf, it devours the patient's physiognomy.

245. What are localized and generalized DLE?
Patients with DLE can present with involvement that is either **localized** (i.e., affecting only the head and neck) or **generalized** (i.e., affecting other areas). The latter is associated with hematologic and serologic abnormalities, has greater progression to SLE, and is more difficult to treat.

246. What are the serologic markers of DLE?
One fifth of patients have positive ANA titers, 1–3% have anti-Ro (SS-A) autoantibodies, and <5% have anti–double-stranded DNA or anti-Sm antibodies. The latter usually reflect SLE.

247. Is skin involvement common in *systemic* lupus erythematosus?
It is present in 85% of patients, both as disease-nonspecific *and* disease-specific manifestations. The latter is acute, subacute, and chronic (discoid) lupus. The first sign of disease is usually an erythematous blush on the cheeks and nose (*butterfly rash*) or a maculopapular eruption above the waistline, similar to a drug reaction. Discoid lesions are also common.

248. What are the disease-nonspecific manifestations of SLE?
They are alopecia, panniculitis (lupus profundus), bullous lesions, urticarial vasculitis, and vasculitic purpura (i.e., palpable purpura that may result in ulceration). Patchy or generalized alopecia can occur independently of other manifestations, and may be associated with flares of disease. Livedo reticularis is also possible (especially in cases of antiphospholipid antibodies), as is mucosal ulceration of the hard palate and nasopharynx, like nasal *septal* perforation. These often reflect active disease. Raynaud's phenomenon occurs in 20–30% of cases.

249. What is lupus profundus?
It is lupus involvement of adipose tissue. This is characterized by multiple subcutaneous nodules, usually with normal skin, but sometimes with overlying discoid lesions of the face, breasts, buttocks, trunk, or proximal arms and legs. These may ulcerate and typically heal with subcutaneous atrophy. Calcification may also occur. Many patients have a positive ANA and antibodies to double-stranded DNA. Yet, lupus profundus also may occur with CDLE or SLE.

250. Who develops lupus?
It depends. DLE affects 25- to 45-year-old subjects, women twice as often as men. SLE peaks instead at 30–40 years, although it may occur in children and even elderly patients. Women are eight times more affected, and so are African Americans. One tenth of patients have a genetic predisposition.

251. Can drugs trigger lupus erythematosus?
Yes. Hydralazine, procainamide, isoniazid, methyldopa, sulfonamides, phenytoin, and penicillamine may all induce a systemic lupus-like illness.

Syphilis

252. What are the primary lesions of syphilis?
They vary depending on stage:
- **Primary syphilis:** Classic lesion is the *chancre*, which occurs within 3 weeks at the site of treponemal penetration—usually the penis or scrotum in men (70%) and the vulva, cervix,

or perineum in women (50%), but also any body region in both genders. The lesion begins as a 1–2 cm, single, round, and firm *papule,* rapidly evolving into a painless nonbleeding *ulcer* (the chancre) with raised indurated borders. Induration is key. In fact, the lesion can almost be flipped between fingers, as if it were a button under the skin. Chancres are highly infectious, but heal in 4–8 weeks—with or without therapy. Painless regional lymphadenopathy is common.

- **Secondary syphilis:** A mucocutaneous eruption that occurs 2–10 weeks after the primary chancre, and becomes most florid at 3–4 months from infection. If untreated, it resolves in the same amount of time, even though relapses may occur. It may be so subtle that 25% of patients are unaware. Lesions are 5–10 mm *macules*, pale-red to pink, circular or ring-shaped, covered by sparse scaling, and diffusely distributed on the trunk and proximal extremities. Over days to weeks, they evolve into red *papules*, which are often necrotic and more widely distributed. Lesions can also affect the palms, soles, and hair follicles, thus resulting in patchy alopecia. One tenth of all patients develop superficial mucosal erosions (of the palate, pharynx, larynx, glans penis, vulva, and even anal canal and rectum). These are circular, silver-gray, and with a red areola. They are highly infectious. Lymphadenopathy is common, as are constitutional symptoms (malaise, anorexia, aching pains, fatigue, fever, headache, and some degree of neck stiffness).

- **Benign tertiary syphilis:** The end-result of the untreated resolution of secondary lesions. It develops 3–10 years after initial infection. Its typical lesion is the *gumma*, which may occur anywhere, although more often in areas of trauma. Cutaneous gummas are nontender and rubbery nodules that range in diameter from less than 1cm to several centimeters and can evolve into papulosquamous or ulcerative lesions. These usually heal with noncontractile scarring, forming characteristic circles and arcs with peripheral hyperpigmentation. Only one third of patients develop tertiary syphilis—divided among cutaneous gummas (16%), cardiovascular involvement (9.6%), and central nervous system disease (6.5%).

253. **Who develops syphilis?**
Early syphilis (primary and secondary disease) may occur in any age group, but more commonly in the sexually active years. Male-to-female ratio is 2:1. Recently, the incidence has increased, initially because of homosexual males, but with anti-HIV changes in sexual practices, because of inner-city, African-American heterosexuals involved in drug use.

254. **What are the other clinical presentations of syphilis?**
- **Syphilis in HIV-infected patients:** Often difficult to diagnose, with negative serology, increased incidence of neurosyphilis, and persistence of disease even after adequate treatment.
- **Congenital syphilis:** Due to transplacental spirochetal transmission. Infection is latent, becoming apparent during childhood and, in some cases, during adult life. The first symptom of *early prenatal syphilis* (before age 2) is rhinitis (snuffles), soon followed by cutaneous lesions. Manifestations of *late prenatal syphilis* (after age 2) include hearing and language abnormalities and vision problems. Facial and dental abnormalities also may be present (*see* Chapter 6, question 125, *Hutchinson teeth and triad*).

Insect Infestations

255. **What are the most common insect infestations?**
The most common are *lice* and *mites*:
- **Pediculosis capitis:** Scalp infestation by the head louse. Characterized by pruritus of the back and sides of the scalp, resulting in excoriation, secondary infection, and cervical adenopathy. Nits (1-mm, oval egg capsules) are firmly attached to hair and number in the thousands. Live lice are few.

- **Pediculosis pubis:** Affects hairy regions, usually the pubis but also the chest, axillae, and upper eyelids. Nits and lice can be seen (1–2-mm, brownish-gray specks in hair and skin). Very pruritic.
- **Scabies:** Infestation by the mite *Sarcoptes scabiei*. From the Latin term for "scratch" (*scabere*), this aptly presents with intractable pruritus, particularly nocturnal, associated with linear ridges, vesicles, nodules, excoriation, and crusting of web spaces, wrist, genitalia, axillae, areolae, inguinal folds, buttocks, waist, and ankles. Close examination with a magnifying lens reveals 1-cm long *serpiginous linear tracts* (burrows). These are made by the mite, which is small and appears as a grayish little dot at the end of the tract. Diagnosis is made by scraping papules, nodules, and tracts, which reveal the mite, the eggs, and the poop (scybala)—with the latter resembling tiny, black footballs.

256. **Who develops insect infestations?**
Any age group. Still, *pediculosis capitis* is more common in children, *pediculosis pubis* in young adults (frequently spread by sexual contact), and *scabies* in nursing homes and hospitals, often as epidemics. They all spread by close physical contact with infected subjects or clothing.

257. **What is Norwegian scabies?**
It is "crusted" scabies, a much more politically correct term, since the only reason the poor Norwegians got stuck with this unfortunate association is a report that came out of their country during the mid-1800s. Whatever the name, this is a separate and very contagious form of scabies, characterized by extensive, widespread, and crusted lesions over the elbows, knees, palms, and soles. Thick, yellowish, and hyperkeratotic scales and plaques may almost suggest *psoriasis*, although the pruritus of scabies is typically much more intense. The condition is characterized by hundreds to millions of adult female mites infesting the host, who is usually immunocompromised (e.g., AIDS), but also elderly, or physically and/or mentally disabled and impaired. Hence, this is a particularly serious problem in institutionalized settings.

SKIN MANIFESTATIONS OF SYSTEMIC DISORDERS

Necrobiosis Lipoidica

258. **What is necrobiosis lipoidica (diabeticorum)?**
A skin disorder associated with diabetes mellitus. First described by Oppehhein in 1929, named *necrobiosis lipoidica diabeticorum* by Urbach in 1932, and eventually simplified as "necrobiosis lipoidica" (NL) since it may occur (albeit rarely) in nondiabetics as well. In fact, 67% of patients *do* have diabetes; 16% have abnormal glucose tolerance; 8% have a family history of diabetes, and only 9% have no diabetic link at all. NL is a disorder of collagen degeneration, with granulomatous response, thickening of the blood vessel walls, and fat deposition. Etiology is unknown, although diabetic microangiopathy probably plays a role, since vascular changes of NL are similar to those of the kidneys and eyes. It is relatively rare (only 0.3% of diabetics), with an average onset at 30 years, although any age can be affected. It is three times more common in women than in men, and its presence or progression does not correlate with glucose control. In fact, NL is rather difficult to treat, with a chronic and indolent course of progression and scarring.

259. **What is the presentation of NL?**
The classic one is a series of asymptomatic and shiny 1–3 mm papules/nodules that are well circumscribed and slowly enlarging over months to years. Usually located over the pretibial areas, they also may affect the face, scalp, trunk, and upper extremities. Lesions eventually form waxy and atrophic round patches, red to brown in color. These may progress into

depressed, atrophic, and yellowish plaques, 2–10 cm in diameter, scaly, and with violaceous borders that are due to skin atrophy, thus making underlying veins more visible. Multiple telangiectasias can also be seen on the thinning epidermis. Plaques may eventually ulcerate, especially after trauma, and occasionally become infected. Lesions tend to be multiple and bilateral, with a pronounced Koebner's phenomenon. In 75% of the cases, they are painless (probably because of concomitant neuropathy), although they also may be extremely painful. Otherwise, the only complaint is usually cosmetic.

Porphyria Cutanea Tarda (PCT)

260. What is PCT?
The most common form of porphyria. Although the mechanism (increased excretion of uroporphyrin, caused by deficiency of uroporphyrinogen decarboxylase) can be transmitted as an autosomal-dominant disorder, most cases are sporadic or acquired. In fact, it has been linked to HIV infection and various forms of liver dysfunction, including hepatitis C, alcoholism, iron overload, hemochromatosis, and even malignancy (especially hepatocellular carcinoma).

261. What is the presentation of PCT?
It is characterized by photosensitive lesions due to increased skin fragility to sun exposure. This results in full-thickness epidermal *erosions and blistering*, with painful indolent sores of sun-exposed areas, like the face, forearms, and back of the hands. These become thickly crusted and secondarily infected, eventually healing with hyperpigmentation and scarring. *Milia* (tiny epidermal white or yellow papules), *hypertrichosis* (over temporal and malar areas), *scleroderma-like plaques,* and *excretion of port-wine urine* rich in porphyrin pigments are other common features.

Sarcoidosis

262. How common is cutaneous involvement in sarcoidosis?
Quite common. It occurs in 20–35% of all patients with systemic disease.

263. What are the skin manifestations of sarcoidosis?
They are either *nonspecific* or *specific*, with only the latter being histologically characterized by noncaseating granulomas. The most common *nonspecific* manifestation is erythema nodosum, whereas the most common *specific* one (especially in African-American women) is a cluster of small, nonscaling, dome-shaped *papules* on the face, periorbital areas, nasolabial folds, and/or extensor surfaces. These may be skin colored or variously hued (violaceous, reddish-brown, or hyperpigmented). They are usually asymptomatic, indurated, and resolving without scarring.

264. What is "plaque" sarcoidosis?
A form of chronic cutaneous involvement (i.e., >2 years), usually reflecting more severe systemic disease. Plaques result from the coalescence of papules into larger lesions, which are round to oval, reddish to purple, flat topped, and infiltrated. They may have an annular appearance (as a result of central atrophy), large telangiectatic vessels, and they may even appear scaly, which often prompts a differential diagnosis with psoriasis or lichen planus. They are usually located on the scalp, back, buttocks, extremities, and face (where they can mimic discoid lupus, especially when central atrophy and scaling are present). They often heal *with* scarring. In fact, scalp plaques lead to alopecia.

265. What is *lupus pernio*?
The most characteristic of all *specific* sarcoid lesions. It is more common in African-American women with long-standing systemic involvement—usually pulmonary. It presents as chronic,

indurated papules or plaques that resemble frostbite (*pernio* in Latin). Like other sarcoid lesions, they are variously hued (red to purple and at times violaceous), and usually located over the bridge and alae of the nose, even though they also can involve the cheeks, ears, and lips (and even the back of the hands, fingers, toes, and forehead). They are commonly associated with chronic uveitis and bone cysts. The course is chronic, often resulting in disfigurement (hence, the term *lupus*). If involving the nasal rim, lupus pernio has been associated with granulomatous disease of the upper respiratory tract and nasal mucosa, resulting in masses, ulcerations, or even life-threatening airway obstruction.

266. What is erythema nodosum (EN)?
The most common *nonspecific* (i.e., *not* granulomatous) cutaneous manifestation of sarcoid. EN is an acute, nodular, and erythematous hypersensitivity reaction that involves the panniculus of the shins. Often self-limited, it resolves with just a residual hyperpigmentation.

267. What are the characteristics of EN?
It afflicts predominantly young women (peak onset 18–34 years), presenting with flu-like symptoms, arthralgias and fever, followed by a painful rash that consists of large (2–6 cm in size), tender, nonscaling, and erythematous nodules/plaques on both pretibial areas (mostly shins and ankles). During the first week of rash, lesions are bright red, hard, tense, and painful. During the *second* week, however, they become bluish to livid and occasionally fluctuant (but never suppurative or ulcerative). Eventually, they fade to a yellowish hue, like a bruise, often leaving residual hyperpigmentation and desquamation of the overlying skin. Although each lesion lasts approximately 2 weeks, new lesions may continue to appear for 3–6 weeks. In one third of the idiopathic cases, the eruption may actually last for more than 6 months. After resolution of all lesions, achiness may persist for weeks.

268. Which sarcoid patients get EN?
Child-bearing women, especially those of North European lineage (particularly Scandinavians).

269. What is Löfgren's syndrome?
A characteristic and febrile form of acute sarcoid that includes:
- EN
- Anterior uveitis
- Hilar adenopathy
- Polyarthritis
Acute and benign, the syndrome resolves spontaneously in 6–8 weeks.

270. Is erythema nodosum exclusive of sarcoid?
No. Currently, the most common cause of EN in children is streptococcal infection, while in adults it is streptococcal infection *and* sarcoid. Still, EN also may occur as a drug reaction, manifestation of systemic diseases, or idiopathic entity. Among *drugs* the usual culprits are oral contraceptives, sulfonamides, iodides, and bromides. Associated *infections* include instead tuberculosis, Mycoplasma pneumoniae, M. campylobacter, Yersinia enterocolitica, and all major mycoses. *Autoimmune diseases* comprise the inflammatory bowel disorders. Finally, other conditions (pregnancy, Hodgkin's disease and lymphoma, Behçet disease) can do it, too.

Behçet's disease

271. What is Behçet's disease (BD)?
A complex and multisystem disease first described in 1937 by the Turkish dermatologist Hulusi Behçet. It typically involves the *skin* (genital aphthae), the *mucosae* (oral aphthae), and

the *eye* (posterior uveitis). The orogenital ulcers can in turn be associated with arthritis and various visceral manifestations, including cardiovascular, renal, gastrointestinal, pulmonary, and neurologic. It is most common in Mediterranean countries, with a prevalence of 1/10,000.

272. What is the presentation of BD?

Systemic symptoms (such as malaise, anorexia, weight loss) often precede the mucosal ulcerations by 6 months to 5 years. Of these, *oral ulcers* are the most common and earliest sign.

273. What is the apperance of *oral ulcers*?

They can be shallow or deep, with a central purulent base characterized by punched-out and clean margins. They are indistinguishable from common aphthae (canker sores), although usually larger (up to 3 cm in diameter), more painful, more frequent, and more rapidly progressing. The most common sites are the tongue, lips, buccal mucosa, and gums, with the tonsils, palate, and pharynx being instead less commonly affected. Ulcers appear singly or in crops, persist for 1–2 weeks, and subside without leaving scars. They tend to recur at least three times over a 1-year period, with the interval between recurrences ranging from weeks to months. Morphologically they can be divided into:

- **Minor aphthae:** 1–5, small and moderately painful, persisting for 4–14 days
- **Major aphthae:** 1–10, very painful, 10–30 mm in diameter, persisting up to 6 weeks, and possibly healing with a scar
- **Herpetiform ulcerations:** recurrent crop of many small and painful ulcers

274. What are the *eye* lesions of BD?

Frequent. Eye involvement occurs in 47–65% of BD patients, occasionally progressing to blindness. The most common manifestation is *posterior uveitis* (i.e., retinal vasculitis), but other manifestations are possible. *Hypopyon*, once considered the hallmark of BD, is now uncommon.

275. Describe the *skin* lesions of BD.

Variously appearing. They occur in 58–97% of patients and include erythema nodosum-like manifestations (the most common), acneiform nodules, erythema multiforme-like lesions, and papulopustular eruptions. Often there is a positive *pathergy test* (*see* question 278).

276. What are the *genital* manifestations of BD?

They are aphthous ulcerations that may accompany oral ulcers in 50–100% of cases, often resembling them. In males, they usually occur on the scrotum, penis, and groin. In females, they occur instead on the vulva, vagina, groin, and cervix. They are recurrent and may heal with scarring.

277. What are the other manifestations of BD?

- Various vascular lesions, often life threatening and causing hemoptysis
- GI involvement
- Arthritis
- Neurologic manifestations, including meningoencephalitis, a multiple sclerosis–like illness, acute myelitis, stroke, or pseudotumor cerebri
- Myocarditis
- Mild glomerulonephritis

278. What is *pathergy*?

The tendency to develop new lesions after minor trauma. Due to nonspecific skin hyperactivity. Although not limited to it, pathergy strongly suggests BD. It consists of an erythematous papule that develops 48 hours after intradermal injection of saline, often evolving into a sterile pustule.

Dermatomyositis

279. How common are dermatologic manifestations in dermatomyositis (DM)?
Skin lesions occur in one half of all patients, yet they do not correlate with the severity of myositis.

280. What are the most typical manifestations?
The two most characteristic (and possibly pathognomonic) are the *heliotrope rash* and the *Gottron papules*. Malar erythema, poikiloderma in a photosensitive distribution, violaceous erythema on extensor surfaces, and periungual and cuticular changes are instead less specific.

281. What is the heliotrope rash?
A symmetric, violaceous to dusky, erythematous rash of the periorbital area—with or without
edema. It can be subtle and only appear as a mild discoloration of the eyelid margins.

282. What are Gottron papules?
Slightly elevated, reddish/violaceous papules and plaques that can be found over bony prominences, especially the dorsal surfaces of knuckles (metacarpophalangeal, proximal interphalangeal, and distal interphalangeal), but also the elbows, knees, and/or feet. At times, these have a slight scale and, occasionally, a thick and psoriasiform one. In addition to psoriasis, they may resemble lesions of lupus erythematosus or lichen planus.

283. What is poikiloderma?
An erythematous disorder, first described by Civatte in 1923, that presents with atrophy, telangiectasia, and mottled pigmentation—both hypopigmentation and hyperpigmentation. It affects the cheeks and lateral sides of the neck of middle-aged women, sparing areas shaded by the chin. In addition to the "V" of the neck, it also may occur on other sun-exposed areas, such as the extensor surfaces of arms or the upper part of the back (shawl sign). It is characteristic but *not* specific of dermatomyositis.

Diabetes Mellitus

284. What other skin manifestations can be observed in diabetes mellitus?
- **Facial erythema**, which must be differentiated not only from the butterfly rash of *LE* (which is better marginated and circumscribed) but also from the malar rash of *rosacea* and *seborrheic/atopic dermatitis*.
- DM also can involve the **scalp**, as an erythematous to violaceous psoriasiform dermatitis. Nonscarring alopecia is, however, rare.
- **Calcinosis of the skin or muscle** is unusual in adults but may occur in as many as 40% of children or adolescents. It presents as firm, yellow or flesh-colored nodules over bony prominences, at times extruding through the skin and leading to secondary infection.

Scleroderma

285. What are the major cutaneous manifestations of scleroderma?
Sclerodactyly and *proximal scleroderma*.

286. What is *sclerodactyly*?
The symmetric thickening, tightening, and induration of the fingers. It has a 10-year survival
rate of 71%.

287. What is *proximal* scleroderma?
Skin involvement proximal to metacarpophalangeal or metatarsophalangeal joints. Induration also may affect the entire extremity, face, neck, and trunk (thorax and abdomen). Proximal

scleroderma that spares the trunk has a 58% 10-year survival, whereas diffuse skin induration has only a 21% 10-year survival.

288. **What are the minor cutaneous manifestations of scleroderma?**
As a result of ischemia, fingertips may be pitted, tapered, and with loss of the digital pad. *Raynaud's phenomenon* also is quite common, with 70% of patients initially presenting with this complaint and 95% eventually developing it during the course of their disease. Skin *pigmentary changes* also are common. These may include a salt-and-pepper appearance, with areas of hyperpigmentation alternating with hypopigmentation, or an overall hyperpigmentation or hypopigmentation. *Telangiectasias* (dilated vessels located just beneath the dermis) are also frequent, and most obvious on the face, perioral area, and neck (but also the upper chest and arms).

289. **What are the characteristics of the hand lesions of scleroderma?**
Early in the disease, the skin of the hands may feel puffy to the patient as a result of edema. This eventually progresses to sclerosis, with rapidity of progression reflecting visceral involvement and severity of outcome. In the sclerotic phase, the skin appears tight and shiny, with loss of hair, decreased sweating, and inability to make folds. Thickening and induration of the skin begin distally on the fingers and advance proximally. *Calcinosis* may occur on the fingers and extremities, including the extensor side of the forearms and the prepatellar areas.

290. **What is *limited* cutaneous scleroderma?**
It is skin thickening of areas that are *distal* to the elbow and knee. It also may involve the face and neck. CREST syndrome (calcinosis, Raynaud's phenomenon, esophageal dysmotility, sclerodactyly, and telangiectasias) is an older term for this subset of limited cutaneous scleroderma.

291. **What is *diffuse* cutaneous scleroderma?**
It is skin thickening of *proximal* aspects of the extremities plus the trunk and face. Reduced oral aperture (microstomia) due to perioral involvement may occur. Measure incisor-to-incisor distance.

292. **What about Raynaud's phenomenon?**
Raynaud's phenomenon of the digits (but also the lips, nose, and ears) occurs in 5–15% of the general population and quite commonly in postmenopausal women. Of these, only 5% develop a connective tissue disease. In scleroderma, it may precede obvious skin changes by months or even years (*see* also Chapter 22, questions 5–9).

Hyperthyroidism

293. **What are the skin manifestations of hyperthyroidism?**
It depends. Graves' disease is associated with a typical *pretibial myxedema*, characterized by thickened, bumpy, and colored plaques over the lower pretibial areas. It is usually asymptomatic. In addition, patients with hyperthyroidism tend to have *thin hair*. They also may have *onycholysis* of the fingernails, *clubbing* (thyroid acropathy), and even areas of *vitiligo* (5–10% of patients).

Pyoderma gangrenosum

294. **What is pyoderma gangrenosum (PG)?**
A painful and ulcerating skin disorder often linked to systemic diseases, including malignancy.

295. How does PG look?

It usually begins as a tender erythematous nodule or a hemorrhagic pustule, which eventually undergoes necrosis, forming ulcers with tender, raised borders that extend into the dermis. These are often solitary, but if multiple may coalesce into a single large ulcer that can be very painful, with irregular and dusky margins and satellite lesions. Progression is often rapid. Lesions are mostly distributed over the lower extremities, but also can appear on the trunk, abdomen, and rarely the head and neck. There is also *pathergy*. Systemic symptoms of fatigue and fever may also occur.

296. What are the causes of PG?

About 25–50% of cases are idiopathic. The rest are associated with systemic disorders, such as ulcerative colitis, Crohn's, various arthritic disorders, neoplasms, but also myelodysplastic syndromes, polycythemia vera, myelofibrosis, and essential thrombocythemia. All present with an atypical PG, often bullous and in unusual sites (such as the face and arms).

Sweet's Syndrome

297. What is Sweet's syndrome?

An acute febrile neutrophilic dermatosis that can be idiopathic or paraneoplastic. It was first described in 1964 by the British dermatologist Robert D. Sweet, who reported eight patients with fever, leukocytosis, and tender, erythematous plaques. Diagnostic criteria were eventually proposed in 1986 by Su and Liu, and subsequently modified by von den Driesch and colleagues. Both major criteria and at least two minor criteria are necessary for diagnosis (Table 3-7).

298. What are the skin lesions of Sweet's syndrome?

They are edematous, tender, beefy-red or violaceous plaques or nodules that suddenly erupt over the face, neck, and extremities (Fig. 3-38). They often have a purulent base, with central clearing and ultimately ulceration. They also may be papular, pustular, vesicular, or bullous. Systemic signs and symptoms (such as fever, myalgias, arthralgias, or ocular involvement—like conjunctivitis) usually accompany the skin eruption. Neutrophilic leukocytosis and elevated sedimentation rate are common, too. Less common are pulmonary infiltrates and hepatic and renal involvement.

299. What do these lesions appear like histopathologically?

They have a diffuse, neutrophilic infiltrate in the dermis *without* leukocytoclastic vasculitis. This is similar to erythema multiforme, but caused by a neutrophilic infiltrate.

TABLE 3-7. CRITERIA FOR SWEET'S SYNDROME DIAGNOSIS	
Sweet's Syndrome	
Major Criteria	**Minor Criteria**
• Abrupt onset of tender or painful erythematous or violaceous plaques or nodules • Predominantly neutrophilic infiltration in the dermis without leukocytoclastic vasculitis	• Preceding fever or infection • Accompanying fever, arthralgia, conjunctivitis, or underlying malignant lesion • Leukocytosis, increased erythrocyte sedimentation rate • Good response to systemically administered corticosteroid but not to antibiotics

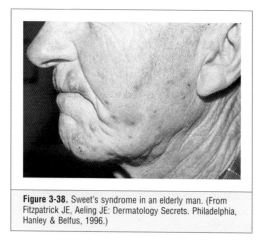

Figure 3-38. Sweet's syndrome in an elderly man. (From Fitzpatrick JE, Aeling JE: Dermatology Secrets. Philadelphia, Hanley & Belfus, 1996.)

300. **How often is Sweet's syndrome associated with an underlying malignancy?**
In 20–50% of the cases. Hematologic disorders account for 90% of all cancers, with acute myelogenous leukemia being the most common, followed by lymphoma, multiple myeloma, and myelodysplastic syndromes. Association with solid tumors is rare, and most are genitourinary.

301. **Is there anything unique in the Sweet's syndrome of cancer?**
Its cutaneous features are more severe, and lesions are more often bullous and on atypical sites, such as the trunk, mucosae (i.e., conjunctivitis), and internal organs (i.e., lungs, kidneys, and liver). Patients have less neutrophilia while having instead platelet abnormalities and anemia.

302. **Which cancers *metastasize to the skin*?**
Breast, GI, prostate, kidney, and head and neck. Melanomas, of course, and leukemias also may metastasize to the skin. Overall, autopsy studies reveal that 2–4% of all patients with internal cancer develop skin metastases. Once these have occurred, prognosis is generally poor.

303. **How do skin metastases present?**
As firm and rapidly growing skin nodules, often covered with fine telangiectasias (due to the neoplastic angiogenesis) and even ulcers (due to inability of the vasculature to catch up with the rapid growth of the tumor). Lesions are subcutaneous or intradermal, skin-colored but occasionally reddish and even bluish. Common on the anterior trunk, but also anywhere else.

304. **What are the unusual patterns of skin metastases?**
One interesting pattern is the ability of lesions to form a zosteriform pattern, with clusters of tumorlets merging into a zoster-like plaque. Other unusual presentations include:
- **Metastatic disease to the scalp** (which can cause localized alopecia, often with a nodular appearance—alopecia neoplastica). Common in renal cancers.
- **Periumbilical nodules** (which are part of the Sister Mary Joseph's nodules—also *see* Chapter 18, questions 45 and 46).
- **Carcinoma en cuirasse**, which may occur in patients with breast cancer, typically presenting as a leathery and infiltrated plaque caused by neoplastic invasion of the lymphatics, with resulting fibrosis of thoracic dermis and subcutaneous tissues. The chest wall fibrosis may be severe enough to interfere with respiration.

ACKNOWLEDGMENT

The author gratefully acknowledges the contributions of Debra J. Grossman, MD, MPH; Cynthia Guzzo, MD; and Scott Bennion, MD, FAAD, FACP, to this chapter in the first edition of *Physical Diagnosis Secrets*.

SELECTED BIBLIOGRAPHY

1. Abbasi NR, Shaw HM, Rigel DS, et al: Early diagnosis of cutaneous melanoma: Revisiting the ABCD criteria. JAMA 292:2771–2776, 2004.
2. Arnold HL, Odom RB, James WD: Andrews' Diseases of the Skin, 8th ed. Philadelphia: W.B. Saunders, 1990.
3. Conn RD, Smith RH: Malnutrition, myoedema and Muehrcke's lines. Arch Intern Med 116:875–878, 1965.
4. Daniel CR III, Osment LS: Nail pigmentation abnormalities. Cutis 25:595–607, 1980.
5. Daniel CR, Sams WM, Scher RK: Nails in systemic disease. Dermatol Clin 3:465–485, 1985.
6. Fawcett RS, et al: Nails as clues to systemic disease. Am Fam Physician 69:1417–1424, 2004.
7. Katta R: Cutaneous sarcoidosis: A dermatologic masquerader. Am Fam Physician 8:1581–1584, 2002.
8. Lynch PJ: Dermatology for the House Officer. Baltimore, Williams & Wilkins, 1982.
9. Mathur SK, Bhargava P: Insulin resistance and skin tags. Dermatology 195:184, 1997.
10. Muehrcke RC: The finger-nails in chronic hypoalbuminaemia. Br Med J 1:1327–1328, 1956.
11. Varma JR: Skin tags—a marker for colon polyps? J Am Board Fam Pract 3:175–180, 1990.
12. Whited JD, Grichnik JM, et al: Does this patient have a mole or a melanoma? JAMA 279:696–701, 1998.

CHAPTER 4

THE EYE

Salvatore Mangione, MD

"The eye is the light of the body."

—Matthew 6:22

"To drive away inflammation of the eyes, grind the stems of the juniper of Byblos, steep them in water, apply to the eyes of the sick person and he will be quickly cured. To cure granulations of the eye, prepare a remedy of cyllyrium, verdigris, onions, blue vitriol, powdered wood, mix and apply to the eyes."

—The Ebers Papyrus, 1500 BC

A. GENERALITIES

The eye is often bypassed or cursorily examined. Yet from measurement of visual acuity to funduscopy, *all* components of the exam can unlock important secrets, not only of the eye but also of the body. Some findings are so important that they should be recognized by all practicing physicians.

1. **Who should have visual acuity testing?**
   Anyone. Measuring vision is like taking the *vital signs of the eye:* nothing intelligent can be said without it. Since normal vision requires not only intact ocular function but also integrity of its vascular and neurologic supply, visual acuity is an excellent tool for the evaluation of ophthalmologic complaints. And since it can detect *painless loss of vision* in one or both eyes, it should be part of the screening exam of *all* adults (visual loss is in fact *painless*, except for disorders presenting with a *red eye*). Note that, in children, vision should be measured *early* (usually after the third birthday) to allow early detection of amblyopia.

2. **What is needed to measure visual acuity?**
   Snellen chart, pinhole occluder, and pocket-size near-vision test card. All are readily available.

3. **What is a *Snellen chart*?**
   A standard, wall-mounted eye chart imprinted with lines of black characters (letters, numbers, or illiterate Es), ranging in size from smallest (bottom) to largest (top).

4. **Who was Snellen?**
   Hermann Snellen (1834–1908) was a Dutch ophthalmologist who graduated from (and later taught at) the University of Utrecht. He created his famous chart in 1862 as a first attempt to standardize visual acuity measurements.

5. **How is the Snellen chart used?**
   By asking the patient to cover one eye at a time and then read from a well-illuminated chart at a distance of 20 feet (6m). Testing starts by convention with the right eye and is carried out with reading or distance glasses. Visual acuity is the smallest line on which the patient can distinguish >50% of all letters. The number of letters missed on the same line should also be recorded, such as 20/20 − 1 or 20/40 − 2.

6. **What does 20/20 mean?**
   That the patient can read at a distance of *20 feet* a letter that was indeed designed to be read at 20 feet; conversely, 20/40 means that the patient can distinguish at 20 feet a letter that could normally be read at 40 feet, and so on. The *numerator* of the visual acuity fraction represents the distance at which the chart is placed, whereas the *denominator* represents the distance at which the letter could be recognized by a person with normal acuity. The denominator also identifies the smallest line on the chart where the patient is able to read >50% of all letters.

7. **Can visual acuity be better than 20/20?**
   Yes. Although 20/20 is normal, most people without ophthalmic disorders can do better than that. Hence, their vision should be recorded accordingly, as 20/15, 20/12, and so on.

8. **What is a *pinhole vision*?**
   It is vision through a *pinhole occluder*. If visual acuity is less than 20/20 (i.e., the patient cannot read the 20/20 line), measurement should be repeated after placing a pinhole occluder over the tested eye. This is a device with a very small opening (pinhole), which admits *only* axial light rays while eliminating instead all the peripheral rays that blur vision through either refractive errors or imperfections/opacities of the cornea and crystalline (see also strabismus and diplopia). Hence, the occluder improves vision in refractive or ocular media problems, but does nothing for retinal or neurovisual disorders. Once *distant visual acuity* has been measured in both eyes, *near visual acuity* should be evaluated, too. This can be done with a modified Snellen chart, such as the *Rosenbaum Pocket-Size Visual Screener*. Hold the card 14 inches (35cm) away from the patient's eyes, one at a time, covering the other with your hand. Reading/distance glasses should be kept on. Visual acuity is the fraction notated at the right of the smallest legible line.

9. **How do you measure vision in patients who cannot read any letters on the chart?**
   By reducing the distance between patient and chart. This should be recorded as the numerator of the new visual acuity measurement (e.g., 5/70), and the fraction then translated into a more conventional recording (e.g., 20/280). If the patient cannot read the largest letters on a Snellen chart at 3 feet, vision may then be measured in terms of *counting fingers* (the examiner records the distance at which counting is accurate). If even this measurement is not possible, vision may be measured as *ability to see hand motions* (HM) or *a flashlight* (light perception [LP]), or finally as *no light perception (NLP)*.

10. **How is vision measured in illiterate patients or children?**
    By using the single "E" chart and asking patients to designate the strokes' direction.

11. **How is vision measured in *bedridden* patients?**
    By using the *Rosenbaum card*, which can be found at any medical supply store.

12. **What is the significance of reduced visual acuity?**
    It may indicate any of the following ocular processes:
    - **Refractive and correctable errors** (myopia, astigmatism, and presbyopia)
    - Treatable and reversible **blinding disease** (cataracts or uveitis)
    - Manifestations of **systemic disorders**, progressive if untreated (diabetes or hypertension)
    - Vision-impairing and possibly life-threatening **CNS disease** (multiple sclerosis, gliomas)
    - **Congenital disorders** (rubella or toxoplasmosis)
    - **Infectious diseases** (cytomegalovirus, retinitis, or toxoplasmosis)

13. **How can one confirm the cause of reduced visual acuity?**
    - **Uncorrected refractive errors** of the eye are usually suspected whenever vision improves with a pinhole occluder.
    - **Opacities of the light-transmitting media** are diagnosed by either ophthalmoscopy or by simply examining the red reflex.
    - **Neurologic or retinal disorders** are revealed by ophthalmoscopy, the swinging flashlight test, or visual field testing.
    - **Amblyopia** is suggested by a childhood history of reduced visual acuity often accompanied by strabismus.

14. **What are the refracting problems that can be corrected by glasses?**
    - **Hyperopia** (in which the axial length of the eye is too *short*)
    - **Myopia** (in which the axial length is too *long*)
    - **Astigmatism** (in which the refracting power of the eye is different in one meridian than another)

15. **When should you refer a patient with subnormal visual acuity?**
    - Presence of visual symptoms
    - No symptoms, but visual acuity of 20/40 (or worse) in one or both eyes
    - A visual acuity difference between eyes of two lines or more
    - Middle-aged or elderly patients with presbyopia, *even if distance visual acuity is preserved* (for prescription of reading glasses)
    - Presence of an afferent pupillary defect
    - Glaucoma screening

B. COLOR VISION

16. **What are color vision screening plates?**
    They are *pseudoisochromatic* tables (i.e., pseudo-similarly colored) that present numbers or figures against a background of colored dots. This color combination is confusing and illegible to a person with abnormal color discrimination.

17. **How is color vision tested?**
    By consecutively presenting color plates to the patient, one eye at a time, and by then recording results as a fraction, with the numerator indicating the number of correct responses and the denominator the number of total plates presented. In testing for unilateral *dyschromatopsia*, a simpler but still reliable method is to ask the patient to cover the affected eye and look at a red object, such as the cap of a mydriatic solution bottle. Then the patient looks at the same object with the *other* eye (while the unaffected one is covered) and reports whether the red color appears the same. In *dyschromatopsia*, the affected eye will see the color red as being gray or washed-out.

18. **What is dyschromatopsia?**
    From the Greek *dys* (abnormal), *chroma* (color), opsis (*vision*), this is an acquired deficiency in color vision, as opposed to congenital color blindness.

19. **What causes dyschromatopsia?**
    Optic nerve diseases or toxic/degenerative processes of the macula.

C. VISUAL FIELDS

20. **Why is visual field testing important?**
    Because it may reveal significant neurologic or ocular diseases. Terminology and interpretation, however, are often confusing.

21. Describe the normal anatomy of the visual pathways.

This is quite complex and yet fundamental for the understanding of visual field defects (Fig. 4-1). Our visual world (i.e., *visual field*) is divided into right and left *hemifields*. Each eye gets information from both.

After originating in the photoreceptors of the *retina*, vision is transmitted via the *optic nerve* axons. These partially cross at the *optic chiasm* and then emerge as *optic tracts*, wrapping around the midbrain to finally reach the *lateral geniculate nucleus* (*LGN*), where they stop for synapsis. From the LGN, axons fan out through the deep white matter of the

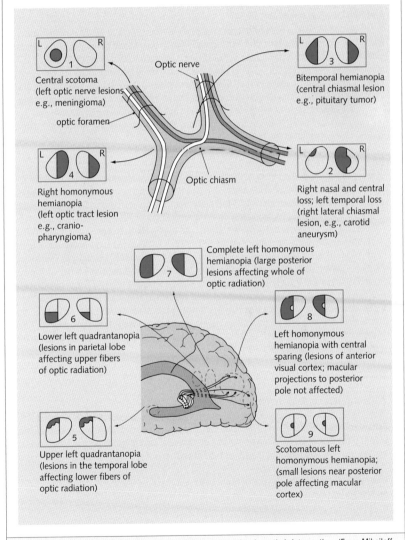

Figure 4-1. Neurologic visual pathways, and diseases originating from their interruption. (From Mihailoff G: Crash Course Nervous System. St. Louis, Mosby, 2005.)

brain (parietal and temporal lobe) as *optic radiations*, ultimately reaching the *primary visual cortex* in the occipital lobes. The crucial aspect of this entire pathway is its inversion of images, insofar as the *nasal* retina of the right eye sees the right half of the world (i.e., the *temporal* half of the visual field), whereas the *temporal* retina of the right eye sees the left half of the world (i.e., the *nasal* half of the visual field). As a result, the *right* nasal retina and *left* temporal retina see very much the same aspect of the outside world: the *right hemifield* (i.e., if you drew a line through the world at your nose, they would see everything to the right of that line).

Because of all these crossings, a *prechiasmal* lesion will be very much akin to losing one eye (i.e., it will affect only *one eye* but *both hemifields*). Conversely, *chiasmal* lesions will affect parts of *both eyes* and *both hemifields* (i.e., inputs from the nasal retinas will be lost, thus causing loss of peripheral vision on both sides). Finally, *postchiasmal* lesions will affect parts of *both eyes*, but *only one hemifield*.

The anatomic distribution of the *optic radiations* follows a wide three-dimensional arc, which first dives into the temporal lobe (*Meyer's loop*), then heads back though the parietal lobe, and finally terminates into the occipital lobe. Lesions involving Meyer's loop (i.e., temporal lobe) cause loss of vision in the upper visual world, but only in the left hemifield. Lesions involving the parietal portion of the optic radiations cause loss of vision in the lower visual world, but only on one side (the left hemifield in this case). Finally, lesions affecting the occipital (visual) cortex cause loss of vision in one hemifield, but with *macular sparing* (i.e., notched hemifield). This sparing results from either overlapping blood supply or large cortical representation of the fovea.

22. **How do you test visual fields?**
By using either a *static* or a *dynamic* technique. Diagnostic accuracy for visual field defects is similar, with high specificity but low sensitivity, especially for anterior or chiasmal lesions (see later).
- **Static testing:** The examiner sits 3 feet away from the patient, who covers one eye with the palm of one hand while fixating on the examiner's opposite eye. While the patient is doing so, the examiner outstretches an arm and briefly holds up one or two fingers. These are then displayed in each quadrant, and the patient is asked to report how many fingers are seen. In fact, the maneuver is often carried out by testing *two* quadrants simultaneously (by presenting *both* examiner's hands to the two quadrants at the same time). This may unmask a parietal lesion that would otherwise allow a patient to see a single object (but not a double) by relying on the contralateral field. The test is then repeated for the opposite eye.
- **Dynamic testing:** This is carried out very much like its static counterpart, except that the examiner continuously wiggles his or her fingers while gradually (and very slowly) bringing them into the patient's visual field from a peripheral angle. The patient is then asked to report when (s)he sees the fingers.

After detecting the field defect, the examiner should then identify whether this defect respects the vertical or horizontal meridian of the visual field (see later).

23. **What are *visual field defects*?**
They are abnormalities of *peripheral vision*, reflecting lesions at various levels of the visual pathways. They are described as *hemianopias* (from the Greek *hemi*, half; *an*, lack of; and *opsis*, vision) if the loss of vision involves one half of the visual field of each eye; *quadrantanopias* if it instead involves one fourth of the visual field of each eye.

24. **How are visual fields defects classified?**
As anterior or posterior:
- **Anterior (or prechiasmal) defects** are *ocular* lesions, since they involve the retina and optic nerves.
- **Posterior defects (chiasmal and postchiasmal)** are instead *neurologic* lesions, since they involve optic tracts, radiations, and the cortex.

25. **What is the difference between *anterior* and *posterior* visual field defects?**
   - **Anterior** defects are unilateral (*monocular*)—typically crossing the vertical meridian.
   - **Posterior** defects are instead *bilateral*, with borders aligned to (and *not* crossing) the vertical meridian of the visual field. They are referred to as *chiasmal* if the defect is bitemporal and *retrochiasmal* if homonymous (see later).

26. **What are the causes of visual field defects?**
   It depends on their location:
   - **Prechiasmal defects** are due to ocular lesions (glaucoma, retinal emboli, optic neuritis).
   - **Chiasmal defects** are due to pituitary lesions (mostly neoplastic).
   - **Postchiasmal defects** are due to *cortical* lesions (temporal, parietal, or occipital).
   - **Optic tracts lesions** are instead rare, representing only 5% of all *postchiasmal defects*.

27. **What is the most important step after finding a monocular visual field defect?**
   To test the visual field of the other eye. Monocular field defects are usually due to problems in the affected eye (prechiasmal), whereas *binocular* defects are usually caused by intracranial (neurologic) processes, either chiasmal or postchiasmal.

28. **What are the other characteristics of *prechiasmal* (ocular) defects?**
   They typically affect only one eye, compromise vision, and may have an abnormal pupillary/retinal exam (such as an afferent pupillary defect, cupping or atrophy of the disc, drusen, and retinal findings). In addition, prechiasmal visual defects typically *cross the vertical meridian*. This is because retinal nerve fibers draining the temporal retina arch across the vertical meridian in order to exit through the optic disc and nerve (which are located on the *nasal* side of the retina).

29. **What are the main types of prechiasmal defects?**
   (1) "Arcuate defects" of the visual field, shaped indeed like an arch, and caused by small lesions of the nerve fibers, and (2) "altitudinal defects," typically characterized by a sharp horizontal border in the visual field and caused instead by larger lesions of the nerve fibers.

30. **What are *severely constricted visual fields*? What are their causes?**
   They also are a form of *anterior* defect, characterized by a concentric "cut" of the most peripheral vision (in this regard they are exactly the opposite of a *central scotoma*, which is characterized by loss of central vision with preservation of the peripheral one). Note that both these prechiasmal defects are monocular; typically cross the vertical meridian; and are usually due to advanced glaucoma, retinitis pigmentosa, and other more uncommon conditions (even though they also may be related to malingering.) A *central scotoma* is instead usually caused by damage to nerve fibers originating in the macula.

31. **What are *chiasmal* defects?**
   They are bitemporal hemianopias.

32. **What is a *bitemporal* hemianopia?**
   It is the loss of vision of one half of the visual field of *both* eyes (from the Greek *hemi*, half; *an*, lack of; and *opsis*, vision), more specifically, the temporal fields of both eyes (bitemporal). This is typical of chiasmal tumors (gliomas and craniopharyngiomas in children, pituitary adenomas in adults).

33. **What are *postchiasmal* defects?**
   Homonymous *hemianopias* or *quadrantanopias*. These typically involve both eyes but preserve vision and pupillary and retinal exam (*see* below).

34. **What is *homonymous* hemianopia?**
   A visual defect affecting the same side (*homonymous*) of visual space in both eyes. For example, if the defect in the left eye involves the *temporal* region (the left portion of the left eye's visual field), the defect in the right eye will affect the *nasal* region (the left portion of the right eye's visual field). Homonymous hemianopia is typical of retrochiasmal lesions (optic tracts, optic radiations, and especially, the visual cortex).

35. What are the causes of inferior and superior quadrantanopias?

Diseases of either the parietal (causing *inferior* quadrantanopia) or temporal cortex (causing instead *superior* quadrantanopia). Still, lesions of the temporal and parietal cortex cause more commonly dense *hemianopias*. Note that the most common cause of an *isolated* homonymous *hemianopia* is a lesion to the *occipital* cortex, usually an ischemic stroke. In patients with other neurologic findings (hemiparesis, aphasia and, especially, an asymmetric optokinetic nystagmus), the most common cause is a *parietal* lesion.

36. What is an *asymmetric optokinetic nystagmus*?

A horizontal nystagmus that can be elicited by having patients look at a vertically striped tape that rapidly moves in front of their eyes, first toward one direction and then toward the other. Amplitude of horizontal nystagmus should be similar in the two directions. If not, it indicates a *parietal lobe* injury, since this typically reduces the nystagmus amplitude triggered by tape moving *toward the same side* of the lesion.

D. PUPILS

37. Why is examination of the pupils important?

Because attention to pupillary shape, size, and response to external stimuli provides extremely valuable clinical information. Figures 4-2 and 4-3 summarize the most common pupil abnormalities.

38. What is the size of a normal pupil?

It depends on age. Pupils are larger in children (7 mm of diameter at 10 years of age), but progressively smaller with aging (5 mm at 50, 4 mm at 80). In addition to being important for amateur astronomers and late-evening bird watchers, this pupillary characteristic also may explain why children are "cute," something cunningly exploited by Japanese cartoonists, who always draw their characters with big eyes and humongous pupils. Big and cute pupils are also nature's way to prevent us from killing our young, especially when the young are crying, incontinent, and totally dependent. Conversely, crying, incontinent and totally dependent *octogenarians* have *small* pupils. Hence they are not cute, and that is why we put them in nursing homes. Italian Renaissance women also were quite aware of this important property of the eye, since they used to dilate their own pupils with atropine (aptly named *belladonna* [i.e., nice-looking woman]) before going out on dates. This, however, often backfired since loss of accommodation led to embarrassing accidents and, ultimately, to the discontinuation of the practice.

39. How does one examine the pupils?

In a darkened room. Ask the patient to fixate the gaze on something in the distance while you shine a penlight from below to ascertain that the pupils are round and equal.

40. What major features should be identified in the pupil?

(1) Shape, (2) size, and (3) responses to external stimuli. These, in turn, include response to *accommodation* and *light*, both direct and consensual. "Direct reaction" is the ipsilateral response to a light stimulus; "consensual reaction," the contralateral response.

41. What is unique about the light reflex?

It contains crossed pathways, which means that both pupillary sphincters receive the same input from the midbrain.

42. What is *anisocoria*?

Pupillary asymmetry—from the Greek *an* (lack of), *iso* (equal), and *core* (pupils). Anisocoria reflects *asymmetric* diseases of either iris of *efferent* connections (i.e., third nerve or sympathetic nerves). The latter causes different signals to reach the two pupillary sphincters. A flip side to this rule is that anisocoria is absent in *afferent* disorders (i.e., affecting the optic nerve or retina) because crossed *efferent* pathways supply both eyes with the same signal.

	Reaction to light (direct)	Associated signs
Unilateral (dilated)		
Third nerve palsy	None	Ptosis (partial or complete), external ophthalmoplegia
Holmes-Adie syndrome	Slow	Better response to accommodation, lower limb areflexia
Marcus Gunn pupil	Slow and incomplete	Normal consensual response, optic atrophy, central scotoma, impaired colour vision
Local lesion of the iris	Variable depending on extent of local damage	Irregular pupil
Unilateral (constricted)		
Horner's syndrome	Reduced dilatation to shade	Ptosis (partial), ipsilateral facial anhidrosis, "enophthalmos"
Bilateral (dilated)		
Midbrain lession	None	Mid-position pupils; impaired vertical gaze
Iatrogenic (atropine, tricyclic antidepressants)	None or reduced	
Bilateral (constricted)		
Senile	None or reduced	
Iatrogenic (opiates, pilocarpine drops)	None or reduced	
Pontine lesion	None	Pin-point pupils, coma, Cheyne-Stokes respiration
Argyll-Robertson	None	Irregular pupils, normal accommodation

Figure 4-2. Pupil abnormalities. (From Liporace J: Crash Course Neurology. St. Louis, Mosby, 2006. Fig. 6.3.)

Unilateral			Reaction to light	Associated signs
Third nerve palsy			Negative	Ptosis (partial or complete) external ophthalmoplegia
Horner's syndrome			Poor reaction to shade	Ptosis (always partial) anhydrosis endophthalmus
Holmes-Adie syndrome			Slow reaction	Constriction to pilocarpine (0.1%) lower limb areflexia
Bilateral				
Argyll Robertson			Negative	Depigmented iris normal accommodation neurosyphilis
Midbrain compression			Negative	Coma lateralizing signs
Pontine stroke			Negative	Coma hyperventilation hyperpyrexia

Figure 4-3. Additional pupil abnormalities. (From Mihailoff G: Crash Course Nervous System. St. Louis, Mosby, 2005.)

43. **What is *accommodation*?**
    A reflex that allows the subject to focus on a near object by activating three effectors:
    (1) the *pupillary sphincters* (causing constriction of the pupils); (2) the *medial recti muscles* (causing convergence of the eyes); and (3) the *ciliary bodies* (causing accommodation of the lens). It is typically spared in the Argyll-Robertson pupil.

44. **What are the most common abnormalities in pupillary *shape*?**
    - The most common is probably the irregular, pear-shaped contour of pupils that have undergone an intraocular surgical procedure, such as cataract excision. There also are other causes of *oval* pupils, such as an incipient transtentorial uncal herniation (before the pupil becomes dilated, fixed, and fully round) and Adie's pupil.
    - Blunt trauma to the eye. This may tear the iris sphincter, making the affected pupil larger and slightly irregular.
    - Inflammation of the iris (iritis). This may cause adhesions (synechiae) of the iris to the anterior capsule of the lens, thus making the pupil irregular.
    - A *coloboma* of the iris. This is a congenital defect characterized by incomplete closure of the embryonic fissure of the optic cup. The involved iris usually has a keyhole shape, with the defect being most commonly in an inferonasal position.

45. **What is *hippus*?**
    A physiologic and synchronous oscillation in pupillary size. This may occur spontaneously or in response to light shined directly onto the eye. The term derives from the Greek *hippos* (horse), chosen to convey the up-and-down movements of a galloping horse. Note that hippus is *not* an *afferent pupillary defect* (i.e., a Marcus-Gunn pupil).

> **Pearl:**
> The response to a back-and-forth swinging of a penlight is initial dilation in afferent pupillary defect and initial constriction in hippus (*see* also question 60).

46. **How is the pupillary diameter controlled?**
    By a dual mechanism: *parasympathetic* (through the third nerve) for the *constrictor* muscle, and *sympathetic* (through the cervical chain) for the *dilator*. Hence, parasympathetic denervation will cause dilation (*mydriasis*), whereas sympathetic denervation will cause constriction (*miosis*).

47. **What are the most common causes of anisocoria?**
    ■ **Simple (physiologic) anisocoria:** A normal variant characterized by a physiologic difference of at least 0.4 mm between the two pupils, due, in turn, to an imbalance in muscular tone of the right and left sphincters. It is the most common anisocoria, present at *all* times in 3% of the population and at some times in up to 20%, with presence or absence depending on day of observation. In contrast to *pathologic* anisocoria, the physiologic form is characterized by a pupillary difference that does *not* change with various levels of illumination. Moreover, physiologic anisocoria is chronic, rarely >1 mm, and *always* isolated (i.e., *never* associated with ptosis, double vision, or light-near dissociation; *see* later). Hence, presence of concomitant findings makes anisocoria a much more ominous condition.
    ■ **Pharmacologic dilation:** Another common and benign cause. This can be due to conscious or inadvertent instillation of mydriatic drops (like in Italian Renaissance women) or even to improper nebulization of anticholinergic agents. The latter may create a diagnostic dilemma in intensive care unit patients, whose mental status often waxes and wanes. A response to cholinergic eye drops (such as pilocarpine) may help separating *pharmacologic paralysis* (which will remain unresponsive) from either *Adie's pupil* or a *third nerve palsy* (which, instead, will constrict in response to topical cholinergics—previously discussed).
    ■ **Third cranial nerve palsy** (i.e., parasympathetic denervation): This is characterized by (1) ipsilateral mydriasis plus; (2) *ptosis* (from paralysis of the levator palpebrae); and (3) *weakness of all extraocular muscles*, with the exception of the lateral rectus and superior oblique (which are the only ones not controlled by the third cranial nerve). Hence, the affected eye will be deviated outward and downward, thus resulting in diplopia. Note that the dilated pupil will still constrict if a cholinergic drop is instilled in the eye. Moreover, due to defective constriction, the anisocoria of third-nerve palsy is greater in bright illumination.
    ■ **Horner's syndrome** (Fig. 4-4): First described in 1860 by the Swiss ophthalmologist Johann Friedrich Horner, this is characterized by miosis of the affected pupil (from paralysis of the pupillodilator muscle) plus dysautonomic findings, including (1) ipsilateral *ptosis* (from

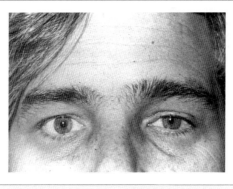

Figure 4-4. Horner's syndrome, with ptosis and miosis on the left. Note that the left lower lid is higher than the right lower lid. This inverse ptosis is due to interruption of the sympathetic innervation to the analog of Mueller's muscle in the lower lid. (From Vander JF, Gault JA: Ophthalmology Secrets. Philadelphia, Hanley & Belfus, 1998.)

paralysis of the superior tarsal muscle), and (2) *anhidrosis* (from damage to sudomotor fibers). In contrast to physiologic anisocoria, the difference between pupils in Horner's varies with illumination: greater in the dark (revealing defective dilation) and smaller in bright light (demonstrating intact constriction). Response to cocaine drops is also different: Horner's worsens, whereas simple anisocoria improves. This has strong predictive value, with sensitivity and specificity > 95%, a positive likelihood ratio (LR) of 96.8, and a negative LR of 0.1. Horner's should always prompt a search for lesions of (1) the *first-order neuron* (such as a *brainstem stroke*, the most common cause of Horner's on a neurology service; hence, the need for a thorough neurologic exam, with special attention to a lateral medullary syndrome); (2) the *second-order neuron* (usually a tumor of lung or thyroid, the most common cause of Horner's on a *medical* service; hence, the need for a thorough neck/supraclavicular/respiratory exam); or, finally (3) the *third-order neurons*. These are less common causes of Horner's, usually due to vascular headache (migraine), trauma or inflammation of the orbit, and cavernous sinus syndrome. Lesions of third-order neurons *may* preserve facial sweating.

- **Miscellaneous:** These include (1) inflammatory processes (e.g., unilateral iritis), (2) old trauma, (3) acute angle closure glaucoma, (4) various neurologic disorders, and (5) previous intraocular surgery (i.e., cataract extraction). In case of the *red eye* (see later), presence of anisocoria argues in favor of a more serious disease.

48. **What is the most common cause of a *third-nerve palsy*?**
Nerve compression against the free edge of the tentorium. This can be due to either a rapidly expanding aneurysm of the posterior communicating artery or *herniation of the ipsilateral uncus* (Hutchinson's pupil). The latter typically occurs with a change in mental status, plus ptosis and ophthalmoplegia. Note that the expanding mass responsible for herniation is usually *ipsilateral* to the mydriasis (and also to the ptosis and ophthalmoplegia, since they all originate in the compression of the ipsilateral third). Ipsilateral is also the hemiplegia, which, however, derives from damage to the *contralateral* cerebral peduncle.

49. **What is a *posterior communicating artery aneurysm*?**
The most common of all cerebral aneurysms. As many as 96% of these patients will have either a partial or *complete* third-nerve palsy (i.e., mydriasis, ptosis, and ophthalmoplegia); 20–60% will just have ipsilateral mydriasis. This provides an important localizing clue for surgery, which is key for preventing rupture.

50. **Who was Hutchinson?**
Sir Jonathan Hutchinson was an English surgeon and pathologist (1828–1913) who described his homonymous pupil in 1865. A devout Quaker, Hutchinson became involved with many philanthropic missions, and in fact even planned a career as a medical missionary. Instead, he gained the friendship of Sir James Paget and became one of the most versatile clinicians of 19th-century medicine. Besides being an ophthalmologist, he was also a venereologist, a clinician to the City of London Chest Hospital, and a general surgeon to the London and Metropolitan hospitals. He developed a special interest in congenital syphilis and was said to have seen more than 1 million patients. He published 1200 medical articles, with contributions in congenital syphilis and skin diseases (he also was among the first to describe sarcoidosis in 1877). Although his intellectual attributes were unchallenged, he had his critics, too. One commented: "He was totally devoid of any sense of humour, and like most humourless men, incredibly obstinate in clinging to his opinions long after they had been demonstrated to be untenable." Another added: "There was nothing scintillating about it, but nonetheless you felt he was speaking out of immense knowledge." In his private life, Hutchinson had 31 years of happy marriage and many children but kept his family in a country home while spending most of his week in London. He died at 85, choosing as an epitaph: "A Man of Hope and Forward-Looking Mind."

51. **What is the pupillary response to a close-up target?**
Constriction, but less than that resulting from a bright light suddenly flashed onto the eye. To test for it, ask the patient to look at a far-away point and then focus rapidly on a much closer object, such as your finger. The pupil should constrict 1–2 mm.

52. **What is the pupillary response to light being suddenly directed onto the eye?**
Constriction of 2–3 mm. The contralateral pupil will constrict by the same amount, provided there are no abnormalities in the parasympathetic innervation of the sphincter.

53. **What are Argyll Robertson (AR) pupils?**
Pupils that do *not* constrict in response to light, but do so when shifting fixation from a distance to a near target—i.e., accommodation. This phenomenon is called "light-near dissociation" and is typical of tertiary (neuro) syphilis. Still, it also can occur in diseases of the dorsal midbrain that present as Parinaud's syndrome (vertical gaze palsy, lid retraction, and convergence-retraction nystagmus; typical of patients with multiple sclerosis, basilar artery strokes, and pinealomas). Light-near dissociation also may present in traumatic injury to the orbital ciliary ganglion or ciliary nerves, or in viral infections of those structures (Adie's pupil, see later). It also can occur in diseases of either retina or optic nerve (which, in contrast to other causes of an AR pupil will also impair vision). Nowadays, a light-near dissociation is mostly encountered in diabetes, neurosarcoidosis, or Lyme disease. The location of the lesion that produces AR is unsettled, although most likely is somewhere in the dorsal midbrain (which would spare the nuclei of Edinger-Westphal that are responsible for accommodation).

54. **What is "near-light" dissociation?**
The opposite of *light-near dissociation*. It describes pupils that *do* constrict in response to light, but not in response to accommodation. It used to be typical of von Economo's encephalitis lethargica, but nowadays reflects mostly an unwillingness of the patient to focus on close objects. Hence, the maneuver should only be tried for absent pupillary light reactions.

55. **Who was Argyll Robertson?**
Douglas M.C.L. Argyll Robertson (1837–1909) was a Scottish surgeon. An avid golfer who studied in Berlin with Von Graefe, he eventually returned to Scotland, where he founded ophthalmology at the University of Edinburgh, mentored Marcus Gunn, and described his homonymous pupil in 1868.

56. **What is Adie's tonic pupil?**
A pupil that, like AR, responds *not* to direct light, but to near targets. Yet, unlike AR, Adie's constricts to near vision only *very slowly* (over seconds), and similarly *slowly* redilates when fixation is shifted to a distant target. Hence, the term *tonic pupil*, which indicates its long-lasting constriction. Adie also is *dilated* at rest and mostly unilateral, whereas AR is instead small and usually bilateral. Moreover, Adie's may create subjective problems with accommodation and is often *oval* (because of the segmental impairment of the iris sphincter). Finally, Adie's *constricts in response to* diluted pilocarpine (0.125% eye drops), a supersensitivity phenomenon that is absent in the normal eye.

57. **What is the significance of Adie's pupil?**
Dubious. Although permanent, Adie's usually offers no disturbance of vision and is unassociated with other important neurologic abnormalities. It usually reflects a lesion to the ciliary ganglion and postganglionic fibers, with aberrant regeneration toward the eye. Normally, the ciliary ganglion sends 30 times more fibers to the ciliary body (*accommodation*) than to the iris (*light reflex*), but after injury the regeneration tends to prioritize the iris. Hence, the preservation in Adie's of pupillary response during near vision (albeit sluggishly), but its loss to light stimulation.

58. **What are the causes of Adie's pupil?**
The most common is idiopathic. Still, various injuries to ciliary ganglion and fibers can cause it, too: orbital trauma, tumors, and viral infections (ophthalmic zoster).

59. Who was Adie?
William J. Adie (1886–1935) was an Australian who studied medicine in Edinburgh and then graduated just in time for World War I. He fought with honor in France, where he even saved his platoon by improvising a gas mask with cloth soaked in urine. Then, thanks to a well-timed measles attack, he also managed to survive the subsequent slaughter of his entire regiment, thus returning to England, where he taught and practiced until his death. His name is linked not only to the description of the homonymous pupil (in 1931) but also to the first description of *narcolepsy*. Adie was a brilliant teacher, an avid skier, and an amateur ornithologist. He died prematurely at 49 of a myocardial infarction.

60. What is the *swinging flashlight test*?
A test of response to light used to screen for an *afferent* pupillary defect. It was introduced by Levatin in 1959 and is carried out by asking the patient to gaze at a fixed target in the distance. A penlight is then shone first in one eye, and then into the other, back and forth, holding it in front of each eye for no more than 1–2 seconds. In normal subjects, as the light swings from one eye to the other, each pupil remains unchanged or constricts very slightly. If one eye has an *afferent* defect (optic nerve lesion or massive retinal damage), the pupil will dilate as the light strikes it (*Marcus Gunn pupil*). Note that it is important to keep swinging the light between the two eyes, since lingering on the affected eye may bleach the retina and thus produce a spurious Marcus Gunn. To avoid this, use the mnemonic, *one two switch, one two switch* to provide an adequate lilt to the swinging.

61. What is a Marcus Gunn (MG) pupil?
The most common abnormal pupillary response, more than all others combined. It is characterized by a normal *efferent,* but an abnormal *afferent* optic circuitry. Because the stimulus from the contralateral eye is coming in much stronger than that from the affected eye, shifting the light from the unaffected to the affected eye will release the urge to constrict (since this is only provided by the good eye). Hence, shifting light from the normal to the affected eye will cause the affected pupil to *dilate*. The relatively reduced input of MG is due to an optic nerve or retinal lesion. In fact, it involves *both* eyes (the damaged and normal contralateral one), even though it is normally described as Marcus Gunn pupil (or an afferent pupillary defect, APD) *only in reference to the eye the light shines on*.

62. What is the response of an MG pupil when the light is shone on it first?
It depends. If the light is shone on the affected pupil *first* (step 1 of the swinging flashlight test), the MG pupil will constrict, albeit poorly. As the light is then swung back and forth, the MG pupil will dilate.

63. What is a common cause of an *afferent pupillary defect* (MG pupil)?
Any *optic neuropathy* (i.e., neuritis, ischemic neuropathy, or optic nerve compression by tumor) that causes problems with the *afferent* pathway. In these patients, the test has a sensitivity of 92–98%, higher than any other test of afferent dysfunction, such as evoked potentials, visual acuity, or funduscopy. *A massive and unilateral retinal lesion*, like a central retinal artery occlusion, also may cause this phenomenon. Conversely, cataracts do not produce MG, since the ipsilateral retina is still able to receive light. Because afferent lesions spare the light reflex, only the presence of MG will be able to identify them.

64. Who was Marcus Gunn?
Robert Marcus Gunn was a Scottish ophthalmologist and a contemporary of another famous Scot, Robert Louis Stevenson, whom he personally knew and befriended. He was inspired to study ophthalmology by Argyll Robertson and then became highly regarded for his ophthalmoscopic skills. He reported his finding in 1904, even though it was probably already known.

65. What are the pupillary manifestations of *diabetes*?
Beside evidence of dysautonomic control (small and sluggishly reacting pupils), diabetes may occasionally induce an AR pupil. It also reduces the amplitude of hippus.

E. EXTERNAL EYE

66. Summarize the examination of the external eye.

Much of the external exam can be done with penlight and thoughtful observation of orbits, eyelid position, conjunctiva, anterior portion of the globe, and corneal/light reflex.

(1) Tear Film

67. What is *Schirmer's test*?

A measurement of tear production, devised by the German ophthalmologist Otto W.A. Schirmer (1864–1917). It can be used to assess patients with Sjögren's syndrome, a disorder consisting of dry eyes and dry mouth (keratoconjunctivitis sicca), often accompanied by other autoimmune manifestations.

68. How is Schirmer's performed?

After anesthetizing the eyes with a topical anesthetic, insert a small strip of filter paper into the fornix (i.e., the recess of the lower lid). Place the strip either medially or laterally, but *not* in the center of the eyelid. Remove the strip after 5 minutes. Measure in millimeters the wetting produced by the tears. Normal wetting distances are 10 and 15 mm for subjects, respectively, above or below the age of 40. A distance <5 mm is usually diagnostic of decreased tear production, whereas a 5–10 mm distance is suspicious

(2) Eyebrows

69. What is the significance of thinning or absence of the lateral eyebrows?

It is a traditional sign of *hypothyroidism* (often referred to as Queen Anne's sign from the name of a celebrity patient), but it also may be a normal variant. In addition, thinning of the eyebrows may represent personal cosmetic practices (such as plucking). Other etiologies include drugs, skin diseases, and lupus erythematosus.

(3) Eyelids and Orbit

70. What are *xanthelasmas*?

From the Greek *xanthos* (yellow) and *elasma* (beaten metal plate), these are yellowish deposits over the eyelids. Most patients have no lipid abnormalities, even though xanthelasmas are encountered in as many as 25% of type III hyperlipoproteinemias, and also in other more common types (such as II and IV). If representing a major cosmetic issue, they can be surgically removed.

71. What is an *ectropion*?

The *eversion* (i.e., outward rolling) of the lower eyelid, not uncommon in the elderly. This exposes a rim of tarsal conjunctiva to external stimuli, causing keratinization, corneal exposure, and eye irritation.

72. What is an *en*tropion?

The *inversion* (i.e., inward rolling) of the lower eyelid. This may mechanically irritate the eye through contact with eyelashes. Often due to trachoma, but also to simple aging.

73. What is a *sty* (hordeolum)?

A focal, *acute*, and painful inflammation of either hair follicle glands (*external* hordeolum) or one of the sebaceous meibomian glands in the eyelid inner margin (*internal* hordeolum). Usually infectious (with *Staphylococcus aureus* being responsible of >90% of cases), hordeolum presents with the typical findings of redness, swelling, and eyelid tenderness. Given the different location, internal hordeola suppurate on the eyelid's conjunctival surface, whereas external hordeola exude mostly from the eyelash rim.

74. **What is a *chalazion*?**
A painless and slowly enlarging eyelid nodule, due to *subacute* inflammation of the meibomian glands. This is a sequela of *blepharitis*, eventually causing glands' obstruction by secretions, with formation of a lipogranulomatous cyst. Chalazions differ from hordeola insofar as they are slower and painless processes. They may spontaneously disappear, although usually they require treatment—even slower and excision.

75. **What is *blepharitis*?**
A diffuse inflammation of the eyelid margin, which becomes swollen, crusted, erythematous, and tender. Due to *S. aureus* (or *S. epidermidis*), blepharitis also may have a hypersensitivity component. There is often ciliary cuffing and a dry eye sensation.

76. **What is *ptosis*?**
It is the unilateral or bilateral drooping of the upper eyelid (from the Greek term for *falling*). This is usually due to neurogenic or myogenic causes.

77. **What are the causes of ptosis? How can they be differentiated?**
The most common are *myogenic* reasons, such as (1) aging, (2) surgery, (3) trauma, and (4) congenital ptosis. The less common, but more ominous, are instead *neurogenic* reasons, and include (1) myasthenia gravis, (2) Horner's syndrome, and (3) third-nerve palsy. Less common reasons usually can be identified by their associated clinical findings, such as ophthalmoplegia and diplopia (third-nerve palsy), myosis (Horner's syndrome), and weakness (myasthenia). Overall, an isolated ptosis does not need to be referred, but a ptosis with diplopia, myosis, or weakness has to be.

78. **What is *proptosis*?**
From the Greek term for falling *forward,* proptosis (or exophthalmos) is the abnormal protrusion of one or both eyeballs. This, too, may be unilateral or bilateral.

79. **What is the most common cause of *exophthalmos in adults*?**
Graves' ophthalmopathy (Fig. 4-5). The next most common reason is a space-occupying lesion, such as a metastatic or primary tumor (benign or malignant). *Unilateral* exophthalmos is instead almost always due to a *tumor*. For other ocular manifestations of Graves' ophthalmopathy, also *see* Chapter 8, The Thyroid, questions 70 and 71.

80. **What is the most common cause of <u>unilateral exophthalmos in children</u>?**
Orbital cellulitis. Still, the most common *space-occupying lesion* responsible for unilateral exophthalmos in children is a rhabdomyosarcoma.

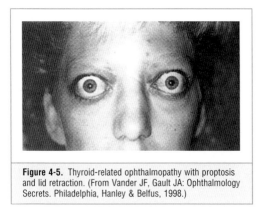

Figure 4-5. Thyroid-related ophthalmopathy with proptosis and lid retraction. (From Vander JF, Gault JA: Ophthalmology Secrets. Philadelphia, Hanley & Belfus, 1998.)

81. **What is the difference between *preseptal and orbital cellulitis*?**
    - **Preseptal cellulitis** involves only the eyelids, which are erythematous and swollen. Hence, the process violates neither the orbital septum nor its contents. Patients with preseptal cellulitis do not appear systemically ill. Vision, pupils, conjunctiva, and ocular motility are entirely normal.
    - **Orbital cellulitis** is instead a medical emergency, since it involves not only the eyelids but also the orbital contents. Patients look systemically ill and have a host of symptoms and signs, including (1) pain on eye movement, (2) erythema and edema of the eyelids, (3) conjunctival injection and chemosis (swelling), (4) limitation of ocular motility on the affected side, (5) proptosis, (6) decreased vision, and possibly, (7) an afferent pupillary defect.

82. **What is a *blow-out fracture*?**
    A fracture of the orbital floor (which is also the roof of the maxillary sinus). This may entrap the inferior rectus muscle, thus making the patient unable to fully look up or down and causing diplopia in those gaze positions. Orbital floor fracture also may damage the infraorbital branch of the trigeminus, thus causing numbness on the ipsilateral cheek.

83. **What is *en*ophthalmos?**
    The opposite of exophthalmos (literally, a falling *inward*). The eye is sunken into the orbit, rather than protruding from it. Enophthalmos may result from a large blow-out fracture.

(4) Extraocular Movements

84. **How valuable is testing of extraocular movements?**
    Valuable primarily when the patient reports new double vision. However, a subtle ocular misalignment of neurologic importance may be present even if the eye movements appear normal. These patients still merit prompt referral to the appropriate consultant. For strabismus and pseudostrabismus, *see* the *Corneal Light Reflex* (questions 119–123).

85. **What is diplopia?**
    It is double vision. Due to ocular misalignment, typically from paralysis of one or more of the external ocular muscles (usually because of lesions of cranial nerves III, IV, or VI, but also myasthenia gravis or extraocular myopathy; *see* question 89). Note, however, that more than one half of all diplopias actually have *no* cranial nerve lesions.

86. **What are the main forms of diplopia?**
    Three quarters are *binocular* (and thus resolve with occlusion of the "good" eye); one quarter is instead *monocular* and thus causes double vision in one eye that persists after the opposite is covered. Note that binocular diplopias tend to be much more serious than monocular diplopias, since they reflect a true neuromuscular misalignment of the eye. Binocular diplopias can be *esotropic* (when the involved eye is deviated toward the nose); *exotropic* (when the involved eye is deviated toward the temple); and *hypertropic* (when the involved eye is deviated upward). Finally, diplopia can be *horizontal* (when the two images are side by side) or *vertical* (when one of the two images is higher than the other).

87. **What is *hetero*tropia?**
    It is *strabismus* (i.e., a condition characterized by visual axes that are not parallel) (*see* later).

88. **What are the causes of *monocular* diplopia?**
    They are either *ocular* or *extraocular*.
    - **Ocular** causes may involve the eyelids (sty), cornea (astigmatism, keratitis), or lens (early cataract). They typically resolve by asking the patient to look through a pinhole card (which eliminates stray rays caused by abnormalities in the media).
    - **Extraocular** causes instead include problems with glasses or contact lenses and typically resolve by removing the lenses or adjusting the glasses.

89. **What is the approach to the patient with *binocular* diplopia?**
The first step is to recognize diplopias that are *not* due to cranial nerve lesions, but instead to eye muscle disease (15% of all binocular diplopias). These include (1) the diplopia of *myasthenia gravis* (which typically worsens with progression of the day and may be associated with ptosis); (2) the diplopia of *thyroid myopathy* (which typically occurs with other signs of Graves' disease, such as proptosis and lid edema–retraction lag); (3) the diplopia of *orbital fracture* (14% of all binocular diplopias) should be easily recognizable by the history of trauma; and (4) finally, presence of ptosis should suggest third-nerve palsy or myasthenia gravis, whereas presence of other neurologic findings would argue in favor of *supranuclear causes* (such as internuclear ophthalmoplegia and skew deviation, responsible for 7% of all binocular diplopias). Once these conditions have been eliminated, the physician should identify the weak ocular muscle(s) caused by *cranial neuropathy* (i.e., third-, fourth-, or sixth-nerve palsy), which is responsible for 40% of all binocular diplopias. Note that a third-nerve palsy can be the presenting manifestation of a posterior communicating artery aneurysm, which has suddenly expanded and is about to rupture (*see* questions 48 and 49).

90. **How can one identify the weak ocular muscle(s)?**
By asking the patient to track an object (usually the examiner's finger) across the eight cardinal directions of gaze: up, down, right, left, left up, right down, right up, left down. One rule that can help interpret this simple maneuver (and narrow down the search of the weak muscle from 12 to two) states that *diplopia (and strabismus) will worsen whenever the patient is looking toward the weak muscle.* Hence, if the weak muscle is the left lateral rectus, diplopia and strabismus will worsen when the patient looks toward the left (the same will occur if the weak muscle is the *right* medial rectus).

(5) Nystagmus

91. **What is nystagmus?**
An oscillation of the eyes on either the horizontal or vertical plane. It is characterized by both a quick and a slow phase and derives from the Greek term for *"nodding."*

92. **How do you classify nystagmus?**
Based on the direction of eye movement. Hence, nystagmus may be horizontal, vertical, and rotatory. Physiologic nystagmus is instead the quick-and-slow eye movement of travelers (typically *train* travelers), whose gaze is fixed on rapidly approaching objects, such as telephone poles. It is entirely normal and can be triggered by asking the patient to look at a rapidly rotating drum covered with vertical stripes (optokinetic nystagmus).

93. **What is the clinical significance of nystagmus?**
Congenital nystagmus often indicates a disorder of vision. *Acquired* nystagmus indicates instead dysfunction of the brain stem (cerebellum, vestibularis, or oculomotor system). Common causes are multiple sclerosis, tumors, medication toxicity, infections, and neurodegenerative and toxic-metabolic states.

(6) Sclera

94. **What are *blue* sclerae?**
The hallmark of *osteogenesis imperfecta*, Toulouse-Lautrec's alleged illness. Still, bluish sclerae may be seen in other patients, too, including 7% of anemics (and 87% of those with iron-deficiency anemia); 3% of Marfan's; and 15% of pseudo-pseudohypoparathyroids. Blue sclerae also may be encountered in healthy subjects. In fact, they are the norm in newborns and small children.

95. How much bilirubin is needed to produce *scleral icterus*?

It depends on the amount of natural light illuminating the patient's eyes. In bright daylight, one can probably detect icterus for bilirubin levels as low as 1.5–1.7 mg/dL. In artificial light, however, levels >4 mg/dL are necessary. The same is true for other areas of the body normally checked for jaundice, such as the roof of palate or the palm of the hands. Of note, the term "scleral" icterus is histologically inaccurate, and one that found its way into textbooks only during the mid-1940s, thanks to German studies published a decade earlier that had shown strong affinity of bilirubin for elastin. In reality, the sclera *per se* contains very little elastic tissue. Instead, it is the innermost layer of the *conjunctiva* (and its contiguous aspect of the sclera, i.e., the episclera) that has elastic fibers. Hence, scleral icterus is *conjunctival* icterus. As Osler had defined it in all the editions of his book: a yellow "tinting of the skin and conjunctivae."

96. Does conjunctival icterus look any different in dark-skinned patients?

No. It is important, however, not to interpret as icterus the brownish color normally present in the bulbar conjunctiva of dark-skinned individuals. This is usually the result of sunlight exposure and should not be confused with hyperbilirubinemia. To separate the two, ask the patient to look upward, then inspect the inferior conjunctival recess. This should be entirely white in nonicteric subjects.

(7) Conjunctiva

97. What is a pingueculum?

A small, rounded, and yellowish collection on the conjunctiva (from the Latin *pinguiculus*, fattish). This degenerative lesion of the bulbar conjunctiva is secondary to sunlight (actinic) exposure and is almost always found in the nasal canthus.

98. What is a pterygium?

From the Greek *pteros* (wing), this is an excessive conjunctival growth, more extensive than the pingueculum, but similar in etiology and histology (albeit more vascular). A pterygium probably starts as pingueculum, since they are similarly located over the temporal or nasal aspect of the bulbar conjunctiva. Both may result from long-term exposure to ultraviolet light and thus be more frequent in the Sun Belt. And both may cause mild irritation, dryness, and a foreign body sensation. Yet, if advanced, they can compromise vision, especially if growing into the visual axis and cornea. If removed, they often grow back.

99. What is a *subconjunctival hemorrhage*?

A well-demarcated hemorrhage in the subconjunctival layer. Although often an impressive sight (and a common cause of red eye, too), a conjunctival hemorrhage remains a rather trivial problem, destined to turn yellow in a few days and eventually resolve. Note that the redness of a subconjunctival hemorrhage is typically *confluent*, and thus easily distinguishable from other forms of red eye.

100. What causes subconjunctival hemorrhage?

Mostly trauma, but sudden increase in venous pressure (like a coughing spell) can do it, too. Yet many cases remain unexplained, usually reflecting defects in hemostasis or fragility of the vessel wall (from aging or diabetes).

101. How does *conjunctivitis* present?

With vessel dilation, and conjunctival swelling, and discharge. Discomfort (usually a scratchy feeling of sand in the eye) is common, but true pain is typically absent (*itchiness*, on the other hand, is typical of *allergic conjunctivitis*, which in contrast to the purulent or viral forms is always binocular). Vision is always spared.

102. **What is the significance of a palpable *preauricular lymph node*?**
It indicates *viral* conjunctivitis. It is just anterior to the tragus and usually tender.

103. **Can conjunctival discharge differentiate the various forms of conjunctivitis?**
Yes, since it is typically purulent in the *bacterial* forms, watery in the *viral* (or chemical), and stringy/white/mucoid (but overall scanty) in the *allergic ones*. Conversely, "pus" is so common in the bacterial forms that its absence questions the diagnosis.

104. **How can one differentiate the injected vessels of uveitis from those of conjunctivitis?**
By looking for prominent *pericorneal* vessels at the *limbus* (i.e., the interface between cornea and sclera). This phenomenon is known as "ciliary flush," and it is typical of uveitis (*see* questions 111–114). By contrast, conjunctivitis causes *diffuse* vascular prominence, plus a typical discharge.

105. **What is *chemosis*?**
It is edema of the bulbar conjunctiva. This may be severe enough to cause the conjunctiva to protrude anteriorly, thus encroaching on the cornea. From the Greek *chemos*, which means not only yawning but also cockle. Indeed, the opening of the affected eye is often reduced to a slit, like the gaping shell of a cockle. Chemosis is typical of allergic conjunctivitis.

(8) Iris

106. **What is *iris heterochromia*?**
A different pigmentation of the two irides. From the Greek *eteros* (different) and *chroma* (color), heterochromia is rare in humans, often suggesting ocular disease, such as chronic iritis or diffuse iris melanoma. Yet, it also may occur as a normal variant. In fact, Alexander the Great and Anastasios the First were both dubbed *dikoros* ("with two pupils") for their very visible *heterochromias*. Patches or sectors of strikingly different colors in the same iris are instead less rare (variegated iris), and in fact the norm in some species, such as Siberian huskies, Australian sheep dogs, and even horses.

107. **Can heterochromia occur in Horner's syndrome?**
Yes, and it usually indicates *congenital* Horner's, with the affected iris being lighter than the other; in *acquired* Horner's syndrome, on the other hand, heterochromia is rare to absent. Other less frequent causes include a ferrous intraocular foreign body, which causes the affected iris to appear darker, and Waardenburg syndrome (*see* Chapter 3, The Skin, question 123).

108. **Can iris color be used as a paternity test?**
Not really. There is no simple Mendelian inheritance in iris color. Hence, no valid paternity test can be based on it, except for being aware that blue eyes are usually phenotypically recessive, so that a brown-eyed child of two blue-eyed parents is a bit unusual but may still happen.

(9) Cornea

109. **What is arcus senilis?**
A stromal lipid deposition near the *limbus* (i.e., the boundary between cornea and sclera). This appears as a bilateral line in the peripheral cornea, starting usually as an arc (hence the name, *arcus cornealis*), but eventually growing into a complete *ring* around the limbus, with a clear and lucid zone separating the two, and a grayish/whitish color—occasionally yellowish.

110. **What is the significance of arcus?**
In subjects older than 50, it is probably minimal, since prevalence simply increases with age (arcus *senilis*). In younger patients, on the other hand, it suggests the presence of type 2 and 3 hyperlipoproteinemia, and thus a higher risk for cardiovascular death.

(10) Anterior Portion of the Globe

111. What is uveitis?
Inflammation of the uvea, the eye's middle coat (from the Greek *uvea* = grape). When the eye's *outer* coat (i.e., the sclera) is peeled away, the middle or vascular coat appears as a dark and grape-like layer. Inflammation of the uvea is usually autoimmune, occurring either in isolation or as part of a systemic rheumatologic disease.

112. How is uveitis classified?
As anterior, intermediate, and posterior. The anterior form also is termed "*iritis*" (if only the iris is involved) or "iridocyclitis" (if both the iris *and* ciliary body are involved). The intermediate form is sometimes called "pars planitis," and the posterior form "choroiditis."

113. What is a *ciliary flush*?
A congestion of conjunctival and episcleral vessels over the corneal rim. It is a feature of *anterior* uveitis, but also keratitis and acute glaucoma. Never seen in conjunctivitis.

114. What are the symptoms of uveitis?
It depends. In *anterior* uveitis the affected eye may have a smaller pupil, yet the predominant symptom is aching ocular pain and photophobia, often requiring the use of dark glasses. Uveitis is different from keratitis since its pain is unrelieved by topical anesthetics; it also is different from conjunctivitis since it has no discharge, and it is different from glaucoma since it has lower intraocular pressure. Note that *intermediate or posterior* uveitis causes *no* pain but rather blurred vision and *floaters* (*see* also questions 139 and 226).

115. What is a *hypopyon*?
A layer of white cells (in Greek *pyon*, pus) in the bottom (in Greek *upo*, lower) of the anterior chamber. This may be seen in infectious processes (such as endophthalmitis after cataract surgery) and *non*infectious inflammatory conditions (such as Behçet's disease).

116. What is a hyphema?
It is blood in the *anterior chamber*, typically from trauma (from the Greek *hyphaimos*, suffused with blood). When bleeding is significant, blood can even be seen with a penlight, as a dark red layer in the inferior portion of the anterior chamber (*see* also question 132).

117. What is an eight-ball hyphema?
A hyphema that entirely fills the anterior chamber, so that the eye appears black like an eight-ball. This does not clear with conservative management but requires evacuation.

118. What is the value of gauging the depth of the anterior chamber with a penlight?
Little. This procedure is extremely inaccurate without special instruments like a slit lamp biomicroscope. Fortunately, very few patients have anterior chamber depths shallow enough to predispose to acute angle closure glaucoma. Hence, it is safe to dilate the pupils without making any attempt to gauge the depth of the anterior chamber.

(11) Corneal Light Reflex

119. What is the corneal light reflex?
The reflection of light shone onto the cornea. If the corneal surface is normal, the reflex will appear as a clear white spot, with smooth and round borders. If the surface is *not* smooth (because of scarring, drying, or edema), the reflection will be irregular or broken up.

120. **What is the *Hirschberg test*?**
   A bedside assessment of ocular alignment, devised by the Baltimore neurologist Leonard K. Hirschberg. To carry it out, ask the patient to fixate a light at a distance of 2–3 feet. Then see whether the corneal light reflex is deviated from the center of the pupil in one eye or both. If so, the eyes are misaligned.

121. **What is strabismus?**
   A misalignment of the eyes. *Congenital* strabismus is often uncertain in origin, whereas the *acquired* form is due to cranial nerve dysfunction, neuromuscular disease, or myopathy.

122. **What is *pseudo*strabismus?**
   An *apparent,* but not true, misalignment of the eyes. This often arises in children with prominent epicanthal skin folds that obscure part of the nasal sclera, thus making the eyes look like they are turned in.

123. **How do you tell strabismus from pseudostrabismus?**
   By examining the corneal light reflection in both eyes (Hirschberg test). If the reflection is centered in the two eyes, then the diagnosis is *pseudostrabismus.*

F. OPHTHALMOSCOPY

124. **Is ophthalmoscopy an important skill?**
   It is a *fundamental* skill. Practice, as always, is paramount.

(1) Technique

125. **What is the clinical value of ophthalmoscopy?**
   Tremendous. If properly used, ophthalmoscopy provides outstanding information about the various structures of the fundus, such as (1) the anterior end of the optic nerve (optic disc), and (2) the retina and its blood supply (retinal vessels and choroids). Ophthalmoscopy also helps to evaluate the *red reflex*, thus providing information on all clear media of the eye, such as (1) cornea, (2) anterior chamber, (3) lens, and (4) vitreous.

126. **Who should undergo ophthalmoscopy? When?**
   All comprehensive examinations should include ophthalmoscopy, especially in patients (1) complaining of altered vision, (2) older than 40 (because of the higher incidence of glaucoma with age), (3) suffering from neurologic disorders that may lead to increased intracranial pressure, or (4) with systemic diseases (such as diabetes and hypertension) that may be associated with vascular degeneration.

127. **How does one perform ophthalmoscopy?**
   By dimming room lights and dilating the patient's pupils. Contact lenses may stay in place, but glasses should always be removed (including your own). As patients gaze at a target straight ahead, approach their eyes from the temporal side (never from the front). This is necessary to avoid direct (and painful) stimulation of the macula. Look into the patient's *right* eye by holding the ophthalmoscope in your right hand and using your right eye. Afterwards, view the patient's left eye by using your left eye (and left hand).

128. **How close should one get?**
   Start 2–3 feet away from the eye, so that you can visualize the red reflex and any abnormalities of the clear media. For proper viewing of the fundus, you should follow Robert Capa, the famous World War II photographer who once said, "If a picture is not good enough, it is because you did not get close enough." Hence, to adequately see the fundus, get as close to the patient as possible. In fact, if you are not uncomfortably close, you are not close enough. As a measure of proximity, place your hand on the patient's forehead, and then touch your

hand with your head. While doing so, continuously adjust the focus of your ophthalmoscope, dialing the knob until the retina is in focus. Then, follow the vessels inward (using the natural "arrows" formed by their bifurcations), until they merge into the optic disc. Departing from the optic disc, explore the four quadrants of the eyeground (superior temporal, superior nasal, inferior nasal, and inferior temporal). Finally, examine the macula. Remember that ophthalmoscopy is a dynamic process, requiring continuously refocusing and repositioning.

129. **What is the best way to examine the macula?**
The traditional method consists in asking patients to look *into the light*. Yet this is not only painful (it causes intense photophobia) but also wrong, since the corneal glare is so bright that it interferes with macular inspection. Instead, approach the macula from the disc, by rotating the ophthalmoscope a few degrees temporally. Since this area is light sensitive (and its inspection always a bit painful), examine it at the end, and quickly.

130. **How can one dilate the pupils?**
By applying mydriatics. The two most commonly used are *tropicamide* (Mydriacyl), 0.5% or 1%, and *phenylephrine* (Neo-Synephrine), 2.5%. Phenylephrine *10%* is no longer used because it may raise blood pressure or cause arrhythmias.

131. **Do mydriatics have systemic effects?**
Yes. All topically administered ophthalmic drugs are absorbed into the systemic circulation via the conjunctival, lacrimal, nasal, or oropharyngeal mucosa. Hence, the hypertensive effects of phenylephrine, an alpha$_1$-adrenergic agonist. If concerned about a cardiovascular reaction, use *tropicamide* (a short-acting antimuscarinic agent).

132. **Are there any *local* contraindications to dilation of the pupils?**
Very few. The *absolute* contraindication is the need to monitor pupillary signs in patients with suspected neurologic disease or trauma. Another one is the presence of an old intraocular lens implant in patients who have undergone cataract extraction (such implants, no longer used, were supported by the iris and thus tended to dislocate after pharmacologic mydriasis). A *relative* contraindication is narrow-angle glaucoma. Yet the precipitation of an attack of acute angle closure glaucoma may actually *help* a previously undiagnosed patient, since it may unmask an important but treatable condition.

(2) Red Reflex

133. **What is the red reflex?**
It is light being reflected by the retina, "red" because of its rich vascular supply. It looks like the red eye of flash photography. It is important clinically because it indicates transparency of all light-transmitting media.

134. **How is the red reflex viewed?**
Through an ophthalmoscope, by observing the pupils from a distance of 1–2 feet, focusing the instrument until a bright red pupil is clearly visualized.

135. **What is *leukocoria*?**
From the Greek *leukos* (white) and *core* (pupils), this is a condition characterized by total loss of the red reflex—hence, a *white* pupil. In children, it usually indicates a serious underlying condition, like a retinoblastoma, even though it also might result from a cataract, severe intraocular inflammation, retinopathy of prematurity, and other congenital lesions. Leukocoria also can be seen in retinal detachment. Its detection should prompt immediate referral to an ophthalmologist.

136. **What common conditions may cause an *abnormal* red reflex?**
All those causing opacity in the light-transmitting media of the eye. Of these, the most common affect *anterior eye structures* (lens or cornea). Posterior opacities are instead rare.

(3) Anterior Eye Structures

137. What are the most common opacities of the anterior eye?
Those affecting the crystalline lens, called *cataracts*. Corneal opacities, such as scars or abrasions, are instead much less common.

(4) Posterior Eye Structures

138. What is the *vitreous*?
A clear, gel-like substance (consisting of hyaluronic acid, collagen, and water) that fills the cavity between lens and retina.

139. What are the most common *opacities* of the vitreous?
Hemorrhages and white blood cell clusters. A *vitreous hemorrhage* usually results from *proliferative retinopathy* (due to diabetes, hypertension, blood dyscrasias like thrombocytopenia and sickle cell disease, retinopathy of prematurity, and many other conditions) or from *tearing of a retinal vessel*. It may appear acutely and be either massive (totally obliterating the red reflex) or subtle (consisting of only a few erythrocytes, presenting usually as "floaters" in the vitreous gel). A vitreous hemorrhage is a reason for immediate referral to an ophthalmologist because it may accompany serious disorders, such as *retinal detachment*. White blood cell clusters result instead from inflammation of the choroid or retina, and may be part of an intraocular infection.

140. After visualization of the red reflex, which eye structures should be examined?
The optic disc, retinal blood vessels, retinal background, and macula.

G. OPTIC DISC

141. What is the optic disc?
It is the point where axons of retinal ganglion cells form the optic *nerve* (nerve head).

142. How does one find the optic disc?
By closely approaching the patient's eye while focusing the ophthalmoscope on the retina. Then follow its blood vessels toward the disc. To find it, you may need to refocus throughout, and also rotate the scope slightly around its vertical axis.

143. In following vessels toward the disc, how do you know the direction is right?
By noticing that the caliber of the vessels *increases*. Another way is to follow the "arrowheads" formed by the bifurcations of the retinal vessels (Fig. 4-6).

144. What does a normal optic disc look like?
Like an oval, with sharp margins and a yellowish-pinkish color.

145. Are there any optic disc anatomic variants?
Some people may have a *hypopigmented crescent* surrounding the optic disc

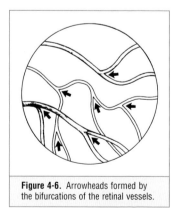

Figure 4-6. Arrowheads formed by the bifurcations of the retinal vessels.

(particularly in its temporal side, as commonly encountered in myopic patients). This is usually caused by the failure of pigmented layers (retina and choroid) to extend onto the optic disc margin. Other people may have an *excess* of pigment, which usually appears as a darker rim surrounding the disc.

146. **What is the optic *cup*?**
The whitish central excavation of the disc. It is also the site where the retinal vessels enter and exit the eye. The diameter of this physiologic cup should not be greater than 50% of the diameter of the optic disc. If greater than that, suspect glaucoma.

147. **What pathologic changes can be detected in the disc?**
Changes in (1) color (either pallor or hyperemia); (2) size of the cup (i.e., cupping, as in glaucoma); (3) elevation of the disc (papilledema or papillitis); and (4) the presence or absence of retinal venous pulsations.

(1) Changes in Color

148. **What causes *redness* of the disc?**
Vascular engorgement, due to retinal vein occlusion, papilledema, or polycythemia. Redness also may result from neovascularization of the disc.

149. **What causes *pallor* of the disc?**
Usually the death of retinal ganglion cells' axons. The paleness is due to loss of supplying blood vessels, which, no longer needed after the axons' demise, die too.

150. **Does pallor of the disc always suggest a disorder of the optic nerve?**
No. It often represents a normal variant, particularly in myopic eyes.

> **Pearl:**
> A diagnosis of unilateral disc neuropathy should be based not only on presence of pallor, but also on abnormal *function* (decreased visual acuity, visual field defect, or afferent pupillary defect).

151. **What are the common causes of *optic atrophy*?**
Conditions causing damage to the retina, optic disc, optic nerve, optic chiasm, or optic tracts, which eventually result in axonal death. These include (1) previous optic neuritis (such as that of multiple sclerosis); (2) previous ischemic optic neuropathy (e.g., from temporal arteritis); (3) compression of the nerve by a mass (tumor, meningioma, or aneurysm); and (4) drug toxicity or toxins (e.g., ethambutol, ethylene glycol, methanol).

(2) Changes in Cup Size

152. **What is the *aqueous humor*?**
The fluid produced by the ciliary body. This normally flows through the pupil, bathes the anterior chamber, and drains into the venous system via the trabecular meshwork and Schlemm's canal.

153. **What is the normal intraocular pressure?**
Between 10 and 21 mmHg.

154. What is *glaucoma*?
A condition characterized by inadequate drainage of aqueous humor at the trabecular meshwork, resulting in increased intraocular pressure. This eventually causes neuronal death in the optic disc, and thus, loss of vision.

155. Why "*glaucoma*"?
The term was first introduced to indicate the peculiar shining of the eyegrounds in patients blinded by the disease (*glaukos* means sparkling in Greek), as opposed to the eyegrounds' opacity (from loss of the red reflex) in blinding by a cataract.

156. What is *chronic* (or *open-angle*) glaucoma? What are its symptoms?
It is a different condition from acute (closed-angle) glaucoma, since the angle here is *not* closed, but simply not working well. This results in a slow drainage that is typically *chronic* and with *no symptoms in its early stages*. In this (most common) form of glaucoma, visual loss progresses *slowly*, compromising initially only the peripheral field, so that patients do not usually notice the deficit. Hence, the need to screen for glaucoma. The diagnosis is made by finding pathologic optic disc *cupping* (*see* question 159) and characteristic visual field loss. Elevated intraocular pressure also may be present.

> **Pearl:**
> A thorough funduscopic exam (coupled with intraocular pressure measurement and possibly visual field testing) is the only way to ensure an early diagnosis.

157. What are the symptoms of *acute* (or *angle-closure*) glaucoma?
Pain (because of increased intraocular pressure), nausea, abnormal visual acuity, and a red, teary eye. Patients may even have vomiting, and often report seeing *halos* around lights. Vision is usually foggy (because of corneal swelling). All these manifestations result from rapid build-up in intraocular pressure, as the iris blocks the aqueous outflow channel (the trabecular meshwork).

> **Pearl:**
> The visual complaint of halos (rainbow-colored fringes around points of light), due to corneal edema, is an important symptom for the diagnosis of acute glaucoma.

158. What are the eye *findings* in acute glaucoma?
Mostly a *red eye,* with decreased vision, a cloudy and hazy cornea with an irregular light reflex (all due to edema), injection of the deep conjunctival and episcleral vessels that surround the cornea (*ciliary flush*), and a pupil that is mid-dilated and unresponsive. All these findings are due to extremely high intraocular pressure, causing the globe to feel rock-hard on palpation. The mid-dilated, unresponsive pupil is a very important sign. In fact, a briskly reactive pupil argues strongly against the diagnosis of acute angle closure glaucoma.

159. How does the *optic disc* look in glaucoma?
It has an abnormally increased cup-to-disc ratio, a phenomenon commonly referred to as *pathologic cupping*. In the normal disc, the diameter of the physiologic cup should be <50% that of the entire optic disc. Anything greater suggests pathologic cupping. This usually extends in a vertical or oblique direction (hence creating an *oval* cup), and it is due to chronic compression of the optic nerve head. Asymmetry between the two eyes' cupping is also common.

> **Pearl:**
> An optic cup >50% the entire disc diameter is suggestive of glaucoma until proven otherwise. A cup >70% strongly suggests the diagnosis.

160. How accurate is funduscopy in diagnosing glaucoma?
It depends on the examiner's skills. Studies have shown sensitivities and specificities of, respectively, 48–89% and 73–93%.

161. Who should be screened for glaucoma?
The American Academy of Ophthalmology recommends screening by an ophthalmologist as follows: (1) age 65 or older, every 1–2 years; (2) age 40–64, every 2–4 years; (3) age 20–39 (African Americans, in whom glaucoma has higher incidence and earlier onset), every 3–5 years. Others can be screened less frequently.

162. What is the utility of Schiotz tonometry?
It is no longer recommended in glaucoma screening, since it produces inaccurate results unless frequently used. Moreover, many glaucomatous patients do not have elevated intraocular pressure. Monitoring of pressure should always be done by an ophthalmologist.

(3) Changes in Disc Size

163. What is papilledema?
It is the swelling (edema) of the head of the optic nerve (the optic disc or papilla) in a setting of increased intracranial pressure.

164. What are the fundus findings of papilledema?
(1) Blurred disc margins; (2) disc swelling, with narrowing/loss of physiologic cupping; (3) disc hyperemia; (4) peripapillary hemorrhages (splinter hemorrhages surrounding the papilla); (5) engorgement of retinal veins; (6) loss of spontaneous retinal venous pulsations; and (7) cotton-wool spots (nerve fiber layer infarcts). Not all are present.

165. What are *spontaneous retinal venous pulsations* (SRVPs)?
They are the visible collapse and refilling of the largest branches of the central retinal vein. SRVPs are usually detected where vessels emerge from the cup and cross the disc.

166. What is the clinical significance of *absent* SRVPs?
One fifth of normal people lack SRVPs; hence, their absence does not represent a significant finding. *Presence,* on the other hand, is much more helpful, since it suggests that the patient's intracranial pressure (ICP) is normal. Note that SRVPs cease whenever the ICP goes above 200 ± 25 mmH$_2$O. Thus, in patients suspected of papilledema (because of blurred optic disc margins), presence of SRVPs indicates a probably normal ICP.

> **Pearl:**
> Whereas papilledema may take 1–2 days to develop after a rise in ICP, SRVPs disappear in *seconds* (and return just as quickly after prompt management of ICP).

167. Is there any loss of visual activity in papilledema?
No. Unless the papilledema is long standing, visual acuity is usually well preserved.

168. **How important is papilledema?**
It is one of the most important funduscopic findings, since it reflects both life- and vision-threatening conditions. Hence, it should be identified by all practicing physicians.

169. **What are the most common causes of papilledema?**
Conditions associated with increased ICP, such as tumors, abscesses, meningitis, hematomas, subarachnoid or intracranial hemorrhages, and pseudotumor cerebri (idiopathic intracranial hypertension).

170. **What else can make the optic disc swell?**
Many entities cause the optic disc to swell *without* a concomitant increase in ICP. For example, swollen discs may be congenital (anomalous discs); due to local eye disease (e.g., central retinal vein occlusion); metabolic (e.g., thyroid ophthalmopathy); inflammatory; infiltrative (e.g., secondary to lymphoma); related to systemic diseases (e.g., malignant hypertension); or caused by local vascular problems (e.g., ischemic optic neuropathy).

171. **What is *optic neuritis*?**
An inflammation of the optic nerve. This may occur in isolation or as part of inflammatory disorders, such as multiple sclerosis. Its two forms are papillitis and retrobulbar neuritis.

172. **What is *papillitis*?**
A form of optic neuritis characterized by *visible swelling of the disc*. As in other optic neuritides, the chief complaint is *acute and unilateral loss of vision*, accompanied by eye pain, an *afferent pupillary defect* (due to the fact that one eye is more involved than the other; *see* questions 60–63), and an acquired impairment in color vision (i.e., *dyschromatopsia, see* questions 18 and 19).

173. **What is *retrobulbar optic neuritis*?**
An inflammatory condition of the optic nerve in which the inflammation occurs *behind the globe*. Hence, it is characterized by a scotoma (i.e., blind spot, from the Greek *skotos*, darkness) but *no* visible optic disc findings (no disc swelling). As with all optic neuritides, the retrobulbar variant also presents with impaired color vision and an afferent pupillary defect.

174. **What is *anterior ischemic optic neuropathy* (AION)?**
An infarction of the optic nerve head or disc. It is the most common cause of acute optic neuropathy in older age groups. It can be *nonarteritic* (nonarteritic anterior ischemic optic neuropathy [NAION]) or *arteritic*. NAION is not usually associated with life-threatening conditions, although it commonly coexists with various vasculopathies, such as hypertension (46.9%), diabetes (23.9%), and myocardial infarction (11%). Smoking may also play a facilitating role. Conversely, the arteritic form of AION is typically associated with a serious and much more ominous condition, giant cell (cranial) arteritis.

175. **What are the manifestations of AION?**
Acute, painless, and monocular loss of visual acuity, visual field cut, and an afferent pupillary defect (i.e., Marcus Gunn pupil) on the affected side. Loss of vision can often be complete and irreversible. Ophthalmoscopy reveals a pale, *swollen* optic nerve head. Dyschromatopsia also may be present (*see* questions 18 and 19).

176. **What causes AION?**
An infarction of the optic nerve head. This occurs most commonly in case of small vessel arteriosclerosis (i.e., the NAION of diabetes and hypertension), but in patients older than 65 it also may be due to *giant cell arteritis,* a granulomatous inflammation of medium-sized arteries. This is a particularly feared type of AION because visual loss is sudden, severe, and *unilateral* but eventually becoming *bi*lateral if unrecognized and untreated. Once blindness has occurred, there is no remedy. Hence the need for early detection. The triad of scalp tenderness, headache, and jaw claudication may often be the only warning symptom.

H. RETINAL CIRCULATION

177. What is the normal organization of the retinal circulation?
The retinal circulation includes branches of the central retinal artery and central retinal vein. The arterial branches originate at the optic disc, move centrifugally toward the four retinal quadrants, and distribute themselves in the superficial nerve fiber layer. The venous branches are arranged similarly but follow an opposite direction, converging *centripetally* toward the optic disc. Because there is a blood–eye barrier, just as there is a blood–brain barrier, retinal vessels autoregulate flow in response to changes in blood pressure, just like vessels in the central nervous system.

178. How can one differentiate retinal veins from retinal arteries?
Retinal veins are darker and larger than arteries (the normal vein-to-artery diameter ratio is 3:2). Arteries, on the other hand, have a more glistening light reflex.

179. Can the retinal arterial light reflex predict disease?
Yes. Changes in light reflex (and arterial width) may result from hypertensive changes or the arteriosclerosis of aging. As hypertension becomes more chronic, the anterior walls progressively thicken, causing the walls to reflect more light (increased light reflex), resembling at first copper wires and eventually silver wires.

180. What is *hypertensive retinopathy*?
The effect on retinal vessels of either acute or chronic hypertension. In poorly controlled hypertension, the vessels leak *serum* (hard exudates) and *blood* (dot, blot, and flame hemorrhages), eventually closing off and thus causing retinal microinfarcts (cotton-wool spots). In a hypertensive crisis, the leakage from optic disc vessels also may cause the optic disc to swell. In *chronic* hypertension, on the other hand, the arterial walls thicken, taking on first a *copper* and later a *silver wire* appearance. As walls thicken, they may indent and thus deviate retinal veins at arteriovenous crossings ("AV nicking").

181. Does AV nicking revert with control of hypertension?
No, it is permanent. Hence, it provides valuable and indelible information about the patient's medical history. AV nicking also may help understand the timing of a hypertensive disease. For example, since the changes take years to develop, a hypertensive patient presenting with renal failure *but no AV nicking* is more likely to have primary nephropathy with secondary hypertension than primary hypertension with secondary renal failure.

182. What are the manifestations of *central retinal artery occlusion* (CRAO)?
Profound and painless loss of vision in one eye. On funduscopy, there is retinal pallor and swelling, except for the macula, which appears instead cherry-red. This bright red spot is a diagnostic finding, caused by visualization of the preserved choroidal circulation through the fovea. The affected eye also demonstrates an *afferent pupillary defect*.

183. What are the causes of CRAO?
The most common is an embolus from the carotid artery or the heart, although giant cell arteritis or local thrombosis can do it, too, albeit less commonly.

184. What are the manifestations of central retinal *vein* occlusion (CRVO)?
CRVO also may cause an acute, painless loss of vision in one eye. Common fundus findings include (1) venous engorgement and dilation, (2) multiple intraretinal dot or flame hemorrhages splattered in all quadrants of the retina, (3) microaneurysms close to the retinal veins, (4) multiple cotton-wool spots, and even (5) optic disc edema.

185. **What causes CRVO?**

Usually a *central retinal vein thrombosis* at the level of the lamina cribrosa. This is often accompanied by atherosclerotic and hypertensive changes, but hyperviscosity syndromes (e.g., blood dyscrasias and dysproteinemias) also may cause CRVO.

186. **What are the funduscopic findings in *branch* retinal vein occlusion (BRVO)?**

Presence of flame hemorrhages and cotton-wool spots, *but only over the retinal quadrant corresponding to the occluded vein.* The vein distal to the occlusion is dilated and tortuous.

187. **What causes BRVO?**

Arterial compression of the vein (e.g., from *arteriovenous crossings*) is believed to be the main cause of BRVO. This would lead to turbulent flow, which, in combination with preexisting endothelial vascular damage (from hypertensive, atherosclerotic, inflammatory, or thrombophilic disease) would result in intravenous thrombus formation. Up to two thirds of BRVOs occur in the supertemporal quadrant, and the condition is not rare. In fact, retinal vein occlusions (branch and central) are the second most common retinal vascular diseases in the United States after diabetic retinopathy.

188. **What is a *Hollenhorst plaque*?**

A bright yellow, refractile arteriolar deposit usually wedged at the bifurcation of a peripheral arteriole (and thus causing a *branch* retinal artery occlusion). This often appears larger than the artery where it sits, and at times may even be seen migrating down the vessel. Migration may be facilitated by gently massaging the eyeball. It represents an arterial cholesterol embolus originating from the ulceration of an atheromatous plaque in a more proximal artery, usually the internal carotid.

189. **What is the clinical significance of a Hollenhorst plaque?**

It indicates severe generalized atherosclerosis. In fact, Hollenhorst patients are much more likely to die of stroke or myocardial infarction, with 10-year survival rates that are only half of age-matched controls. Hollenhorst plaques also are a complication of carotid endarterectomies, occurring in 14% of the cases.

190. **What is retinal *neovascularization*?**

The formation of new retinal vessels. It is always pathologic. New vessels tend to cluster around the disc but also may begin in the peripheral retina. They are often friable and may bleed into the vitreous.

191. **What conditions cause neovascularization?**

The most common is diabetes mellitus (*see* questions 216–222). In addition, other conditions that lead to retinal ischemia (such as hemoglobinopathies) also may cause neovascularization.

I. RETINAL BACKGROUND

192. **What retinal lesions can be identified by ophthalmoscopy?**

Three groups: (1) yellow-white spots, (2) red spots, and (3) brown-black spots.

(1) Yellow-White Retinal Spots

193. **What are *yellow-white* retinal spots?**

The most common types are (1) cotton-wool spots, (2) hard exudates, (3) drusen, (4) chorioretinal scars, and (5) myelinated nerve fiber layer.

194. What are *cotton-wool* spots?
Often misnamed *soft exudates,* these are round or oval patches on the superficial (inner) retina. They are white, ill-defined, and with indistinct borders. Since they are superficial, cotton-wool spots may obscure nearby vessels. They represent small retinal infarcts (and swellings) of the nerve fiber layer of the retina, due to microvascular disease.

195. What are the causes of cotton-wool spots?
Usually, conditions that damage the retinal microvasculature, such as (1) diabetes; (2) hypertension; (3) leukemias/lymphomas; (4) collagen vascular diseases (e.g., systemic lupus erythematosus); (5) infections (including bacterial endocarditis and, rarely, cytomegalovirus retinitis in patients with AIDS); (6) increased intracranial pressure with papilledema; (7) microembolic disease; and (8) severe anemia. As for the latter, cotton-wool spots are encountered in as many as one third of all patients with hemoglobin <7 gm/dL.

196. What are *hard* exudates?
They are small, yellowish/whitish, and well-demarcated retinal lesions. They are *deeper* in the retina than cotton-wool spots and are always due to microvascular retinal disease. As opposed to cotton-wool spots, however, they are not produced by microinfarcts, but instead by leaky and damaged vessel walls. Leakage of serum residues and various lipid aggregates eventually causes accumulation of lipoproteins in the middle retinal layers; hence, the waxy and often glistening look of these lesions.

> **Pearl:**
> Soft and hard exudates *always* indicate an underlying pathologic process.

197. What are the causes of hard exudates?
The same ones causing cotton-wool spots (i.e., processes affecting the retinal microvasculature, such as [1] diabetes and [2] hypertension).

198. What are *drusen*?
From the German term for *geode* (due to their glittering appearance), drusen are discrete, round, and yellowish lipoproteinaceous deposits in the retinal pigment epithelium (RPE, Fig. 4-7). First described by Donders in 1854, they are a normal byproduct of aging, often located in the macular region, but rarely causing visual disturbances. Yet, when in great number and large size, they are the earliest finding of age-related macular degeneration. They are totally unrelated to *Optic Disc Drusen*, which are instead globular deposits located on the optic nerve

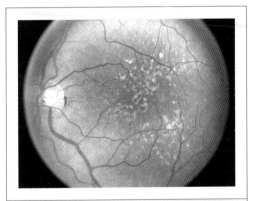

Figure 4-7. Drusen are the byproduct of retinal metabolism and manifest as focal yellow-white deposits deep to the retinal pigment epithelium. They serve as a marker of nonexudative, age-related macular degeneration. (From Vander JF, Gault JA: Ophthalmology Secrets. Philadelphia, Hanley & Belfus, 1998.)

head (optic disk), found in 1–3% of the population, made of mucoproteins and mucopolysaccharides, often calcifying, and possibly representing a clue to the presence of retinitis pigmentosa.

199. **What are *chorioretinal scars*?**
Lesions of the retina and choroid, but *not* of the sclera. They may result from inflammations, trauma, surgery, or laser photocoagulation, although more typically they are encountered as sequelae of toxoplasmosis.

200. **What are *myelinated nerve fibers*?**
They are congenitally myelinated (i.e., *medullated*) axons of retinal ganglion cells. Myelination of these fibers is normally present only posterior to the lamina cribrosa, but *not* on the retinal surface. Occasionally, however, patches of the nerve fiber layer *within the eye* become myelinated. These have a bright white color and varying size; they also have feathery borders and, since they are superficial, often obscure blood vessels. They represent a congenital variant, with no pathologic significance.

(2) Red Spots

201. **What are the most common red lesions of the retina?**
(1) Microaneurysms; (2) blot and dot hemorrhages; (3) flame and splinter hemorrhages; and (4) preretinal hemorrhages, including the subhyaloid variety.

202. **What causes *retinal hemorrhages*?**
Leaky and damaged retinal capillaries, as may be encountered in chronic microvascular diseases like diabetes.

203. **What other lesions may be associated with red spots?**
Yellow-white spots, especially hard exudates in the perimacular region. These are due to damaged retinal vessels, leaking not only *blood* (responsible for red spots) but also *plasma* (causing hard exudates—*see* questions 196 and 197).

204. **Why do red lesions have different shapes and sizes?**
Shape and size depend on the location of the hemorrhage:
- When the hemorrhage occurs in the *superficial (nerve fiber) layer* of the retina, it follows the orientation of nerve fibers and assumes a linear shape (*flame* or *splinter* hemorrhage). Red lesions of this type are most common in hypertension.
- When the hemorrhage occurs in the *middle retinal layer*, it obeys the vertical orientation of that part of the retina, assuming a circular shape (*dot* hemorrhage if the border is sharp, *blot* hemorrhage if indistinct). Red lesions of this type are most common in diabetes mellitus.

205. **What are *microaneurysms*?**
They are small, round, well-demarcated, red dots representing saccular outpouchings of the retinal capillaries (from the Greek *aneurysma* = dilation). They may be seen in association with other manifestations of microvascular disease and are almost always associated with diabetes mellitus.

206. **What diseases present with *dot-and-blot* hemorrhages?**
The most common is diabetes; but these lesions also may be encountered in (1) severe hypertension, (2) collagen vascular diseases, (3) infections, and (4) various hematologic disorders (leukemias or severe anemia).

207. **Which processes are associated with *flame* and *splinter* hemorrhages?**
It depends on location. When clustered *around* the disc, splinters and flames usually suggest a major ophthalmologic or neurologic emergency, such as (1) increased intracranial pressure with papilledema, (2) intracranial hemorrhage, or (3) poorly controlled glaucoma. When localized *outside* the disc, they have instead the same differential diagnosis of dot-and-blot hemorrhages, albeit linked more to hypertension than diabetes.

208. **What are *white-centered* hemorrhages?**
Red spots with white centers, often called *Roth spots* (even though Roth did not really describe them). They represent hemorrhagic microinfarcts of the retina with a fibrinous (e.g., whitish and pale) center. They are typical of endocarditis, even though they also may occur in diabetes, intracranial hemorrhage, anemia, thrombocytopenia, leukemia, and various infectious processes.

209. **Who was Roth?**
Moritz Roth was a Swiss pathologist (1839–1914) who studied and taught in his native Basel. In addition to his retinal spots, he wrote a well-received biography of the Renaissance pathologist Andreas Vesalius.

(3) Brown-Black Spots

210. **What are brown-black retinal lesions?**
Abnormal melanin proliferation. The most common pigmented retinal lesions are (1) retinitis pigmentosa, (2) retinal pigment epithelium hypertrophy, and (3) melanomas/benign choroidal nevi. Black borders often occur around the yellow-white lesions of chorioretinal scars (*see* question 199).

211. **What is *retinitis pigmentosa*?**
A degenerative disease of the retina. In the United States, 19% of all cases are autosomal dominant; 19% are autosomal recessive; 8% are X-linked; 46% are isolated, and 8% are undetermined. Only a few cases are due to known diseases and thus treatable. Among these is retinitis pigmentosa from vitamin A deficiency.

212. **How does retinitis pigmentosa present on funduscopy?**
With aggregations of pigment on the retina, usually arranged in a *bony spicule* formation. The pigment, however, may not always be present. In fact, 10% of the cases have no pigment at all. Note that bony spicules are usually in the midperipheral retina and thus difficult to visualize under direct ophthalmoscopy.

213. **What is *retinal pigment epithelium hypertrophy*?**
A congenital "grouped" pigmentation that results from hypertrophy of *pigment cells* in the retinal pigment epithelium (the same cells responsible for the red-orange color of the retinal background). Note that the color of the normal retinal background is also the result of choroidal blood and pigment. In fact, the darker fundus of pigmented races is due to the increased choroidal pigment of their fundi. Still, retinal pigment epithelium hypertrophy is often seen in Gardner's syndrome, for which multiple bilateral pigmented lesions have a 78% sensitivity and a 95% specificity.

214. **How does retinal pigment epithelium hypertrophy present ophthalmoscopically?**
With many (>4) and bilateral retinal pigmented lesions. These have different sizes and shapes and are never larger than an optic disc. Hence, they usually do not compromise vision. Their typical grouping resembles animal tracks (bear track lesions). Their number is key to the diagnosis of retinal pigment epithelium hypertrophy, since normal subjects never have more than four pigmented lesions. These are usually in the *peripheral* retina and thus difficult to see ophthalmoscopically.

215. **What are *choroidal melanomas* and *benign nevi*?**
- **Melanomas** are the most common malignancies of the eye. They appear as raised and highly pigmented and are often asymptomatic.
- **Benign nevi** consist instead of clumps of choroidal melanocytes, presenting ophthalmoscopically as flat, grayish/greenish pigmented lesions with indistinct borders. They do not compromise vision.

J. DIABETIC RETINOPATHY

216. What is the relevance of diabetic retinopathy?
It is the most severe of all ocular complications of diabetes. A major cause of blindness.

217. Is there any correlation between diabetic retinopathy and nephropathy?
A strong one. Diabetic nephropathy (i.e., the glomerular disease of Kimmelstiel-Wilson) is almost always associated with diabetic *retinopathy*. Thus, absence of retinal disease in patients with changes suggestive of diabetic nephropathy should call into question the very diagnosis. Conversely, patients with diabetic retinopathy may *not* have glomerulopathy, since retinopathy usually *precedes* nephropathy.

218. What are the findings of diabetic retinopathy?
It depends on whether the patient is in the earlier and preproliferative stage (previously referred to as *background*) or in the full-blown proliferative stage. The difference between the two is that nonproliferative changes occur *within* the retina, whereas proliferative changes occur *on* the retina (or *in* the vitreous). *Earliest signs* of nonproliferative involvement include *microaneurysms* and *dot* intraretinal hemorrhages, occurring in nearly 80% of type 2 diabetics after 20 years of disease and in nearly all type 1 diabetics of the same duration. Both lesions reflect *incompetent capillaries*, resulting in bleeding and exudate formation. Progression of *nonproliferative retinopathy* is then characterized by an increase in number and size of intraretinal hemorrhages (both *dot* and *blot*), often accompanied by *hard* and *soft exudates*. Eventually, patients will develop *venous beading* (retinal veins resembling a string of beads) and *intraretinal microvascular abnormalities* (IRMA) (i.e., new or preexisting tortuous vessels that are contained within the retina).

> **Pearl:**
>
> Microaneurysms are so typical of diabetic retinopathy that diagnosis should be considered until proven otherwise. Conversely, absence of microaneurysms argues against the diagnosis, even in the presence of retinal hemorrhages and exudates.

219. What is *proliferative diabetic retinopathy (PDR)*?
The most advanced stage of diabetic retinopathy. It consists of *chronic retinal ischemia* resulting in new vessel formation (neovascularization) on the inner surface of retina, optic disc, or vitreous (Fig. 4-8). If untreated, this may lead not only to preretinal or vitreous hemorrhage, but also to tractional retinal detachments. The new vessels appear tiny, irregular, and often with a fibrous component. They may

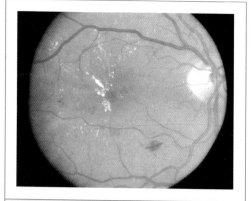

Figure 4-8. Background diabetic retinopathy with exudate, hemorrhages, and edema. (From Vander JF, Gault JA: Ophthalmology Secrets. Philadelphia, Hanley & Belfus, 1998.)

develop quite rapidly, even within 1 year after the initial appearance of an isolated cotton-wool spot. They often resemble the spokes of a wheel, insofar as they radiate outward toward a circumferential vessel. Neovascularization of the disc carries a worst prognosis than new vessel formation in other areas. Yet, all patients with PDR are at risk of losing vision, and thus should be candidates for photocoagulation. Patients with diabetes should be referred at least once a year for ophthalmologic evaluation.

220. What are the *late* manifestations of PDR?
New vessels may extend into the drainage system of the anterior chamber angle of the eye, and thus lead to *neovascular glaucoma*.

221. What are the best predictors of proliferative retinopathy?
Intraretinal microvascular abnormalities, venous beading, and the extent of microaneurysms and hemorrhages. Soft exudates are not as predictive, and hard exudates even less. The extent of retinopathy at the initial visit is instead a good predictor of disease *progression* (and so is pregnancy, which accelerates progression). Note that all PDR changes can be detected by retinal examination. Yet, in the hands of generalists, ophthalmoscopy has only a 53–69% sensitivity, even when carried out with dilation (91–96% specificity; positive likelihood ratio [+LR] = 10.0). Since detection of proliferation is higher for specialists (particularly macular edema, which is almost never detected by the direct ophthalmoscopy of generalists), current guidelines call for referral of diabetics to an ophthalmologist, with frequency of follow-up to be determined by stage of disease.

222. What is *macular edema*?
Another important manifestation of progressive diabetic retinopathy. It is characterized by the breakdown of the blood–retinal barrier, with leakage of plasma into the central portion of the retina (macula), resulting in swelling. Hence, patients will *not* lose vision entirely, but only its *central* component. Resorption of plasma *fluid* by the vessels (but not of lipoproteins and lipids) will subsequently lead to their deposition as *hard exudates*. In a large population-based study, the incidence of macular edema over a period of 10 years is 20.1% in type 1 diabetics, 25.4% in type 2 diabetics on insulin, and 13.9% in type 2 diabetics *not* on insulin. Tighter blood glucose control may decrease its incidence. Macular edema is almost never detected by generalists when using direct ophthalmoscopy; hence, the need for subspecialists' evaluation. Indirect clues to its presence include rings of hard exudates (often surrounding the edematous area) and diminished visual acuity. Note, however, that normal visual acuity should not rule out macular edema, since vision may often be spared.

K. RETINAL DETACHMENT

223. What is retinal detachment?
The shearing of the retina into two layers: (1) an outer one (composed of the retinal pigment epithelium), and (2) an inner one that represents the sensory retina. Embryologically there is only a virtual space between the two, yet under certain circumstances, this may actually widen, thus resulting in separations of the layers.

224. What are the causes of retinal detachment?
- The most common is a *degenerative tear in the sensory retina*, which, in turn, allows the entry of fluid from the vitreous cavity and subsequent separation of the sensory layer from its underlying pigmented epithelial layer.
- The second most common cause is *mechanical traction on the retina*, as in diabetics with PDR, whose contracting neovascular membranes pull the retina away from the retinal pigment epithelium.

225. **Who is at risk for retinal detachment?**
Usually middle-aged patients (peak incidence: 55–65 years), especially if severely myopic. Still, retinal detachment may occur at any age.

226. **How does retinal detachment present?**
With three "F's": floaters, flashes, and field loss. The most common initial complaint is the sudden appearance of *f*loaters (i.e., opacities that float in the vitreous of the affected eye). These represent either clusters of red cells released at time of retinal tear or a fibrous condensation in the vitreous. Subsequently, there will be *f*lashes of light (i.e., phospheni, from the Greek *phos*, light, and *phaino*, to show). These "shows of light" represent mechanical activation of the sensory retinal layer, stretched by traction from the vitreous. Eventually, with progression of the detachment, a "curtain" will gradually obscure the vision (*f*ield loss). This may occur as early as few hours or as late as few weeks since the initial event (*see* Fig. 4-9).

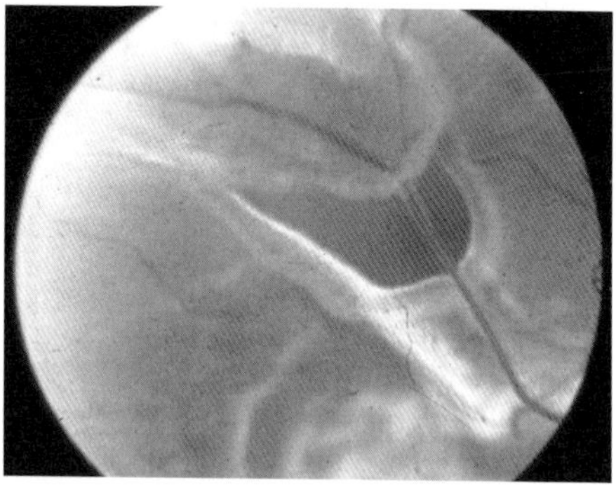

227. **What are the ophthalmoscopic findings in retinal detachment?**
It depends. If the entire retina is detached, there will be loss of the red reflex. Conversely, if only part of the retina is detached, the affected section will appear *whiter*, with fine folds on its surface. Most often, however, retinal detachment is difficult to visualize under direct ophthalmoscopy, except when performed with special instruments that allow better visualization of the peripheral retina (*see* Fig. 4-10).

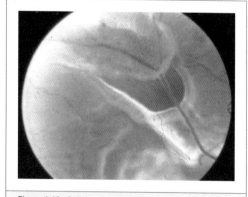

Figure 4-9. Horseshoe retinal tear with a bridging vessel. (From Vander JF, Gault JA: Ophthalmology Secrets. Philadelphia, Hanley & Belfus, 1998.)

L. MACULA

228. **How does a normal macula look?**
Like a little spot (*macula* in Latin). This is temporal to the optic disc and approximately one fourth its size, darker than the surrounding retina (macular cells are taller and more heavily pigmented), with small vessels converging toward it (but not entering it), and with a little dipping in the center (the *fovea centralis*). The central depression of the

Figure 4-10. Bullous rhegmatogenous retinal detachment with mobile, corrugated appearance. (From Vander JF, Gault JA: Ophthalmology Secrets. Philadelphia, Hanley & Belfus, 1998.)

fovea may function as a concave mirror and thus reflect the light of the ophthalmoscope (foveal reflex). In some people, the macula may even appear yellowish (macula lutea) because of the presence of a yellow retinal pigment. Note that the macula is the site of *central vision*.

229. What are the most common macular abnormalities?
In addition to edema (*see* question 222), they are drusen, hemorrhages, exudates, and scars.

230. What is *macular degeneration*?
The leading cause of severe visual loss in people older than 50, typically presenting with loss of central vision (which is concentrated in the macula) but preservation of peripheral vision. Thus, patients with age-related macular degeneration cannot read but can ambulate normally. Alternatively, they may complain of *metamorphopsia* (a distortion in perceived shape of objects—from the Greek *meta*, after; *morphe*, shape; and *opsis,* vision) or of *micropsia* (a reduction in perceived size of images—from the Greek *micros,* small, and *opsis*, vision).

231. How many types of macular degeneration are there?
Two major types: (1) a *dry* form, characterized by drusen and degeneration of the retinal pigment epithelium but no choroidal neovascularization, and (2) a *wet* form, characterized instead by formation of new choroidal vessels.

232. How does macular degeneration appear ophthalmoscopically?
- The **dry type** has drusen as precursors, followed by loss of pigment in the retinal pigment epithelium. This may be total, causing choroidal vessels to show through.
- The **wet type** is associated with thickening of the retinal pigment epithelium and a choroidal neovascular membrane, which appears as a gray-green area deep to the retina. Hemorrhage and exudates may emanate from the choroidal membrane, leading to a disciform scar in the macula.

M. RED EYE

233. What is a red eye?
A hyperemic (congested) eye. Vascular congestion may be due to involvement of any of the major ocular layers. Although a red eye is usually the result of trivial disorders, most commonly viral conjunctivitis. In a few cases, though, it may herald serious and possibly vision-threatening conditions. Hence, the need for a thorough evaluation.

234. What causes a red eye?
All the major eye layers, if involved, may produce a red eye. The most important are:
- **Conjunctiva:** Conjunctivitis, allergic, bacterial, and especially viral, is the most common (and usually benign) cause of a red eye. The same is true for *subconjunctival hemorrhage*. Note that allergic conjunctivitis is always binocular, while viral and bacterial conjunctivitis are often *monocular*.
- **Cornea:** Inflammation of the cornea or *keratitis* (from the Greek *keras*, horn or cornea) is also common but potentially a much more serious disorder. This is because *keratopathies* violate the corneal epithelium, enter the corneal stroma, and result in scarring that may cause blindness. This is common in herpes simplex keratitis, but also may occur in Graft-versus-host disease, and also in conditions producing an excessive drying of the cornea (Sjögren's syndrome, rheumatoid arthritis). In herpetic keratitis a fluorescein stain of the basement membrane of the cornea (made possible by the injury of its superficial layer) will demonstrate the typical dendritic ulcer. Finally, a surface keratopathy may also result from *corneal abrasion*, its classic symptom being a foreign body sensation.
- **Episclera:** Episcleritis is inflammation of the connective tissue between the sclera and conjunctiva. It is a less-common and usually benign condition.

- **Sclera:** Inflammation of the sclera (scleritis) is also less common but more serious. It usually indicates an underlying systemic process, such as connective tissue disease.
- **Iris and ciliary body:** These structures belong to the *uvea*, the synovium of the eye. The iris represents its anterior region, the ciliary body its intermediate, and the choroid its posterior. Acute iridocyclitis (from the Greek *irid*, iris, and *kyklos*, circle or ciliary body) is inflammation of both the iris *and* ciliary body. *Photophobia* is the hallmark of uveitis (like in keratopathy, but without the foreign body sensation). The iris is typically irregular, because adherent through synechiae to the lens (*see* question 235), and there may even be residual blindness, especially when the *choroid* is involved (posterior uveitis). *Anterior* uveitis may instead result in glaucoma. Overall, uveitis can be part of a systemic disease (like sarcoidosis), but it is much more commonly idiopathic and recurrent.
- **Adnexal structures:** This may include a tear or sebaceous glands. Dacryocystitis and sties are common disorders.

> **Pearl:**
>
> In addition to the previously mentioned conditions, a red eye should always prompt consideration of *acute angle-closure glaucoma* (*see* questions 157–160).

235. **What other ocular *signs* may accompany a red eye?**
The most important include the following:
- **Ciliary flush.** This is dilation or hyperemia (which ophthalmologists refer to as "injection") of the deep conjunctival and episcleral and pericorneal vessels, which appear as a deep red ring encircling the cornea. Ciliary flush is a serious sign, usually indicating one of three disorders: (1) iridocyclitis, (2) acute glaucoma, or (3) keratitis. It is typically absent in more benign conditions, such as conjunctivitis. Hence, always refer it.
- **Corneal opacities.** These are always serious findings in patients with a red eye. Corneal opacities may be either *localized* (as in keratitis or corneal ulcers) or *diffuse* (as in acute glaucoma, in which the edema of the cornea creates a haze that obscures the iris). They also may result from cellular deposits on the cornea (as in iridocyclitis).
- **Disruption of the corneal epithelium.** This is usually the result of trauma. Corneal abrasions are easily visualized under cobalt blue light and after application of fluorescein. They can even be detected by noticing a distortion of the corneal light reflex.
- **Anisocoria.** This is usually a sign of iridocyclitis, and overall argues in favor of more serious disease (such as corneal abrasion or foreign body, keratitis, and uveitis), rather than benign processes (such as conjunctivitis—19% sensitivity, 97% specificity, +LR 6.5, and −LR 0.8. The pupil of the involved eye is *smaller* (because of a reflex constriction of the iris sphincter muscle) and may be distorted (because of inflammatory adhesions between lens and iris).
- **Proptosis.** This is usually a serious sign, indicating swelling or a mass in the orbit or cavernous sinus.
- **Eye discharge.** This is instead a *benign* finding, most commonly associated with a process such as conjunctivitis. A watery, clear discharge usually indicates *viral* conjunctivitis, whereas a purulent discharge is the hallmark of a bacterial etiology.
- **Preauricular lymph node enlargement.** This is much more common in *viral* than bacterial conjunctivitis. Hence, it may provide a clue to the etiology of the process.

236. **What other ocular *symptoms* may accompany a red eye?**
Several symptoms may be present in patients with a red eye. Five important ones almost always indicate serious ocular emergencies:
- **Blurred or reduced vision.** This is always absent in conjunctivitis but frequently present in disorders such as keratitis, iridocyclitis, or acute glaucoma. The key maneuver is to have

the patient blink. An improvement in vision indicates the cleaning of inflammatory debris from the cornea (as in the case of conjunctivitis), whereas persistent blurring indicates a much more serious disorder.

- **Pain.** This is always absent in conjunctivitis (in which patients usually complain of a scratchy, itchy feeling but never of pain) but common in three serious conditions associated with ciliary flush: keratitis, iridocyclitis, or acute glaucoma. Conversely, *itchiness* is so typical of allergic conjunctivitis to become almost a sine qua non.
- **Halos.** These are indicative of corneal edema, usually resulting from a sudden increase in intraocular pressure (as in acute glaucoma). Patients with this complaint describe a rainbow-like ring surrounding a point of light (i.e., the halo).
- **Photophobia.** This is also absent in conjunctivitis but common in serious conditions like iritis.
- **Mid-dilated and unreactive pupil.** This is typically associated with acute angle closure glaucoma.

ACKNOWLEDGMENT

The author gratefully acknowledges the contributions of Sylvia R. Beck, MD, and Richard Tipperman, MD, to this chapter in the first edition of *Physical Diagnosis Secrets*. He also wishes to express his thanks to Dr. Jonathan Trobe for his kind and helpful review of the current edition.

SELECTED BIBLIOGRAPHY

1. Aiello LM, Cavallerano J: Diabetic retinopathy. Curr Ther Endocrinol Metab 6:475–485, 1997.
2. Alio J, Hernandez I, Millan A, et al: Pupil responsiveness in diabetes mellitus. Ann Ophthalmol 21:132–137, 1989.
3. American Diabetes Association: Diabetic retinopathy. Diabetes Care 21:547–549, 1998.
4. Buxton MJ, Sculpher MJ, Ferguson BA, et al: Screening for treatable diabetic retinopathy: A comparison of different methods. Diab Med 8:371–377, 1991.
5. Capo H, Warren F, Kupersmith MJ: Evolution of oculomotor nerve palsies. J Clin Neuroophthalmol 12:12–15, 1992.
6. Cogan DG, Mount HTJ: Intracranial aneurysms causing ophthalmoplegia. Arch Ophthalmol 70:757–771, 1963.
7. Dacso CC: The Argyll Robertson pupil in clinical medicine. Am J Med 86:199–202, 1989.
8. David NJ: Optokinetic nystagmus: A clinical review. J Clin Neuroophthalmol 9:258–266, 1989.
9. Early Treatment Diabetic Retinopathy Study Research Group: Fundus photographic risk factors for progression of diabetic retinopathy. Ophthalmology 98:823–833, 1991.
10. Enyedi LB, Dev S, Cox TA: A comparison of the Marcus Gunn and alternating light tests for afferent pupillary defects. Ophthalmology 105:871–873, 1998.
11. Federman J, Gouras P, Schubert H, et al: Retina and vitreousPodos S, Yanoff M (eds): Textbook of Ophthalmology Vol. 9. St. Louis, Mosby, 1991.

CHAPTER 5

THE EAR

Salvatore Mangione, MD

> *"People need to have things trumpeted into their ears several times and from all directions—the first sound pricks up the ear, the second shakes it, and with the third it goes in."*
> —René Théophile Hyacinthe Laennec, 1821; letter to his cousin Menadec

> *"The ears should be kept perfectly clean; but it must never be done in company. It should never be done with a pin, and still less with the fingers but always with an ear-picker."*
> —St. John Baptiste de la Salle (1651–1719), *The Rules of Christian Manners and Civility, I*

GENERALITIES

The ear is an important site for physical examination; abnormalities may reflect either *local* or *systemic* disease. It also is an important sensory organ, whose function can be assessed (albeit in a rudimentary manner) with basic bedside tools.

1. **What are the components of the ear?**
   - External ear (comprising the auricle and the external auditory canal)
   - Middle ear
   - Inner ear
   - Nervous supply

A. EXTERNAL EAR

2. **What is the external auditory canal?**
   It is a 1-cm–long conduit, opening outside through the *auricle* and delimited inside by the *eardrum*. It is made by bone in its inner two thirds and cartilage in its outer third. The latter is also rich in sebaceous glands, ceruminous glands (responsible for the production of wax, or "cerumen"), and hair follicles.

3. **What is "wax" made of?**
   Of a combination of desquamated keratin, debris, and secretions by ceruminous glands (which, in turn, are responsible for the wax color). Usually soft and brownish, wax can also become abundant and inspissated.

4. **What is the best way to remove cerumen?**
   There are various schools of thought. The first relies on a number of proprietary substances, all purportedly able to soften the wax when instilled as a solution into the external canal. Another method relies instead on removing the cerumen *mechanically*, bit by bit through a metal loop. Its effectiveness depends in great part on the examiner. Our favorite method is to flush the canal with warm tap water using a syringe with a 14- to 16-gauge plastic IV catheter. Remember that wax removal is not easy, and serious complications (even hematomas) may result from inexperienced insertion of various wax-removing probes, especially the infamous cotton-tipped swabs—particularly if carried out by patients or their associates.

5. **What is the nervous supply of the external canal?**
   Mostly *trigeminal*—hence, exquisitely sensitive. Still, the innermost part of the canal is supplied by the *vagus* (and its stimulation may indeed cause a vagal response, often just a dry cough).

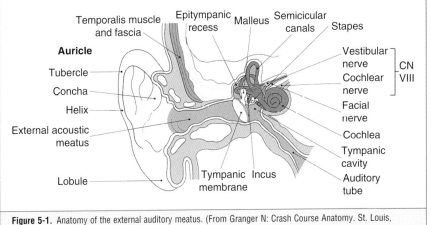

Figure 5-1. Anatomy of the external auditory meatus. (From Granger N: Crash Course Anatomy. St. Louis, Mosby, 2007.)

6. **What is the auricle (or pinna)?**
   It is the part of the external ear that is outside the canal (Fig. 5-1). Made of cartilage and skin, it is highly flexible.

7. **What are auricular bumps? What causes them?**
   Auricular papules or nodules are common. Most are benign, but some represent early neoplasms or clues to underlying systemic disorders. Specific etiologies include:
   - **Darwin's tubercle** (Fig. 5-2): Benign and congenital nodule near the auricular apex (on the helix, at the junction of upper and middle thirds). Nontender and rarely bilateral, it was first described by the British sculptor Thomas Woolner, a founding member of the Pre-Raphaelite Brotherhood and a spare-time anatomist. Woolner depicted it in his statue of "Puck," and Charles Darwin was so impressed that he named it the *Woolnerian tip*. It is an atavistic feature (i.e., a trait typical of our mammalian ancestors—more specifically, monkeys).
   - **Keloids** (Fig. 5-3): Smooth and flesh-colored papule(s) on one or both sides of the earlobe. They indicate an exuberant and fibrotic response to injury.
   - **Tophi:** One or more nontender nodules on the auricular edges. They are named after the Latin *tufa* (a calcareous and volcanic deposit) and may indeed be mildly hard. They can occur on both helix and antihelix, and usually indicate hyperuricemia and gout.
   - **Chondrodermatitis nodularis chronica helicis (CNH):** This is a common, benign, and painful condition of the most prominent projection of the ear, usually the apex of the helix, but it also may affect the antihelix. It is typical

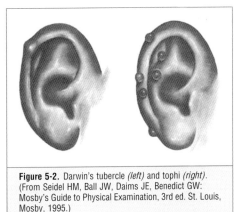

Figure 5-2. Darwin's tubercle *(left)* and tophi *(right)*. (From Seidel HM, Ball JW, Daims JE, Benedict GW: Mosby's Guide to Physical Examination, 3rd ed. St. Louis, Mosby, 1995.)

of the right ear of middle-aged to older men, usually fair-skinned individuals with cutaneous sun-damage. In 10–35% of cases, it may also affect women. It is rather common (in a series, the most frequent external ear condition seen in an ear-nose-throat clinic) and is probably due to prolonged and excessive pressure, leading to inflammation, edema, and ischemic necrosis. This eventually degenerates into *secondary perichondritis* due to the vascular characteristics of the ear. Onset may be precipitated by pressure, trauma, or cold. Sleeping on the affected side is also common. The nodule appears spontaneously and painfully, rapidly enlarging to a maximum size of 4–8 mm, after which it remains stable. It is firm, tender, skin-colored, sharply demarcated, and round to oval in shape. The edge is usually raised, with a central ulcer or crust. It is not associated with systemic disorders.

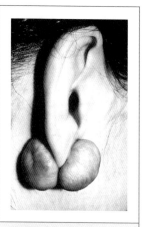

Figure 5-3. Keloids of the earlobe. (From Fitzpatrick JE, Aeling H: Dermatology Secrets. Philadelphia, Hanley & Belfus, 1996.)

8. **Can I really diagnose gout by looking at the ear?**

    Yes. Presence of tophi should prompt questions about *podagra*, *chiragra*, or *gonagra*—medieval monikers for monoarticular arthritis of the great toe, hand, or knee, a frequent nuisance of the well-fed (and drunk) aristocracy of old. Similar nodules over extensor surfaces of elbows, hands, or feet are also consistent with tophaceous gout. Since urate crystals precipitate more easily in colder areas of the skin, auricles and nasal cartilages are often the first tophi sites.

9. **What are the causes of itching of the ear?**

    Usually local disorders, often infectious (hence, use otoscopy). Still, *systemic* disorders may present this way too—for example, diabetes, hepatitis, or lymphoma.

10. **What is *otorrhea*?**

    It is diarrhea of the ear. In other words, the ear "runs" (which is indeed the meaning of *reo* in Greek). A discharge from the ear always argues for infection, either in the *middle* (see later) or *external* ear. These infections are often associated with pruritus and pain (otalgia).

11. **How can the color of the discharge provide clues to its origin?**

    - A *bloody* discharge suggests trauma or cancer.
    - A *clear and serous* discharge suggests leakage of cerebrospinal fluid—often posttraumatic.
    - A *purulent* discharge suggests either infection of the middle ear with perforation of the drum (otitis interna) or infection of the external ear (otitis externa).

12. **Why is otitis externa "maligna" so malignant?**

    Because it occurs only in patients with impaired neutrophil function from either quantitative or qualitative disorders (such as leukemia, poorly controlled diabetes, or treatment with corticosteroids and chemotherapy). This leads to a *Pseudomonas aeruginosa* infection that usually spreads directly into adjacent structures (causing a diffusely swollen and exquisitely tender auricle) and eventually spills into the bloodstream. If missed, it can cause gram-negative sepsis, shock, and even death. Hence, prognosis is guarded, and diagnosis/treatment imperative.

13. **What is instead garden variety "otitis externa"?**
Simple otitis externa per se is a rather common inflammation of the external canal, seen in subjects who suffer from eczema, psoriasis, or dermatitis, but also individuals with narrow ear canals. The skin can become so swollen as to close the ear canal and thus cause temporary deafness. It also can be so painful as to impede sleep. Discharge from the ear is usually scanty. Once again, the main symptom is *otalgia*—typically exacerbated by manipulation of the tragus.

14. **What is *swimmer's ear*?**
An otitis externa of swimmers, wherein removal of wax and maceration by water cause a common (but not serious) nuisance.

15. **How do you tell an earache due to otitis media from one due to otitis externa?**
By pulling up and down the auricle (or tragus). In otitis media, this is painless, whereas in otitis externa, it is painful.

16. **What is the value of pushing over the mastoid process?**
Tenderness suggests suppurative mastoiditis—an ominous complication of ear infections.

17. **Is otalgia always due to ear problems?**
No. Ear pain can be referred from other sites too—for example, the teeth, pharynx, and spine. In fact, any process affecting the territory of distribution of trigeminal, facial, glossopharyngeal, vagus, and even C2 and C3 cervical nerves can cause ipsilateral otalgia.

18. **Distinguish among *vesicles*, *bullae*, and *pustules***
Vesicles are blisters that contain clear fluid; *bullae* are blisters larger than 0.5 cm in diameter, and *pustules* are blisters that contain purulent fluid.

19. **What may induce vesicles in the auricle?**
Not too many causes: (1) severe *contact dermatitis* (such as poison ivy); (2) *varicella/zoster*; and (3) *Ramsay Hunt syndrome* (painful and vesicular rash of the inferior portion of the auricle, due to herpetic infection of the geniculate ganglion and treated with acyclovir. See questions 48 and 49).

20. **What are the causes of auricular *red spots*?**
   - **Trauma:** This also may result in auricular ecchymoses and even hematomas (see question 22).
   - **Port wine stain:** Usually congenital and of only cosmetic importance. One of the most famous port wine stains in history was on the forehead of Soviet President Michail Gorbachev.
   - **Sturge-Weber disease:** Port wine nevus on the upper part of the scalp, associated with intracranial vascular abnormalities that may cause cerebellar calcifications and seizures.

21. **Who were Sturge and Weber?**
William A. Sturge (1850–1919) was a native of Bristol, England. A devout Quaker, a passionate liberal, and a strong supporter of women's rights (including free access to medical education), he married a physician named Emily Bovell, with whom he shared a practice in London. An excellent speaker, teacher, and compassionate physician, Dr. Sturge contracted rheumatic fever at age 44, eventually abandoning medicine and moving to the French Riviera. Still, he found the energy to look after Queen Victoria during her four visits to France. After his second marriage to a young archeologist, he studied early Greek art and became the founder and first president of the East Anglia Society of Prehistoric Archaeology, collecting more than 100,000 archeologic pieces, which upon his death were donated to various museums. Throughout his life, he wrote only four medical papers.
Frederick Parkes Weber (1863–1962) is the English physician associated with Rendu-Osler-Weber disease. In addition to these two conditions, he also described Weber-Klippel syndrome and Weber-Christian disease. An enthusiast of physical exercise and an avid climber (like his father), he lived well into his 90s, spending the last part of his life collecting ancient coins and vases, which he eventually donated to the British Museum.

22. **What is a tender and swollen auricle?**
It is an uncommon but dramatic event. A diffusely swollen auricle is usually due to:
- **Trauma:** Easily identifiably by a history of recent altercation, especially if supported by other evidence of trauma, like a broken nose or a black eye. In fact, a "cauliflower" ear auricle is a time-honored occupational hazard of boxers, first portrayed in a beautiful Hellenistic statue of a resting fighter (Fig. 5-4). Unless evacuated, auricular hematomas heal with fibrosis and deformity and may even result in hearing loss. For instance, it has been suggested that Edison's deafness was the result of having been picked up by the ears as a child. Still, there is no evidence that he had a cauliflower ear. President Johnson, on the other hand, contributed to our advance in veterinary medicine by demonstrating that cauliflower ears do not occur in dogs, especially beagles. In fact, he used to pick up his pooch by the ears and then toss him around in front of the press corps. LBJ, however, had no ear problems we know of, with the possible exception of selective deafness to war protesters in nearby Lafayette Park.
- **Relapsing polychondritis:** May affect all facial cartilages, including the alar of the nose and the auricular of the ear(s).
- **Otitis externa maligna** (see question 12).

23. **Why should one palpate the pulse anterior to the tragus?**
Because this pulse, so often overlooked, corresponds to the *temporalis artery*, a branch of the external carotid. This supplies the lateral area of the scalp and can be compromised in polymyalgia rheumatica or temporal arteritis (a vasculitis of all branches of the external carotid). Hence, it must be palpated in all patients with proximal muscle weakness and jaw claudication, since tenderness of the vessel and/or nodularity may be an important diagnostic clue.

24. **Why should one inspect (and palpate) the *postauricular space*?**
To rule out *mastoiditis* in patients complaining of earache. In this case, there will be exquisite tenderness in the 1-cm crescent-shaped depression immediately behind the external auditory canal (and also on the mastoid tip, see question 16). In addition, there may be (1) a palpable *posterior auricular node* (presenting as a nodule in the area of the mastoid process); and (2) a positive *Battle's sign* (ecchymosis over the mastoid, most often due to trauma and indicative of basilar skull fracture).

25. **When does Battle's sign occur?**
It usually occurs approximately 48 hours after the traumatic event.

26. **Where are preauricular and postauricular *lymph nodes*? What may cause their swelling?**
The *preauricular* lymph node is immediately anterior to the tragus; its tender swelling usually reflects conjunctivitis or periorbital inflammation. The *postauricular* node is instead over the mastoid process; its tender swelling indicates otitis externa or mastoiditis.

27. **Can I diagnose coronary artery disease by looking at the auricle?**
Maybe. Earlobe creases in adults are an acquired phenomenon and thus different from the folds occasionally present in normal children or the congenital creases of newborns with Beckwith syndrome (gigantism, macroglossia, and umbilical abnormalities in a setting of hepatosplenomegaly, renal hyperplasia, and microcephaly). Still, the possible association between diagonal earlobe fissures and coronary artery disease was indeed described by the American Sanders T. Frank and then reported in the 1990s by William J. Elliott. In an 8-year study of 108 patients, Dr. Elliott found greater cardiac mortality rates in patients with a crease in at least one earlobe and suggested that loss of elastin could explain both crease(s) and arteriosclerosis. In a follow-up study of 1000 patients admitted to a medical service, he found that 74% of those with a crease had coronary artery disease as compared to 16% of the creaseless ones. Since then, more than 30 studies have found, with a few exceptions, similar results. Overall, except for Asians and Native Americans, creases appear to be a significant independent variable for coronary artery disease. They are associated with higher rates of

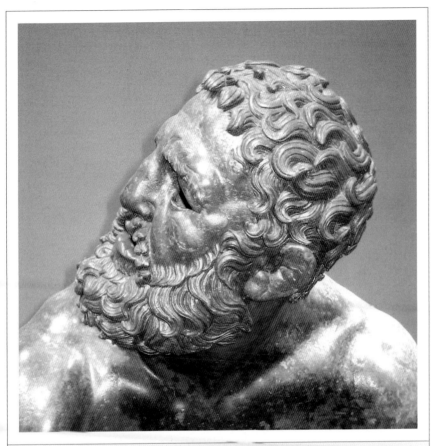

Figure 5-4. *The Resting Boxer* (Museo Nazionale Romano, Rome; photo by the author). Bronze seated statue of a battered fighter, with cauliflower ear and copper inlays to portray blood running from cuts. First century copy of an original second century work by Apollonius the Athenian. Found in Rome during the 1885 excavations of the once opulent Baths of Diocletian (300 AD). The Baths had fallen into ruin after the Goths destroyed the supplying aqueducts during their 537 AD siege. To escape being melted down for metal as all other bronze statues, the Boxer had been hidden beneath the foundations of Aurelianus' Temple of the Sun. Covered in finely sifted earth to avoid damage, he hybernated for 1350 years, until being finally brought to light, seated upright, and so dignified that Italian archeologist Rodolfo Lanciani wrote: "I have witnessed in my long career many discoveries. I have experienced surprise after surprise. I have sometimes, and most unexpectedly, met with real masterpieces, but I have never felt such an extraordinary impression as the one created by the sight of this magnificent specimen of a semi-barbaric athlete, coming slowly out of the ground, as if awakening from a thousand year–long sleep after long and terrible struggles."

cardiac events in patients hospitalized for suspected ischemia and are also significantly correlated with male gender, cigarette smoking, cardiac familiarity, hypertension, and age. In fact, some authors have suggested that skin creases and heart disease might simply share an equally higher prevalence in older subjects without being pathogenetically associated. Hence, the jury is still out on the subject. A related but even more interesting sign is *hair in the canal*, which also seems to be associated with coronary artery disease in retrospect, without any relationship to its pathogenesis.

28. **Why should a clinician auscultate over an auricle?**
Because it may reveal a bruit consistent with arteriovenous malformation of the carotid artery. In patients presenting with unilateral tinnitus (often paroxysmal and without associated vertigo,

nausea, nystagmus, abnormal audiogram, or magnetic resonance imaging of the posterior fossa), auscultation of the ear during episodes of tinnitus may reveal the bruit. Whenever the symptom disappears, so does the bruit. This is a clue that may require a magnetic resonance arteriogram or angiogram.

29. **How is auscultation of the auricle performed?**
By placing the diaphragm of the stethoscope over the auricle. Listen for *bruits* (clues to arteriovenous fistulas) and *crepitus* (clues to temporomandibular disease).

B. MIDDLE EAR (TYMPANIC CAVITY)

30. **What are the boundaries of the middle ear?**
The eardrum on the outside and the cochlea on the inside.

31. **What are the functions of the middle ear?**
1. To house the three auditory ossicles (so that they can transfer the mechanical stimulation produced by sound from the eardrum to the cochlea).
2. To connect with mastoid antrum and rhinopharynx. The latter connection is secured through the eustachian tube.

32. **What is the function of the Eustachian tube?**
To equalize pressure on both sides of the eardrum. Although usually closed, the "tube" serves this function by reopening upon yawning or swallowing (and, forcefully, through the Valsalva maneuver, which incidentally was developed by Antonio Valsalva exactly for this reason, since the stethoscope had not been invented yet).

33. **Does the middle ear house anything else?**
Two muscles, both of which are supposed to contract whenever loud noise requires some dampening of sound transmission: (1) *stapedius* (which attaches to the neck of the stapes and is supplied by the facial nerve); and (2) *tensor tympani* (which attaches instead to the malleus and is supplied by the trigeminal nerve).

34. **How can the tympanic membrane be examined?**
Through otoscopy.

C. OTOSCOPIC EXAMINATION

35. **What is the best way to otoscopically visualize the tympanic membrane?**
Ask the patient to turn the head slightly to the side. Then grasp the superior aspect of the auricle (the helix), and gently pull it up and out (i.e., posteriorly). This reduces the curvature of the external canal and eases the speculum insertion (if examining a child, straighten the canal by pulling instead the auricle down and back). These maneuvers may also elicit pain, thus alerting the clinician to inflammatory processes in the canal. Once this part has been completed, gently insert the speculum. To examine the right ear, hold the otoscope up in your right hand; to examine the *left* ear, hold it instead in your left hand. If cerumen obstructs the view, remove it (previously discussed). To minimize discomfort, always choose the appropriate speculum size.

36. **Other than cerumen, what else may prevent visualization of the tympanic membrane?**
- **Otitis externa (also called swimmer's ear):** Swelling and erythema of the ear canal (see questions 13 and 14).
- **Exostosis:** Bony protuberance(s) covered by normal skin and projecting into the canal's lumen making visualization difficult. Often bilateral.
- **Furuncle(s):** Exquisitely tender, erythematous, and inflammatory nodule(s) on the canal's wall.

37. How should the external canal appear otoscopically?
It should be neither red, nor swollen, nor tender. And, of course, there should be no foreign bodies. This is especially important in children.

38. What does the normal tympanic membrane look like?
As pale, gray, translucent, and surrounded by a ring (*anulus* in Latin). Always inspect it carefully, since this may be the site of tiny perforations. The normal tympanic membrane also includes visible projections of the *malleus* (hammer in Latin), the largest of the three auditory ossicles, and actually more of a "club" than a hammer. It comprises a head (caput), a neck (collum), and a handle (manubrium) (Fig. 5-5). From the base of the manubrium arises the short lateral process. The manubrium and lateral process are attached firmly to the tympanic membrane, with the lateral process projecting anteriorly and superiorly. The head articulates instead with a saddle-shaped surface on the body of the incus. Otoscopically the only visualized structures are (1) the short lateral process and the manubrium; (2) the umbo of the malleus (from the Latin *umbo*, boss of a shield, knob), which coincides with the head of the hammer and presents as an inferior and posterior projection through the tympanic membrane; (3) a reflective triangular cone of light, located inferiorly and anteriorly to the umbo; (4) the flaccid portion of the tympanic membrane (*pars flaccida*), located anteriorly and superiorly to the manubrium; and (5) the *pars tensa*, which is located just posteriorly to the manubrium. "Flaccida" and "tensa" reflect, respectively, areas of greater or lesser mobility of the tympanic membrane.

39. What are the distinguishing otoscopic features in *purulent* otitis media?
Purulent otitis media (usually bacterial) is more common in children than adults, where it presents with a rim of redness, prominent vessel dilation (injection), and outward bulging of the eardrum. Other findings include loss of markings for the umbo, loss of the light reflex, and decreased mobility on *pneumatic otoscopy* (see questions 52–54). At times, spontaneous perforation of the eardrum may cause purulent discharge into the canal. Symptoms include earache, fever (often quite high), and hearing loss of the conductive type.

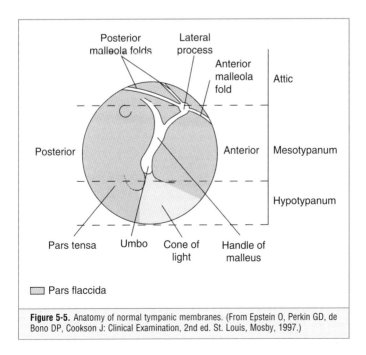

Figure 5-5. Anatomy of normal tympanic membranes. (From Epstein O, Perkin GD, de Bono DP, Cookson J: Clinical Examination, 2nd ed. St. Louis, Mosby, 1997.)

40. **What are the distinguishing otoscopic features in *serous* otitis media?**

Serous otitis media (usually viral) presents instead with an air/fluid level and at times even bubbles behind the eardrum due to retromembrane fluid, usually amber in color. Bulging from the fluid may lead to loss of the cone of light and retraction of the tympanic membrane. As a result, the malleus becomes prominent and white, while the eardrum acquires a yellowish hue. Symptoms include earache, low-grade fever, and conductive hearing loss.

41. **What does *bulging* indicate?**

Presence of fluid behind the eardrum, pushing it outward and causing loss of markings for the umbo and disappearance of the light reflex. This is a nonspecific sign of fluid accumulation, independent of its nature, which can be purulent or serous.

42. **What does "retraction" indicate?**

A drop in pressure of the tympanic cavity (i.e., the middle ear). This is usually due to obstruction of the eustachian tube.

43. **What is a *hemotympanum*? What are the other manifestations of basilar skull fracture?**

Hemotympanum is the presence of blood behind the tympanic membrane, usually due to a basilar skull fracture. It was first described by the English surgeon William H. Battle (1855–1936), along with a plethora of other signs of similar significance, including (1) Battle's sign (hematoma over the mastoid process; see questions 24 and 25); (2) periorbital ecchymoses; and (3) rhinorrhea and otorrhea (i.e., leakage of cerebrospinal fluid through the fractured planes).

44. **What does a perforation of the tympanic membrane look like?**

Like a hole in the center of the eardrum (i.e., pars tensa), with a diffuse and nonerythematous loss of tympanic membrane markings. The edges of the hole are usually smooth if the perforation was *traumatic* (in which case bloody material also may be present) and ragged if it was instead *infectious* (in which case pus may also be present). Traumatic or infectious ruptures can be easily differentiated from *iatrogenic* perforations (such as tympanoplasty tubes), since the latter have a plastic or metallic orifice in the inferior aspect of the eardrum, just below the tip of the umbo.

45. **What is *Angel's sign*?**

A finding described by Rick Angel in 1994, consisting of an otoscopy performed while the patient is blowing against a pinched nose. In case of a perforated eardrum, this maneuver elicits a rivulet of fluid (or pus) in the external canal, thus increasing the sensitivity of the exam.

46. **What does chronic otitis media look like?**

Like an eardrum perforation in the presence of chronic, painless, and usually foul-smelling discharge. Associated bony erosion may often lead to conductive hearing impairment.

47. **What is *bullous myringitis*?**

An inflammation of the tympanic membrane (from the Greek *myrinx*, tympanum) characterized by the presence of one or more vesicles, each filled with fluid (clear, blood-tinged, or even purulent), usually associated with one or more petechiae near the base, and at times large enough to form a bulla. This is usually part of a localized form of external otitis, presenting with severe earache, hearing loss, and bloody discharge. Although traditionally attributed to *Mycoplasma pneumoniae*, bullous myringitis also may result from various viral or bacterial infections and even occur in a setting of Ramsay Hunt syndrome. It is usually self-limited.

48. **What is Ramsay Hunt syndrome?**

It is herpes zoster infection of the geniculate ganglion, with facial paresis, hyperacusis, and unilateral loss of taste. Other symptoms include reduced salivation and tear formation, earache, and vesicles on the ear canal and drum.

49. **Who was Ramsay Hunt?**
Ramsay Hunt (1874–1937) was a Philadelphia neurologist. A graduate of the University of Pennsylvania, he studied in Paris, Vienna, and Berlin and eventually settled at Cornell University in New York, where in 1907 he described the eponymous syndrome.

50. **What is a *cholesteatoma*? What does it look like?**
From the Greek *chole* (biliary-like mass), *steat* (tallow), and *toma* (tumor), this is a pearly, benign, and tumor-like mass of cholesterol and keratinizing squamous epithelium, typically located in the middle ear and usually the result of chronic otitis media. Otoscopically, it presents as an exophytic papular lesion of yellow-white color and keratin-like composition. Histologically, it consists of squamous metaplasia (or an inward extension of squamous epithelium), lining an expanding cystic cavity. Cholesteatomas are often adjacent to a posterosuperior perforation of the tympanic membrane and may grow into the external canal or the mastoid.

51. **What is the significance of dense, white, and horseshoe-shaped eardrum plaques?**
It is a clue to the presence of tympanosclerosis, a condition characterized by hyalinization and calcification of the drum—often resulting from previous insertion of ventilation tubes. Although quite impressive, these calcifications do not usually impair hearing, unless they extend to the middle ear.

D. PNEUMATIC OTOSCOPY

52. **Is there any reason to perform pneumatic otoscopy?**
Although not part of the routine exam, it can differentiate pathologic from normal eardrums, especially in children, whose tympanic membrane is often reddened by crying. In this case, a mobile eardrum (even if red) is more likely to be normal than the result of otitis media, and vice versa. In fact, reduced eardrum mobility increases the likelihood of middle ear infection by 40%. Reduced eardrum mobility also is quite serious in children, since it may impair hearing and language.

53. **How is pneumatic otoscopy performed?**
First visualize the tympanic membrane. Then attach a pneumatic bulb to the head of the otoscope, and squeeze it to observe any movement of the tympanic membrane. Since the normal eardrum is mobile (albeit slightly), air pumped into the external canal will make the membrane (and its light reflex) move inward, while air aspirated from the canal will make the membrane move *outward*. Any reduced mobility is therefore abnormal. *Absent* mobility reflects instead perforation, middle-ear adhesions, a blocked eustachian tube, or acute otitis media.

54. **What if I do not have a pneumatic bulb?**
A "poor man's" way to test the mobility of the eardrum is to ask the patient to pinch his or her nose and then swallow. This creates enough of a pressure change to elicit a visible movement.

E. INNER EAR

55. **What is the function of the inner ear?**
To house the receptors for *hearing* (cochlea) and *balance* (semicircular canales and utricle). In addition to hearing loss, damage to these centers will manifest itself with vertigo (a sense of spinning or turning while at rest), unsteadiness of gait, and tinnitus (buzzing or ringing in the ear).

F. BEDSIDE HEARING TESTS

56. How do you test hearing at the bedside?
By using a screening maneuver (such as the *whispered voice test*), followed by a tuning fork assessment in patients who screen positive for hearing impairment.

57. What is the whispered voice test?
It is a validated and standardized screening test. To carry it out:
1. Stand behind the patient at a distance of 2 feet (i.e., around an arm's length). This is important since it prevents lip-reading.
2. Occlude one of the patient's ears by rubbing in a circular fashion a finger over the external auditory canal.
3. After quietly exhaling, whisper three letters (or numbers or combination thereof), and ask the patient to repeat the entire sequence.
4. If the patient can do so, the hearing is normal. If the patient gets one of three items wrong, whisper an additional sequence by using the same technique. If the patient gets two or more items wrong, the test is abnormal, and the examined ear is then further tested with a tuning fork.
5. Repeat the test for the other ear.

58. How accurate is the whispered voice test?
Quite accurate. It has excellent sensitivity, specificity, and likelihood ratios. Hence, a positive test rules in significant hearing loss, whereas a negative one essentially rules it out.

59. What are the tuning fork tests?
They are simple bedside tests that rely on a tuning fork to differentiate conductive from sensorineural hearing loss:
- Conductive loss involves the *transmission* of sound. This is usually due to problems of the external or middle ear (including the eardrum, often perforated) and is found in patients whose speech is soften than normal.
- Sensorineural loss involves instead the *perception* of sound. This is usually due to problems of the inner ear (cochlea) or its neural connections/centers and is found in patients whose speech is louder than normal. In fact, most neurosensory loss is the result of presbycusis (i.e., the aging-related degenerative loss of the inner ear receptor/auditory nerve).

60. How do these tests work?
By the principle that in patients with hearing loss, sound conducts preferentially through the bone. The two tests most commonly used for this purpose are Weber and Rinne, whose combination can separate conductive from neurosensory deafness (Fig. 5-6).

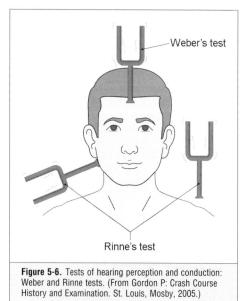

Figure 5-6. Tests of hearing perception and conduction: Weber and Rinne tests. (From Gordon P: Crash Course History and Examination. St. Louis, Mosby, 2005.)

61. **How do you carry out *Weber's* test?**
    Place the base of a vibrating tuning fork over the midline of the skull, at an equal distance between the two ears (alternatively, place it over the forehead or nasal bridge). Then ask the patient where the buzz of the tuning fork is best perceived. Normal subjects hear it better in the midline. Patients with unilateral disease, on the other hand, perceive it best in only one ear (*lateralized Weber sign*). In *conductive hearing loss* (from impacted cerumen, for example), Weber is lateralized to the *bad* ear (which is not distracted by ambient noise), whereas in *sensorineural loss*, Weber is lateralized to the *good* ear. Still, up to 40% of normal subjects can "lateralize" the sound. Hence, to avoid false positives carry out the test only in patients who screen positive for hearing loss (by, for example, failing the whispered voice test).

62. **How do you carry out *Rinne's* test?**
    Press the base of a vibrating tuning fork over the patient's mastoid process, and keep it there until (s)he can no longer hear any sound. At that point, hold the tuning fork as close as possible to the ipsilateral ear. This will test bone conduction (BC) and air conduction (AC). A normal subject can still hear sound (because AC lasts longer than BC, due to the amplifying effects of the eardrum and middle ear). Patients with *conductive deafness* (hearing loss produced by cerumen or middle-ear disease) have normal bone conduction but impaired air transmission and thus cannot hear any sound when the tuning fork is placed close to the ear (i.e., BC is greater than AC; negative Rinne's). Patients with *sensorineural deafness* due to damaged inner ear receptors have instead an equal reduction of AC and BC. This causes the normal pattern to prevail: AC will still last longer than BC (positive Rinne's test). The test is then repeated for the other ear.

Pearl

In conductive disease, Rinne's is negative, whereas Weber is lateralized to the "bad" side. In sensorineural disease, Rinne's is instead positive, whereas Weber is lateralized to the "good" side (but only in patients with severe unilateral loss).

---

63. **How accurate are these tests?**
    Rinne's is quite accurate for detecting conductive hearing loss. Weber's, on the other hand, is much less accurate (it has good specificity but poor sensitivity) because many patients with unilateral hearing loss (of any type) will not exhibit lateralization. Of course, tuning fork tests have other limitations too. For example, they cannot identify bilateral and symmetric hearing loss. They also are unable to separate pure conductive loss from mixed conductive/ neurosensory loss.

64. **Can tuning forks of different frequencies be used for these tests?**
    Probably not. Comparative studies have shown that the 512 Hz tuning fork has better sensitivity for detecting conductive hearing loss than the 1024 Hz. It also has better specificity than the 256 Hz. Tools of even lower frequency (such as the 128 Hz) generate so much vibration to be perceived even by patients with hearing impairment. Note that you should activate the tuning fork by striking it against a soft surface, since hard surfaces may generate multiple overtones. To eliminate these overtones, some tuning forks have added weights to their tines. These do eliminate interference, but they also shorten the tuning fork's vibration; hence, they should not be used.

65. **Who were Weber and Rinne?**
    E.F.W. Weber (1806–1871) was the proponent of the physiology behind the test, even though the test is usually credited to a later German otologist, F.E. Weber-Liel (1832–1891). Heinrich A. Rinne (1819–1868) was another German ear, nose, and throat surgeon.

ACKNOWLEDGMENT

The author gratefully acknowledges the contributions of Katherine Worzala, MD, and Dale Berg, MD, to this chapter in the first edition of *Physical Diagnosis Secrets*.

SELECTED BIBLIOGRAPHY

1. Arbit E: A sensitive bedside hearing test. Ann Neurol 2:250–251, 1977.

2. Brady PM, Zive MA, Goldberg RJ, et al: A new wrinkle to the earlobe crease. Arch Intern Med 147:65–66, 1987.

3. British Society of Audiology: Recommended procedure for Rinne and Weber tuning-fork tests. Br J Audiol 21:229–230, 1987.

4. Browning GG, Swan IRC: Sensitivity and specificity of Rinne tuning fork test. Br Med J 1297:1381–1382, 1988.

5. Burkey JM, Lippy WH, Schuring AG, et al: Clinical utility of the 512-Hz Rinne tuning fork test. Am J Otol 19:59–62, 1998.

6. Chole RA, Cook GB: The Rinne test for conductive deafness: A critical reappraisal. Arch Otolaryngol Head Neck Surg 114:399–403, 1988.

7. Crowley H, Kaufman RS: The Rinne tuning fork test. Arch Otolaryngol 84:70–72, 1966.

8. Doyle PJ, Anderson DW, Pijl S: The tuning fork—An essential instrument in otologic practice. J Otolaryngol 13:83–86, 1984.

9. Eekhof JA, de Bock GH, de Laat JA, et al: The whispered voice: The best test for screening for hearing impairment in general practice? Br J Gen Pract 46:473–474, 1996.

10. Elliot WJ: Ear lobe crease and coronary artery disease. Am J Med 75:1024–1032, 1983.

11. Frank STM: Aural sign of coronary artery disease. N Engl J Med 289:327–328, 1973.

12. Gelfand SA: Clinical precision of the Rinne test. Acta Otorinolaryngol 83:480–487, 1977.

13. Golabek W, Stephens SDG: Some tuning fork tests revisited. Clin Otolaryngol 4:421–430, 1979.

14. Huizing E: The early description of the so-called tuning fork tests of Weber and Rinne: I. The "Weber test" and its first description by Schmalz. Otolaryngol Rel Spec 35:278–282, 1973.

15. Jacob V, Alexander P, Nalinesha KM, et al: Can Rinne's test quantify hearing loss?. ENT J 72:152–153, 1993.

16. Johnson EW: Tuning forks to audiometers and back again. Lanryngoscope 80:49–68, 1970.

17. Johnston DE: A new modification of the Rinne test. Clin Otolaryngol 17:322–326, 1992.

18. Lichtenstein M, Bess FN, Logan SA: Validation and screening tools for identifying hearing-impaired elderly in primary care. JAMA 259:2875–2878, 1988.

19. Macphee GJ, Crowther JA, McAlpine CH: A simple screening test for hearing impairment in elderly patients. Age Ageing 17:347–351, 1988.

20. Nadol JB: Hearing loss. N Engl J Med 329:1092–1102, 1993.

21. Ng M, Tackler RK: Early history of tuning fork tests. Am J Otolaryngol 14:100–105, 1993.

22. Samuel J, Eitelberg G, Habi JI: Tuning forks: The problem of striking. J Laryngol Otol 103:1–6, 1989.

23. Sheehy JL, Gardner C, Hambley WM: Tuning fork tests in modern otology. Arch Otolaryngol 94:132–138, 1971.

24. Stankiewicz JA, Mowry HJ: Clinical accuracy of tuning fork tests. Laryngoscope 89:1956–1973, 1979.

25. Swan IRC, Browning GB: The whispered voice as a screening test for hearing impairment. J R Coll Gen Pract 35:197, 1985.

26. Wilson WR, Woods LA: Accuracy of the Bing and Rinne tuning fork tests. Arch Otolaryngol 101:81–85, 1975.

CHAPTER 6

NOSE AND MOUTH

Salvatore Mangione, MD

"How do you know that I've told a lie?" Pinocchio asked the Fairy.
"Lies, my dear boy, are quickly discovered; because they are of two kinds. There are lies with short legs, and lies with long noses. Yours is clearly of the long-nosed variety."
—Carlo Collodi, *The Adventures of Pinocchio*

A. THE NOSE

(1) Generalities

If you can excuse the pun, it is wise to be nosy about the nose. In fact, examination of this important facial appendix may reveal unsuspected abnormalities that lead to a diagnosis of either systemic diseases or capital sins (such as cocaine abuse).

(2) The External Nose

1. **What are the normal structures of the external nose?**
   They are shown in Fig. 6-1:
   - **Bridge:** Located superomedially and representing the *bony* upper third of the nose
   - **Alae** (*wings* in Latin): Cartilages that make up the inferior, medial, and lateral two thirds of the nose
   - **Nares:** The paired orifices (i.e., the nostrils)
   - **Tip** and **columella**

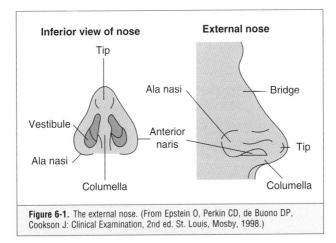

Figure 6-1. The external nose. (From Epstein O, Perkin CD, de Buono DP, Cookson J: Clinical Examination, 2nd ed. St. Louis, Mosby, 1998.)

2. **What is rhinophyma?**
From the Greek *rhino* (nose) and *phyma* (tumor), this is a variety of acne rosacea characterized by a bulbous and rather prominent nose. It is also referred to as copper-, hammer-, or potato-nose since the skin is thickened, erythematous, nontender, and often covered with multiple telangiectasias (*rum* or *gin blossoms*). In fact, other colorful lay terms for this condition include brandy nose, rum nose, and toper's nose—all paying tribute to its alleged association with the bottle, which is actually rather loose. Pathology shows follicular dilation and sebaceous hyperplasia, with fibrosis and hypervascularity. Of note, rhynophima may degenerate into basal cell carcinoma.

3. **What are the causes of rhinophyma?**
The ones conventionally blamed are climatic exposure and alcohol, with the best example of gin blossoms being those of the great comedian W.C. Fields, a man whose nose was directly proportional to his affinity for liquor. Rhinophyma is also rather common among politicians, with an early phase of it noted in the 42nd U.S. president, Bill Clinton. If this prompts you to wonder whether Pinocchio had rhinophyma, too, the answer is *no*. Pinocchio had *variable rhinomegaly*, a peculiarly reversible condition related to his telling lies.

4. **Is there any scientific basis for the "Pinocchio effect"?**
Yes. Recent evidence indicates that liars may indeed experience nasal changes, resulting in a telltale itch that eventually prompts them to unconsciously touch their nose. To corroborate this phenomenon, Alan Hirsch, director of the Chicago-based *Smell and Taste Research Foundation*, gathered 23 giveaway signs (both verbal and nonverbal) of "mendacious speech" and recently used them to analyze Bill Clinton's famous 1998 grand jury testimony on the Lewinsky affair. Overall, Clinton did 20 of the 23 signs, but whenever being particularly untruthful (or "legally accurate"), he consistently touched his nose, which brings us back to Collodi's Pinocchio and science. The nose contains abundant vascular erectile tissue (an unfortunate property it shares with the penis), which involuntarily dilates whenever a person lies, thus making the node redder, bigger, and itchy. Hence, the repetitive nose-touching of liars. Hirsch honored Collodi's insight by naming this phenomenon the "Pinocchio effect." His observation has been confirmed in other famous cases. For example, even O.J. Simpson touched his nose rather frequently during trial when describing Nicole Brown Simpson's murder. Hence, simple observation might allow policemen, attorneys, psychiatrists, and everyone else to tell whether someone is lying. Or, as Yogi Berra used to say, "You can observe a lot by watching."

5. **What is a *saddle nose*? Does it really exist outside of board questions?**
A saddle nose is the congenital (or acquired) erosive *indentation* of the nasal bone, turning the distal tip of the nose upward and outward. A true saddle nose (caused by destruction of the *bony* portion of the nose) is typical of congenital *lues*, but actually more frequent in *Wegener's* granulomatosis. Given the increasing availability of good therapy for both these conditions, a saddle nose has now become less common. A *pseudo-saddle nose* is instead a feature of *relapsing polychondritis,* although the destruction in this case involves *cartilage* and *not* bone.

6. **What are nasal fractures?**
They are the most common trauma-related disorders of the nose. They present with *severe pain* and *anterior epistaxis*, often from both nares. Periorbital ecchymoses invariably develop 24 hours after trauma, along with significant sequelae, such as septal hematoma or septal deviation. Because these fractures are *open*, antibiotics are necessary to prevent osteomyelitis.

7. **What is a septal hematoma? How does it differ from septal deviation?**
A *hematoma* is a purple and painful nodule in the nasal septum, easily spottable through the nostril. Conversely, traumatic displacement of the nasal septum (i.e., *septal deviation*) may be

difficult to see until later, since edema of the early posttraumatic stages makes physical exam difficult to perform. Both of these complications require referral to an ear-nose-throat (ENT) specialist for drainage or reduction. If undrained, the hematoma may cause the septal cartilage to become ischemic and necrotic, with a resulting permanent nasal deformity.

8. **What is *lupus pernio*?**
    It is a chronic, nonblanching, diffuse, and purple skin discoloration of the external nose, in the absence of true nasal enlargement (Fig. 6-2). Hence, it differs from rhinophyma. A sign of active sarcoid, it may occur with uveitis, erythema nodosum, and pulmonary involvement. It may also coexist with lesions of the ears, cheeks, hands, and fingers. The term *lupus* refers to any disfiguring skin

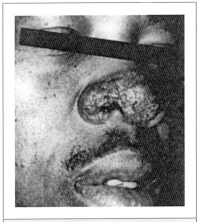

Figure 6-2. Lupus pernio. (From Fitzpatrick JE, Aeling JL: Dermatology Secrets. Philadelphia, Hanley & Belfus, 1996.)

condition that, like a wolf (*lupus* in Latin) "devours" the patient's facial features. It is thus used with modifying terms to designate various disfiguring skin diseases, such as lupus verrucosus, lupus erythematosus, lupus tuberculosis, lupus vulgaris, and, of course, lupus pernio. *Pernio* is Latin for frostbite and refers to the peculiar violet-bluish hue of the condition (*see* Chapter 3, The Skin, question 265).

9. **What did Rudolph of the reindeer story really have?**
    Probably rhinophyma, but that begs the question: Did Santa spill the grog while feeding his reindeer?

(3) The Internal Nose

10. **What are the normal structures of the internal nose?**
    The normal internal structures are shown in Fig. 6-3:
    1. The **vestibules**. As indicated by the term, these are paired internal widenings, immediately beyond each naris. They are delimited:
        - Medially by the *septum*. Like the external nose, this is partly bony and partly cartilaginous. The word *septum* is an anglicized adaptation of the Latin *saepire*, "*to erect a hedgerow.*" Indeed, the function of the septum is to provide a medial boundary to each vestibule.
        - Laterally by a wall of *cartilage*
    2. Deeply beyond the vestibules are the **turbinates**, or **conchae**. These are curving bony structures that project into the internal nose. There are three turbinates (and three corresponding meatuses) in each nasal cavity: superior, middle, and inferior. Their main function is to increase the nasal surface for humidification, temperature control, and filtering of inhaled air. To do so, they are covered by a well-vascularized and erectile mucosa.

Pearl:

On routine examination by either otoscope or Vienna speculum, one can only inspect the vestibule, anterior portion of the septum, and the inferior and middle turbinates.

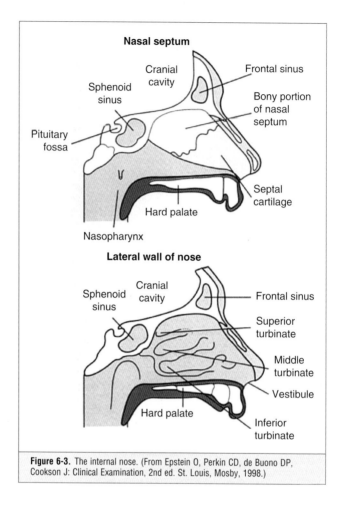

Figure 6-3. The internal nose. (From Epstein O, Perkin CD, de Buono DP, Cookson J: Clinical Examination, 2nd ed. St. Louis, Mosby, 1998.)

11. **What are *paranasal sinuses*?**

They are the frontal, maxillary, ethmoid, and sphenoid sinuses: four hollow and air-filled paired cavities that open through small ostia into recesses of the nasal cavities called *meatuses*. These are covered by bony shelves lined by erectile soft tissue (the turbinates)—three on each side.

12. **And what about the *adenoids*?**

They are aggregates of lymphatic tissue located on the roof of the nasopharynx, just below the sphenoid sinus. They typically regress with puberty and so in adults are usually absent. Yet in infants and children, they may enlarge considerably and cause nasal obstruction, nasal voice, snoring, restless sleep, and mouth breathing. Since mouth breathing in times of facial formation may result in bony changes, affected children often develop an *adenoid facies*, with a high, arched palate; prominent upper teeth; pinched-in nose; shortened upper lip; a staring expression of the eyes; and a slightly elongated and dumb-looking face. Adenoidal hypertrophy also may obstruct the eustachian tubes and thus result in recurrent middle ear effusions and otitis media.

13. **What is the significance of *flaring of the nostrils*?**
Flaring of the nostrils (i.e., of the *alae* of the nose) is a sign of increased work of breathing, typical of impending respiratory failure. It is often associated with other findings of distress, such as *respiratory alternans* and *abdominal paradox* (*see* Chapter 13, Chest Inspection, Palpation, and Percussion, questions 52–58). It also can occur in peritonitis as a result of impaired and painful excursion of the diaphragm.

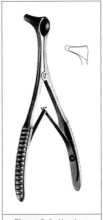

14. **What are the best tools for inspecting nares and internal nose?**
    ■ **Otoscope:** This can be mounted with a nasal speculum (instead of an *ear* speculum) and thus used to shine a light directly into each vestibule.
    ■ **Handheld Vienna nasal speculum:** This is a speculum that opens upon closure of the handles. It is commonly used with a head mirror (Fig. 6-4).
    In the absence of these tools, you may simply use fingers and penlight. Either way, always instruct the patient to first blow the nose (gently but forcibly) to expel any mucus.

Figure 6-4. Handheld Vienna speculum. (Courtesy Chosmic Surgical, Inc., Ellicott City, MD.)

15. **Is inspection of nasal secretions useful?**
Yes. In fact, there is quite some value in *snot*, the colloquial term for excessive flow of nasal mucosa. Although the butt of vulgar jokes, snot is actually noble in origin, going all the way back to the Old English *gesnot*. It also retains diagnostic value, since different diseases tend to produce different snots:
    ■ A **clear** discharge is suggestive of viral or atopic rhinitis.
    ■ A **yellow** discharge may instead indicate an early suppurative process.
    ■ A **green** discharge is quite consistent with purulent sinusitis.
    ■ Obviously, a **bloody** discharge suggests anterior epistaxis.
    ■ A **dark and almost black** discharge (especially in comatose diabetics) argues for mucormycosis.

16. **What is an abscess of the nasal vestibule?**
It is a superficial abscess of hair follicles (*furunculosis*), usually caused by *Staphylococcus aureus* and not uncommonly located in the nasal vestibule or septum. Quite painful, it presents as an erythematous and fluctuant nodule in the septal mucosa. Usually treated with antibiotics and warm compresses, it may require incision and drainage to avoid cavernous sinus thrombosis.

17. **What are the causes of swelling/bumps in the nasal septum?**
    ■ Septal hematoma
    ■ Septal abscess
    ■ Nasal polyps
    ■ Papillomas
    ■ Tumors
    All require ENT referral, since an untreated hematoma (or abscess) may result in septal *perforation*.

18. **What are the most common causes of airflow obstruction in one or both nares?**
In addition to the conditions previously listed, other causes include nasal mucosa edema, septal deviation, and foreign bodies—all diagnosable by exam. Foreign bodies are especially common in children, given their unique penchant for inserting rocks, twigs, and crayons into nares and various body orifices.

19. What are nasal polyps?

They are pedunculated, fleshy, and friable structures that hang from the lateral or septal mucosa. Polyps originate from localized swellings of either sinus or nasal mucosa, initially small, but eventually growing with each recurrence of submucosal edema until they may even protrude from the vestibule and cause nasal obstruction. They are often multiple, clearly visible, easy to move back and forth, and not tender (which differentiates them from other internal nasal structures). They are common in *chronic (atopic) rhinitis* and *aspirin sensitivity* (often in association with asthma) and can be easily removed through endoscopy.

20. What is a papilloma of the nasal vestibule?

It is a *wart* of the inner nose. In contrast to the more common polyp, papillomas are jagged in appearance and more likely to bleed. Like polyps, they can interfere with the sense of smell and cause obstruction. They are easily visible on exam and must *all* be removed since they can undergo *neoplastic degeneration*. Like warts elsewhere, they often recur.

21. What is a nasopharyngeal carcinoma (lymphoepithelioma)?

It is a sequela of Epstein-Barr virus (EBV) infection, rare in Europe but frequent in Southeast Asia, where it represents the third most common cancer. Tumor growth is often asymptomatic, and presentation is late, typically with cervical lymphadenopathy. Hence, the prognosis is poor, even though screening for anti-EBV antibodies may help detect early and treatable disease.

22. What does a nasal septal perforation look like?

Like a hole in the septum. This can be demonstrated on inspection or by shining a light into one nostril and seeing it transilluminate both sides.

23. What are the common causes of a septal perforation?

The traditional four are:

- **Traumatic:** Facial injury or self-induced lesions (nose picking/piercing)
- **Iatrogenic:** Prior septal surgery, nasogastric tube placement, or nasal intubation
- **Inflammatory/malignant:** Often the sequela of untreated septal hematomas or abscesses
- **Cocaine snorting:** One of the most frequent causes today, often presenting with large and expanding perforations. Cocaine contains adulterants that may irritate the mucosa, plus has strong alpha-agonist effects (causing vasoconstriction and ischemia of the nasal cartilage). Nasal obstruction often accompanies perforation.

24. What are the less-common causes of perforation?

- **Chemical irritants** (chromic or sulfuric acid fumes, glass dust, mercurials, and phosphorous)
- **Infections** (tuberculosis, syphilis, and, more rarely, leprosy)
- **Collagen vascular diseases** (Wegener's, midline granuloma, systemic lupus erythematosus, rheumatoid arthritis, mixed connective tissue disease, and progressive system sclerosis)

25. What are the nasal manifestations of a basilar skull fracture?

In addition to the direct facial trauma, patients often show evidence of *nasal* fracture, such as periorbital ecchymoses, swelling/tenderness of the nasal bridge, and anterior epistaxis. There also may be *cerebrospinal fluid rhinorrhea* (leakage of cerebrospinal fluid [CSF] through the fracture site). This is a risk factor for the development of meningitis and thus necessitates prompt surgical attention.

26. How do you recognize CSF rhinorrhea?

By placing a drop of nasal secretions over a paper tissue. In CSF rhinorrhea, this will serve as a "poor man's" paper chromatography, showing a clear halo around "nasal" secretions that represent instead spinal fluid leakage. Alternatively, the glucose content of secretions may be measured at the bedside by using a Chemstrip. In patients with CSF rhinorrhea, this will reveal a high glucose concentration, close to spinal fluid levels of 40–80 mg/dL.

27. What is a cold? What are its nasal manifestations?
The common cold, one of humankind's most frequent afflictions, has a plethora of nasal manifestations: swollen mucosa (to the point of obstruction), stuffy feeling, and serous or purulent nasal discharge. Since it represents a viral infection of the upper respiratory tract, there may be concomitant serous otitis media, nonexudative pharyngitis, and shotty nodes.

28. What results in swelling of the nasal mucosa?
One of three causes:
- **Viral:** Nasal and oropharyngeal infections by either rhinoviruses or adenoviruses
- **Atopic:** Pollen or dander exposure causing nasal congestion, allergic (serous) conjunctivitis, and sneezing
- **Vasomotor:** Response to a specific inhalant, characterized by boggy edema of the mucosa and marked tearing. Inhalants may either be noxious to all (such as tear gas) or only to some. For example, perfumes may elicit an idiosyncratic response in a few predisposed individuals, causing pronounced swelling of the nasal mucosa.

29. Can you diagnose the cause of GI bleeding by peeking into the patient's nose?
Yes, bleeding in the gut may indeed be linked to the nose. The most common reason is *simple epistaxis*, wherein patients swallow nasal blood, resulting in guaiac-positive stools and even melena. More rare are the multiple nasal telangiectasias of Rendu-Osler-Weber syndrome, an autosomal dominant disorder characterized by multiple (and often bleeding) vascular lesions of the gut, mouth, face, extremities, and chest. The tongue and lips also may have telangiectasias.

30. Who was Rendu?
Henry J.L. Rendu (1844–1902) was the grandson of a distinguished Parisian painter and the son of an agricultural inspector. An art lover, he was so fascinated by his father's profession as to pursue a medical career only after a stint in agriculture, geology, and botany. Still, he never lost his passion for plants and eagerly maintained it as a lifelong hobby. At age 43, he finally joined the staff of the Necker Hospital in Paris (the same one where Laënnec had been chief of chest medicine), rapidly gaining fame as a charismatic lecturer and gifted clinician.

31. Who was Weber?
Frederick P. Weber (1863–1962) was a British physician, already encountered in the ear chapter because of Sturge-Weber disease. Educated in Cambridge, Vienna, and Paris, Weber cultivated throughout his life an interest in medical philosophy, the arts, and numismatics, which he then expressed in many books and articles. His father was Herman D. Weber (1823–1918), himself a famous and long-lived physician (he is the same Weber who described the midbrain syndrome that still carries his name). Weber père was a charming man with many interests, who taught himself English so that he could read Shakespeare and befriend, among others, Addison, Carlyle, and several Waterloo veterans (including the famous Sir Peregrine Maitland of Wellington's cry: "Now it's your time, Maitland, now it's your time!"). Increasingly fascinated by England, Weber senior eventually moved there in 1854, married an Englishwoman, and became member of the Royal College of Physicians. Both father and son were avid climbers and advocates of physical exercise as key to long and productive lives (which served them well, since both lived well into their 90s). The older Weber climbed several mountains in the Italian Alps (including one for his 80th birthday) and walked 40–50 miles/week.

32. Who was Osler?
Sir William Osler (1849–1919) is such a legend that a few lines in this chapter will do him a disservice. Born in the backwoods of Canada as son of a missionary, Osler was so spiritual

that early in life he even considered joining the clergy. A charming and compassionate man with a prankish twist, he was a charismatic teacher, a superb bedside diagnostician, and a good person who never lost his respect for patients as fellow humans in need of help. After teaching in Canada and the United States, he moved to England, where he became regius professor of Medicine at Oxford. The last part of his life was unfortunately quite sad, tormented by the memory of his only son, who had died in Flanders toward the end of World War I.

33. What is anosmia?

It is the congenital or acquired absence of smell (from the Greek *an*, lack of, and *osme*, smell).

- **Acquired anosmia** may result from a long list of disease processes, affecting either the central nervous system or nose. Among them are multiple sclerosis, Parkinson's disease, diabetes mellitus, pernicious anemia, liver cirrhosis, chronic renal insufficiency, Cushing's syndrome, cystic fibrosis, sarcoidosis, allergic rhinitis, nasal polyposis, and zinc deficiency. Still, sequelae of a viral infection are often the most common reasons for acquired reversible anosmia.
- **Congenital anosmia** is almost always caused by Kallmann's syndrome. Described by the German psychiatrist Franz J. Kallmann (1897–1965), this consists of familial hypogonadotropic hypogonadism with or without anosmia (usually characterized by congenital absence of olfactory lobes). Kallmann's is inherited through sex-linked recessive or autosomal transmission, with expression mostly in males. It can be treated with gonadotropins.

34. Do smell and taste interact?

Yes. Patients whose olfaction is weakened or absent (hyposmia or anosmia) can only taste the five fundamental sensations of sweet, sour, bitter, salty, and *umami* (i.e., the taste of glutamate). This is because *flavor* results from oral combination of the five basic tastes plus the foodstuff's odor and various chemical characteristics, such as texture, temperature, and other sensations. Hence, flavor is typically absent when olfaction is also absent. Overall, smell disorders are more common than isolated taste disorders (such as *hypogeusia* and *ageusia*). *Perversion* of taste can also occur, with misreadings and distortions, such as foul tastes from otherwise pleasant substances.

35. Is perception of alcohol odor an indication that the sense of smell is intact?

No. Alcohol is an *irritant*. Hence, it stimulates the trigeminal rather than the olfactory endings of the nasal mucosa. That is why even patients without olfactory lobes (such as those with Kallmann's syndrome) can "feel" an alcohol sponge. Same is true for other irritants, such as ammonia and pepper. To test the sense of smell, you should use nonirritating substances with strong odors. Coffee and spices (such as cinnamon, cloves, nutmeg) are excellent choices.

B. THE ORAL CAVITY

Americans may have no identity, but they do have wonderful teeth.
Jean Baudrillard, Astral America

(1) Generalities

If it is true that you should not look a gift horse in the mouth, it is also true that patients are not horses. Hence, always do a good inspection of the oropharynx, since mouth and tongue lesions may provide important clues to systemic disorders. Even the lowly teeth, which represent important risk factors for serious anaerobic infections of the respiratory tract, can hint at an otherwise unsuspected systemic or psychiatric disorder. In fact, lead poisoning, congenital syphilis, and bulimia can all be recognized by an astute dental examination. Unfortunately, far too many patients have gone undiagnosed because of a poor or incomplete mouth exam.

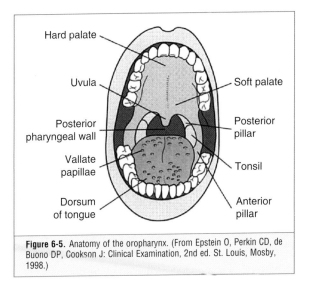

Figure 6-5. Anatomy of the oropharynx. (From Epstein O, Perkin CD, de Buono DP, Cookson J: Clinical Examination, 2nd ed. St. Louis, Mosby, 1998.)

(2) Posterior Pharynx and Tonsils

36. **What are the two main structures of the posterior pharynx?**
The *hard* and the *soft palate* (Fig. 6-5). These are supported by the *anterior* and *posterior pillars*.

37. **What is a cleft palate?**
A congenital deformity that is usually corrected in infancy but may persist into adulthood. It is quite common (1 case in 1000 live births, with or without cleft lip), with greater prevalence in Native Americans (3.6 cases per 1000 live births), and lower in African Americans (0.3 cases per 1000 live births). Of all cases, 20% are an isolated cleft lip; 50% are a cleft lip and palate, and 30% are a cleft palate alone. Cleft lip and palate together are more common in males, whereas isolated cleft palate is more common in females. Bifid uvula occurs in 1 of 80 patients, often in isolation (*see* question 38).

38. **What is the uvula? What disease processes may affect it?**
The uvula (*little grape* in Latin) is the midline structure that projects from the roof of the posterior pharynx, and whose main function is probably to prevent fluids from entering the nasopharynx upon swallowing. Interesting presentations include:
  - **Absent uvula:** Usually due to surgical removal as part of uvulopalatopharyngoplasty (UPPP) for obstructive sleep apnea. May result in inhalation of swallowed fluids.
  - **Bifid uvula:** Fascinating but entirely benign normal variant, wherein the uvula is congenitally forked. Not a sign of lying, it may instead be associated with an occult cleft palate. Look for it.
  - **Bobbing uvula:** Patients with chronic and severe aortic insufficiency may have a *rhythmic pulsatile movement* of the uvula (Mueller's sign). This is the equivalent of the de Musset sign (*see* Chapter 1, Facies, General Appearance, and Body Habitus, questions 51 and 54) and is quite rare nowadays, thanks to timely valvular treatment.
  - **Neoplastic uvula (squamous cell degeneration):** As for many other oropharyngeal structures.

39. What is uvulomegaly? What are its causes?

Uvulomegaly is a swollen and elongated uvula. Causes are mostly two: one quite common (pharyngitis), and the other exceptionally rare (gamma-heavy chain disease). Uvulomegaly of pharyngitis is often associated with oral manifestations, whereas that of heavy chain disease is associated instead with pancytopenia and "B" symptoms of lymphoproliferative disorders. In both conditions, the uvula may become large enough to cause coughing, snoring, and even gagging.

40. What is a *localized reddening* of both anterior pharyngeal pillars? What are its causes?

It is a condition that is different from *diffuse* inflammation of the oropharynx. It was first described by Cunha in association with *chronic fatigue syndrome* (CFS) and dubbed the *crimson crescents*. As many as 80% of CFS patients may indeed present with a peculiar purplish discoloration of the two anterior pharyngeal pillars. These crescents are always bilateral, of a vivid crimson color, and quite briskly demarcated from the rest of the pharynx. There is no pain, no sore throat, and *no other evidence of pharyngitis*. Crescents last for months and gradually fade as disease goes into remission. During exacerbations, however, they may redden again. Although present in 3–5% of nonchronic fatigue patients with nonspecific sore throats, crimson crescents are typically absent in pharyngitis due to group A streptococcus, mononucleosis, cytomegalovirus, or the common viral upper respiratory tract infection.

41. What are the causes of a *diffuse* reddening of the oropharynx?

The most common are viral and bacterial infections:
- **Viral** etiologies include rhinovirus, adenovirus, human immunodeficiency virus (HIV), EBV, cytomegalovirus (CMV), and coxsackievirus.
- **Bacterial** causes include instead group A streptococci, *Neisseria gonorrhoeae*, and, in the olden days, diphtheria.

42. How common is sore throat?

Very common. In fact, it is the third most frequent presenting complaint in office-based practice, accounting for 4.3% of all visits. Identifying patients with group A beta-hemolytic streptococcal pharyngitis (strep throat) is often difficult.

43. What are the causes of an exudate (i.e., *pus*) on the posterior pharynx?

Many agents can cause *exudative pharyngitis* (Table 6-1), the most important being upper respiratory tract viruses, group A beta-hemolytic streptococci, and the EBV.

44. What are the clinical features of viral upper respiratory tract infections?

Pharyngeal vesicles and ulcers. These are so typical as to argue against group A streptococci being the cause of the patient's sore throat (*see herpangina*, questions 87 and 89).

TABLE 6-1. CAUSES OF EXUDATIVE POSTERIOR PHARYNGITIS	
Pathogen	**Probability (%)**
Viral	50–80
Streptococcal	5–36
Epstein-Barr virus	1–10
Chlamydia pneumoniae	2–5
Mycoplasma pneumoniae	2–5
Neisseria gonorrhoeae	1–2
Haemophilus influenzae type b	1–2
Candidiasis	<1
Diphtheria	<1

(Data from Ebell M, et al: Does this patient have strep throat? JAMA 284:2912–2918, 2000.)

45. What are the clinical features of group A beta-hemolytic streptococcal infection?
Marked and *diffuse* pharyngeal swelling and redness, with coating of lymphoid tissue by a punctuated or confluent gray exudate. This eventually causes whitish tonsillar spots (follicles), thus giving the disease its name of *follicular tonsillitis*. Even though the beefy red color of the pharynx typically ends at the soft palate with just a few scattered petechiae, there are often erythema and swelling of the surrounding structures (faucial pillars, uvula, and base of the tongue). Cough and rhinorrhea are usually minimal, but high fever, chills, and mild nausea can be present. Enlarged (and tender) jugulodigastric and anterior cervical lymph nodes are typically palpable, especially at the angle of the jaw. This is particularly true in the early phase of the disease. Throat pain is persistent, often radiating to the ear upon swallowing. In fact, mouth opening is painful and at times difficult. Tongue coating and halitosis can occur too. Local suppurative complications include peritonsillar abscess (<1% of patients treated with antibiotics), retropharyngeal abscess, suppurative cervical lymphadenitis, otitis media, sinusitis, and mastoiditis. More serious complications (such as meningitis, pneumonia, bacteremia, rheumatic fever, and scarlatina) are instead less common.

46. What is scarlatina (scarlet fever)?
It is a *typical scarlatiniform rash*, characterized by fine scarlet-like papules that start on the trunk, spread to the extremities, and spare palms and soles. The tongue is initially coated (and with enlarged papillae), but later may become denuded ("strawberry tongue"). There are also circumoral pallor and rash accentuation in skin folds, especially in the antecubital fossae (Pastia sign). In very young children, there may even be excoriations around the nares. The rash typically blanches to pressure, has a sandpapery feel, and eventually subsides in 6–9 days, to be then followed by desquamation of palms and soles.

47. When should you think of *gonococcal* pharyngitis?
When confronted with an *exudative* and *ulcerative* pharyngitis that is refractory to standard therapy. Inquire about the patient's sexual activities, and do a Thayer-Martin culture of the throat.

48. What is infectious mononucleosis? What are its features?
Infectious mononucleosis, the clinical illness caused by EBV, presents after an incubation of 30–50 days with:
- *Fever*
- Severe *exudative pharyngitis* with tonsillar swelling, sore throat, and often dysphagia. The involved mucosa is swollen, erythematous, coated with a grayish exudate, and typically characterized by small erosions and petechiae. Other features include splenomegaly and hepatomegaly.
- Prominent *cervical lymphadenopathy*. This occurs in >90% of young patients, typically presenting as enlarged, symmetric, and tender *anterior* nodes—which are usually involved in only a few other conditions. Note, however, that *posterior* nodes also may be involved (in 60% of the cases), and that adenopathy is absent in more than 70% of patients older than 40%).
- Severe *constitutional symptoms*, such as fatigue, arthralgias, myalgias, lethargy, functional impairment, and nausea. Hemolytic anemia also may occur. In most patients, acute signs and symptoms resolve within 3–4 weeks, but lethargy can persist much longer—even months.

49. What are the *glandular fever*–like syndromes?
They are infections presenting with illnesses clinically indistinguishable from *glandular fever* (i.e., infectious mononucleosis). These include:
- **HIV** (at time of seroconversion): Since this is an early stage, the patient is viremic (and thus highly infectious), but HIV-antibody negative.
- **CMV:** Compared with *infectious mononucleosis (EBV)*, the lymphadenopathy of CMV is less prominent and the pharyngitis less severe.

- **Toxoplasmosis:** This is acquired through ingestion of either *tissue cysts* in raw or inadequately cooked meat (such as sheep and pig) or *sporocysts* on unwashed fruit or vegetables contaminated with cat feces. Cats are the definitive hosts of the parasite (*Toxoplasma gondii*), excreting it as cysts in their feces. Cysts can remain viable in soil for months, eventually infecting humans and animals (e.g., pigs and sheep). Infection is usually *asymptomatic*, although it can present with a *glandular fever-like syndrome*.

All of these infections share the same *nonspecific* clinical manifestations of EBV, with severity ranging from a flu-like illness to a very debilitating disease. Acute symptoms include sore throat, fever, tender lymphadenopathy, erythematous rash involving the trunk, and various constitutional symptoms (such as malaise, headache, myalgias). Most symptoms only last a few weeks, but lymphadenopathy and malaise may persist for months.

50. **Can strep throat be diagnosed by history and physical examination?**

Not really. Although its various findings have good interobserver reliability (with the possible exception of adenopathy), no single element of history or physical exam is powerful enough to confirm the diagnosis of streptococcal pharyngitis. Findings with the highest positive likelihood ratio (LR) (and thus best at *ruling-in* the disease) are:

- Tonsillar exudates (LR = 3.4)
- Pharyngeal exudates (LR = 2.1)
- Strep throat exposure in the previous 2 weeks (LR = 1.9)

No finding, if absent, can rule *out* the disease. The ones with lowest negative LR are:

- Absence of tender anterior cervical nodes (LR = 0.60)
- Absence of tonsillar enlargement (LR = 0.63)
- Absence of tonsillar or pharyngeal exudate (LR = 0.74)

Routine use of throat cultures or rapid antigen test may lead to overtreatment of low-risk patients (due to false positive results) and undertreatment of high-risk patients (due to false negative results). Hence, you should rely on a *combination* of clinical findings. Those that can best separate patients *with* and *without* strep throat are:

- Pharyngeal or tonsillar exudates
- Fever by history
- Tonsillar enlargement
- Tenderness or enlargement of the anterior cervical and jugulodigastric lymph nodes
- Absence of cough

In addition, strep throat will *not* present with rhinorrhea or earache, but may instead occur with nausea, vomiting, headaches, and moderate to severe sore throat. Still, the pharyngitis of mono can closely resemble "strep-throat," with fever, exudates, and adenopathy.

51. **What are the causes of a nodule in the posterior pharynx?**

- **Human papilloma virus (HPV):** This causes a *warty* lesion on the tonsils, tonsillar pillars, or even buccal mucosa. May degenerate into squamous cell carcinoma.
- **Squamous cell carcinoma:** Presents as a *papule* or *nodule* in the posterior pharynx of 50- to 70-year-old patients, usually males (three to four times), often in association with smoking, tobacco-chewing, heavy ethanol ingestion, and HPV infection. About 90% of tonsillar cancers are squamous cell, 60% presenting with cervical metastases (bilateral in 15% of the cases), and 7% with distant spread. Note that carcinomas of the tonsils are not necessarily exophytic or ulcerated. In fact, they often look identical to lymphomas, distinguishable only by biopsy.
- **Lymphoma:** The second most common type of tonsillar cancer, presenting as a *submucosal mass* in an otherwise asymmetric tonsillar enlargement. Ipsilateral adenopathy is common.
- **Peritonsillar abscess (quinsy):** A *tender nodule* that follows exudative pharyngitis and is associated with erythema and uvular displacement. The term *quinsy* goes back to middle English (from the original Greek *kunankhê,* dog collar), but also brings to mind the fictional television character Dr. Quincy (Jack Klugman), the medical examiner whom a patient inevitably ended up seeing if (s)he did not receive prompt surgical drainage of a quinsy.

52. **What is Vincent's angina of the tonsil?**
It is an acute necrotizing infection of the pharynx caused by the same organisms that cause "trench mouth" gingivostomatitis (i.e., fusiform bacilli and the *Borrelia vincentii* spirochete). Patients present with a few days of rapidly worsening unilateral sore throat, ipsilateral referred earache, and fetid bad breath/bad taste. Exam reveals submandibular lymphadenopathy and an ulcerated tonsil, with a deep, well-circumscribed, and grayish base that easily bleeds upon swabbing. A smear of the exudate confirms the presence of fusobacteria and spirochetes.

(3) Oral Mucosa

53. **What is the magic of "Ahhhh"?**
Saying "Ahhhh" is effective for two reasons:
- It *elevates the soft palate*, thus allowing visualization of the base of the tongue, uvula, tonsillar pillars, and even hypopharynx.
- It permits adequate assessment of the motor division of cranial nerves IX (glossopharyngeal) and X (vagus). In cases of bilateral damage to these nerves, saying "Ahhhh" will *not* elevate the uvula. In cases of unilateral damage, saying "Ahhhh" will instead deviate the uvula toward the intact side (it also will prevent the rising of the soft palate from the paralyzed side).

54. **What are the best sound and tongue positions for the task?**
There are three schools of thought: (1) the traditional falsetto "Ahhhh," with tongue protruded; (2) "Ae" rather than "Ahhhh"; and (3) "Ha," with the tongue maximally pulled in. Although no studies have assessed the predictive values of these sounds, the controversy is best settled by the universal rule: use whatever works best for you, and make sure that by doing so you can visualize the patient's tonsils and oral mucosa. Yet, proper examination of the throat remains challenging. It requires *elevation* of the soft palate and uvula and *depression* of the posterior tongue. Although the tongue blade does help, it also can induce gagging, coughing, and even biting. An alternative consists in asking the patient to pant, or in cases of small children, to imitate a puppy.

55. **What is the descriptive nomenclature of lesions in the oral mucosa?**
One akin to that of dermatology (*see* Chapter 3, question 2), similarly relying on lesions' size and characteristics to classify them as:
- **Macules** (if *flat* and <0.5 cm)
- **Patches** (if *flat* and ≥0.5 cm)
- **Papules** (if *palpable* and <0.5 cm)
- **Plaques** (if *palpable* and ≥0.5 cm)
Other terms, such as *vesicles* and *bullae* for fluid-filled lesions, are similarly used.

56. **What are the colors of oral lesions?**
It depends on the lesion. Colors range from *flesh* to *white*, *black*, and *red* (Table 6-2).

57. **What causes *flesh-covered* palpable lesions in the oral mucosa?**
The most common are normal anatomic structures, such as *Wharton's* or *Stensen's* ducts, which drain, respectively, the submaxillary and parotid salivary glands.
- **Wharton's ducts** are two tiny papules on the floor of the mouth (just under the tongue and 5 mm lateral to the frenulum, representing the opening of the submaxillary glands).
- **Stensen's ducts** represent instead the opening of the *parotid* glands. They are located on both sides of the buccal mucosa, directly opposite to the second upper molar and near the bite line.
- **Ranula**
- **Torus**

TABLE 6.2.   ORAL LESIONS*

Flesh-Colored Lesions	Smoker's melanosis
Wharton's Duct	Hemochromatosis
Stensen's Duct	Addison's disease
Ranula	Melanoplakia
Torus (mandibularis, palatinus)	Malignant melanoma
Buccal exostosis	**Red Lesions**
White Lesions	Pyogenic granuloma
Thickening of oral mucosa (linea alba)	Erythema migrans
Hairy leukoplakia	Palatal petechiae
Oral thrush	Kaposi's sarcoma
Koplik spots	**Ulcerated Lesions**
Fordyce spots	Thermal injuries (burns)
Wickham sign	Aphthous ulcers (canker sore)
Squamous cells carcinoma	Autommimune gingivostomatitis
Pigmented Lesions	Viral gingivostomatitis
Amalgam tattoo	Primary syphilis (chancre)
Peutz-Jeghers syndrome	Squamous cells carcinoma

*See text for further discussion.

58. **What is a *ranula*?**
Latin for *small frog,* a ranula is a unilateral, painful, dome-shaped fluctuant nodule on the floor of the mouth. It is caused by the salivary duct obstruction of a sublingual or submandibular gland, resulting in mucus retention. It may require surgery.

59. **What is a *torus*?**
It is a benign and nontender *exostosis* (i.e., a cartilage-capped and mucosa-lined bony spur). Based on its origin, a torus may be *mandibularis* or *palatinus*. The mandibularis is smaller and located on the lingual surface of the mandible, whereas the palatinus is larger and originates from the midline of the hard palate. The term *torus* is Latin for protuberance, used most commonly to indicate the bony structures of the skull. Tori are benign and require only clinical recognition.

60. **Who were Wharton and Stensen?**
   - **Thomas Wharton** was one of the personal physicians to Oliver Cromwell and an active presence during the 1665 great plague of London.
   - **Niels Stensen** was instead a Danish anatomist and geologist who lived first in Copenhagen, then in Leiden and Montpellier, and finally in Paris, where he investigated heart, brain, muscles, and glands. Stensen described the tetralogy of Fallot more than two centuries before Fallot himself and in 1661 discovered the homonymous excretory duct of the parotid gland. His anatomic studies eventually brought him to Florence, as court physician to Grand Duke Ferdinand II. There he was converted to Catholicism by a nun and became a priest. In his new

devotion (and much to the dismay of his scientific colleagues), he completely abandoned science and spent the rest of his life ministering to Roman Catholics in northern Germany. His homonymous ducts are often called Steno's ducts, from the Latinized version of Stensen into *Nicolaus Stenonis*, or, more simply, *Steno*.

61. What is a buccal exostosis?

It is a benign and painless bony spur (which is the literal meaning of the term "exostosis"), very much like the *torus* (previously discussed), except that its location is different: on the facial surface of either the upper, or less commonly, lower jaw. It originates in the alveolar bone during early adulthood and may slowly enlarge over the years. Yet, it is more commonly self-limited, never undergoes neoplastic degeneration, and usually requires no treatment, other than a differentiation with other mucosal-colored lesions.

62. What are the two most common causes of *white* spots in the oral mucosa?

- **Thickening of oral mucosa:** This is the most common cause of oral white spots. It is usually due to recurrent trauma, such as biting of the sides of the mouth, and may manifest as a horizontal white line (*linea alba* in Latin) in the buccal mucosa, stretching between Stensen's duct and the angle of the mouth. It is created by the juxtaposition of upper and lower teeth. It is also called *occlusal* (or *bite*) line. Whitish thickenings of buccal mucosa also can occur near broken teeth or ill-fitting dentures.
- **Squamous cell carcinoma:** The second most common cause of oral white spots, referred to in the past as *leukoplakia* (Fig. 6-6).

  Less common causes of white spots in the oral mucosa include:
- Hairy leukoplakia
- Oral thrush
- Koplik's spots
- Fordyce's spots

63. What is hairy leukoplakia?

A distinctive lesion of the lateral aspects of the tongue and, occasionally, of the buccal mucosa of the cheeks (*see* also question 100).

64. What is oral thrush?

Candidal infection of oropharyngeal mucosa. This presents as multiple whitish papules and plaques, often surrounded by an erythematous rim. Unlike *hairy leukoplakia* (which is part of the mucosa, and not an overlay), candidal lesions are

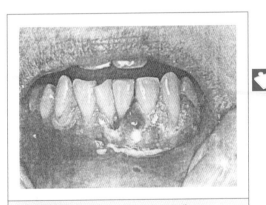

Figure 6-6. Squamous cell carcinoma presenting as leukoplakia with erythematous and verrucous areas. (From Sonis ST: Dental Secrets, 2nd ed. Philadelphia, Hanley & Belfus, 1999.)

easily scraped off with a tongue blade, leaving an underlying mucosa that is highly inflamed and often bleeding. Diagnosis is confirmed by potassium hydroxide (KOH) preparation. Oral thrush patients are either immunocompromised (as a result of AIDS, high-dose steroids, chemotherapy) or on inhaled corticosteroids.

65. What are Koplik's spots?
They are less-common causes of white oral lesions, presenting as a cluster of tiny white macules on the buccal mucosa, near the first and second molars. Consistent with early *rubeola*, they precede the skin rash by a day.

66. Are Koplik's spots specific for rubeola?
No. They also may be seen in echovirus and adenovirus infections. Hence, they are an interesting, albeit minor, feature of systemic viral infection.

67. Who was Koplik anyway?
Henry Koplik (1858–1927) was an American pediatrician. Born in New York and trained in Berlin, Vienna, and Prague, he eventually practiced at the Mt. Sinai Hospital of New York. In addition to being one of the founding fathers of the *American Pediatric Society,* Koplik also was instrumental in developing the first sterilized milk deposit for American infants.

68. What are Fordyce's spots?
They are tiny, whitish (or more often yellowish) dots, 1 mm in size. They are found on lips, cheeks, or tongue and represent normal *mucosal sebaceous cysts*. They were described in 1896 by the American dermatologists John Fordyce.

69. What is Wickham's sign?
Wickham's sign (or Wickham's striae) is a lacy, white, reticulated pattern on the surface of lesions in patients with *lichen planus*. Lesions are flat topped, shiny, pruritic, whitish/grayish, streaky, and with a violaceous background. They are located not only on the buccal mucosa but also on flexor surfaces and male genitalia. At times, they may form linear groups and thus give a patterned configuration that resembles lichens on rocks.

70. Who was Wickham?
Louis F. Wickham (1860–1913) was a French dermatologist and one of the early promoters of radium as treatment of skin cancer. His name also is linked to a special knife that he designed for the scarification of lesions in lupus vulgaris.

71. Why is leukoplakia a "garbage can diagnosis" that should be abolished?
All white lesions used to be termed *leukoplakia*, since the word, quite conveniently, means *white lesions* in Greek (*leukos*, white, and *plax*, patch). Subsequently, the term was unjustly elevated to the rank of diagnosis. Since it is absolutely impossible to differentiate benign from malignant white lesions solely on the basis of inspection and palpation, the term leukoplakia should be returned to its original *descriptive* meaning. Hence, suspicious white lesion *must* be biopsied.

72. What features of a white lesion increase its chance of being malignant?
- Being palpable, indurated, bleeding, and associated with a concurrent ulcer (*see* Fig. 6-6). The risk is even higher in patients with satellite lymphadenopathy.
- Having concomitant risk factors for malignancy, such as the past or present use of ethanol or tobacco (smoking and chewing). Of interest, in a large review of oropharyngeal carcinomas, neoplastic lesions were more frequently *red* than white (64% versus 11%). Thus, *erythroplasia* rather than leukoplakia could be a better clue to a diagnosis of malignancy.

Pearl:

In the final analysis, the only way to differentiate a malignant from a benign oral lesion is to perform an excisional biopsy.

73. **List the causes of *pigmented* spots in the oral mucosa.**
   - Amalgam tattoo (blackish-grayish stain in the buccal mucosa, adjacent to an area of tooth restoration; caused by accidental mucosal exposure to dental amalgam)
   - Peutz-Jeghers syndrome
   - Smoker's melanosis
   - Hemochromatosis (bluish-gray pigmentation of the hard palate and, to a lesser degree, of the gums; seen in 15–25% of patients with hemochromatosis)
   - Malignant melanoma (pigmented lesion with irregular borders; often palpable and ulcerated)
   - Addison's disease
   - Melanoplakia (*black spots* in Greek); consists of one or more pigmented patches on the buccal mucosa of healthy, dark-skinned individuals; normal and of little clinical significance

74. **What is Peutz-Jeghers syndrome?**
   Named after the Dutch John Peutz and the American Harold Jeghers, this is an autosomal dominant disease characterized by pigmented and hamartomatous intestinal polyps. It is associated with multiple melanin deposits on the mucocutaneous junctions of the mouth and, occasionally, anus. Pigmented spots (1–5 mm in diameter) appear shortly after birth or in very early childhood. They also may be seen on the lips, oral mucosa, and dorsal aspects of fingers and toes. Perioral lesions usually fade with age, whereas lesions on fingers, toes, and oral mucosa become more prominent. Peutz-Jeghers carries a slightly higher risk of gastrointestinal malignancies, albeit not as high as Gardner's syndrome

75. **What is smokers' melanosis?**
   A benign focal pigmentation that presents as multiple, irregularly shaped, flat, and brownish macules, <1 cm in diameter, and mostly localized over the maxillary (and mandibular) anterior labial gum, buccal mucosa, and floor of the mouth and soft palate. Smoker's melanosis requires prolonged exposure to cigarette smoke and thus occurs only after the third decade of life. It is *not* due to local stains, but to a benign increase in melanocytic activity. Since melanocytes are stimulated by estrogens and progesterone, smoker's melanosis is much more common in women. It is also associated with yellow staining of the teeth and fingernails and with an increased risk of oral carcinoma. Differential diagnosis includes physiologic pigmentation (usually in dark-skinned individuals), Peutz-Jeghers syndrome, Addison's disease, and melanoma.

76. **How are skin and mucosae in Addison's disease? Who was Addison?**
   Skin and mucosae are hyperpigmented. Buccal mucosa (as well as lips, tongue, and gingiva) may also have a few scattered melanotic spots. The disease is named after Thomas Addison (1793–1860), a contemporary of Bright and Hodgkin. Born in Newcastle and educated in Edinburgh, Addison taught and practiced at Guy's Hospital in London, gaining a reputation as a brilliant teacher and an astute clinician. Yet his shy and introverted personality, plus his emphasis on diagnosis more than treatment, adversely affected his popularity. Even his work on primary adrenal insufficiency (published in London in 1855) was almost discounted as fiction. Plagued by recurrent bouts of depression, Addison eventually jumped to his death at age 67.

77. **How do you distinguish Peutz-Jeghers syndrome from plain freckling?**
   The pigmented spots of Peutz-Jeghers are not only more prominent on the lips than the surrounding skin but also are *present in the buccal mucosa.* This is not the case with freckling (*see* question 113).

78. **List the common causes of red spots in the oral mucosa.**
   - Pyogenic granuloma
   - Erythema migrans
   - Palatal petechiae
   - Kaposi's sarcoma

79. What does *pyogenic granuloma* look like?
As a red, small, well-defined, and rounded nodule composed of highly vascular granulation tissue. This projects from the buccal mucosa and frequently ulcerates. Histologically, it resembles a capillary hemangioma.

80. Describe the lesions of *erythema migrans*.
They are multiple, flat, irregularly shaped red patches with raised white rims, usually located on the buccal mucosa, ventral tongue, and gum. Erythema migrans is often associated with a geographic tongue, which is in fact also referred to as erythema migrans *lingualis*(i.e., *benign migratory glossitis,* geographic tongue. *See* question 97).

81. What are *palatal petechiae*?
They are scattered lesions near the border of the hard and soft palate. These are highly suggestive (but not pathognomonic) of infectious mononucleosis, where they may be seen in two thirds of patients toward the end of the first week of illness.

82. What do the oral lesions of *Kaposi's sarcoma* look like?
As raised or flat purplish lesions. These typically affect the palate of AIDS patients, while instead sparing the elderly, nonimmunocompromised patients of Mediterranean origin who have the classic form of the disease.

83. What are the causes of *ulcers and erosions* in the oral mucosa?
The most common are (1) *thermal injuries* (such as burns from hot coffee), and (2) *aphthous ulcers* (canker sore, from the Greek *aphthae,* ulcerations). Less common (but more ominous) causes include (1) *autoimmune gingivostomatitis* (pemphigus, pemphigoid, and Stevens-Johnson syndrome), which causes a tender, painful, inflammatory sloughing of mucosa, usually preceded by vesicles or bullae; (2) *carcinoma* or *primary syphilis*, both of which produce a painless and solitary ulcer; and (3) *viral gingivostomatitis* (from either herpes or coxsackievirus).

84. What are *aphthous ulcers*?
They are among the most *painful* mucosal erosions: round or oval, with a whitish-yellowish color and a reddened rim. Aphthous ulcers come in three different types: minor, major, and herpetiform:
- **Minor aphthae** are extremely common and usually involve the labial or buccal mucosa, soft palate, tongue, and mouth floor. They are usually shallow, <1 cm in diameter, and either isolated or multiple.
- **Major aphthae** are instead large and deep. Hence, they often heal with scarring.
- **Herpetiform aphthae** tend to be more numerous and vesicular in morphology.
  Patients with benign aphthous ulcers should have no fever, adenopathy, gastrointestinal symptoms, arthritis, or other skin or mucous membrane involvement (such as uveitis, conjunctivitis, or genital ulcerations). If present, these manifestations suggest an underlying systemic disease and thus should always prompt a thorough diagnostic search. Otherwise, minor aphthae are benign, idiopathic, and spontaneously healing, albeit often recurring.

85. How do you differentiate between a *canker* and a *chancre*?
Although both may result in oral mucosal ulcers, there is considerable difference between these two terms:
- **Canker** (Middle English term for a malignant, spreading, invading, and ominous lesion) has now become a modern colloquialism for *canker sore*, a quite painful but entirely benign aphthous ulcer (previously discussed in question 83).
- **Chancre** (an Old French term, subsequently adopted by modern French language) still refers to the much more serious, painless ulcer of *primary syphilis*.

Both terms actually derive from the Latin *cancer* (crab), or the Sanskrit *karkata* (crab) and *karkara* (hard). Their gloomy connotation reflects the time-honored and ominous significance of having a mouth ulcer, often the first manifestation of the "French disease": syphilis. Note that the link between syphilis and France was initiated by the Italian physician, astronomer, wine connoisseur, and philosopher extraordinaire, Girolamo Fracastoro, who in 1530 wrote a poem titled: *Syphilis, sive Morbus Gallicus* ("Syphilis, or the French Disease"). Ironically, the French had acquired syphilis during their 1494–1515 invasion of Italy (and, indeed, tried to dub it *the Italian disease*, a term that never took). The Italians, in turn, had acquired it from the Spanish sailors who had visited their ports after returning from America. Considering where syphilis probably originated, a more appropriate term would have been *the American disease*. As for the poem that started it all, its protagonist was indeed Syphilis, a shepherd and, presumably, the first victim of the disease. Fracastoro used the term *syphilis* again in his medical treatise *De Contagione*, published in 1546—a true landmark in the history of infectious disease, since it proposed a scientific germ theory that predated Pasteur and Koch by more than 300 years. The term *syphilis* was eventually adopted into English in 1718.

86. **Can the vermilion border of the lip identify the cause of oral mucosal ulcers and vesicles?**
Yes. Lesions that cross the vermilion border of the lip and involve the skin are due invariably to *herpes simplex*. Conversely, lesions that do not cross the border (and are thus limited to the lip) are more likely due to *coxsackievirus* infection or an *autoimmune disease*.

87. **Where is Coxsackie? Who there has the disease?**
Coxsackie is a city in New York state, the proud hometown of patients in whom the virus of *herpangina* (infection of the oropharynx) was first isolated. This virus is also responsible for aseptic meningitis, pericarditis, myocarditis, and pleurodynia. Of course, coxsackie viruses are not limited to Coxsackie, New York, but cross both interstate and international borders.

88. **What is Bornholm and why is it in geographic competition with Coxsackie?**
Bornholm is a Danish island in the Baltic Sea, where the syndrome of *epidemic pleurodynia* (aptly called *Bornholm disease*) was first described. The intriguing aspect of this syndrome (characterized by sore throat, cough, and paroxysms of pain, usually pleuritic but also abdominal) is that it is caused by a virus named after *another* geographic location, Coxsackie, New York.

89. **Why should you examine the palms and soles of patients with oropharyngeal vesicles/erosions?**
Because these patients (especially children with coxsackie herpangina) may indeed present with vesicles on palms and soles, both important clues for explaining a particularly vexing sore throat.

C. TONGUE

90. **Describe the anatomy of the tongue.**
It consists of skeletal muscle covered with mucosa. On its *dorsum* are many exophytic structures (the *papillae*) that increase surface area and, more importantly, contain taste buds for gustatory sensation. These come in different types: *filiform, fungiform,* and *circumvallate*. Filiform and fungiform papillae are small and cover the entire dorsal surface of the organ; circumvallate papillae are instead larger and only located on the posterior dorsum, in semicircular arrangement.

91. **What is *dysgeusia*?**
It is the altered perception of taste (from the Greek *dys*, abnormal, and *geusis*, taste). It may reflect either *local* (i.e., involving the tongue) or *central* abnormalities (involving the nervous system).

92. **What is the best way to inspect the tongue?**
By achieving its effective protrusion. This is best accomplished by asking the patient to say the infamous "Ahhhh" (or "Aeee," but probably not "Ha"—as previously discussed) while at the same time protruding and curling the tongue upward, which allows access to the sublingual surface of the organ. Examination of the far interior and lateral aspect can be accomplished by placing gauze on the tip of the tongue, gently grasping it, and pulling it out. Note that a unilateral paralysis of cranial nerve XII (hypoglossal) is associated with asymmetric protrusion of the tongue.

93. **Summarize the abnormalities of the tongue.**
See Table 6-3.

94. **What is *macroglossia*? What are its causes?**
Macroglossia (*large tongue* in Greek) is a rare finding. The patient presents with indentations on the sides of the tongue (caused by pressure from the lateral teeth), and may also have a history of thickened speech, snoring, or full-blown sleep apnea. Although politicians are at greater risk for developing an *occupational* variety of this condition, macroglossia is often associated with systemic disorders, such as acromegaly, hypothyroidism, Down syndrome, amyloidosis, and various thesaurismoses. In all these conditions, the enlargement of the tongue is caused by either proteinaceous infiltration or hypertrophy of the muscle. The exception, of course, is politicians (whose macroglossia is due to idiopathic tongue-in-cheek), and some normal people, who present instead with simple lateral indentations, without clear-cut macroglossia or systemic illness.

95. **What is a *scrotal tongue*?**
A relatively common finding in the elderly. The tongue has many ugly-looking fissures (hence, the colorful term, *scrotal*) of otherwise little or no clinical significance.

96. **What is a *hairy tongue*?**
Another common condition, characterized by an abnormal desquamation of the *filiform papillae*, which, instead of being 1 mm long, can become 15 mm in length, thus giving the tongue its characteristic "hairy" coating, plus a brownish-to-blackish

TABLE 6-3. TONGUE ABNORMALITIES[*]
Atypical Tongues
Macroglossia
Scrotal tongue
Hairy tongue
Geographic tongue
Median rhomboid glossitis
Tongue-tie
Discolorations
White Tongue
Geographic tongue
White hairy tongue (= hairy leukoplakia)
Oral thrush
Squamous cell carcinoma
Red Tongue
Atrophic glossitis
Black Tongue
Hairy tongue
Use of charcoal for gastrointestinal decontamination
Ingestion of dark-colored candy or black licorice
Ingestion of bismuth-containing products (Pepto-Bismol)
Colonization by *Aspergillus niger*
*See text for further discussion.

discoloration (*lingua villosa nigra, or "black hairy tongue"*). Note that a hairy tongue also may appear brown, white, green, or pinkish, depending on its etiology and secondary factors (such as the use of colored mouthwashes, breath mints, candies). Common causes include radiation therapy to the head and neck and certain medications, especially broad-spectrum antibiotics. The condition, however, may often be idiopathic, and in this case usually results from inadequate tooth brushing, or a diet with too little roughage to mechanically débride the dorsum of the tongue. Prevalence is high, and usually higher with age (from 8.3% in children and young adults to 57% in IV drug abusers and prison inmates), probably because of the high frequency among older subjects of practices that predispose to the condition. Although there is no racial predilection, a hairy tongue is more prevalent in males. It is also more prevalent in HIV patients, smokers, and tea/coffee drinkers. It is usually asymptomatic, although patients may complain of tickling (and at times gagging) upon swallowing. Overgrowth of *Candida* sp. may result in a burning feeling (*glossopyrosis*), while retention of oral debris between the elongated papillae (and its associated bacterial and fungal overgrowth) may cause halitosis. Yet, like the scrotal tongue, a hairy tongue is usually of little clinical significance. Differential diagnosis includes oral candidiasis and the much more ominous *hairy leukoplakia*. Treatment consists in using a tongue scraper to remove elongated papillae and retard the growth of additional ones.

97. What is a *geographic tongue*?

A benign inflammatory condition, often referred to as *benign migratory glossitis* (i.e., *erythema migrans lingualis*; *see* also question 80). This is characterized by multiple, smooth, red, and glossy patches of glossitis, each surrounded by a serpiginous rim of a whitish/hyperkeratotic border (Fig. 6-7). The patches resemble the islands of an archipelago (hence, the nickname of *geographic*), and primarily affect the tongue's *dorsum*, even though they may often extend to the lateral borders. Histologically, they are caused by atrophy of the filiform papillae and may even

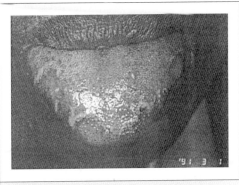

Figure 6-7. Geographic tongue. (From Sonis ST: Dental Secrets, 2nd ed. Philadelphia, Hanley & Belfus, 1999.)

wax and wane with time. Hence, the adjective of *migratory*. Eventually, they resolve spontaneously only to reappear at different sites (if lesions occur in other mucosae, the condition is instead termed *erythema migrans*). A geographic tongue often runs in families and is relatively common, being present in up to 3% of the general population. It has no racial or ethnic predilection, but does affect adults more than children and women more than males (2:1). In fact, exacerbations have often been linked to hormonal factors. Still, unlike atrophic glossitis, a *geographic tongue* is *not* associated with nutritional deficiency, but is instead idiopathic. A psychosomatic relation has even been suggested. Histologically, lesions are quite similar to those of psoriasis, or to the mucocutaneous presentations of Reiter's syndrome. In fact, a geographic tongue is four times more prevalent in psoriatics. It remains, however, asymptomatic (although some patients report increased sensitivity to hot and spicy foods), quite benign, and usually self-limited. Differential diagnosis includes candidiasis, contact stomatitis, chemical burns, lichen planus, and psoriasis. Given the typical clinical presentation, reassurance (and not biopsy) is the best management.

98. **What is a *median rhomboid glossitis* (MRG)?**

It is another benign involvement of the dorsum of the tongue, inflammatory or infectious in nature, and often mistaken for cancer. Rather uncommon (estimated prevalence <1% of adults), it presents as a rhomboidal patch of reddened mucosa on the midline of the dorsum, just anterior to the "V" region of the circumvallate papillae (*sulcus terminalis*). This patch is sharply circumscribed, flat or raised, and with a firm texture. It is either asymptomatic or associated with a slightly burning sensation after spicy foods. The etiology is unknown, although candidiasis has been implicated, especially given the frequency of positive cultures and histologic examinations.

99. **Can the tongue be *white*?**

Yes. Although it may often appear whitish as a result of foodstuffs ingested, several entities may result in a tongue that is *really* white—the same entities causing white oral lesions.

100. **What is a white hairy tongue *(hairy leukoplakia)*?**

A serious condition characterized by multiple white, warty, corrugated, and painless plaques, full of hair-like projections of keratin growth (Fig. 6-8). These are usually on the lateral margins of the tongue, but can occasionally involve the buccal mucosa of the cheeks and other oral sites. Unlike thrush, hairy leukoplakia *cannot* be scraped off. The lesion is typically associated with HIV infection, even though it also can occur in severely immunocompromised *organ transplants*. Caused by the Epstein-Barr virus, it is

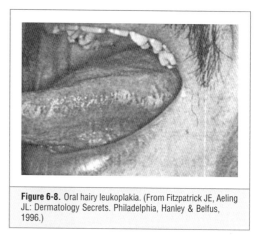

Figure 6-8. Oral hairy leukoplakia. (From Fitzpatrick JE, Aeling JL: Dermatology Secrets. Philadelphia, Hanley & Belfus, 1996.)

neither painful nor dangerous. In fact, most patients are unaware of it. May even regress in response to antiviral therapy, yet it does carry a worse prognosis for HIV progression. Clinical appearance is distinctive enough to yield a diagnosis. When in doubt, biopsy.

101. **What is the cause of a *smooth, red tongue*?**

The most common is *atrophic glossitis,* the final stage of *glossitis*. This is an entity characterized initially by papillary hypertrophy, then by papillary flattening, and finally by loss of all but the circumvallate papillae. As a result, the initially shiny red color (*beefy tongue*) changes to a paler hue, in a tongue that is often smooth and sore (because of *atrophy*).

102. **What causes atrophic glossitis?**

Usually, a profound deficiency of B-complex vitamins, such as niacin, pyridoxine, thiamine, riboflavin, folate, and B_{12}. Physical examination may help differentiating folate from B_{12} deficiency by testing of proprioceptive sensation. In folate deficiency, the patient has glossitis but normal proprioception; in B_{12} deficiency (and, therefore, in pernicious anemia), the glossitis is instead accompanied by abnormal proprioception. Other causes of glossitis include regional enteritis, iron-deficiency anemia, alcoholism, severe malnutrition (protein-calorie), and malabsorption. Glossitis often presents with *cheilitis (see* question 108).

103. What causes palpable lingual *nodules* and *papules*?

Many entities, with most being variants of normalcy, but some being harbingers of malignancy.

- **Circumvallate papillae:** These may become so prominent at times to appear suspicious. Easily visualized by having the patient protrude the tongue, they are entirely normal.

- **Lingual thyroid:** Another benign but more unusual entity, this is the vestigial remnant of the thyroid's embryologic site, before the gland migrated down to the front of the neck during the first trimester of pregnancy (failure to migrate causes a lingual thyroid; excessive migration causes instead a mediastinal/substernal thyroid). It presents as a smooth, round, and red midline nodule at the base of the tongue. Lingual thyroids are four times more common in females, typically asymptomatic, and rarely >1 cm (even though at times they may exceed 4 cm). Larger lesions may interfere with swallowing and respiration, and even present with a typical "hot potato speech." Also, up to 70% of patients may have hypothyroidism, and 10% cretinism. A lump of this sort in a teenage or young adult should never be removed, but instead diagnosed by confirming iodine uptake on radionuclide scan.

- **Lingual tonsils:** Reddish and smooth-surfaced nodules/papules on the posterior lateral border of the tongue in the foliate papilla area. Normal, albeit hypertrophic, lymphatic tissue.

- **Papilloma:** Soft, well-circumscribed, and pedunculated nodule that originates in the lingual mucosa and may achieve relatively large size. Caused by the human papilloma virus.

- **Carcinoma:** Any nontender, firm, and whitish plaque, papule, or nodule (even ulcer) should be considered neoplastic until proven otherwise. Carcinomas, especially squamous cell, tend to involve the lateral aspects of the tongue; hence, they may be missed by haphazard examinations.

104. Is an indurated tongue ulcer neoplastic?

Not necessarily. A *midline,* indurated ulcer of the dorsum of the tongue is unlikely to represent cancer, but suggests instead a *granulomatous disorder* (tuberculosis or histoplasmosis). Conversely, an ulcer located on the *lateral* or *inferior* surface of the tongue suggests a diagnosis of *Behçet syndrome* (first described by the Turkish dermatologist Hulusi Behçet in 1937, and consisting of orogenital ulcers plus joint and ocular manifestations). Finally, a nonindurated peripheral ulcer unassociated with systemic manifestations is a simple aphtha.

105. What is a tongue-tie?

Not what happens to shy people when out on a date, but a congenital condition characterized by a short lingual frenulum. This prevents protrusion of the tongue *(ankyloglossia)* and may occasionally interfere with breast-feeding. Usually requires surgery.

106. What are sublingual varicosities? What is their significance?

They are enlarged and purplish veins of the tongue's undersurface. They resemble little drops of purple-black caviar, and thus are often referred to as *caviar lesions*. Varicosities of this type tend to be an entirely normal by-product of age, due to loss of elasticity in the venous wall, resulting in venodilation and tortuosity, often resembling a hemangioma. Still, in some patients they may indicate a chronic increase in right-sided cardiac pressure, and thus suggest a diagnosis of either superior vena cava syndrome or congestive heart failure.

107. What is the significance of tongue-biting?

In patients presenting with a history of syncope, it represents an insensitive but highly specific clue to the diagnosis of generalized tonic-clonic seizures, especially when the biting involves the side of the tongue. In a study of 106 consecutive patients admitted to an epilepsy monitoring unit, tongue-biting had a sensitivity of 24% and a specificity of 99% for the diagnosis of generalized tonic-clonic seizures. *Lateral* tongue-biting had a specificity of 100%.

D. LIPS

108. **What is the difference between cheilosis and cheilitis?**
Unfortunately, *cheilosis* and *cheilitis* are often used interchangeably (as in the hybrid term, "angular cheilosis"), thus generating a bit of confusion. They should be distinguished as follows:

- **Cheilosis** (*cheilos*, lip in Greek) is reddening and cracking of one or both angles of the mouth—hence, the term of angular cheilosis, or angular *stomatitis*. This is usually encountered in edentulous patients with ill-fitting dentures, where it is caused by recurrent leakage of saliva, maceration of surrounding tissues (hence, the French term *perlèche*, excessive licking), and superimposed infection by endogenous organisms. These include *Candida* for patients with dentures and *S. aureus* for dentate individuals. Concomitant nutritional deficiencies (such as B_{12}, pyridoxine, riboflavin, or folate) as well as HIV, iron deficiency anemia. and Plummer-Vinson syndrome, also may contribute to its development.
- **Cheilitis** results instead from accelerated tissue degeneration, usually from excessive exposure to wind, especially sunlight (*actinic cheilitis*). It is characterized by dry scaling of the lips with painful vertical fissures. These are typically perpendicular to the vermilion border and tend to predominate in the lower lip. Cheilitis is a risk factor for squamous cell carcinoma, and also an early sign of Crohn's disease. Causes are ultraviolet radiation and the same nutritional deficiencies previously listed. Prevention includes use of sun blockers in lipstick and balm.

109. **What are the causes of lip *ulcers* or *erosions*?**
The most common are *squamous cell carcinoma* and *Herpes labialis*. Carcinoma usually presents as a solitary, nontender, and firm ulcer involving the lip; *Herpes labialis*, on the other hand, results in a cluster (*herpes* means indeed "cluster" in Greek) of tender vesicles and erosions.

110. **What causes a diffusely enlarged lip?**
Other than trauma (i.e., "fat-lip"), the most common cause is *angioedema*.

111. **What is angioedema (angioneurotic edema)?**
It is a painless, nonpruritic, nonpitting, and well-circumscribed edema caused by increased vascular permeability. This may come and go rather quickly (over a period of hours), typically involving the head and neck (the face, lips, floor of the mouth, tongue, and larynx), but also other regions of the body. In fact, it may involve the gastrointestinal tract, causing intestinal wall edema with colicky abdominal pain, nausea, vomiting, and diarrhea. In more serious cases, it may even cause life-threatening *laryngeal* edema, with stridor, upper airway obstruction, and respiratory failure. Although nonpruritic, angioedema is usually allergic in origin, triggered by medications, foods (berries, shellfish, fish, nuts, eggs, and milk), pollen, animal dander, insect bites, environmental exposure (water, sunlight, cold or heat),and emotional stress. It may even follow infectious illnesses or be associated with autoimmune disorders and leukemia.

112. **What is *hereditary* angioedema?**
A more rare (and serious) genetic condition that affects up to 1/10,000 individuals. It is characterized by recurrent episodes of edema, involving the intestinal wall (and thus causing abdominal pain, nausea, and vomiting), but also the hands, feet, face, and *upper airways*.

113. **What is the cause of pigmented areas on the lips?**
The most esoteric, of course, is Peutz-Jeghers syndrome (previously discussed). Yet, a much more common occurrence is simple *ephelides* (i.e., *freckles*). These are pigmented macules, 2–3 mm in diameter, that may indeed involve the lips as solitary or multiple lesions. Ephelides are benign but should always be excised if changes occur.

114. **What lip lesion may result in an ophthalmologic emergency?**
Herpes keratitis. In fact, any red and painful eye in a patient with antecedent or concurrent herpes labialis should indeed suggest the possibility of ocular extension. Diagnosis is confirmed by a positive corneal uptake of fluorescein with a characteristic dendritic pattern.

E. GUMS AND TEETH

115. **What is a *parulis*?**
A sessile nodule on the gingiva at the site of drainage of a fistulous tract originating from a tooth infection.

116. **What is an *epulis* fissuratum (denture-induced hyperplasia)?**
It is an exuberant response of the gum to recurrent trauma (*epulis*, gumboil in Greek), usually from ill-fitting dentures. It presents as *folds* of hyperplastic mucosa that encompass the border of the denture flange, and usually has a normal mucosal color. At times, however, it may also present as a sessile or pedunculated nodule, purplish-brown in color, and with more of a pyogenic granuloma-like appearance. This is due to capillary proliferation, and may result in easy bleeding. Since the epulis is due to trauma from denture flanges, it is usually observed in the maxillary or mandibular vestibule, typically in the anterior portion of the jaws. It is more common in women than men, Caucasians than African Americans, and older than younger individuals—probably because of greater use of dentures in these three groups. It is typically slow growing and asymptomatic. It must be differentiated from squamous cell carcinoma and pyogenic granuloma.

117. **What is a *pyogenic granuloma*?**
A rather common and benign *vascular* lesion of the skin of the head, neck, digits, and upper trunk, but also of the various mucosae, including gums and lips, gastrointestinal tract, nose, larynx, conjunctiva, and cornea. Despite its name, it is neither infectious (hence, no "pyogenic") nor granulomatous. Instead, it has unknown etiology, although it can present as a "pregnancy tumor" in 5% of all pregnancies (or more rarely after use of oral contraceptives). The lesion typically presents in children and young adults as a solitary and shiny, bright red nodule, friable and polypoid, slowly evolving over a period of a few weeks. This often bleeds spontaneously, may ulcerate, and can even be associated with bony erosion. Surgical excision may be indicated for control of local symptoms. If untreated, lesions eventually atrophy into a soft fibroma.

118. **What is the most common cause of a diffuse thickening of the gums? What are the other possible causes?**
The most common cause is *gingivitis vulgaris*, usually associated with periodontal disease. This represents not only a local problem, but also an important clue to the possible presence of coronary artery disease (CAD). In fact, patients with periodontal infections are twice as likely to have CAD, probably because of increased plasma levels of inflammatory mediators, such as fibrinogen, C-reactive protein, and several cytokines. Periodontal pathogens also may cause atherosclerosis by entering the bloodstream and invading the blood vessel wall. Other causes of gum thickening include:

- Scurvy
- Medications (the two most common are phenytoin and cyclosporine)
- Leukemic infiltration

119. **What is scurvy?**
The result of vitamin C deficiency, and an important cause of gum hypertrophy and bleeding. It is also an important (albeit rare) cause of morbidity and even mortality. Scorbutic gums are diffusely swollen, friable, thickened, and bleeding. There also may be concurrent petechiae in the perifollicular areas and dysmorphic, corkscrew-like hair. All these manifestations can be

prevented (and reversed) by vitamin C—something well known to the British sailors of old, whose fondness for citrus fruits even earned them the nickname of "limeys."

120. **What is the most ominous cause of gum hypertrophy and bleeding?**
Leukemic infiltration. This is often due to acute monomyelocytic leukemia, where gum disease may even be the presenting manifestation.

121. **What are the local complications of gingivitis vulgaris?**
The most common is tooth loss. The patient may also develop recurrent aspiration (with anaerobic pneumonias and abscesses) and severe gingival infections, with pain, fever, gum erosions (*acute necrotizing ulcerative gingivitis* or *trench mouth*), and halitosis "paramaligna."

122. **What does "long of tooth" mean?**
It refers to the observation that teeth tend to look longer over the years. This used to be viewed as a normal feature of aging but is actually due not to teeth *lengthening* (as in sharks) but to *gum regression* (as in gingivitis). Hence, anyone *long of tooth* may rapidly become *short of teeth*.

123. **What causes tooth loss?**
Not so much tooth *extraction* (or *fracture*) but rather:
- **Tooth abrasion:** From localized grinding (*bruxism*, from the Greek word *brucho*, or "grinding") and recurrent trauma due to toothpicks or pipes, which may notch the occlusal surface of the affected tooth.
- **Tooth attrition:** From decades of mastication, resulting in diffuse wearing down of teeth—as if they had been filed (like Nurse Diesel in Mel Brooks' *High Anxiety*). Because of attrition, the yellow-brown dentin becomes surrounded by only a rim of worn-down enamel. Hence, the yellowish hue of the tooth.
- **Tooth erosion:** Diffuse wearing down of teeth caused by recurrent exposure to corroding chemicals. It is often seen in people who consume large quantities of freshly squeezed citrus fruits or even sugar-sweetened carbonated beverages. It is, however, much more common in *bulimic patients,* whose enamel is exposed to regurgitated gastric acid, causing dental erosion in two thirds of subjects. These usually affect the posterior (lingual) aspect of the teeth, particularly the incisors. Similar erosions also may occur in nonbulimic patients because of simple acid reflux disease. Thinning of the enamel results in exposure of the yellow-brown dentin, with yellow discoloration of teeth and cavity formation.

124. **If you plumb a sulcus and it is normal, can the patient still have plumbism?**
Yes. A dentist plumbs a gingival sulcus to detect the severity of gingivitis. An inappropriately deep sulcus indicates moderate to severe gum disease, but certainly not *plumbism,* which is chronic lead intoxication. Although rarer than gingivitis, plumbism can be diagnosed by examining the tooth gingival *margin*: chronically and markedly elevated serum levels of lead will cause *lead lines* (also called *Burton's lines* from Henry Burton, a physician at St. Thomas Hospital in London and a victim of the great cholera epidemic of 1849). These lines are dark blue in color and formed by a series of tiny dots circling the tooth at its point of gum insertion. They are produced by tartar bacteria synthesizing lead sulfide (which is bluish black). Hence, they are absent in patients with no concomitant gingival infection (such as edentulous subjects). Note that similar dark lines also may be seen with chronic exposure to bismuth. Other manifestations of plumbism include renal insufficiency, peripheral neuropathy, saturnine gout (monoarticular arthritis), and, in younger individuals, a cognitive delay that may be quite profound.

125. **What are Hutchinson's teeth?**
They are part of Hutchinson's triad of congenital syphilis (interstitial keratitis, labyrinthine deafness, and Hutchinson's teeth). The upper incisors are smaller than normal and *notched*.

126. **What is halitosis?**
It is bad breath (*halitus* is Latin for breath, and *osis* is a Greek suffix indicating an abnormal condition). In the olden days, physicians used to differentiate "*fetor oris*" (a smell originating from the rhinopharynx or oropharynx, including the paranasal sinuses) from true *halitosis*, intended as a systemic odor exhaled from the lungs. This difference, however, is entirely disregarded today.

127. **What is the diagnostic importance of halitosis?**
Aside from its social and psychologic implications, halitosis is an important sign of underlying disease awaiting recognition and treatment. Although usually unrecognized by the patient, it is rarely missed by the unfortunate innocent bystander. Hence, unless you are blessed with Kallmann's syndrome (previously discussed), you cannot escape it—both medically and socially.

128. **What nonpathologic factors may cause halitosis?**
   - Age-related changes
   - So-called morning breath (due to reduced nocturnal wash-out by the saliva)
   - Hunger breath
   - Menstrual breath (mostly quoted by German texts from the late 1800s)
   - Tobacco breath
   - Various "breaths" from miscellaneous foods and drugs, such as garlic, onions, fish, metronidazole, and paraldehyde

129. **What are the pathologic causes of halitosis?**
Pathologic causes may be either local or systemic. The most common *local causes* include:
   - *Disorders of the oral cavity,* such as retained food, stomatitis, glossitis, periodontal disease, poorly cleaned dentures, and even decreased saliva with development of dry mouth (xerostomia)
   - *Disorders of the nose and sinuses,* such as atrophic rhinitis, chronic sinusitis, nasal septal perforation, ozena (an atrophic disease involving the nose and turbinates), and retained foreign bodies (especially in children)
   - *Disorders of the tonsils and pharynx,* such as recurrent infections of the tonsils and adenoids, pharyngitis, and especially Zenker's diverticulum
   - *Disorders of digestive organs* (esophagus, stomach, and small intestines), such as achalasia and gastroesophageal reflux
   - *Disorders of the lungs,* such as anaerobic lung abscesses, bronchiectasis, pneumonia, and empyema

   Systemic conditions presenting with a particular odor of the breath include:
   - The fruitish, sweet smell of acetone in diabetic ketoacidosis
   - The ammoniacal odor of fetor hepaticus and uremia

130. **What about psychiatric conditions that may be related to halitosis?**
In psychiatric conditions, the "bad smell" is *not* real, insofar as it is only felt by the patient and not by others. Psychiatric patients may perceive bad odors as emanating from either an *external* source or themselves. Causes of extrinsic olfactory hallucinations include schizophrenia and temporal lobe epilepsy. Conversely, a common cause of intrinsic olfactory hallucinations is the *olfactory reference syndrome* (ORS). This is a hypochondriacal psychosis characterized by excessive preoccupation with body image. Patients with ORS are sensitive, insecure, mildly paranoid, compulsive, and depressive. They also are convinced of smelling badly (especially of having bad breath). In fact, they are so obsessed with this idea that they

eventually isolate themselves. Providing reassurance is usually not enough, since patients often seek confirmation of their smells from a different doctor.

ACKNOWLEDGMENT

The author gratefully acknowledges the contributions of Dale Berg, MD, and Katherine Worzala, MD, MPH, to this chapter in the first edition of *Physical Diagnosis Secrets*.

SELECTED BIBLIOGRAPHY

1. Benbadis SR, Wolgamuth BR, Goren H, et al: Tongue-biting in seizures. Arch Intern Med 155:2346–2349, 1995.

2. Cunha BA: Crimson crescents and chronic fatigue syndrome. Ann Intern Med 116:347, 1992.

3. Drinka PJ, Langer E, Scott L, Morroe F: Laboratory measurements of nutritional status as correlates of atrophic glossitis. J Gen Intern Med 6:137–140, 1991.

4. Ebell MH, Smith MA, Barry HC, et al: Does this patient have strep throat?. JAMA 284:2912–2918, 2000.

5. Eisenberg E, Krutchkoff D, Yamase H, et al: Incidental oral hairy leukoplakia in immunocompetent persons: A report of two cases. Oral Surg Oral Med Oral Pathol 74:332–333, 1992.

6. Friedman IH: Say "ah" [letter]. JAMA 251:2086, 1984.

7. Johnson BE: Halitosis, or the meaning of bad breath. J Gen Intern Med 7:649–656, 1992.

8. Jones RR, Cleaton-Jones P: Depth and area of dental erosions, and dental caries, in bulimic women. J Dent Res 68:1275–1278, 1989.

9. Kidd DA: Collins Gem Dictionary: Latin-English, English-Latin. Williams Collins Sons, London, 1979. As quoted in JD Sapira: The Art and Science of Bedside Diagnosis. Baltimore, Urban & Schwarzenberg, 1990.

10. Mashberg A, Feldman LJ: Clinical criteria for identifying early oral and oropharyngeal carcinoma: Erythroplasia revisited. Am J Surg 156:273–275, 1988.

11. Moore, MJ: Say "ah" [letter]. JAMA 251:2086, 1984.

12. Redman RS, Vance FL, Gorlin RJ: Psychological component in the etiology of the geographic tongue. J Dent Res 45:1403–1408, 1966.

13. Roenigk RK: CO_2 laser vaporization for treatment of rhinophyma. Mayo Clinic Proc 62:676–680, 1987.

14. Savitt JN: "Say ae." N Engl J Med 294:1068–1069, 1976.

15. Schroeder PL, Filler SJ, Ramirez B, et al: Dental erosion and acid reflux disease. Ann Intern Med 122:809–815, 1995.

CHAPTER 7

THE NECK

Salvatore Mangione, MD

". . . the privilege of decapitation should no longer be confined to nobles, and the process of execution should be as painless as possible."

−1789 French law proposed by Joseph-Ignace Guillotin—a physician and member of the Revolutionary Constituent Assembly. A mild-mannered and polite man, Dr. Guillotin had been born prematurely after his mother saw a man publicly tortured on the wheel.

A. NECK FEATURES AND SWELLINGS

(1) Generalities

The neck is an important crossroad of anatomic structures and organ systems, the most important of which is the *thyroid* (discussed in Chapter 8).

1. **What neck features should be identified during inspection?**
   The most important is the *contour*. Abnormalities include:
   - A **buffalo hump** at the base of the neck.
   - A **short neck**, which is suggestive of Klippel-Feil syndrome or sleep apnea syndrome.
   - **Pterygium colli** (from the Greek *pterygion*, wing). A *webbed* neck is seen in Turner's syndrome, Noonan's syndrome, and Bonnevie-Ullrich syndrome.

2. **What is *Turner's syndrome*?**
   A syndrome characterized by ovarian dysgenesis in phenotypic females with X-monosomy, short stature, low-set ears, shield chest, heart defects (especially coarctation), café-au-lait spots, freckles, and a webbed neck. It was first described in 1938 by Henry H. Turner, founder of the Endocrine Society and a University of Oklahoma endocrinologist.

3. **What is *Noonan's syndrome*?**
   A syndrome characterized by congenital heart defects (usually pulmonic stenosis) in a setting of pectus carinatum, short stature, mental retardation, hypertelorism, and a webbed neck. Females are fertile, but males tend to be cryptorchic with high gonadotropins. Bleeding and dermatologic abnormalities are common. It was first described in 1963 by U.S. cardiologist Jacqueline Noonan and pediatrician Dorothy Ehmke.

4. **What is *Bonnevie-Ullrich syndrome*?**
   A syndrome characterized by skeletal and soft tissue abnormalities, such as lymphedema of the hands and feet, nail dystrophy, skin laxity, short stature, and, of course, a webbed neck. It was first described by U.S. geneticist Kristine Bonnevie (1872–1950) and German pediatrician Otto Ullrich (1894–1957). When associated with Klippel-Feil syndrome, it goes under the name of Nielsen disease.

5. **What is *Klippel-Feil syndrome*?**
   First described in 1912 by the French neurologists Maurice Klippel and André Feil, this syndrome consists of congenital fusion of two or more cervical vertebrae, producing a low posterior

hairline and a short neck that often causes retroflexion of the head (opisthotonos). This may even lead to neurologic compromise, such as *platybasia* (a developmental anomaly of the skull causing the floor of the posterior cranial fossa to bulge upward into the foramen magnum), cord compression, cervical instability, and motility impairment. There also may be cardiac defects, ocular malformations, and various urogenital anomalies (renal agenesis).

6. **With what syndrome is a buffalo hump at the base of the neck most commonly associated?**
   Cushing's syndrome.

7. **What are the anterior and posterior triangles of the neck?**
   They are important regions of the lateral neck, separated from each other by the sternocleidomastoid muscles (SCMs) (Fig. 7-1). These can be easily located through inspection and palpation, especially if tensed against resistance. The remaining borders of **the posterior triangle** are the anterior margin of the trapezius and the upper margin of the clavicle, whereas the remaining borders of the **anterior triangle** are the mandible and midline.

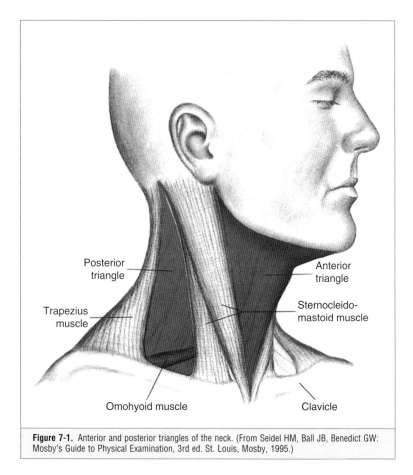

Posterior triangle

Anterior triangle

Trapezius muscle

Sternocleido-mastoid muscle

Omohyoid muscle

Clavicle

Figure 7-1. Anterior and posterior triangles of the neck. (From Seidel HM, Ball JB, Benedict GW: Mosby's Guide to Physical Examination, 3rd ed. St. Louis, Mosby, 1995.)

8. **What are the contents of the cervical triangles?**
   - In the **anterior triangle,** one can often palpate the jugulodigastric node. Other nodes are instead undetectable, unless enlarged by infection, inflammation, or malignancy. The anterior triangles also may harbor important embryologic remnants, such as thyroglossal duct/cysts, branchial cysts, and dermoids.
   - In the **posterior triangle,** there are many undetectable nodes that can become enlarged after a pharyngitis or a viral upper respiratory illness (URI).
   - The **subclavian artery** may be felt pulsating at the base of the neck, just above the clavicle.
   - The **transverse process of the atlas** may be palpated high in the neck, between the mandibular angle and mastoid process. It may be misinterpreted as a cervical mass.
   - The pulsatile **common carotid artery** (and its prominent bifurcation) is usually felt more laterally, along the SCM.

9. **Which swellings may be encountered during inspection of the neck?**
   Many. Classification and origin depend on location (posterior or anterior triangle; and for the latter, *midline* or *lateral* aspect) and nature (inflammatory or neoplastic) (Table 7-1).

(2) Swellings of the Anterior Triangle (*Midline*)

10. **What is the origin of midline swellings of the anterior cervical triangle?**
    They are mostly *thyroidal* (goiters or nodules). Less commonly, they represent remnants of embryonic structures, such as *dermoids* or *thyroglossal duct cysts* (Fig. 7-2). Since only thyroid and laryngeal structures ascend with deglutition, nonthyroidal masses can be easily identified by asking the patient to swallow.

11. **What is a thyroglossal (duct) cyst?**
    A swelling in the remnant of the thyroglossal *duct*, which in the embryo connects the thyroid to its point of origin at the base of the tongue. The duct usually disappears in the adult, leaving only a pit at its site of departure (the *foramen cecum* of the tongue). In some subjects, however, it may persist as an anomalous tract connecting the foramen cecum to the thyroid isthmus. In a few patients, this tract may even harbor a cyst or a fistula.

TABLE 7-1. NECK MASSES
Anterior triangle
Midline
■ Mostly thyroidal—goiter/nodule(s)
■ Thyroglossal (duct) cyst
■ Thyroglossal fistula
■ Dermoid (cyst)
Lateral aspect
■ Branchial cleft cyst
■ Branchial fistula
■ Branchial hygroma
■ Cystic hygroma
■ Laryngocele
■ Masseter muscle hypertrophy
Posterior triangle
Neoplastic
■ Lymphomas
■ Metastatic
■ Neurogenic
■ Paragangliomas/glomus tumors
■ Miscellaneous (ectopic salivary)
Inflammatory: localized
■ Tuberculous lymphadenitis (scrofula)
■ Bacterial lymphadenitis (abscess)
■ Suppurated branchial or thyroglossal cyst
Inflammatory: diffuse
■ Ludwig's angina

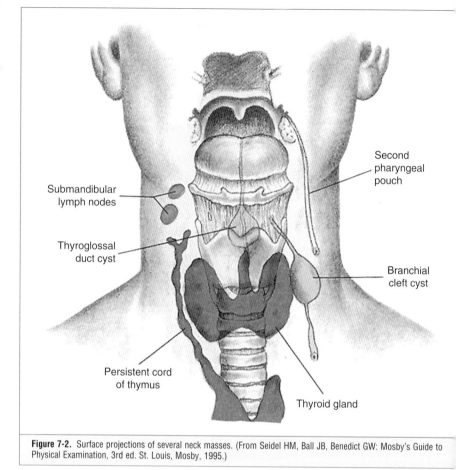

Figure 7-2. Surface projections of several neck masses. (From Seidel HM, Ball JB, Benedict GW: Mosby's Guide to Physical Examination, 3rd ed. St. Louis, Mosby, 1995.)

Although a *thyroglossal cyst* can occur anywhere along the path of the duct, most are found near the hyoid bone and thyrohyoid membrane (i.e., under the deep cervical fascia). These usually present as a tense, nontender, mobile, and nonlobulated midline mass, with acute tenderness and fluctuation, suggesting spontaneous hemorrhage or infection. Thyroglossal cysts may at times be just off the midline, pushed laterally by the convexity of the underlying thyroid cartilage and hyoid bone.

Still, since they are thyroidal in origin, they typically ascend with swallowing. Hence, they can be differentiated from the thyroid by their unique ability to rise with *protrusion of the tongue* (because of their firm attachment to the tongue's base). A lingual protrusion can be carried out by holding the suspected cyst between the thumb and index finger and then asking the patient to stick out the tongue as forcefully as possible. Alternatively, one can ask the patient to try to touch the chin with the tongue.

12. **Do thyroglossal cysts transilluminate?**
No—which is counterintuitive, considering their cystic nature.

13. **How common is a thyroglossal cyst?**
Quite common. In fact, of all congenital neck masses, 75% are thyroglossal duct cysts.

14. **What accounts for the other 25% of congenital neck masses?**
Branchial cleft cysts, typically located more laterally, just between the SCM and hyoid.

15. **What is a thyroglossal *fistula*?**
A fistulous opening of the thyroglossal duct—a less-common entity than a thyroglossal *cyst*.
It presents as a midline pit over the cricoid, intermittently draining and recurrently infected.

16. **What is a *dermoid* (cyst)?**
A bizarre and usually benign tumor that may occur in any line of embryologic fusion. In the neck,
it presents as a midline swelling of the anterior triangle, typically in the submandibular region
(just above the hyoid) but occasionally in the lower and suprasternal region. It also may cause
swelling in the mouth floor, typically pushing the tongue upward. Dermoids are remnants of
embryonic skin and thus may contain hair and cheesy epithelial debris, especially when located
in the gonads. They are usually small (<2 cm), soft, and occasionally fluctuant. They are not
attached to the skin and do not move with swallowing, but they *do* transilluminate. They present
in young adults or children as asymptomatic and slow-growing masses.

(3) Swellings of the Anterior Triangle (*Lateral Aspect*)

17. **What are branchial cleft cysts?**
Rather common congenital (and familial) masses of the lateral aspect of the anterior triangle.
Usually absent at birth, they become evident later on in life, at times bilaterally. They can be
associated with a sinus tract, and if so, can open onto either the skin or pharynx.

18. **Where do branchial cleft cysts originate?**
From failed closure of the second branchial cleft. During the fourth week of embryonic life, five
paired pharyngeal ridges (called the branchial *arches*) form the lateral and ventral walls of the
embryo's pharynx. These are separated externally by the branchial *clefts* and internally by the
pharyngeal *pouches*. Both arches and clefts will ultimately participate in the formation of the
various head and neck structures. With time, the second arch grows downward, ultimately
covering the third and fourth arches, thus burying clefts, which eventually disappear around the
seventh week of development. In some individuals, however, a remnant of the second branchial
cleft may persist, leading to the formation of an epithelium-lined cyst (*branchial cleft cyst*), with
or without a sinus tract to the overlying skin (*branchial fistula*). Note that, phylogenetically, the
branchial system is related to the gill slits of fish and amphibians. Hence, the name *branchial*,
which is Greek for gills.

19. **Where are branchial cysts located?**
Usually between the upper and lower two thirds of the *anterior* border of the SCM (hence, in the
lateral aspect of the anterior triangle). They also may continue deep into the muscle.

20. **What does a branchial cyst look like on exam?**
As a solitary, painless, and tense globular swelling, just below the angle of the jaw. As the
swelling enlarges, the cyst bulges—characteristically (and exclusively) around the *anterior border*
of the SCM. Still, a branchial cyst is *never* superficial to (or posterior to), the muscle per se.
Hence, it's never in the posterior triangle. Cysts neither transilluminate nor move with deglutition,
tend to be smooth, nontender, and usually asymptomatic. Yet, they may cause compressive
symptoms, and, if infected, even result in a neck abscess or draining fistula. Note that intermittent
swelling and tenderness is not uncommon during URIs.

21. **Is adenopathy common in branchial cysts?**
No. If present, consider either tuberculous adenitis (scrofula) or a complicating abscess.

22. **How does a branchial *fistula* present?**
As a pit over the anterior border of the SCM, usually exiting at the level of the hyoid, but at times even superiorly (anteroinferior to the earlobe) or inferiorly (near the lower part of the SCM)—still, *always anterior to the muscle*. Note that fistulas also may open *internally*. Hence, they can cause a mucopurulent discharge onto either the skin or pharynx.

23. **What is a branchial hygroma?**
A fluid-filled bursa or sac originating from branchial formations. It is usually cervical but may be thoracic, too.

24. **What is a cystic hygroma?**
A multiloculated and benign cyst composed primarily of budding lymphatics. It may occur anywhere, although neck (75%) and axilla (20%) are the preferred sites. Evident at birth in 65% of the cases (and by age two in the remainder), cystic hygromas present as large and soft structures with no clear margins. Complications include airway obstruction, infections (16%), and hemorrhages (13%).

25. **What is a laryngocele?**
A laryngeal hernia (from the Greek *kele*, hernia). This typically presents as an air-filled cervical outpouching, usually chronic and asymptomatic. Yet, at times it may present acutely, with hoarseness, stridor, or infection.

26. **How does a laryngocele form?**
Like a colonic diverticulum: through increased intraluminal pressure. Hence, it is typical of patients who recurrently "blow" their laryngeal walls, either because of disease (patients with [chronic obstructive pulmonary disease] COPD resorting to pursed-lip respiration) or profession (glass blowers and trumpet players—such as frog-mouthed Dizzy Gillespie). Laryngoceles start as an outpouching of the laryngeal ventricle, at times bilateral. As the exterior of the larynx expands through the constrictor muscles, the air-filled diverticulum becomes visible as a swelling in the lateral wall of the larynx, between hyoid and thyroid cartilages. This may eventually cause a change in voice, and, if complicated by infection, lead to abscess and encystation.

27. **What bedside maneuver can be used to identify a laryngocele?**
The Valsalva maneuver. Forced expiration against a closed glottis will inflate the laryngocele by increasing intra-airway pressure. This can be easily carried out by asking the patient to "bear down" as if having a bowel movement.

28. **How does congenital hypertrophy of the masseter present?**
Like a parotid mass. Differentiation can be easily accomplished by palpation.

29. **What is torticollis?**
An acute spasm of the sternocleidomastoid muscle. This typically presents as lateral prominence and deviation of the neck.

(4) Swellings of the *Posterior* Triangle

30. **What are the most common swellings of the posterior triangle?**
Lymphonodal swellings, either neoplastic or inflammatory (infectious).

31. **What are the most common *neoplastic* swellings?**
    - **Lymphomas:** These commonly present with cervical adenopathy.
    - **Metastatic lymphadenitis:** Most commonly from thyroid, nasopharynx, and the postcricoid region. Neoplastic nodes may compress or invade the sympathetic chain, thus causing Horner's syndrome (ptosis and miosis of the affected side).
    - **Neurogenic tumors:** These include neurofibromas and neuroblastomas, which, along with lipomas and cystic hygromas, are not uncommon in children.
    - **Paragangliomas or glomus tumors:** Rare in the neck—usually at the carotidal bifurcation, or higher up in the parapharyngeal region. May have a pulse and a bruit.
    - **Miscellaneous parapharyngeal tumors:** Mostly ectopic salivary neoplasms, which, like neurogenic tumors and lymphomas, cause not only neck swelling, but also medial displacement of the pharyngeal wall and tonsil.

32. **How can lymphadenitis be differentiated from other inflammatory neck swellings?**
    It depends on whether it is acute or chronic. *Acute* lymphonodal inflammation is easily identified by the presence of localized swelling and tenderness, plus the occasional systemic symptoms (fever and malaise). Still, it can be confusing. An acutely inflamed node over the mastoid process, for example, may simulate mastoiditis, while instead being just the result of a banal scalp infection. Occasionally, an acute lymphadenitis may progress to a localized abscess and thus become *fluctuant*. Knowledge of nodal drainage can help in identifying the primary infection site (scalp, nose, sinuses, oral cavity, throat, or larynx).

33. **What are the causes of *chronic* enlargement of a cervical node?**
    The most common is chronic infection, although a persistent and hard node should always raise the suspicion of malignancy. Protracted painless cervical adenopathy may occur with tuberculosis, lymphomas, HIV or EBV infection, and sarcoidosis. It can be differentiated from a thyroid mass because of its inability to ascend upon swallowing.

34. **How does a tuberculous cervical abscess typically present?**
    As a chronic, firm, and nontender lump, with a draining sinus tract in the posterior triangle of the neck (although a tuberculous abscess also may present *without* sinus formation). Relatively common in developing countries (especially Asia), *cervical tuberculous lymphadenitis* has become rare in the United States, thanks to pasteurization of milk.

35. **Where do neck abscesses typically originate?**
    From suppurative inflammation of lymph nodes. These may grow large and tender, especially in children. Other causes of cervical abscesses are branchial or thyroglossal cysts, also presenting as superficial and fluctuant masses. Identification relies on specific location.

36. **Do neck abscesses always present as localized fluctuant masses?**
    No. When suppuration is not well contained (as in the deeper fascial spaces of the neck), there may be neither fluctuance nor obvious port of entry. This is typical of *Ludwig's angina*.

37. **What is Ludwig's angina?**
    An acute submandibular cellulitis of normal hosts due to extension of a mouth infection into the deep spaces of the neck. Spread is eventually limited by the attachment of the fascial planes to the mylohyoid muscle. This results in a tense and rapidly expanding edema of the cervical soft tissues, ultimately leading to tongue elevation and fatal airway compression.

38. **What is the role of dental ailments in Ludwig's angina?**
    Major, with 80% of Ludwig's patients reporting recent dental work or pain. Tooth extraction often precedes it, especially when involving lower molars because the second and third molars

have deep roots that reach down into the attachment of the mylohyoid muscle (and usually below it), whereas first molars and anterior teeth have much more superficial roots.

39. **How does Ludwig's angina spread?**
Through the interrelation of the various potential spaces of the neck. These are formed by the attachment of the fascial layers to the neck structures and consist of:

- The **submandibular space**. This is the primary site of infection in Ludwig's. It is subdivided into two spaces that communicate posteriorly: (1) the *sublingual space,* which is bound superiorly by the mouth floor, posteriorly by the tongue base, anterolaterally by the mandible, and inferiorly by the mylohyoid muscle; and (2) the *submaxillary space,* which is bound superiorly by the mandibular ramus and inferiorly by both the hyoid and the posterior belly of the digastric muscle. Note that the anterior and lateral borders of the entire submandibular space are formed by the outer investing fascia's attachments to the mandible.
- The **pharyngomaxillary space**. This is bound superiorly by the base of the skull, posteriorly by the prevertebral fascia, laterally by the outer investing fascia, anteriorly by the pterygomandibular raphe, and inferiorly by the hyoid bone. It communicates laterally with the parotid and mas-ticator spaces, and posteriorly with the *retropharyngeal space.*
- The **retropharyngeal space**. This is contained between the middle and deep cervical fascia. It begins superiorly at the base of the skull and extends inferiorly to the upper mediastinum.

An infection that reaches the *submandibular space* can spread among *all* potential spaces of the neck, with different presentations depending on the area of involvement:

- "Woody" swelling of the neck for *submandibular* edema
- Elevation and protrusion of the tongue for *sublingual* infection
- Inability to open the mouth (*trismus*) for irritation of the muscles of mastication

Infection of the submandibular space may eventually spread posteriorly along the stylo-glossus muscle and into the *pharyngomaxillary space*, and from there enter the retropharyngeal space, and, ultimately, the mediastinum.

40. **How does Ludwig's angina present on exam?**
As bilateral swelling of submental, sublingual, and submaxillary spaces. Bimanual palpation reveals a characteristically "woody" firmness of the normally soft tissues of the mouth floor. Other common signs include a *nonfluctuant* (i.e., brawny, indurated) and tender neck swelling around the floor of the mouth, which is red, hard, and accompanied by trismus and tongue protrusion. Death from Ludwig's angina is usually the result of suffocation (from edema of the mouth, tongue, glottis, and upper airways) or spread of the infection (pneumonia, mediastinitis, and septicemia). Hence, any toxic-appearing and drooling patient with a brawny cervical swelling should be thought of as having Ludwig's until proven otherwise.

41. **Who was Ludwig?**
Wilhelm Frederick von Ludwig (1790–1865) was a German surgeon who served in the Allied Army that invaded Russia with Napoleon. Captured at the battle of Vilna, he spent 2 years in a Russian prison before returning to Tubingen, where he became physician to the royal family. There he described in 1836 the angina that was to become his ticket to fame, in Queen Catherine of Würtemberg and four other patients, all presenting with indurated edema of the submandibular and sublingual areas, minimal throat inflammation, and no lymphonodal involvement or suppuration. The swelling eventually spread to the muscles between the larynx and mouth floor, killing the patients. It was Ludwig's only important observation. A successful physician, he left at his death most of his fortune to a hospital for the poor.

42. **What is a submental sinus?**
A sinus of chronic granulation tissue, just around the apical infection of a lower incisor tooth. On exam, it presents as a midline pit under the chin.

43. What other inflammatory condition may occur in the neck?
- An inflamed **sebaceous** or **intradermal cyst**. This may occur anywhere, presenting as a smooth subcutaneous mass with a central visible punctum. Its superficial location easily differentiates it from other neck swellings.
- **Cellulitis**. A superficial soft tissue infection different from Ludwig's—although it also may result from a lower molar dental abscess. Yet there is no localized swelling or masses.

B. SALIVARY GLANDS

44. Which salivary glands are palpable?
The submaxillary, sublingual, and parotid glands.

45. Where are the *parotids*?
In front of and below the ears, just behind the mandibular angles. The largest of the salivary glands, they can be easily palpated bilaterally. The *facial nerves* (and their branches) pass through the parotid glands, as do the *external carotid arteries* (and their branches).

46. Where are the *submaxillary* glands?
Medially and anteriorly to the angles of the mandible. They have the size and shape of a walnut and are best appreciated upon swallowing. They can be difficult to palpate in young individuals with firm tissues.

47. Where are the *sublingual* glands?
In the mouth floor, just under the tongue. They *are* palpable but not routinely assessed.

48. What is the submandibular triangle of the neck?
The triangle delimited by the mandibular angles. Swellings in this area usually arise from the submaxillary glands or structures directly extending into the triangle, like the parotid tail or an upper cervical node. Differential diagnosis should include cancer and infections (Ludwig's angina).

49. What are the causes of salivary gland swelling?
It depends on whether the swelling is unilateral or bilateral. **Unilateral swelling** is usually due to a ductal calculus and its infectious complications (most commonly *Staphylococcus* sp. or *Streptococcus Viridans*). Inspection of the Wharton's duct (under the tongue, just lateral to the frenulum) for the submaxillary glands and Stensen's duct for the parotids may reveal the stone or simply pus. More rarely, unilateral painless swelling of one salivary gland may indicate tumor.
Bilateral swelling carries a much wider differential diagnosis:
- *Malnutrition*, such as starvation, kwashiorkor, and anorexia nervosa. Painless salivary swelling may occur even in bulimics, who are malnourished but do not look cachectic.
- *Sjögren's syndrome*. This is a keratoconjunctivitis sicca, characterized by dry eyes (xerophthalmia) and dry mouth (xerostomia). It is caused by a lymphocytic infiltration of salivary and lacrimal glands, associated with an autoimmune arthritis. It was first described in 1933 by Henrik Sjögren, the same surgeon who in 1935 developed corneal transplants.
- *Mikulicz's syndrome*. Chronic dacryoadenitis with bilateral painless swelling of lacrimal and salivary glands and decreased-to-absent lacrimation/salivation—not autoimmune but otherwise identical to Sjögren's. Causes include tuberculosis, Waldenström's syndrome, systemic lupus erythematosus, and infiltration by sarcoid and lymphoma. It was first described by Johann von Mikulicz (1850–1905), a pioneering Polish-German surgeon and spare-time pianist, who studied under Billroth, taught at Krakow, and was among the first to use gloves during surgery.
- *Alcoholism* (with or without cirrhosis). May cause fatty infiltration of the salivary glands and painless enlargement, very much like in the pancreas.
- *Diabetes mellitus*

- *HIV infection*
- *Thyrotoxicosis*
- *Leukemic infiltrates* and *lymphomas*
- *Drugs.* Painless (or painful) swelling may result from sulfonamides, propylthiouracil, lead, mercury, and iodide.
- *Acute parotitis.* Usually infectious, most commonly viral (mumps). Still, bacterial parotitis also may cause acute swelling and tenderness of the parotids, but this is usually unilateral and limited to debilitated patients with uncontrolled diabetes, renal failure, dehydration, or severe electrolyte imbalances. Often due to staphylococcal infection, it may progress to abscess, causing the overlying skin to become deeply red.

50. How do the parotids feel in acute parotitis?
They become swollen and easily palpable, to the point of pushing the earlobes forward and laterally. In severe cases, the swelling may limit jaw mobility.

51. Is parotitis exclusively limited to the parotids?
Not necessarily. In fact, most conditions causing swelling of the parotids also tend to cause swelling of the other salivary glands.

52. What do parotid tumors look like?
Like a rapid and uncomfortable swelling of the parotideal region, usually with facial palsy. *Pleomorphic adenomas* are the most common parotid tumor; *mucoepidermoid carcinomas* cause skin ulceration; whereas *lymphomas* typically present with facial palsy.

53. How common is a pleomorphic adenoma?
It accounts for 70–80% of all benign parotid tumors, even though 15% of all pleomorphic adenomas occur *outside* the parotid (in the submandibular and minor salivary glands).
It presents in middle-aged women as a painless, well-demarcated, solitary, and slowly growing mass. Irregularity of the tumor usually indicates hemorrhage, calcification, or necrosis. Sarcomatous degeneration is rare, and only in lesions present for 10–15 years.

54. What is Frey's (auriculotemporal) syndrome?
A syndrome due to a lesion of the *auriculotemporal nerve*, a frequent sequela of parotid trauma or surgery. It is characterized by recurrent episodes of localized facial flushing and/or sweating in the ipsilateral cutaneous distribution of the nerve (i.e., the cheek and the area anterior to the ear), usually triggered by eating and eventually subsiding within minutes after discontinuation of the food. It also has been termed *gustatory sweating syndrome.*

55. Who was Frey? When did she describe her syndrome?
Although auriculotemporal syndrome was first described in 1757 by Duphenix, it was not popularized until 1923, when Lucja Frey started researching it. She was a Polish physician and one of the first female academic neurologists in Europe. When her country was invaded by the Russians, Dr. Frey's husband (a prominent lawyer) was arrested and killed by Soviet police. Then, when Poland was occupied by the Germans, she herself, being Jewish, was "resettled" in the Lwów ghetto. She worked in a Ghetto poliklinik until August 20, 1942, when the entire facility was raided by the Nazis, and all patients and staff were immediately murdered.

C. TRACHEA

56. Describe the physical exam of the trachea.
It consists primarily of an assessment for shifts and mobility (*see* Chapter 13, questions 136–147).

ACKNOWLEDGMENT

The author gratefully acknowledges the contributions of Janice Wood, MD, to this chapter in the first edition of *Physical Diagnosis Secrets*.

SELECTED BIBLIOGRAPHY

1. Allard RHB: The thyroglossal cyst. Head Neck Surg 5:134–146, 1982.
2. Bailey H: Thyroglossal cysts and fistulae. Br J Surg 12:579–589, 1925.
3. Bounds GA: Subphrenic and mediastinal abscess formation: A complication of Ludwig's angina. Br J Oral Maxillofac Surg 23:313–321, 1985.
4. Ellis P, Van Nostrand AW: The applied anatomy of thyroglossal tract remnants. Laryngoscope 87:765–770, 1977.
5. Ewing CA, Kornblut A, Greeley C, et al: Presentations of thyroglossal duct cysts in adults. Eur Arch Otorh 256:136–138, 1999.
6. Girard M, Deluca SA: Thyroglossal duct cyst. Am Fam Physician 42:665–668, 1990.
7. Guarisco JL: Congenital head and neck masses in infants and children. Ear Nose Throat J 70:40–47, 1991.
8. Hawkins DB, Jacobsen BE, Klatt EC: Cysts of the thyroglossal duct. Laryngoscope 92:1254–1258, 1982.
9. Himalstein MR: Branchial cysts and fistulas. ENT 159:2329, 1980.
10. Juang YC, Cheng DL, Wang LS, et al: Ludwig's angina: An analysis of 14 cases. Scand J Infect Dis 21:121–125, 1989.

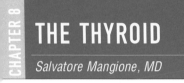

CHAPTER 8

THE THYROID

Salvatore Mangione, MD

"New York, the nation's thyroid gland."

—Christopher Morley (1890–1957)

A. GENERALITIES

The thyroid may not be the most important organ in a busy general practice, but in physical diagnosis it is second only to the heart in number of examination errors and lack of physician's confidence. This is unfortunate, since better skills may guide a more intelligent use of costly scans and better assessment of the likelihood of hyperthyroidism in anxious young patients.

B. ANATOMIC REVIEW AND THYROID GLAND INSPECTION

1. **What are the thyroid's landmarks?**
   They are the *laryngeal prominence* and *cricoid cartilage*. Start your exam by identifying the *hyoid bone,* a horseshoe mobile structure just under the mandible, so called because of its "upsilon" like shape. Immediately below it, you will find the *thyroid cartilage,* which can be readily identified by its V shape, the midline notch on the superior edge (*laryngeal prominence*), and its being the most prominent structure in the anterior neck (*Adam's apple*). Just below it, separated by a little gap (the cricothyroid recess), is the horizontal ring of the *cricoid cartilage*. The thyroid *isthmus* lies immediately below, 4 cm from the laryngeal prominence. It connects the two lateral lobes of the gland by crossing the trachea over the second, third, and sometimes even the fourth ring. Note that while the distance between isthmus and landmarks (cricoid cartilage and laryngeal prominence) is constant in all individuals, the distance between laryngeal prominence and suprasternal notch is variable. This may result in glands that are either *low lying* or *high lying* in the neck (*see* Fig. 8-1).

2. **Where are the thyroid lobes in relation to other neck structures?**
   The lateral lobes fan out from the midline isthmus just below the cricoid cartilage, curve posteriorly around the sides of trachea and esophagus, and then ascend backwards and upward like the two branches of a V (Fig. 8-2). Each lobe is 3–5 cm long, so that the lower margin reaches down to 2 cm above the clavicle (and fifth to sixth tracheal ring), whereas the upper margin extends instead upward to the middle of the thyroid cartilage. Except for its isthmus, the thyroid is covered by thin, strap-like muscles, of which only the sternocleidomastoid muscles (SCMs) are visible. Since the fascial envelope of the gland is continuous with the pretracheal fascia of both the hyoid and cricoid, the isthmus will ascend and descend with the larynx upon swallowing. This is important because it helps in distinguishing the thyroid from other neck structures.

3. **What is the pyramidal lobe?**
   An upward extension of one of the lobes, usually the left, present in up to 50% of autopsies. Rarely palpable in the normal-sized gland, it is detectable in 10–15% of nontoxic goiters.

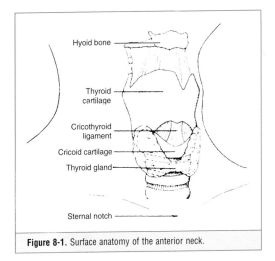

Figure 8-1. Surface anatomy of the anterior neck.

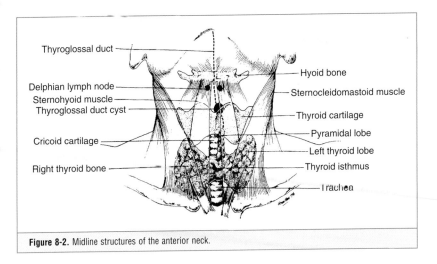

Figure 8-2. Midline structures of the anterior neck.

4. **What is the best way to *Inspect* the thyroid?**

By having the patient either stand or sit, with the head slightly tipped backward (around 10 degrees), and the cervical muscles as relaxed as possible. Neck extension is beneficial for two reasons:

- It raises the trachea further up from the suprasternal notch, thus moving upward any low-lying thyroid, too.
- It tightens the skin over the gland, thus enhancing visualization. Slight contralateral flexing of the neck also may accentuate a mass, nodule, or gland asymmetry.

Once the patient is well positioned, inspect the midline, 2–3 cm above the clavicles. Look within the SCMs for the inferior margins of the thyroid lobes, and then locate the isthmus (just below the cricoid cartilage). Finally, inspect the *superior* margins of the lobes (which should barely touch the sides of the thyroid cartilage). Look also for any possible pyramidal lobe. Use cross-illumination with a penlight to better accentuate shadows and nodules. Observing the gland from the side also may help detect possible protrusions. Note that *unless a goiter is present, there should be no bulging between cricoid cartilage and suprasternal notch.* Hence, a goiter is effectively ruled out if the gland is not visible *on lateral view* of an *extended neck*. Once inspection is complete, assess the associated venous structures of the neck, and record any possible abnormality (Figs. 8-3 and 8-4).

5. **How helpful is swallowing during inspection or palpation?**
Quite helpful. According to some authors, it may raise the sensitivity of inspection to that of inspection and palpation *combined*. Although its role has not been formally studied, most skilled examiners *do* ask patients to swallow during inspection (and even palpation) for the following reasons:
- Swallowing modifies the shadows of thyroid irregularities or masses, thus enhancing their visual detection.
- It *raises the gland*, thus making it more accessible to both inspection and palpation.
- It slides the gland (or its irregularities) against the examiner's hands, thus improving tactile discrimination and recognition.
- Most importantly, it allows the examiner to *localize* the abnormality because only the thyroid, lower trachea, and larynx move with swallowing. Deglutition lifts up both the trachea and thyroid by 1.5–3.5 cm. This movement culminates in a brief moment of hesitation, followed by a return of both the larynx and thyroid to their original location. Any mass that does not follow this triple sequence is not in the thyroid.

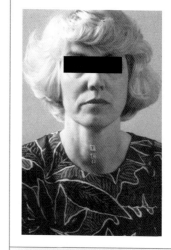

Figure 8-3. Nodule in the left lobe of the thyroid.

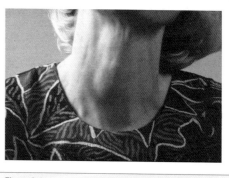

Figure 8-4. Accentuation of the thyroid nodule with lateral flexion.

6. **Should the patient be given a glass of water?**
Probably yes, since the extent to which laryngeal and thyroid structures move upward is proportional to the amount of swallowed bolus. Give patients a glass of water and ask them to hold a sip in their mouth until given the command to swallow. Repeat as needed.

7. **How much information can be gained by inspection?**
Quite a bit, thanks to the gland's superficial position in the anterior neck. Inspection can tell us about location, size, shape, symmetry, and surface. It also can teach us about mobility with swallowing, thus distinguishing the thyroid from other neck structures.

8. **What is *Marañón's sign*?**
It is the red (and at times itchy) skin overlying the thyroid of Graves' patients. It was first described by the Spanish endocrinologist, Gregorio Marañón (1887–1960).

C. THYROID GLAND PALPATION

9. **What are the goals of palpation?**
   To confirm size, location, shape, symmetry, and mobility of the gland—all previously identified through inspection. Palpation also can assess *texture* and *consistency* as well as fluctuance or tenderness—focal or diffuse. A *hard* thyroid, for example, suggests cancer, whereas a *rubbery* one is typical of Hashimoto's disease. Palpation also can identify a *solitary* nodule or the multiple bumps of a *multinodular* goiter. It can detect the diffuse, fine, and rounded protuberances of Graves' disease, whose gland is as bosselated as a raspberry. In these patients, a diffusely enlarged and *soft* goiter (i.e., one with the consistency of surrounding tissues) suggests a hypervascular Graves' thyroid, whereas a *firm* goiter argues instead for an infiltrated gland, as in the later phases of the disease. Finally, tenderness in a firm and diffusely nodular gland argues for subacute thyroiditis, whereas *tracheal deviation* and cervical *adenopathy* suggest cancer.

10. **What does the normal gland feel like?**
    Like the meat of an almond. In fact, each lobe is the size of a whole almond, no larger than the distal phalanx of the thumb ("rule of thumb").

11. **Should a normal thyroid be palpable?**
    Not necessarily. Glands of 15–20 gm (upper limit of normal) are barely palpable, whereas smaller ones (10–15 gm) are almost never detectable. Since thyroid size in a population is largely determined by dietary iodine supply, glands tend to be larger in deficient areas. Iodine supplementation has lately reduced the upper limit of normal from 35 to 20 gm in the United States, even though it remains 35 in iodine-deficient regions. This means that even a palpable thyroid may be "normal" in some parts of the world.

12. **What is the average size of the gland?**
    Lobes are 2 cm wide, 4–5 cm high, and 2.5 cm deep. The isthmus is 1.25–2 cm wide (and high) and <0.6 cm deep. Weight is 10–20 gm, and volume <20 mL. Still, it is more convenient (for both physician and patients) to categorize thyroids as *normal and palpable* or *normal and nonpalpable*. Experienced examiners can easily palpate small goiters of up to 1.5 times normal (25–30 gm). In fact, in some iodine-deficient regions, glands of this sort may be considered nongoitrous. Thyroids weighing 40 gm (i.e., twice normal) are usually large enough to be appreciated even by a first-year student.

13. **How do you palpate a thyroid?**
    Unlike inspection, palpation comes in many forms, including bimanual or single hand and anterior or posterior. None has been shown to be better.
    - Start with **proper positioning**. In contrast to inspection, a slight *ipsilateral* flexion and rotation of the neck may allow you easier access to a mass, nodule, or gland asymmetry. Hence, to palpate the right lobe, ask the patient to flex and rotate the neck toward the *right*. Do the opposite for the left lobe. Yet, as for inspection, a slight neck extension (10 degrees) may help, too, by lifting the top of a substernal goiter into a more accessible position. Still, most experts recommend flexion over extension. Finally, ask the patient to swallow repeatedly while you palpate the moving gland.
    - The **posterior bimanual approach** is the most commonly used. While standing behind the patient, place the index and middle fingers of both hands along the midline of the neck, just below the chin. These should be 2 cm above the suprasternal notch, and 0.5 cm inside the medial margin of the SCM. From that position, locate first the thyroid cartilage, then slide gently down to the horizontal groove that separates it from the cricoid cartilage. This is covered by the cricothyroid membrane, which overlies the first tracheal ring and represents the reference point for emergency tracheostomy (cricothyroidotomy) in upper airway

obstruction. Continue sliding down until you reach the next well-defined tracheal ring. At this point, you are on the thyroid isthmus, which lies between the cricoid cartilage and suprasternal notch, and is almost never palpable. Slide your fingers laterally on the isthmus, and go around for approximately 2–3 cm along each side: you will be touching the two main lobes of the gland. Use a soft touch to minimize discomfort and maximize yield. If the gland is enlarged, evaluate its consistency. Then ask yourself whether the enlargement is asymmetric or bilateral, nodular or diffuse, with movable overlying layers associated with adenopathy. Use one hand to fix the trachea and the other to palpate one lobe at a time (Figs. 8-5 and 8-6). You can practice by placing the second and third fingers of both hands over your own sternal notch. Move them up 2 cm above the clavicles (toward the lower thyroid poles), then palpate each lobe in detail.

- The **anterior single-hand approach**. Face the patient and use the thumb plus the index finger of one hand to palpate each lobe. Do this just inside the SCMs (Fig. 8-7).

14. **What are the normal variants in size and location?**
    - Women have larger and more easily palpable glands.
    - In 1% of the population, the entire left lobe (or its lower half) is absent.
    - The right lobe is often larger than the left.

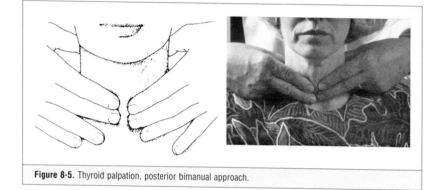

Figure 8-5. Thyroid palpation, posterior bimanual approach.

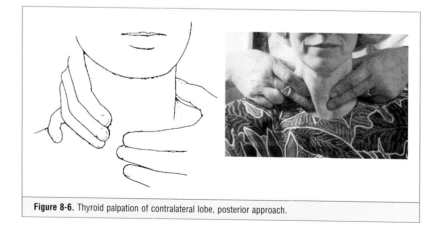

Figure 8-6. Thyroid palpation of contralateral lobe, posterior approach.

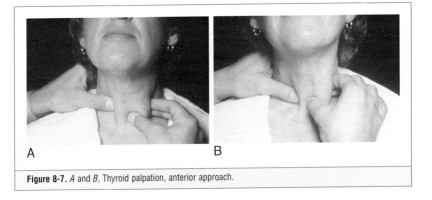

A   B

Figure 8-7. *A* and *B,* Thyroid palpation, anterior approach.

- A pyramidal lobe presents as a triangular projection, arising from the isthmus and extending up toward the hyoid. It feels like thyroid, and it moves with deglutition.
- Posterior, extracapsular, and ectopic tissue can occur in 5% of normal glands. This usually extends from the posterior aspect of the tongue toward the pyramidal lobe, and occasionally down into the mediastinum (*see* Chapter 6, Nose and Mouth, question 103).

D. ADDITIONAL COMPONENTS OF THE FOCUSED THYROID EXAMINATION

15. **What other aspects of the general exam should be emphasized?**
    If you suspect an autoimmune disorder (such as Graves'), search for extrathyroidal signs—especially in the eyes and integument (nails and skin). Search also for findings of dysthyroidism.

16. **What additional aspects of the neck exam are important in thyroid evaluation?**
    - Scars indicative of previous thyroid surgery
    - Redness at the base of the neck (Marañón's sign)
    - Venous engorgement (especially after Pemberton's maneuver)
    - Tracheal shift
    - Lymphadenopathy (especially Delphian node[s]—*see* Chapter 18, Lymph Nodes, question 30)
    - Transillumination of nodules and cysts

17. **What are the potential complications of a large goiter?**
    Mostly *obstructive*, with impaired venous return (facial plethora) and a compression of the esophagus and trachea that may result in dysphagia and dyspnea. Stridor occurs in 10% of substernal goiters; tracheal deviation in one third. Although Graves' glands may be up to two times normal (i.e., 40 gm), multinodular goiters are usually the most prominent offenders. When a large mediastinal or substernal thyroid obstructs the superior vena cava, there will be venous engorgement over the anterior chest and neck and possible impairment of cerebral venous return (Fig. 8-8). If reversible, all these findings can be unmasked by the Pemberton's maneuver.

18. **What is the *Pemberton's maneuver*?**
    A reversible superior vena cava (SVC) obstruction caused by a substernal goiter being "lifted" into the thoracic inlet as a result of arm raising. This makes the goiter behave like a "thyroid cork," blocking the inlet and thus preventing venous return. To carry out the maneuver, ask the patient to elevate the arms above the level of the head, as if surrendering ("elevat[ing] both arms

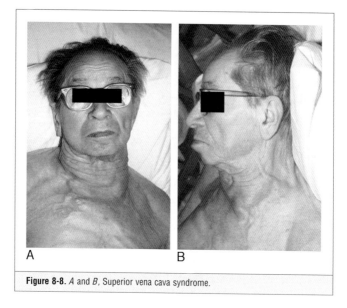

Figure 8-8. *A* and *B*, Superior vena cava syndrome.

until they touch the sides of the head," in Pemberton's words). If the sign is present, "after a minute or so, congestion of the face, some cyanosis, and lastly distress become apparent." In fact, the test is considered positive when the patient experiences either facial plethora (blue or pink suffusion of the neck and/or face due to venous stasis) or head congestion, dizziness, and stuffiness. If severe, the "thyroid cork" may even cause dyspnea and hypotension. The test is negative if nothing happens after *3 minutes* of arm elevation (Fig. 8-9).

19. **What is the significance of a positive Pemberton's maneuver?**
Facial plethora after arm raising (Pemberton's *sign*) is diagnostic of increased pressure in the thoracic inlet. It is also *prognostic*, since these patients often have more severe disease, with airway compromise, reduced peak expiratory flow, and thrombosis of right subclavian and axillary veins. Hence, the maneuver should be used in all patients with:
   - Goiter *and* positional head and neck symptoms
   - A large cervical goiter
   - Evidence of substernal extension of the gland
   Note that venous obstruction is *not* uncommon in substernal goiters, which present with distended neck and thoracic veins in 10–20% of the cases. Although rare, full-blown SVC syndrome also may occur. Still, many patients usually have few physical signs—with the possible exception of the inability to palpate the lower pole of the gland. This should serve as a clue to the presence of a *substernal goiter*. When in doubt, have the patient swallow, extend the neck, or carry out maneuvers that increase intrathoracic pressure—such as coughing or Valsalva's or Pemberton's.

20. **Is Pemberton's sign specific for a substernal goiter?**
No, it may be encountered in other patients with reversible SVC syndrome because of lymphomas or upper mediastinal tumors. It also may occur in thoracic outlet obstruction.

21. **Who was Pemberton?**
Hugh Spear Pemberton (1890–1956) was a graduate of Liverpool University, and to Liverpool he returned after serving in WWI, practicing at Northern Hospital till his sudden death in January

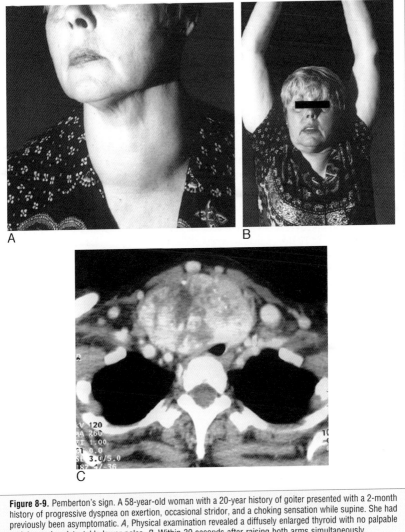

Figure 8-9. Pemberton's sign. A 58-year-old woman with a 20-year history of goiter presented with a 2-month history of progressive dyspnea on exertion, occasional stridor, and a choking sensation while supine. She had previously been asymptomatic. *A,* Physical examination revealed a diffusely enlarged thyroid with no palpable nodules and undetectable lower poles. *B,* Within 30 seconds after raising both arms simultaneously (Pemberton's maneuver), marked facial plethora (Pemberton's sign) developed, indicating compression of the jugular veins. Serum thyrotropin and free thyroxine concentrations were normal. *C,* Computed tomography of the neck revealed a large goiter extending into the anterior superior mediastinum and causing compression and deviation of the trachea. The patient underwent thyroidectomy, and her symptoms resolved. Pathologic examination revealed a multinodular goiter. (From Basaria R. Pemberton's sign. N Engl J Med 350:1338, March 25, 2004, with permission.)

1956 (just a year after retirement). An endocrinologist with an interest in diabetes, he also published on thyrotoxicosis, peripheral vascular disease, and hospital planning. The description of his homonymous sign appeared in a brief letter to *The Lancet* in 1946. Within 3 years the maneuver was on Bailey's 1949 *Demonstration of Physical Signs in Clinical Surgery*, and then in most physical examination textbooks.

22. **When should one auscultate the thyroid?**
    Whenever a goiter presents with signs of hyperthyroidism. A *bruit* reflects the gland's increased vascularity—rare in simple thyrotoxicosis, but common in Graves'.

23. **How do you distinguish a thyroid bruit from other neck sounds?**
    By location:
    - A **venous hum** is heard lower in the neck than a thyroid bruit. It is also suppressed by compression of the ipsilateral neck veins. Note that the continuous character of a "hum" cannot reliably differentiate it from a bruit, since 20–36% of all hyperthyroid patients have indeed a *continuous* bruit (due to arteriovenous communications within the hyperplastic gland). Compression of neck veins will help differentiate the two.
    - A **carotid bruit** is heard higher and lateral to the gland than a thyroid bruit.
    - A **thyroid bruit** can be differentiated from the transmitted murmur of *aortic stenosis* or *aortic sclerosis* through a complete cardiac exam, very much like the *stridor* and *hoarseness* that often accompany thyromegaly.

24. **What is *Berry's sign*?**
    An absent carotid pulse in patients whose cancer has invaded the vascular bundle. Always a sign of malignant thyromegaly.

25. **Who was Berry?**
    Sir James Berry (1860–1946) was a Canadian surgeon who contributed extensively to the field of thyroid resection. During World War I, he also was a philanthropist, assembling with his first wife a medical team, and then traveling to Serbia. Captured by the Hungarians, he was forced to repatriate, but eventually returned to Eastern Europe to continue his humanitarian work. Berry died in 1946, at the age of 86.

26. **How can one categorize thyroid abnormalities?**
    By assessing both physical findings and endocrine function (Table 8–1).

E. GOITER

27. **What is the normal thyroid size?**
    "Normal" depends on iodine supply in the local diet. In the not-too-distant past, for example, thyroids became progressively larger as one ascended from the sea to the mountains. In fact, euthyroid goiters were so common in the Swiss and Italian Alps that they became part of the local folklore. For example, one of the most colorful of the *Commedia dell'Arte* masks was Gioppino, an Alpine mountaineer whose trademark sign was a gigantic goiter (Fig. 8-10). The very word *cretin* (in reference to endemic and congenital hypothyroidism) also has something to do with mountaineers and goiters. Sapira reminds us that some early Christians ran to the Pyrenees to escape persecution. They escaped successfully, but also acquired hypothyroidism, and the mental slowing associated with it. When traveling to different villages, they were easily recognized and immediately referred to as *cretins* (*Chretien* is French for Christian). Huge goiters still occur, but only in mountainous regions (like the Himalayas), where iodinated salt is not routinely instituted.

28. **Which physical examination techniques can help establish thyroid size?**
    - Detection of surface abnormalities by either inspection or palpation

TABLE 8-1. PHYSICAL FINDINGS AND DISEASE PROCESSES

Thyroid Finding	Function	Disease Process
Diffuse Enlargement		
Diffuse, smooth goiter	Normal	Simple goiter, endemic goiter
Multiple nodules	Normal/hyper/hypo	Multinodular goiter
Diffuse, bosselated goiter	Hyper	Graves' disease
Firm, small, nontender goiter	Hypo	Chronic thyroiditis (Hashimoto's)
Firm, diffuse tenderness	Hyper/hypo	Subacute thyroiditis
Firm, hard, fixed, unmovable gland	Normal	Malignancy
Firm, hard, with lymphadenopathy	Normal	Malignancy
Focal tenderness	Normal/hypo	Abscess
Focal Enlargement		
Toxic with thyroid nodule	Hyper	Functional adenoma (Plummer's)
Transilluminated nodule	Normal	Thyroid cyst
Nontoxic with thyroid nodule	Normal	Malignancy
Focal tenderness, hyperthyroid	Normal	Hemorrhage in functional adenoma

- Estimated glandular volume or weight
- Visible thyroid prominence on lateral neck exam
- Neck circumference, as recorded by tape measure
- Maximal width of the lower poles, as measured by calipers or rulers
  Still, little validation supports one method over another.

29. **How precise are inspection and/or palpation in estimating thyroid size?**
    Quite precise. For *interobserver variability,* agreement among physicians in determining presence or absence of goiter (and in categorizing glandular size into one of three/four groups) is usually very good. The *k* for combined data from four studies is a respectable 0.77 (k ranges from +1.0 [two clinicians are in perfect agreement] through 0.0 [chance agreement] to −1.0 [two clinicians are in perfect disagreement]). Agreement is better among examiners with greater experience. It is also slightly better for palpation (k = 0.74) than inspection (k = 0.65). Data are good even for *intraobserver* variability. In this case, however, inspection (k = 0.73) seems to be slightly better than palpation (k = 0.65).

30. **Why is estimating size clinically important?**
    Because in patients with suspected or known disease, size can:
    - Confirm thyroid involvement
    - Help with differential diagnosis
    - Guide and interpret laboratory testing
    - Guide selection of therapy
    - Help monitoring
      For example, in patients presenting with symptoms of hyperthyroidism, an enlarged gland increases the likelihood of thyrotoxicosis, whereas a normal-sized gland makes anxiety more likely. Moreover, Graves' disease patients presenting with a larger goiter are less likely to undergo immunologic remission during antithyroid therapy, thus favoring radioactive iodine

(whose dose is also based on the size of the gland). Finally, evaluation of size can help monitor response to treatment. For example, shrinking of a large goiter after hormonal replacement suggests effective suppression.

31. **What is a goiter?**
From the Latin *guttur* (throat), this is a chronic enlargement of the gland (Fig. 8-11). Goiters occur endemically in iodine-deficient areas and sporadically elsewhere. As Sapira reminds us, the Latin for goiter is *struma*, a term still occasionally used, even though originally it did not indicate an enlarged thyroid, but instead a *scrofula* (i.e., the widening of the neck that makes the patient resemble a sow [*scrofula* in Latin]). Although this was mostly due to tuberculous lymphadenopathy, it eventually became linked to the thyroid after the Struma river of Bulgaria, an area of endemic goiter.

32. **What is the threshold for a goiter?**
Some authors have suggested the "rule of thumb," which defines as *enlarged* a lobe the size of the thumb's distal phalanx. Alternatively, one could calculate the volume of each lobe by multiplying width by depth by length, and then multiplying the result by 2.

33. **Are goiters neoplastic?**
No. Cancers are usually *nodular*, even though at times they may be goitrous.

34. **So what is the nature of goiters? Are they euthyroid?**
Goiters are neither neoplastic nor inflammatory, but rather *hypertrophic* or *degenerative*. They do not reflect functional status either, since enlargements may occur in both euthyroid and dysthyroid states (either hypo- or hyper-). Overall, most goiters are *eu*thyroid (80%); 10% are *hypo*thyroid, and 10% *hyper*thyroid. Hence, they usually present as asymptomatic masses.

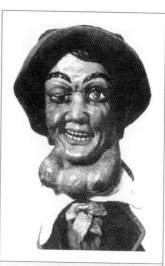

Figure 8-10. Goiter in the Commedia dell'Arte. The beginning of the 19th century saw the appearance of *Gioppino* in the Northern Italian area of Bergamo, even if little is known about its precise origins. The mask was first used onstage in 1820, by the puppeteer Battaglia, although many scholars believe it goes back even earlier, substantiating their claims with illustrations that clearly show its trademark three-hump goiter. Gioppino is a typical peasant character, full of common sense with a unique penchant for wine and good food. He invariably manages to get himself out of tricky situations by adhering to the popular motto: "big feet but a clever mind." He sports a giant and trilobulated goiter (presumably euthyroid in function, since it has not slowed down its owner's brain) and Horner's syndrome (probably due to sympathetic compression by the goiter).

35. **What are the three most common forms of a goiter?**
Multinodular goiter, Hashimoto's thyroiditis, and Graves' disease. In euthyroid subjects, think of multinodular goiter and Hashimoto's; in hypothyroid patients, think of Hashimoto's; and in hyperthyroid patients, think of Graves' and multinodular goiters (Graves' also will have unique skin and eye manifestations).

36. **What about subacute thyroidits?**
It usually presents with *tenderness*, which can often mimic pharyngitis. Thyromegaly is otherwise modest (1.5–3 times normal). Note that the differential diagnosis of a painful and tender gland also should include spontaneous hemorrhage into a cyst or nodule.

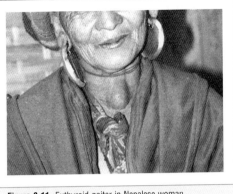

Figure 8-11. Euthyroid goiter in Nepalese woman.

37. Is goiter common in pregnancy?

No. Usually, there is a silent and postpartum thyroiditis that may manifest itself as goiter, although only half of the patients present as such (most are instead *hyper*thyroid). Otherwise, a true goiter is rather uncommon in pregnancy. Yet, mild hypertrophy is frequent, especially because of the changed hormonal milieu. In the past, this was even used as a "poor man's" (or woman's) pregnancy test. For example, overbearing Roman fathers used to keep a keen eye on their daughter's neck by periodically measuring its circumference, so to detect, as early as feasible, any possible "loss of purity."

38. What is the prevalence of goiter in iodine-replete countries?

Very low. If we define as "normal" a thyroid <10 gm (with an upper limit of 20), the prevalence of goiter in iodine-replete countries is about 2% in men and 10% in women.

39. Can goiters be easily differentiated from normal glands?

Yes. Normal thyroids are barely visible and only slightly palpable due to interference by various surrounding structures, especially the SCMs. Hence, the first sign of goiter is usually an increase in size of the lateral lobes, which become easily palpable. This is followed by a visible enlargement of the *entire gland*, first on lateral neck inspection and then on frontal view (with the neck extended). By the time the goiter is large enough to become palpable, it can be spotted from both front and sides.

40. So how can physical examination help identify a goiter?

Siminoski recommends the following strategy:

1. Examine the thyroid through inspection *and* palpation.
2. Categorize it as either normal or goitrous. If a goiter is present, subcategorize it as small (1–2 times normal) or large (>2 times normal).
3. If the goiter is *small*, consider the possibility of overestimation. Look for prominence in the neck profile and for visibility on frontal view while the neck is extended.
4. Finally, place the patient into one of the following three categories:
   - Goiter ruled *out* (normal thyroid size, or gland not visible with neck extended)
   - Goiter ruled *in* (large goiter or lateral prominence >2 mm)
   - Inconclusive (all other findings)

41. What may lead to false-positive and false-negative results of goiter detection?

(a) False-positive thyroid enlargement (pseudogoiter)

1. *Accentuated prominence of a palpable but in reality normal gland*:

- Thin patients whose thyroid is uniquely and misleadingly accessible.
- Patients with long and curving neckline that makes the thyroid quite prominent in spite of its normal location and size. Such pseudogoiters have been dubbed the Modigliani syndrome, after the Italian artist's penchant for long and lordotic necks. They are the most common cause of referral for possible goiter.
- Patients whose thyroid is higher than usual in the neck. These account for 10% of all referrals. Important clues are a negative thumb sign and a laryngeal prominence that is more than 10 cm above the suprasternal notch.

2. *The presence of a fat pad in the anterolateral neck* (common in young women and obese patients). In contrast to the thyroid, the fat pad does not rise with swallowing.
3. *Anterior neck masses.* These can be easily differentiated from goiters by using swallowing. Branchial cleft cysts, cervical lymphadenopathy, and pharyngeal diverticula are all less likely to adhere to laryngeal structures, and thus will not rise with deglutition. Goiters instead will. One important exception is the thyroglossal duct cyst, which not only rises with swallowing, but also does so upon forced tongue protrusion (*see* Chapter 7, The Neck, questions 10–15).

(b) False-negative thyroid enlargement

1. *Inadequate examination skills.* The most common reason for a false-negative exam.
2. *Short and thick-necked patients,* especially if obese, elderly, or with COPD
3. *Atypical or ectopic placement of the thyroid.* Instead of being *cervical*, the goiter may be substernal or retroclavicular. Laterally placed lobes, obscured by the SCMs, also may yield false-negative results.

42. **What is the overall accuracy of physical examination in detecting a goiter?**
    Good. Combining data from nine separate studies, *sensitivity* is 70% and *specificity* 82%.

43. **What is the clinical significance of a *positive* exam for goiter?**
    It depends. Goiters detected by inspection of the extended neck *and* palpation are unreliable. Conversely, goiters detected by inspection of the neck *in normal position and* palpation argue strongly in favor of thyromegaly (positive [likelihood ratio] LR = 26.3).

44. **What is the significance of a *negative* exam?**
    Negative inspection, palpation, or a combination thereof *does* argue against the presence of goiter (LR of 0.4). Yet, it does *not* exclude it (*see* question 41). In fact, as many as half of all ultrasonically proven thyromegalies will remain undetected on exam.

45. **What is the accuracy of physical examination in assessing thyroid size?**
    Quite good. The accuracy of exam in assigning thyroid size to the three categories of *normal* (0–20 gm), *small goiter* (1–2 times normal [i.e., 20–40 gm]), and *large goiter* (>2 times normal [i.e., >40 gm]) has positive likelihood ratios of 0.15, 1.9, and 25, respectively. Overall, glands that are 1–2 times normal tend to be overestimated in size, whereas glands that are 2.5 times normal tend to be underestimated.

46. **Is the accuracy of detecting a goiter modified by the presence of thyroid nodules?**
    No, but it is increased by the examiner's experience. As a result, senior physicians tend to have better accuracy than their more junior counterparts.

F. THYROID NODULES

47. **How common are nodules?**
    Rather common, being present in half of all sonographic exams or autopsies. Yet most are clinically occult, being seen (or palpated) in only 5% of women and 1% of men. When detected on exam, single nodules often turn out to be multiple on ultrasound.

48. **Why are nodules so commonly missed?**
Same reasons as why *goiters* are missed: neck too short or thick, nodules too deep or small, and physicians too inept or cursory in their exams.

49. **What is the average size of a palpable nodule?**
3 cm. In fact, the larger the nodule, the more likely its detection (with <1 cm nodules being missed 90% of the time; <2 cm nodules 50% of the time).

50. **Are thyroid nodules necessarily neoplastic?**
No, only 5% are malignant. The rest are degenerative or adenomatous. Most are euthyroid.

51. **And so, what is the significance of a thyroid nodule?**
It should still be considered neoplastic until proven otherwise. Hence, it must be pursued with a fine needle aspirate. Ominous findings (such as vocal cord paralysis, cervical adenopathy, and fixation of the nodule to the surrounding tissues) argue in favor of malignancy, but are present in only one third of all thyroid cancers.

G. GRAVES' DISEASE

52. **What is hyperthyroidism?**
A constellation of signs and symptoms due to increased blood levels of thyroid hormone.

53. **How common is hyperthyroidism?**
It affects 4% of women and 0.2% of men.

54. **What are its most common causes?**
In addition to excessive administration of thyroid supplement, causes are mostly three: *Graves' disease* (60–90%), *toxic nodular goiter,* and *thyroiditis* (subacute, silent, or postpartum).

55. **How does hyperthyroidism present?**
   - **Hypermetabolism** is evidenced by weight loss, preference for colder temperatures, diarrhea, and amenorrhea or scant flow.
   - **Goiter** is present in 70–90% of all hyperthyroid patients—nodular and asymmetric in toxic nodular goiter, symmetric and diffuse in thyroiditis or Graves' disease. Two thirds of Graves' and one third of toxic nodular goiters may have a bruit on thyroid exam.
   - **Skin.** Some manifestations are *specific* (pretibial myxedema of Graves' disease), whereas others relate instead to increased metabolism and thus are *nonspecific* (warm, moist, velvety skin; fine, silky hair; palmar erythema; hyperpigmentation at pressure points; thin, breakable nails; onycholysis).
   - **Changes in the eyes** include lid lag, lid retraction (with widened palpebral fissures), and Graves' ophthalmopathy.
   - **Cardiovascular effects** include tachycardia, wide pulse pressure, palpitations, and systolic flow murmur.
   - **Neurologic symptoms** include (1) anxious appearance, restlessness, fidgety behavior; (2) fine tremor on outstretched arms due to increased sympathetic tone; (3) neuromuscular weakness; (4) decreased exercise tolerance in two thirds of cases (as a result of both proximal muscle wasting and the inability of the cardiovascular system to adequately increase output); and (5) hyperreflexia in one fourth of patients.

56. **What are the findings most suggestive of hyperthyroidism?**
Lid retraction (LR = 31.5), lid lag (LR = 17.6), fine finger tremor (LR = 11.4), moist and warm skin (LR = 6.7), and tachycardia (LR = 4 .4). Findings more likely to rule *out* hyperthyroidism

are normal thyroid size (LR = 0.1), heart rate <90/min (LR = 0.2), and no finger tremor (LR = 0.3). A cumulative score of 19 symptoms and signs (Wayne index) has an LR for hyperthyroidism of 18.2 (if >20) and of 0.1 (if <10). Older hyperthyroid patients exhibit more anorexia and atrial fibrillation, more frequent lack of goiter, and overall *fewer signs*, with tachycardia, fatigue, and weight loss in more than 50% of patients (and all three in 32%).

57. **And so, how does hyperthyroidism present in the elderly?**
Mostly with *cardiac* or *neurologic* manifestations, often subtle:
- Apathy and depressed mood
- Myopathy
- Proximal muscle weakness
- Cardiomyopathy or cardiomegaly with high-output failure
- Atrial arrhythmias
- Means-Lerman scratch (high-pitched pulmonic sound similar to pericardial friction rub—*see* Chapter 11, Heart Sounds and Extra Sounds, question 52)
- Flow murmur (increased intensity)
  Hence, any older patient presenting with new-onset heart failure, atrial fibrillation, or depression should be thoroughly evaluated for hyperthyroidism.

58. **What are the three major manifestations of Graves' disease?**
- Hyperthyroidism with a diffuse goiter
- Dermopathy
- Ophthalmopathy
  When all three are present, the diagnosis is rather simple. But since manifestations may follow an independent course, the diagnosis is often more challenging.

59. **What is the frequency of Graves' disease?**
It depends on gender and age, being higher in women and in the third to fourth decade of life.

60. **Who was Graves?**
Robert Graves was an Irishman (born in Dublin in 1797) who studied and practiced in Ireland and England and eventually became a superb clinician and teacher with a sarcastic sense of humor. In addition to medicine and painting (his main hobby), he had a knack for languages (he once was jailed in Austria as a possible Prussian spy because the border guards did not believe that a foreigner could speak such good German) and was also a born leader. During a trip in the Mediterranean, for example, he once saved a ship and its mutinous crew by assuming command in the middle of a storm. Besides linking his name to the association of goiter and exophthalmos, Graves also reported scleroderma, angioneurotic edema, and the pin-sized pupils of pontine hemorrhage. Note that in German-speaking countries, Graves' disease is still referred to as von Basedow's disease, in honor of Karl A. von Basedow (1799–1854), the German physician who in 1840 described the triad of goiter, exophthalmos, and palpitations. This eventually became known as the Merseburg triad, after the German town where von Basedow practiced medicine.

61. **What is the dermopathy of Graves?**
It is the result of a local infiltrative process, present in 4% of cases and usually involving the shins (*pretibial myxedema*). Histologically, it is characterized by dermal thickening, with presence of lymphocytes, various inflammatory cells, and lots of mucopolysaccharides. Although hyperthyroid signs may also be present, pretibial myxedema (like the ocular involvement of Graves', which is also infiltrative) is *not* due to hyperthyroidism. In fact, it is independent of, and unrelated to, the functional state of the gland. Hence, patients may be completely euthyroid, with an asymptomatic and diffusely bosselated goiter, and yet still carry the classical infiltrative manifestations of skin or eyes. Nonetheless, half of all dermopathy cases *do* coincide with the active state of Graves' and thus are commonly associated with hyperthyroidism.

62. **What does pretibial myxedema look like?**
The most common presentation is a localized, nonpitting edema of the shins. The more classic examples are instead well-demarcated, raised, and bilateral pinkish/brownish nodules on the anterior aspects of the shins (Fig. 8-12). These lesions may progress into a plaque or be located elsewhere on the legs, although they rarely involve the feet. Finally, pretibial myxedema may be pruritic or hyperpigmented.

63. **How do you distinguish pretibial myxedema from the myxedema of hypo-thyroidism?**
Pretibial myxedema is *localized*, whereas the hypothyroid form is more generalized.

64. **What is thyroid *acropachy*?**
It is the clubbing plus new periosteal bone formation that can occur in 5% of Graves' patients. Unlike the bony enlargement of *pulmonary hypertrophic osteoarthropathy*, thyroid periostitis occurs in the hands and feet, but *not* the long bones. It also is typically asymptomatic and *painless*. The cause is long-acting thyroid-stimulating hormone (LATS). Hence, it is absent in other causes of thyrotoxicosis.

65. **What other autoimmune findings can occur in Graves' disease?**
Premature graying, vitiligo, and hyperpigmentation.

66. **What are the *ocular* manifestations of Graves'?**
In addition to the nonspecific sympathetic manifestations of *lid lag* and *lid retraction*, Graves' disease is associated with a unique infiltrative disease of the eyes, characterized by edema and lymphocytic penetration of ocular fat, connective tissue, and extraocular muscles. This may manifest with discomfort, a tearing/gritty sensation in the eyes, and diplopia. Eventually, congestion of multiple layers of the eyeball will cause *proptosis* of the involved eye (i.e., an abnormal forward protrusion of the eyeball from the orbit—more than18 mm in extent) and *ophthalmoplegia* (*see* Figs. 8-13 and 8-14).

67. **Can proptosis be unilateral?**
Yes, but rarely. Although Graves' is the most common cause of proptosis in adults, this involves one eye in only 5% of the cases. Hence, unilateral proptosis should always be considered neoplastic (primary or metastatic) until proven otherwise.

68. **How do you detect and assess the degree of proptosis?**
The "poor man's" test is to have the patient bend the head forward while you look down on the orbits and estimate the distance to the corneal surface. This usually allows you to assess whether the distance is indeed greater than normal. For a more accurate measurement, you can use a Hertel exophthalmometer (Fig. 8-15), a hand-held device designed to quantitate the distance between the lateral orbital rim and anterior corneal surface.

69. **Does the degree of proptosis predict optic nerve involvement and loss of vision?**
No. Only lid edema and extraocular motion defects predict involvement of the optic nerve and impending loss of vision.

70. **What are the characteristics of Graves' congestive ophthalmopathy?**
It is characterized by the following (Fig. 8-16):
- Lid and periorbital edema
- Chemosis (conjunctival edema and injection)
- Ophthalmoplegia

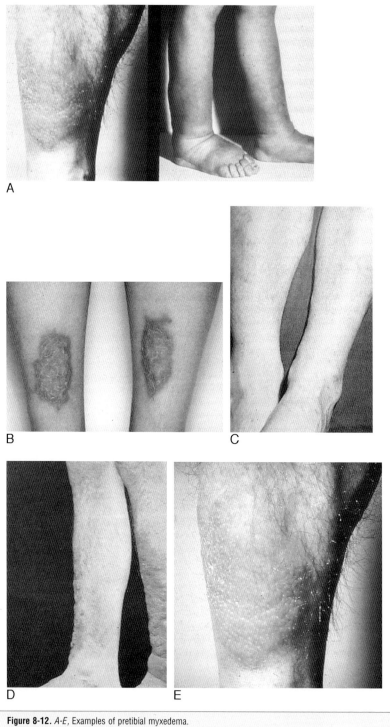

Figure 8-12. *A-E*, Examples of pretibial myxedema.

- Optic nerve compression, resulting in optic nerve edema (papilledema), atrophy, and visual loss

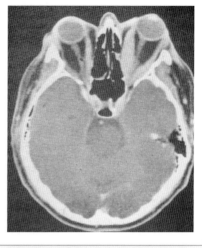

Figure 8-13. CT image of exophthalmos.

71. **What is ophthalmoplegia?**
    It is the inflammation, infiltration, engorgement, and paralysis of extraocular muscles in patients with Graves' disease (often referred to as *exophthalmic* or *congestive* ophthalmoplegia). It preferentially affects the medial and inferior recti but may result in many extraocular motion defects and impairments, including muscle weakness and amblyopia, impaired upward gaze, impaired convergence, strabismus, visual field defects, and restriction of gaze and visual acuity. Described mostly in the past century by various German and Austrian physicians (plus a couple of Frenchmen, two Britons, a Swiss, and a Russian), these signs carry a plethora of eponyms. Note that lid retraction and lid lag can occur in *any* hyperthyroid patient, since they are caused by the sympathetic hyperactivity of the Mueller's muscle (the same responsible for ptosis in Horner's syndrome). Rosenbach's sign is also the result of sympathetic hyperactivity. All other signs are instead typical of Graves' infiltrative ophthalmopathy, occurring in 25–50% of patients (*see* Table 8-2).

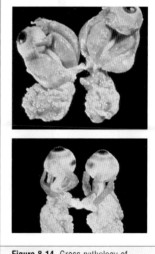

Figure 8-14. Gross pathology of exophthalmos.

72. **What is onycholysis?**
    It is the *partial* separation of the nail plate from the nail bed at its more distal and lateral attachments (*total* separation is termed *onychomadesis*). Onycholysis is an uncommon finding of hyperthyroid states that typically involve the ring finger, wherein the free edge of the nail becomes undulated, upturned, and often so loose as to collect debris beneath it. Onycholysis can also involve all other fingernails. It is due to sympathetic overactivity and thus represents a nonspecific manifestation of hyperthyroidism. When associated with Graves' disease, it is termed *Plummer's nails* (Fig. 8-18). It can also occur with psoriasis, fungal nail infection (usually candidal), trauma, Raynaud's disease, phototoxic reaction to tetracyclines, and constant wetting of the hands, as in dishwashers (*see* Chapter 3, The Skin, question 20).

73. **Who was Plummer?**
    Henry Plummer was an American internist. Born in Hamilton, Minnesota, in 1874, he studied at Northwestern University and practiced at the Mayo Clinic from 1901 until his death in 1936. His creativity and innovation led him to redesign the medical records of Mayo and to develop the

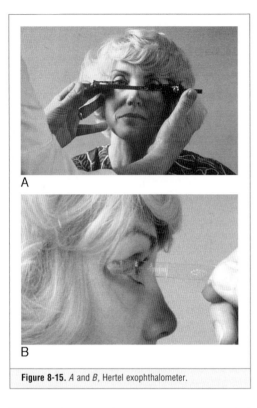

Figure 8-15. *A* and *B*, Hertel exophthalometer.

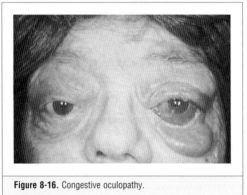

Figure 8-16. Congestive oculopathy.

examination beds that are still commonly used throughout North America. Outside medicine, his interests included literature, music, and especially gardening. Plummer's name also is linked to a thyroid nodule associated with hyperthyroidism but *no* ocular manifestations. The condition is sometimes called Plummer-Vinson adenoma in memory of Porter Vinson, a fellow in medicine at the Mayo Clinic and a junior associate of Plummer. This should not be confused with Plummer-Vinson *syndrome* (sideropenic dysphagia, iron deficiency anemia, dysphagia, esophageal web, and atrophic glossitis), which is *not* associated with onycholysis, but with the *koilonychia* of iron deficiency (*see* Chapter 3, The Skin, question 23).

TABLE 8-2. THYROTOXICOSIS EYE MANIFESTATIONS

Sign	Discoverer	Finding
Dalrymple's* (lid retraction [i.e., "thyroid stare"])	John Dalrymple (1803–1852). British ophthalmologist who also played a role in the identification of the Bence-Jones protein. Died at 49 of renal failure.	Abnormal widening of the palpebral fissure. Normally, the margin of the upper lid covers 1 mm of the iris, but in lid retraction the upper eyelid is pulled backward, thus displaying a bit of sclera and giving the patient a typical scared/staring look. *May result in corneal exposure with ulceration.*
Von Graefe's* (lid lag)	Friedrich Wilhelm Ernst Albrecht von Graefe (1828–1870). German physician and founding father of modern ophthalmology. Died at 42 of tuberculosis.	On downward gaze, the globe moves briskly while the upper lid lags behind, thus disclosing the sclera between the corneal limbus and lid (Fig 8-17).
Rosenbach's*	Ottomar Rosenbach (1851–1907). German physician and controversial promoter of the psychosomatic origin of many diseases.	Fine tremor of the gently closed eyelids. Especially the upper.
Möbius'	Paul Julius Möbius (1853–1907). German neurologist and student of Von Strümpell.	Failure of ocular convergence following close accommodation at 5".
Stellwag's	Karl Stellwag von Carion (1823–1904). Austrian ophthalmologist.	Infrequent (and incomplete) blinking, plus proptosis.
Kocher's	Emil Theodor Kocher (1841–1917). Swiss surgeon and strong promoter of antisepsis. Nobel laureate for his contribution on thyroid physiology, pathology, and surgery.	On upward gaze, the upper lid retracts briskly while the globe lags behind (counterpart to Von Graefe's).
Joffroy's	Alexis Joffroy (1844–1908). French neuropsychiatrist and student of Charcot.	Absent wrinkling of the forehead when the eyeballs are rolled upward.
Sainton's	Paul Sainton (1868–1958). French physician and chair at the Hôtel-Dieu Hospital in Paris.	On upward gaze, the frontalis muscle contracts *after* the upper lid has completely retracted.
Jellinek's	E. H. Jellinek. British neurologist of the 19th century.	Brownish pigmentation of eyelids, especially the upper.
Topolansky's	Russian physician.	Pericorneal congestion in patients with Graves', with conjunctival edema (chemosis) and hyperemia.

*Nonspecific signs of hyperthyroidism. All others are typical of Graves' ophthalmopathy.

H. HYPOTHYROIDISM

74. **What is hypothyroidism?**
A constellation of signs and symptoms due to inadequate levels of thyroid hormone.

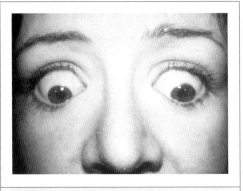

Figure 8-17. Von Graefe's sign (lid lag).

75. **What is its frequency?**
In countries that use iodine supplements, it affects 9% of women and 1% of men. The two most common causes are Hashimoto's thyroiditis (two thirds of the cases) and radioiodine gland ablation (one third of the cases).

76. **What is the value of physical exam in hypothyroidism?**
It helps to separate patients with *overt* disease from those with the subclinical form, who have neither symptoms nor signs. It also helps to estimate pretest probability, prior to the inevitable hormonal measurement that remains the *sine qua non* for diagnosis.

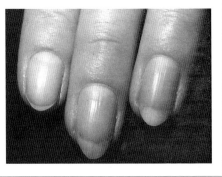

Figure 8-18. Plummer's nails (onycholysis).

77. **How does hypothyroidism present?**
With a reduced metabolic rate, tissue accumulation of mucopolysaccharides, and a series of neurologic/cardiovascular repercussions.

78. **What are the manifestations of hypothyroidism?**
See Table 8–3.

79. **What is the clinical significance of hypothyroid findings?**
They can only *suggest* the diagnosis, since confirmation of hypothyroidism depends exclusively on a highly sensitive thyroid-stimulating hormone (TSH) assay. Still, prevalence of symptoms and signs of overt *hypothyroidism* is remarkably different today from the old reports in the literature. To this end, Zulewski et al. have recently revisited the 1969 Billewicz index by quantifying each of its 14 signs and symptoms (Table 8–4) as +1 if present and 0 if absent. Using as gold standard modern thyroid function tests (absent in Billewicz's time) they defined as *hypothyroid* patients with a cumulative score >5; as *euthyroid* those with score ≤2; and as *intermediate* (or borderline hypothyroid) those with scores 2–5. By doing so, they were able to identify 62% of overt hypothyroid and 24% of subclinical

TABLE 8-3.   MANIFESTATIONS OF HYPOTHYROIDISM

Skin and Soft Tissues

- Mostly due to accumulation of water-binding mucopolysaccharides (hence, the term *myxedema*)
- Coarse, dry, scaling, and cool skin (dryness from reduced sebum production, coolness from diminished blood flow)
- Sallow and yellowish color due to accumulation of carotenoids; in contrast to jaundice, also involves palms and soles
- Periorbital puffiness with facial edema
- Doughy, nonedematous swelling
- Thick nails
- Coarse hair that breaks easily
- Missing lateral eyebrow (Queen Anne's sign). Present in one third of hypothyroid patients but also may occur in normal subjects; hence, of limited clinical value.

Neurologic Manifestations

- Disinterested, complacent, lethargic
- Good muscle strength (but lethargic)
- Paresthesias
- Deafness
- Prolonged contraction and relaxation of the Achilles ("hung-up" reflex)—this can separate hypothyroid from euthyroid patients, but when assessed by the naked eye can be absent in three fourths of cases.
- Hypothyroid speech (low-pitched, slow, and deep voice that has been compared to a 45 RPM record playing at 33 RPM); it can occur in up to 40% of patients and is due to accumulation of polysaccharides in the vocal cords.

Cardiovascular Manifestations

- Bradycardia

Other Manifestations

- *Goiter* (more specific than sensitive: +LR, 2.8; −LR, 0.6)
- Weight gain—not as common as traditionally claimed, and in some studies not any more frequent in hypothyroid than euthyroid patients
- Constipation
- Menorrhagia

hypothyroid patients, as compared to 42% and 6%, respectively, when using Billewicz's definition. As for hyperthyroidism, clinical scores of *hypothyroidism* may perform less well in the elderly. Overall, findings more strongly suggestive of hypothyroidism are: bradycardia (+LR = 3.88), abnormal ankle reflex (+LR = 3.41), and coarse skin (+LR = 2.3). Cool *and* dry skin also has high likelihood ratio. Still, no single finding, when absent, can effectively rule *out* hypothyroidism (−LR = 0.42–1.0). Even the combination of signs with the highest likelihood ratios (coarse skin, bradycardia, and delayed ankle reflex) is only modestly accurate (+LR = 3.75; −LR = 0.48).

TABLE 8-4. FREQUENCY OF HYPOTHYROID SIGNS AND SYMPTOMS IN PATIENTS AND CONTROLS

Sign/Symptom	Patients (%) (n = 50)	Controls (%) (n = 80)
Ankle reflex	77	6.5
Dry skin	76	36.2
Cold intolerance	64	36
Coarse skin	60	18.3
Puffiness	60	3.7
Pulse rate	58	57.5
Sweating	54	13.8
Weight	54	22.5
Paresthesia	52	17.5
Cold skin	50	20
Constipation	48	15
Movements	36	1.3
Hoarseness	34	12.5
Hearing	22	2.5

(Data from Zulewski H, Muller B, Exer P, et al: Estimation of tissue hypothyroidism by a new clinical score: Evaluation of patients with various grades of hypothyroidism and controls. J Clin Endocrinol Metab 82:771–776, 1997.)

ACKNOWLEDGMENT

The author gratefully acknowledges the contributions of Janice Wood, MD, to this chapter in the first edition of *Physical Diagnosis Secrets*.

SELECTED BIBLIOGRAPHY

1. Bahn RS, Heufelder AE: Pathogenesis of Graves' ophthalmopathy. N Engl J Med 329:1468–1475, 1993.
2. Bartley GB: The differential diagnosis and classification of eyelid retraction. Ophthalmology 103:168–176, 1996.
3. Bartley GB, Fatourechi V, Kadrmas EF, et al: Clinical features of Graves' ophthalmopathy in an incidence cohort. Ant J Ophthalmol 121:284–290, 1996.
4. Basaria R: Pemberton's sign. N Engl J Med 350:1338, 2004.
5. Berghout A, Wiersinga WM, Smits NJ, et al: Determinants of thyroid volume as measured by ultrasonography in healthy adults in a non-iodine deficient area. Clin Endocrinol 26:273–280, 1987.
6. Berghout A, Wiersinga WM, Smits NJ, et al: The value of thyroid volume measured by ultrasonography in the diagnosis of goiter. Clin Endocrinol 28:409–414, 1988.
7. Bicknell PG: Mild hypothyroidism and its effects on the larynx. J Laryrngol Otol 87:123–127, 1973.
8. Billewicz WZ, Chapman RS, Crooks J, et al: Statistical methods applied to the diagnosis of hypothyroidism. Q J Med 38:255–265, 1969.
9. Blum M, Biller BJ, Bergman DA: The thyroid cork. Obstruction of the thoracic inlet due to retroclavicular goiter. JAMA 227:189–191, 1974.
10. Brander A, Viikinkoski P, Tuuhea J, et al: Clinical versus ultrasound examination of the thyroid gland in common clinical practice. J Clin Ultrasound 20:37–42, 1992.

CHAPTER 9

THE BREAST

Salvatore Mangione, MD

"Thy two breasts are like two young roes that are twins, which feed among the lilies."
—Song of Solomon, 4:5

A. GENERALITIES

The *clinical breast examination* (CBE) is an effective screening tool for breast cancer; its accuracy depends on methodology and operator. Most of the research data stress palpation over inspection.

1. **Why do a clinical breast examination (CBE)?**
   For either *diagnosis* of breast complaints (and primarily to rule out cancer) or for *screening* (to detect cancer in asymptomatic women). In primary care, CBEs are more screening than diagnostic (73% and 27%, respectively). They also get intertwined with medical litigation, since failure to detect breast cancer is a leading reason for malpractice claims, and primary care clinicians account for one half of all indemnities made.

2. **Who should undergo a screening CBE? How frequently?**
   According to the American Cancer Society, CBEs should be carried out every 3 years in women between 20 and 39 years, and annually in women 40 and older. In this age group, the CBE can detect at least 50% of asymptomatic cancers and possibly contribute to a mortality reduction. A well-conducted exam cannot only detect potentially curable cancers, but also add to the yield of mammography, especially in women older than 70 (since fatty changes in their breast make lump detection easier).

3. **What is the precision of CBE?**
   Hard to say, since CBEs are often carried out in nonstandardized fashion. Hence, their high interobserver variability. For example, 37 to 74 of 100 women screened by four different surgeons were found to have abnormal findings, and yet for only 25 of these women did all four surgeons agree on the findings. Agreement also varied by lesion: 13.5% for nipple discharge, 22.1% for dilated veins, 24.2% for "peau d'orange," 59.4% for the lump per se, 61.5% for ulceration, and 68.1% for finding visibility.

4. **What is the accuracy of CBE?**
   Hard to say, too, since to determine its screening accuracy the CBE should be compared to a standard criterion, which mammography cannot be, since cancers missed by mammograms can be found on CBE. Having said that, CBE sensitivity on pooled data is rather low (54%), but specificity is much stronger (94%). Overall, CBE has high false positive rates and even higher false negative rates. In silicone models, it has a sensitivity similar to that of population studies (40–71%), but a much lower specificity (41–77%).

5. **What is the value of breast examination as compared to mammography?**
   CBE alone can detect 3–45% of cancers that screening mammography missed, with randomized clinical trials demonstrating reduced mortality rates in women screened by both

techniques. Hence, CBE is an effective screening tool for breast cancer. Although unable to rule *out* disease when used alone, detection of certain abnormal findings by CBE can greatly increase the probability of breast cancer. Sensitivity of both professional and lay examiners can be improved by learning the correct examination method, and then practicing it on silicone breast models. Overall, for lesions of similar size, both examiner and patient factors can affect CBE's accuracy.

6. **What *examiner's* factors are associated with CBE's greater accuracy?**
   - Longer duration of exam
   - Higher number of correct steps (a systematic search pattern, thoroughness, varying palpation pressure—fingers, finger pads, and circular motion)
   - Examiner's experience (previous training with silicone models)

7. **What *patient's* factors can adversely affect CBE's accuracy?**
   Age. Denser breasts (typical of younger women) are harder to examine than fatty breasts (typical of older women), thus making lump detection more difficult. Larger breasts are also difficult, and so are fibrocystic breasts, which tend to be rather lumpy.

8. **What is the bottom line for CBE modifiers?**
   Duration of exam, number of correct techniques, patient's age, and the size/lumpiness of the breast may all affect CBE's sensitivity. Size and hardness of the cancer can do it, too.

(1) Inspection

9. **Which areas should be examined?**
   Breast tissue is contained in an imaginary pentagon, whose *lateral border* follows the midaxillary line, from the middle of the axilla down to the inframammary (or bra) line (fifth to sixth interspace); the *lower border* crosses along the inframammary fold toward the xiphoid process; the *medial border* ascends the midsternal line toward the suprasternal notch; and the *upper border* follows the clavicle before turning down toward the midaxilla. This pentagon can then be divided into four quadrants (Fig. 9-1). Most cancers originate in the upper outer quadrant of the breast, and also below the areola and nipple, two areas containing a large amount of glandular tissue. Always inspect first and palpate later.

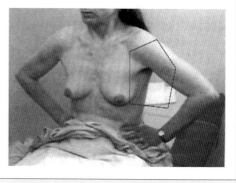

Figure 9-1. Breast anatomy—glandular area.

10. **What is the best way to inspect the breasts?**
    By examining the patient supine and then seated. Look for the breasts' size, shape, and contour. Identify asymmetries, swelling, erythema, increase in venous pattern, and skin dimpling. Also search for nipple changes, including deviation, retraction, and inversion.

11. **Which bedside maneuver can help to detect breast abnormalities on inspection?**
The most commonly taught and used maneuvers include a change in position of the patient's
arms and hands, first described by Haagensen (Fig. 9-2). To do so, ask the patient to carry out
the following sequence:

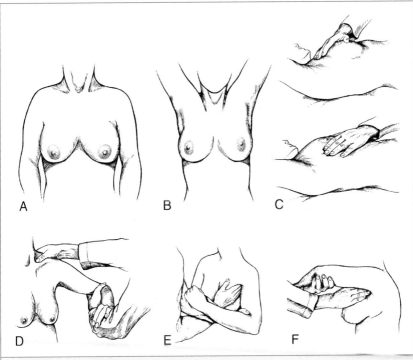

Figure 9-2. Physical examination of the breast. *A*, Observation with patient sitting and arms resting at side. *B*, Observation with arms raised above the head. *C*, Systematic palpation with palm side of hand and fingers while patient is supine. *D*, Palpation of supraclavicular region of sitting patient with examiner supporting and elevating arm. *E* and *F*, Examination of axillae with volar surface of fingers by examiner standing on opposite side and totally supporting patient's arm. (From James EC, Corry RJ, Perry JF: Principles of Basic Surgical Practice. Philadelphia, Hanley & Belfus, 1987.)

1. Rest the hands on the lap (to *relax* the pectoralis muscles).
2. Press them over the hips (to *tense* the pectoralis muscles and make dimpling and retraction more visible).
3. Raise them above the head, clasping them behind it (to also trigger skin dimpling, an important harbinger of cancer).
4. Lean forward (to allow the breasts to hang out pendulous from the chest).
   Although these positions are commonly taught and practiced, they *do* take time. Moreover, the *screening* value of positioning (and even inspection) remains largely unproven. In a series of 296 breast cancers found on exam, 96% were discovered by palpation, 3% by visible nipple abnormalities, and only 1% by retraction alone. Yet, if the patient is symptomatic (or an abnormality is discovered during palpation), then careful inspection should definitely be carried out.

12. **What are the most significant abnormalities that can be detected by *inspection*?**
Noncongenital nipple asymmetry/deviation and retraction/inversion (both valuable clues to an underlying cancer). Nipple inversion may actually be normal, but only if long standing and correctable by manual pulling. Skin inspection also is important. Look for:
- Dimpling
- "Peau d'orange"
- Scaly, red dermatitis of the areola and nipple (which suggests Paget's disease of the breast)
Look for these in each Haagensen's position.

13. **What is skin dimpling?**
A slight depression or indentation in the breast's surface (Fig. 9-3). This is an important clue to an underlying infiltrating carcinoma, causing fibrosis and retraction of the breast tissue. The same mechanism is responsible for nipple deviation.

14. **What are the suspensory ligaments of the breast?**
Suspensory (or Cooper's) ligaments are thin, fibrous bands that run through the breast, attaching stroma to skin. Tension on these ligaments produces the characteristic *dimpling* that sometimes occurs over malignant masses.

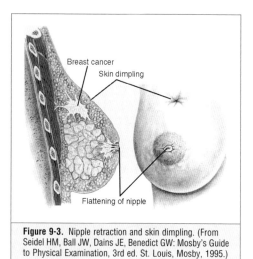

Figure 9-3. Nipple retraction and skin dimpling. (From Seidel HM, Ball JW, Dains JE, Benedict GW: Mosby's Guide to Physical Examination, 3rd ed. St. Louis, Mosby, 1995.)

15. **What is peau d'orange?**
It is French for *orange peel*—an apt description of the skin overlying an infiltrating cancer. It is due to lymphatic blockage by the tumor, resulting in localized lymphedema, with skin thickening and unusually large pores. It typically involves the lower aspect of the breasts.

What is Paget's disease of the breast?
A malignant lesion of the areola and/or nipple, almost always associated with an *in situ* or invasive carcinoma. It is caused by extension of neoplastic cells from the lactiferous ducts into the epidermis, eventually causing it to become irritated. It presents as a scaly dermatitis of the nipple, with itching, crusting, and even erosion. Eventually, it involves the skin extensively, possibly without any palpable underlying mass. It may resemble other scaly and excoriative nipple diseases, such as eczema or the trauma of nursing.

> **Pearl:**
> Redness and thickness of the nipple should always be considered suspicious. When appropriate, biopsy must be carried out to exclude Paget's disease.

17. **Who was Paget?**
Sir James Paget (1814–1899) was a British surgeon who spent his entire career at the St. Bartholomew's Hospital of London. A tall, brilliant, and charming man, he was so much enamored with clear and concise language to often quip, "To be brief is to be wise." His fame

grew to the point that Prime Minister Gladstone remarked that people are divided into two classes, "those who had, and those who had not heard of James Paget." His name is linked to the first demonstration of trichinosis in humans (which he reported while still a medical student), osteitis deformans (described the same year in which he was made a baronet), the aforementioned breast disease, and a skin cancer of the apocrine glands presenting with the same cells as Paget's disease of the breast.

(2) Palpation

18. What is the best way to palpate the breast?

One that uses (1) proper patient position; (2) awareness of breast boundaries; (3) adequate examination patterns; and (4) correct finger position, movement, and pressure. *Duration of palpation* is also crucial to success, with longer exams having overall a better yield. Note that a careful examination of an average-sized breast takes at least 3 minutes (6 minutes for both breasts), which is much more than the average 1.8 minutes physicians usually spend teaching breast self-examination (BSE) and examining *both* breasts.

19. Describe the proper patient position.

Since CBE requires flattening of the breast tissue against the chest, the patient must be supine. To further flatten the breast, one could try bedside maneuvers, especially in women with larger breasts. For example, to flatten the lateral part of the breast, you can ask the patient to roll onto her contralateral hip, rotate the shoulders back into a supine position, and place her ipsilateral hand on the forehead. Conversely, to flatten the medial part of the breast, you can ask the patient to lie flat on her back and raise her elbow until it is at the same level with her shoulder.

20. What should the examiner remember about breast boundaries?

Since breast tissue extends *laterally* toward the axilla (axillary tail) and *superiorly* toward the clavicle, you should cover a rectangular area that is bordered superiorly by the clavicle, medially by the midsternum, laterally by the midaxillary line, and inferiorly by the bra line. This will ensure that you examine all breast tissue.

21. What is meant by an adequate examination pattern?

Although two fifths of physicians may use no discernible pattern, proper technique is key for lesion detection. The two traditional methods are the radial spoke pattern and the concentric circles pattern (Fig. 9-4). However, the *vertical strip pattern* has been found to be more thorough. Begin your palpation in the axilla, and extend it in a straight line *down* the midaxillary line toward the bra line. Then move your fingers medially, continuing palpation *up the chest*, and in a straight line to the clavicle. Cover the entire breast, going up and down between the clavicle and bra line in a vertical strip pattern (or lawnmower technique). To cover all breast tissue, overlap rows.

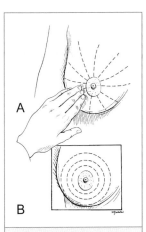

Figure 9-4. Traditional patterns of breast palpation. *A*, Spokes of a wheel approach. *B*, Concentric circles approach. (From Swartz MH: Pocket Companion to Textbook of Physical Diagnosis, 3rd ed. Philadelphia, WB Saunders, 1997.)

22. Describe the correct finger position, movement, and pressure.

The MammaCare method is a breast palpation technique that combines vertical strip pattern and specific finger techniques to allow detection of a soft 2-mm lump in simulated breast tissue. In this technique, the three middle fingers are held together, with the metacarpal–phalangeal joint slightly flexed, and the surface examined by the finger *pads* (*not* tips). Each area is palpated by:

- *Making small circles*, as if following the edge of a dime
- *Making three circles at each spot*, using three different *pressures*—*light* for superficial structures (skin and subcutaneous tissue), *medium* for the breast per se, and *deep* for the chest wall. This ensures that all levels of tissue are reached.
- *Examining each area carefully*, all the way down to the thoracic wall. Pay attention to the tactile quality of skin, subcutaneous fat, and breast tissue
- Then moving on to the next area, always using a consistent pattern

23. **What are the final steps in the CBE?**

    Complete the exam by palpating for adenopathy in the supraclavicular and axillary fossae (Fig. 9-5). Then examine the nipple, through palpation and a squeeze. Although search for adenopathy is a routine component of the CBE, breast cancer is present in only 10–30% of women with isolated axillary lymphadenopathy and an otherwise normal CBE.

24. **What is the bottom line of the breast exam?**

    Use a vertical strip pattern to cover all tissue. Make circular motions with the *pads* of the middle three fingers. Examine each area with thee different pressures. Spend 3 minutes per breast.

25. **How does normal breast tissue feel?**

    It depends on the phase of the menstrual cycle. Premenstrual and perimenstrual breasts, for instance, are swollen, tender, and with prominent glands. Tenderness is usually (but not always) a sign of benignity, being common in mastitis or fibrocystic disease.

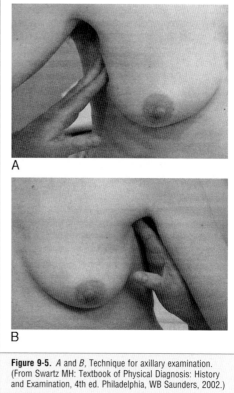

Figure 9-5. *A* and *B*, Technique for axillary examination. (From Swartz MH: Textbook of Physical Diagnosis: History and Examination, 4th ed. Philadelphia, WB Saunders, 2002.)

26. **How should a breast lump (or nodule) be described?**

    - **Size:** Assess it by using a ruler, tape measure, or, even better, plastic calipers. Remember that larger lumps (>2 cm) are more likely to be neoplastic.
    - **Location:** Describe it in relation to the breast's four quadrants and the distance from the areolar rim. Report the finding by using the clock analogy.

- **Tenderness:** Usually a sign of benignity
- **Consistency or firmness:** Rock-hard in cancers; soft, compressible, and at times even cystic in benign lesions
- **Shape:** This should include an assessment of regularity/irregularity and contour. Lesions with indistinct and irregular margins are more likely to be malignant.
- **Relation to surrounding tissue:** Use Haagensen's maneuvers to evaluate mobility over superficial and deep planes. Fixed lesions are more likely to be malignant.
- **Character of the overlying skin:** Look for warmth, redness, swelling, or retraction.

27. **What are the characteristics of malignant breast tissue?**
    A carcinomatous lesion is typically painless, irregular in contour and shape, hard in consistency, not mobile, and not well demarcated from the surrounding tissues. Retraction signs are usually a late phenomenon. A serous (or serosanguineous) nipple discharge can be an important sign of intraductal carcinomas (*see* questions 37–40).

28. **Are *lumps* ever normal?**
    Yes. In fact, normal breasts are often lumpy, but these lumps are typically movable, regular, and soft or cystic. They also may change with the menstrual cycle. Neoplastic lumps are instead hard, fixed, and irregular. Nonmovable and large lesions (>2 cm) are especially ominous (likelihood ratio [LR] = 2.4). Yet many cancers do not read the books. In fact, one half of all breast lesions in one study were well circumscribed, soft, and movable. The opposite is also true, with benign masses often resembling cancer. Correlation with presence or absence of risk factors can further increase/decrease the likelihood of disease. Still, since the characteristics of neoplastic and benign lumps often overlap, breast cancer is rarely diagnosed on CBE alone. Instead, the CBE should be used to locate abnormalities and guide further evaluation.

29. **How common is breast cancer? What are its risk factors?**
    Breast cancer will occur in approximately 12% of American women over their lifetimes, with risk affected by age (annual incidence at age 70 being 20 times higher than at age 30) and family history (having two first-degree relatives with breast cancer at an early age quadruples the risk). Other risk factors include genetic mutations (*BRCA1* and *BRCA2* genes) and estrogen exposure (age of menarche, first pregnancy and menopause, parity, and estrogen replacement therapy). Strong risk factors increase the likelihood of any neoplastic abnormality detected on exam.

30. **How accurate is physical exam for the detection of a breast lump?**
    Variable, depending not only on examiner's skills but also on the size and location of the lesion. For example, tumors <1 cm are difficult to palpate (unless very superficial), whereas 2–3 cm lesions are easily detectable. In silicone models, the sensitivity of exam ranges between 17% and 83%, increasing not only with examiner's experience but also with the exam's *duration*. In real patients, the sensitivity of the breast exam for detecting a neoplastic lesion can be as low as 24% and as high as 62%. Because of its much greater sensitivity, mammography should always supplement (but *not* substitute) physical examination. False negative rates of mammography range from 3% to 63% (usually around 20%). In a study by Hicks, 7% of all cancers detected by exam were misdiagnosed as benign by mammography, whereas as many as one fourth of all detected cancers were picked up during self-examination between mammograms.

31. **How high is the interobserver variability in describing a breast lump?**
    Quite high. For example, in a study of 232 women presenting with a breast lump, two observers disagreed on lesions' consistency and margins in one third of the cases. They also disagreed on the presence of axillary nodes in one half of the cases. In another study, four breast surgeons detected a lump in 32/42 patients and agreed on biopsy in 11/15 patients eventually diagnosed with cancer.

32. **What are the most common benign breast lesions?**
    - **Fibroadenomas:** The most common benign *neoplasms*. They present as solitary, well-demarcated, rubbery, mobile, nontender masses, often round, but also ovoid or oblong. May occur at any time after puberty, but less frequently after menopause.
    - **Benign cysts:** The most common breast *lumps*. Since they are often part of a fibrocystic pattern, they tend to coexist with other cysts. They are round, mobile, soft, and cystic in feel. They vary with the menstrual cycle, becoming tender before menses, and smaller immediately after (hence, to avoid misdiagnosis do a breast exam only in this phase of the menstrual cycle). They regress after menopause.

33. **What is a *florid nipple adenoma*?**
    A benign lesion that presents as an areolar nodule. This often becomes ulcerated and thus may be confused with Paget's disease.

34. **What is the differential diagnosis of an *inflammatory* breast mass?**
    It depends on whether it is diffuse or localized:
    - **Diffuse** inflammatory breast masses include acute mastitis and inflammatory breast carcinoma.
    - **Localized** inflammatory masses are instead the result of an acute breast abscess—a well-localized, tender, swollen, erythematous, and often fluctuant lesion. Patients usually present with systemic signs and symptoms of infection (like fever, malaise, and leukocytosis), usually in a setting of lactation, since abscesses are often the end result of an acute mastitis.

35. **How can one separate acute mastitis from inflammatory breast carcinoma?**
    Both conditions present with diffuse and tender masses:
    - **Acute mastitis** is a glandular infection that involves only a single breast quadrant, usually during lactation. The affected area is red, swollen, tender, and associated with systemic signs of infection (fever, malaise, elevated white blood cell count).
    - **Inflammatory breast carcinoma** involves instead the *entire* breast and is typically associated with axillary adenopathy (usually absent in acute mastitis). Lack of association with lactation and lack of response to antibiotics should raise the suspicion for neoplasm and prompt a biopsy.

36. **Describe the *lymphatic drainage* of the breasts.**
    - The **superficial and central areas** are drained by lymphatics that radiate from the areola and then converge toward the low/central axillary nodes and the subclavian nodes.
    - The **deep tissue** is drained instead by pectoral, subclavian, and internal mammary nodes. These eventually drain into mediastinal stations.
    - Finally, **other breast lymphatics** drain into hepatic and subdiaphragmatic nodes (Fig. 9-6).

B. NIPPLE DISCHARGE

37. **How do you assess for nipple discharge?**
    By applying gentle pressure at the base of the nipple, with the thumb and first or second finger (Fig. 9-7). Note that a discharge that occurs only with nipple compression/squeezing is usually physiologic. In a study of 448 women complaining of discharge, none of the 178 who had it only after expression was found to have cancer. Conversely, cancer was present in 2% (3/151) of those with spontaneous discharge but otherwise normal CBE.

38. **What are the causes of a serous nipple discharge?**
    Both benign and malignant processes. The former include intraductal papilloma, sclerosing adenosis, chronic cystic mastitis, duct ectasia, fibrocystic disease, and tuberculosis. Malignant

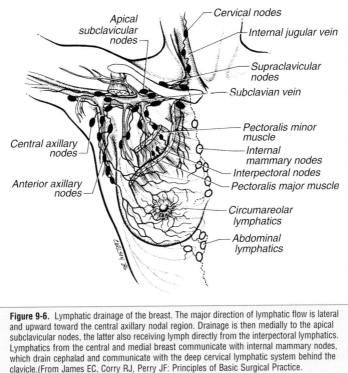

Figure 9-6. Lymphatic drainage of the breast. The major direction of lymphatic flow is lateral and upward toward the central axillary nodal region. Drainage is then medially to the apical subclavicular nodes, the latter also receiving lymph directly from the interpectoral lymphatics. Lymphatics from the central and medial breast communicate with internal mammary nodes, which drain cephalad and communicate with the deep cervical lymphatic system behind the clavicle.(From James EC, Corry RJ, Perry JF: Principles of Basic Surgical Practice. Philadelphia, Hanley & Belfus, 1987.)

etiologies include breast carcinoma, adenofibrosarcoma, fibrosarcoma, malignant melanoma, neurosarcoma, and Paget's disease. Note that a nipple discharge is usually *not* a *presenting* feature of carcinoma (<3% of cases), yet 6–13% of nipple discharge patients eventually get diagnosed as having breast cancer. Discharges may be seen in as many as 13% of nulligravida, and 22% of parous women between the ages of 16 and 50. Hence, a nipple discharge is a common problem in premenopausal women. In half of all cases, there are no definite causes.

39. **How about a *bloody discharge*?**
A discharge positive for occult blood has high sensitivity and high

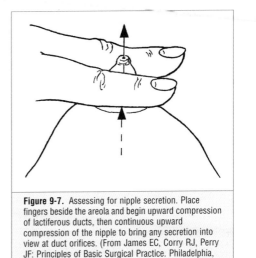

Figure 9-7. Assessing for nipple secretion. Place fingers beside the areola and begin upward compression of lactiferous ducts, then continuous upward compression of the nipple to bring any secretion into view at duct orifices. (From James EC, Corry RJ, Perry JF: Principles of Basic Surgical Practice. Philadelphia, Hanley & Belfus, 1987.)

negative predictive value (but low specificity) for a malignant lesion. In a study by Chaudary et al., 16/16 neoplastic patients tested positive for occult blood, but so did 199/268 with benign lesions. In another study, 27/27 who tested *negative* for blood had benign lesions.

40. How common is a *watery* nipple discharge? What are the causes?
It is not too common, being present in only 2.2% of patients with nipple discharge. In one study, one half of them had cancer.

41. What is *galactorrhea*?
A milky discharge (from the Greek *galacto*, milk, and *rhoia*, flow) in a nonpregnant patient. This results from either local or systemic processes. In local disease, the galactorrhea is usually *unilateral*, whereas in systemic disorders it is *bilateral*. Mechanical stimulation is often a common cause, too. Local etiologies include trauma, surgery, or zoster infection. Systemic causes include hyperprolactinemia; Cushing's syndrome; thyroid diseases; and certain drugs, such as oral contraceptives, phenothiazines, tricyclic antidepressants, and alpha-methyldopa.

42. What is the milk line?
The ridge of embryonic tissue from which the breasts form. This extends from the axillae to the vulva, but normally involutes, leaving on the thorax only the two breasts. Persistence of breast tissue along the milk line results in supernumerary (extra) nipples or breasts.

43. What is *polythelia*?
From the Greek *poly* (many) and *thele* (nipple), this is the presence of supernumerary nipples along the milk line. These often appear as tiny, raised, and pigmented nevi—very rare in the general population (0.22–2.5%). Although in the past extra nipples were considered clues to underlying congenital abnormalities (especially cardiac), they are actually only part of certain renal syndromes, such as duplicate renal arteries and adenocarcinomas—an association almost exclusively of Caucasians.

44. What is *polymastia*?
From the Greek *poly* (many) and *mastos* (breast), this is the presence of supernumerary *breasts*—a condition much less common than polythelia and yet not entirely unheard of. For example, Anne Boleyn (Henry the VIII's unfortunate second wife) was rumored to have a third breast. She is actually much more famous for triggering the separation of Henry from his first wife (did the extra breast do it?), and, as a result, the separation of the Anglican Church from Rome, which eventually led to the separation of Anne's own head from the rest of her body, considering that she was 5'4" at the beginning of her reign and only 4'6" at the end of it. Since she also gave birth to (future Queen) Elizabeth I, we are left to wonder what the history of England (and America) would have been if her anatomy had been a tad more correct. Along the lines of historical incorrectness, Anne Boleyn's breasts should therefore be ranked as high as Cleopatra's nose, which, despite its length, played a major role in causing that civil war between Marc Antony and Octavius that eventually gave birth to the Roman Empire.

45. What is *athelia*?
From the Greek *a* (lack of) and *thele* (nipple), this is the congenital absence of nipples—a condition quite different from the congenital absence of *one* nipple, which can be seen in adults with mitral valve prolapse and children with leukemia. Absence of one nipple also may be part of Poland's syndrome: microsyndactyly (or lack of one hand), atrophy of the ipsilateral pectoralis major, and genitourinary abnormalities.

46. Who was Poland?
Alfred Poland (1820–1872) was an English surgeon and quite an interesting character, too. Utterly disinterested in his own personal appearance, he was once sternly warned by the

treasurer of his hospital to dress more "professionally" (advice that he totally ignored). He won, however, the respect and love of colleagues and students alike for being an excellent surgeon, a charismatic teacher, and a man of encyclopedic knowledge. These qualities, however, did not translate into economic gains (probably because of his habit of scheduling surgery at unusual hours, a custom that kept his practice conveniently small). Afflicted by several bouts of hemoplysis (which did not interfere with his eagerness to teach, and infect, his students), he eventually died of consumption.

47. **What can one learn from examining the chest wall of postmastectomy patients?**
Mostly the possibility of recurrent tumor, especially at the suture line. Generalized induration and tanned skin appearance may also occur as a result of local radiotherapy.

C. BREAST SELF EXAMINATION (BSE)

48. **What is the role of breast self-examination (BSE)?**
It is a useful adjunct to breast cancer screening. Note that the breast has not always been part of the physical examination of the female patient. Only during the 1950s and 1960s did the American Cancer Society start to encourage it, eventually prompting women to request it and physicians to incorporate it in their standard periodic exam. In the 1970s and 1980s, *independent* BSE was born, mostly out of the need for early detection. This is a complex skill that requires continued reinforcing. Women are often ambivalent about it, but should receive excellent instruction and feedback.

49. **What is the value of BSE?**
Often contradictory. Some studies have shown it to be associated with smaller cancers at diagnosis, whereas others have failed to demonstrate this effect. Possible reasons for discrepancy include retrospective design, inconsistent competency and compliance among women, and various tumor sizes. One of the major arguments against BSE is false reassurance, with delay in seeking professional examination (a notion supported, in part, by a study from the United Kingdom that showed delays of more than 1 month in making a diagnosis among women who conducted BSE). Yet, even on this point data are conflicting. A study from the World Health Organization showed less delay in women doing BSE. Evidence for a BSE-induced reduction in mortality is even scantier. In a study of 18,242 women conducting self-examination (classified into good, medium, and poor performers, based on their skill), BSE had, at best, a 17% sensitivity and a 44.5% positive predictive value. Such results are still far from defining it as a good screening test. Yet, there *is* value in teaching patients how to conduct self-examination, and thus increasing their awareness of disease. Both teaching by nurses and training with silicone models can improve the BSE sensitivity, with effects persisting over time.

D. GYNECOMASTIA

50. **What is gynecomastia?**
From the Greek *gyneco* (female) and *mastos* (breast), this is a condition of excessive development of male mammary glands, characterized by ductal proliferation and periductal edema. It is frequently the result of increased estrogen levels or, at least, of an imbalance in the estrogen/testosterone ratio. Hence, mild gynecomastia is often seen in male neonates (due to the persistence of maternal estrogens) or in normal adolescents at puberty (65% of healthy Boy Scouts between 14 and 14.5 years). Its prevalence increases with age, becoming as high as 72% in men between 50 and 69 years of age. The gynecomastia of liver cirrhosis is also related to hormonal imbalance, as is the gynecomastia of hyperthyroid patients (10–40% of cases), which also results from increased load of circulating estrogens, and resolves with restoration of

euthyroidism. Finally, abnormal production of estrogens in males (because of adrenal gland or germ cell tumors) may also cause gynecomastia. In addition to the aforementioned causes, gynecomastia can be iatrogenic, too. Gynecomastia also has been reported in association with diabetes, adrenocortical hyperplasia, a variety of prostatic and testicular disorders, and many drugs—including beta blockers, spironolactone, and cimetidine.

ACKNOWLEDGMENT

The author gratefully acknowledges the contributions of Carol Fleischman, MD, to this chapter in the first edition of *Physical Diagnosis Secrets*.

SELECTED BIBLIOGRAPHY

1. Atkins H, Wolff B: Discharges from the nipple. Br J Surg 51:602–606, 1964.

2. Baines CJ, Wall C, Risch HA, et al: Changes in breast self-examination behaviour in a cohort of 8214 women in the Canadian National Breast Screening study. Cancer 57:1209–1216, 1986.

3. Barton MB, Harris R, Fletcher SW: The rational clinical examination. Does this patient have breast cancer? JAMA 282:1270–1280, 1999.

4. Boyd NF, Sutherland HJ, Fish EB, et al: Physical examination of the breast. Am J Surg 142:307–426, 1981.

5. Chaudary MA, Millis RR, Davies GC, Hayward JL: Nipple discharge: The diagnostic value of testing for occult blood. Ann Surg 196:651–655, 1982.

6. De Gowin RL: Diagnostic Examination, 6th ed. New York, McGraw-Hill, 1994.

7. Egan RL, Goldstein GT, McSweeney MM, et al: Conventional mammography, physical examination, thermography, and xeroradiography in the detection of breast cancer. Cancer 39:1984–1992, 1997.

8. Fletcher SW, O'Malley MS, Bumce LA: Physicians' abilities to detect lumps in silicone breast models. JAMA 253:2224–2228, 1985.

9. Gump FE: Sensitivity and specificity in silicone breast models. JAMA 254:2409, 1985.

10. Hicks MJ, Davis JR, Layton JM, Present AJ: Sensitivity of mammography and physical examination of the breast for detecting breast cancer. JAMA 242:2080–2083, 1979.

11. Mushlin AI: Diagnostic tests in breast cancer. Clinical strategies based on diagnostic probabilities. Ann Intern Med 103:79–85, 1985.

12. Newman HF, Klein M, Northrup JD, et al: Nipple discharge: Frequency and pathogenesis in an ambulatory population. N Y State J Med 83:928–933, 1983.

13. Nydick M, Bustos J, Dale JH Jr, et al: Gynecomastia in adolescent boys. JAMA 178:449–454, 1961.

14. O'Malley MS, Fletcher SW: US Preventive Services Task Force. Screening for breast cancer with breast self-examination. A critical review. JAMA 257:2196–2203, 1987.

CHAPTER 10

THE CARDIOVASCULAR EXAM

Salvatore Mangione, MD

"Just when the lamps were lit, a messenger came and brought me to the Emperor as he had bidden. Three doctors had watched over him since dawn, and two of them felt his pulse, and all three thought a fever attack was coming. I stood alongside but said nothing. The Emperor looked first at me and asked why I did not feel his pulse as the others two had. I answered: 'These two colleagues of mine have already done so, and as they have followed you on the journey, they presumably know what your abnormal pulse is, so they can judge its present state better.'

When I said this, he bade me, too, to feel his pulse. My impression was that—considering his age and body constitution—the pulse was far from indicating a fever attack, but that his stomach was stuffed with the food he had eaten, and that the food had become a slimy excrement. The Emperor praised my diagnosis and said, three times in a row: 'That is it. It is just as you say. I have eaten too much cold food!'

He then asked what measures should be taken. I replied what I knew of a similar case, saying: 'If you were any plain citizen of this country, I would, as usual, prescribe wine with a little pepper. But to a royal patient as in this case, doctors usually recommend milder treatment. It is enough for a woolen cover to be put on your stomach, impregnated with warm spiced salve."

—Galen (129–201 AD), describing his care of Emperor Marcus Aurelius

A. GENERALITIES

Cardiovascular examination is centered on five main components, all essential for making a diagnosis. This section discusses *inspection*, *palpation*, and *percussion*. *Auscultation* is addressed in two separate presentations.

1. **What are the main components of the cardiovascular physical examination?**
   - The *general appearance* of the patient (inspection)
   - The *arterial pulse* (palpation); this component also should include assessment of the arterial blood pressure (discussed separately in Chapter 2, Vital Signs, questions 37–127)
   - The central venous pressure and the jugular venous pulse (inspection)
   - *Precordial impulses and silhouette* (inspection, palpation, and percussion of the point of maximal impulse [PMI])
   - Auscultation

   These five components have been compared to the fingers of a hand, insofar as they are *all* needed to grab a diagnosis. Cardiac exam also could be compared to the evaluation of a pump, starting with the feeding and exit pipes and ultimately focusing on the pump itself: using your *eyes* (inspection of the PMI), your *touch* (palpation of the PMI), and your *ears*. *Auscultation*, the queen of cardiovascular examination, is in fact the longest (and largest) of these metaphoric fingers, and thus capable of reaching the farthest. Still, physical examination is only one of five *more general* components of the cardiovascular assessment. The other four are:
   - History
   - Office-based studies (such as electrocardiogram [ECG] and chest x-ray)
   - Noninvasive laboratory evaluations (such as echocardiography and nuclear medicine)
   - Invasive evaluations (cardiac catheterization)

B. GENERAL (PHYSICAL) APPEARANCE

2. **What aspects of general appearance should be observed in evaluating cardiac patients?**
   As suggested by Perloff, one should sequentially evaluate the following nine areas:
   - General appearance, facies, and body conformation
   - Gestures and gait
   - Face
   - Ears
   - Eyes
   - Extremities
   - Skin
   - Thorax
   - Abdomen
     See Tables 10-1 and 10-2.

C. THE ARTERIAL PULSE

"With careful practice the trained finger can become a most sensitive instrument in the examination of the pulse...from [its] examination we obtain information on three different points: first, concerning the rate and rhythm of the heart's action; second, concerning certain events occurring in a cardiac revolution; third, concerning the character of the blood pressure in the artery...The trained finger can recognize a great variety in the apparent volume of the wave itself. Although the pulse wave occupies such a short space of time, yet the sensitive finger readily recognizes these different features."

—J. MacKenzie, The Study of the Pulse, 1902

Evaluation of the arterial pulse is a time-honored method of bedside examination. It can still provide valuable cardiovascular information. In selective processes (such as tamponade, aortic valve disease, and hypertrophic cardiomyopathy), it can even prove *essential* for securing a diagnosis. Yet, assessment of the characteristics of the arterial pulse requires skill and practice, and at times can be frustrating. It is worth the effort, though, and thus deserves attention, even in our times of intra-arterial monitoring.

3. **Which arteries should be examined during the evaluation of the arterial pulse?**
   It depends on what you are trying to evaluate. If you are simply assessing the presence of peripheral pulses, *all* accessible arteries should be examined. The following points are especially important:
   - *Arteries on both sides* should be compared to detect asymmetries suggestive of embolic, thrombotic, atherosclerotic, dissecting, or extrinsic occlusion.
   - *Arteries of upper* and *lower extremities* should be *simultaneously* examined in hypertensive patients to identify reduction in volume (or pulse delays) suggestive of aortic coarctation.
   - If trying to evaluate the characteristics of the arterial *waveform*, you should examine only *central* arteries—*carotid, brachial,* or *femoral*.
     Since this section focuses on the bedside examination of the arterial wave as part of the cardiovascular exam, we will exclusively discuss evaluation of *central* arteries. Assessment of *peripheral* vessels is discussed in Chapter 22, Extremities and Peripheral Vascular Exam, questions 1–25.

4. **Isn't the radial artery the most commonly used vessel for the evaluation of the pulse?**
   No—and if so, it shouldn't be, since the radial artery is only suited for evaluation of pulse *rate* and *rhythm*, especially in fully clothed patients—a feature that made it quite popular in the

TABLE 10-1.   DIAGNOSTIC CLUES: BODY AND FACIES, GESTURES AND GAIT, FACE AND EARS

Body Appearance and Facies

- The anasarca of congestive heart failure
- The struggling, anguished, frightened, orthopneic, and diaphoretic look of pulmonary edema
- The tall stature, long extremities (with arm span exceeding patient's height), and sparse subcutaneous fat of *Marfan's syndrome* (mitral valve prolapse, aortic dilation, and dissection)
- The long extremities, kyphoscoliosis, and pectus carinatum of *homocystinuria* (arterial thrombosis)
- The tall stature and long extremities of *Klinefelter's syndrome* (atrial or ventricular septal defects, patent ductus arteriosus, and even tetralogy of Fallot)
- The tall stature and *thick* extremities of *acromegaly* (hypertension, cardiomyopathy, and conduction defects)
- The short stature, webbed neck, low hairline, small chin, wide-set nipples, and sexual infantilism of *Turner's syndrome* (coarctation of the aorta and valvular pulmonic stenosis)
- The dwarfism and polydactyly of *Ellis-van Creveld* syndrome (atrial septal defects and common atrium)
- The morbid obesity and somnolence of *obstructive sleep apnea* (hypoventilation, pulmonary hypertension, and cor pulmonale)
- The truncal obesity, thin extremities, moon face, and buffalo hump of hypertensive patients with *Cushing's syndrome*
- The mesomorphic, overweight, balding, hairy, and tense middle-aged patient with coronary artery disease
- The hammer toes and pes cavus of *Friedreich's ataxia* (hypertrophic cardiomyopathy, angina, and sick sinus syndrome)
- The straight lower back of *ankylosing spondylitis* (aortic regurgitation and complete heart block)

Face and Ears

- Pulsatility of the earlobes (tricuspid regurgitation)
- Head bobbing (De Musset's and Lincoln's signs)
- The round and chubby face of congenital pulmonary stenosis
- The hypertelorism, pigmented moles, webbed neck, and low-set ears of *Turner's syndrome*
- The round and chubby face of congenital valvular pulmonic stenosis
- The elfin face (small chin, malformed teeth, wide-set eyes, patulous lips, baggy cheeks, blunt and upturned nose) of *congenital stenosis of the pulmonary arteries and supravalvular aortic stenosis*—often associated with hypercalcemia and mental retardation.
- The unilateral lower facial weakness of infants with *cardiofacial syndrome*—this can be encountered in 5–10% of infants with congenital heart disease (usually ventricular septal defect); often noticeable only during crying.
- The premature aging of *Werner's syndrome* and *progeria* (associated with premature coronary artery and systemic atherosclerotic disease)
- The drooping eyelids, expressionless face, receding hairline, and bilateral cataracts of *Steinert's disease* (*myotonic dystrophy*, associated with conduction disorders, mitral valve prolapse)
- The epicanthic fold, protruding tongue, small ears, short nose, and flat bridge of *Down syndrome* (endocardial cushion defects)
- The dry and brittle hair, loss of lateral eyebrows, puffy eyelids, apathetic face, protruding tongue, thick and sallow skin of *myxedema* (associated with pericardial and coronary artery disease)
- The macroglossia not only of *Down syndrome* and *myxedema*, but also of *amyloidosis* (linked to restrictive cardiomyopathy, congestive heart failure)

Continued

TABLE 10-1. DIAGNOSTIC CLUES: BODY AND FACIES, GESTURES AND GAIT, FACE AND EARS—CONT'D

Gestures, Gait, and Stance

- The *Levine's sign* (clenched fist over the chest of patients with an acute myocardial infarction)
- The preferential squatting of *tetralogy of Fallot*
- The ataxic gait of *tertiary syphilis* (associated with aortic aneurysm and regurgitation)
- The waddling gait, lumbar lordosis, and calves pseudohypertrophy of *Duchenne's* muscular dystrophy (associated with hypertrophic cardiomyopathy and a pseudo infarction pattern on ECG)

Face and Ears

- The paroxysmal facial and neck flushing of *carcinoid syndrome* (with pulmonic stenosis and tricuspid stenosis/regurgitation)
- The saddle-shaped nose of *polychondritis* (associated with aortic aneurysm)
- The tightening of skin and mouth, scattered telangiectasias, and hyperpigmentation/hypopigmentation of *scleroderma* (with pulmonary hypertension, pericarditis, and myocarditis)
- The flushed cheeks and cyanotic lips of *mitral stenosis* (acrocyanosis)
- The gargoylism of *Hurler's syndrome* (associated with mitral and/or aortic disease)
- The short palpebral fissures, small upper lip, and hypoplastic mandible of *fetal alcohol syndrome* (associated with atrial or ventricular septal defects)
- The diagonal earlobe crease as a (questionable) marker of coronary artery disease (*earlobe sign* [also known as Frank's sign])

prudish Victorian times of Dr. MacKenzie. Conversely, the radial artery is *not* suited for evaluation of the wave *contour*, which requires a vessel *large* and *central* enough to retain most of the original characteristics of the aortic waveform. For that, the optimal choice is a carotid, brachial, or femoral artery, because amplitude and upstroke can only be appreciated in large central arteries (such as carotids and brachials), being otherwise missed in small peripheral arteries, like the radials. In fact, some findings (like the bifid pulse of hypertrophic obstructive cardiomyopathy [HOCM]) can only be appreciated on arterial tracing.

5. **What alterations occur in peripheral arteries?**
The major ones are an increase in *amplitude* and *upstroke velocity*. As the distance from the aortic valve increases, the primary percussion wave that is transmitted downward along the aorta begins to merge with the secondary waves that reverberate back from more peripheral arteries. This fusion leads to greater amplitude and upstroke velocity in *peripheral* as compared to central arteries (Fig. 10-1). This phenomenon is similar to that occurring at the shoreline, where waves tend to be taller. It is also the mechanism behind Hill's sign, the higher *indirect* systolic pressure of lower extremities as compared to upper extremities (*see* Chapter 2, Vital Signs, questions 110–115).

6. **Are there any findings that are better evaluated in *peripheral* rather than central arteries?**
Pulsus paradoxus and *pulsus alternans*. Both are best felt over smaller arteries (such as the radial), since the greater amplitude produced by these vessels magnifies the subtle arterial findings of both paradoxus and alternans. Yet, the *contour* of the arterial pulse should not be examined in peripheral vessels, since the normal alterations in amplitude and upstroke of these arteries might make the pulse of aortic stenosis inappropriately (and misleadingly) brisk.

TABLE 10-2. DIAGNOSTIC CLUES: EYES, EXTREMITIES, SKIN, THORAX, AND ABDOMEN

Eyes

- Xanthelasmhas of dyslipidemia and coronary artery disease (CAD)
- The enlarged lacrimal glands of *sarcoidosis* (restrictive cardiomyopathy, conduction defects, and, possibly, cor pulmonale)
- The cataracts and deafness of *"rubella syndrome"* (patent ductus arteriosus [PDA] or stenosis of the pulmonary artery)
- The stare and proptosis of increased central venous pressure
- The lid lag, stare, and exophthalmos of *hyperthyroidism* (tachyarrhythmias, angina, and high output failure)
- The conjunctival petechiae of *endocarditis*
- The conjunctivitis of *Reiter's disease* (pericarditis, aortic regurgitation, and prolongation of the P–R interval)
- The blue sclerae of *osteogenesis imperfecta* (aortic regurgitation)
- The icteric sclerae of *cirrhosis*
- The *Brushfield's spots* (small white spots on the periphery of the iris, usually crescentic and with an outward concavity, frequently but not exclusively seen in Down syndrome— endocardial cushion defects)
- The fissuring of the iris (coloboma) of *total anomalous pulmonary venous return*
- The dislocated lens of *Marfan's syndrome*
- The retinal changes of *hypertension* and *diabetes* (CAD and congestive heart failure)
- The Roth spots of *bacterial endocarditis*

Extremities

- The *cyanosis and clubbing* of "central mixing" (right-to-left shunts, pulmonary arteriovenous fistulas, and drainage of the inferior vena cava into left atrium)
- The *differential cyanosis and clubbing* of PDA with pulmonary hypertension (the reversed shunt limits cyanosis and clubbing to the feet, but spares hands)

- The tightly *tapered and contracted fingers of scleroderma*, with ischemic ulcers and hypoplastic nails (often associated with pulmonary hypertension and myocardial disease, pericarditis, and valvulopathy)
- The *arachnodactyly*, hyperextensible joints (especially knees, wrists, and fingers), and flat feet of Marfan's syndrome (associated with aortic disease and regurgitation)
- The ulnar deviation of rheumatoid arthritis (pericardial, valvular, or myocardial disease)
- The *mainline track lines* of addicts (tricuspid regurgitation, septic emboli, and endocarditis)
- The *liver palms* (thenar and hypothenar erythema) of chronic hepatic congestion

Skin

- The *jaundice* of hepatic congestion
- The *cyanosis* of right-to-left shunt
- The *pallor* of anemia and high output failure
- The *bronzing* of hemochromatosis (restrictive cardiomyopathy)
- The *telangiectasias* of Rendu-Osler-Weber (at times associated with pulmonary arteriovenous fistulae)
- The *neurofibromas, café-au-lait spots, and axillary freckles* (Crowe's sign) of von Recklinghausen's (pheochromocytomas)
- The symmetric *vitiligo* (especially of the distal extremities) of hyperthyroidism
- The *butterfly rash* of SLE (endo-myo-pericarditis)
- The *eyelid purplish discoloration* of dermatomyositis (cardiomyopathy, heart block, and pericarditis)
- The *skin nodules and macules of sarcoidosis* (cardiomyopathy and blocks)
- The *xanthomas* of dyslipidemia
- The hyperextensible skin (and joints) of Ehlers-Danlos (mitral valve prolapse)
- The *coarse and sallow skin* of hypothyroidism
- The skin nodules (sebaceous adenomas), shagreen patches, and periungual fibromas of *tuberous sclerosis* (rhabdomyomas of the heart and arrhythmias)

Continued

TABLE 10-2. DIAGNOSTIC CLUES: EYES, EXTREMITIES, SKIN, THORAX, AND ABDOMEN—CONT'D

Extremities (cont.)

- The *"reversed" differential cyanosis and clubbing* of transposition (aorta originating from the right ventricle): hands are cyanotic and clubbed, but feet are normal
- The sudden pallor, pain, and coldness of *peripheral embolization*
- *Osler's nodes* (swollen, *tender*, raised, pea-sized lesions of finger pads, palms, and soles) and *Janeway lesions* (small, *nontender*, erythematous or hemorrhagic lesions of palms or soles) of bacterial endocarditis
- The clubbing, *splinter hemorrhages* of endocarditis
- The Raynaud's of scleroderma
- The *simian line* of Down's syndrome (atrial septal defect [ASD])
- The hyperextensible joints of *osteogenesis imperfecta* (aortic regurgitation)
- The *nicotine finger stains* of chain smokers (CAD)
- The leg edema of congestive heart failure

Thorax and Abdomen

- The thoracic bulges of ventricular septal defect/atrial septal defect
- The pectus carinatum, pectus excavatum, and kyphoscoliosis of *Marfan's syndrome*
- The akyphotic and straight back of mitral valve prolapse
- The systolic (and rarely diastolic) murmurs of pectus carinatum, excavatum, straight back
- The barrel chest of *emphysema* (cor pulmonale)
- The shield chest of *Turner's syndrome*
- The cor pulmonale of severe *kyphoscoliosis*
- The ascites of right-sided or biventricular failure
- The hepatic pulsation of tricuspid regurgitation
- The positive abdominojugular reflux of congestive heart failure

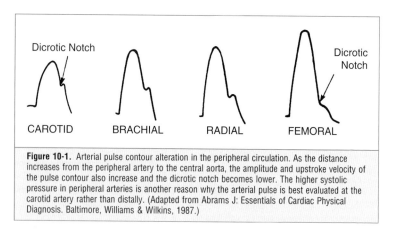

Dicrotic Notch

Dicrotic Notch

CAROTID   BRACHIAL   RADIAL   FEMORAL

Figure 10-1. Arterial pulse contour alteration in the peripheral circulation. As the distance increases from the peripheral artery to the central aorta, the amplitude and upstroke velocity of the pulse contour also increase and the dicrotic notch becomes lower. The higher systolic pressure in peripheral arteries is another reason why the arterial pulse is best evaluated at the carotid artery rather than distally. (Adapted from Abrams J: Essentials of Cardiac Physical Diagnosis. Baltimore, Williams & Wilkins, 1987.)

7. **What alterations result from decreased arterial compliance?**
The same encountered in peripheral arteries: stiffer vessels conduct the waveform with greater velocity, giving the pulse higher *amplitude* and brisker *upstroke*, even though stroke volume might be weak and diminished (as in aortic stenosis). Hence, the arterial pulse of hypertensive, atherosclerotic, and older patients is less reliable for detecting left ventricular outflow obstruction.

8. **What about vasoconstricted arteries?**
Highly constricted arteries may also have a diminished pulse, even when stroke volume is normal or increased.

9. **What is the best technique for evaluating the arterial pulse in carotid arteries?**
First, *inspect* the carotids in the upper triangular spaces, medial to the sternocleidomastoids. Look for the visible and abnormal pulsations of aortic regurgitation. Then listen over the vessel to rule out bruits. If negative, apply the thumb or index finger over the carotids, one vessel at a time. Vary pressure for optimal evaluation of pulse characteristics (especially *amplitude* and *contour*). Remember that *light* pressure is often more valuable. As always, practice and experience are crucial.

10. **What is the best technique for evaluating the arterial pulse in brachial arteries?**
First, use the fingers of your *left* hand to palpate the radial artery of the patient's right arm. Then, use the thumb of your *right* hand to compress the patient's brachial artery until the radial pulse is completely obliterated. At this point, release very gently the pressure over the brachial artery until you feel the radial pulse again. Your thumb has now become like a "poor man's" transducer, allowing you to feel both *amplitude* and *contour* of the brachial pulse.

11. **What should you evaluate when examining the arterial pulse?**
You should evaluate the *upstroke*, the *peak*, and the *downstroke* of the waveform. More specifically, you should focus on the following eight characteristics:
- Rate and rhythm
- Volume and amplitude
- Contour
- Speed (or rate of rise) of the upstroke
- Speed (or rate of collapse) of the downstroke
- Stiffness (or distensibility) of the arterial wall
- Presence of a palpable *shudder* or *thrill*
- Presence of audible *bruits* or transmitted *murmurs*

12. **What are the characteristics of a normal arterial pulse?**
A normal arterial pulse comprises a *primary* (systolic) and a *secondary* (diastolic) wave. These are separated by a *dicrotic notch* (*dikrotos*, double-beating in Greek), which corresponds to the closure of the semilunar valves (S_2) (*see* Fig. 10-2).

13. **Are both the primary and secondary waves palpable?**
No. Neither the dicrotic notch nor the secondary wave is normally felt, only the primary wave. Yet, in certain pathologic conditions, a double-peaked pulse may indeed become palpable. Yet in these cases, the two spikes are usually *systolic*. More rarely, the second spike coincides with diastole.

14. **How are primary and secondary waves generated?**
- The *primary wave* derives from the ejection of blood into the aorta. Its early portion (*percussion* wave) reflects discharge into the *central* aorta, whereas its mid-to-late portion (*tidal* wave) reflects movement of blood from the central to the peripheral aorta. The two portions are separated by an *anacrotic notch*, only visible on tracing and usually not palpable.
- The *secondary* wave is generated instead by the elastic back-reflection of the waveform, from the peripheral arteries of the lower half of the body.

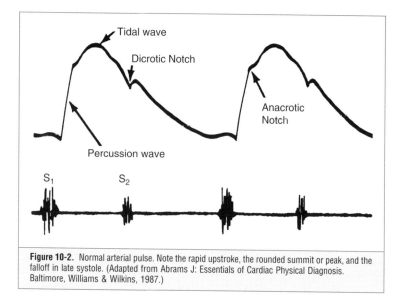

Figure 10-2. Normal arterial pulse. Note the rapid upstroke, the rounded summit or peak, and the falloff in late systole. (Adapted from Abrams J: Essentials of Cardiac Physical Diagnosis. Baltimore, Williams & Wilkins, 1987.)

15. **What is the significance of a *normal rate of rise* of the arterial pulse?**
It argues against the presence of significant aortic stenosis (AS), but only in the young (elderly patients may have spuriously brisk pulses—previously discussed). Hence, a normal rate of rise can be useful in evaluating a benign systolic ejection murmur.

16. **What is the meaning of a slow rate of rise of the arterial pulse?**
A pulse that is reduced (*parvus*) and delayed (*tardus*) argues for *aortic valvular stenosis*. This also may be occasionally accompanied by a palpable thrill.

17. **Is there any correlation between the *slow rise* of the arterial pulse and the severity of AS?**
Yes. If ventricular function is good, a slower upstroke correlates with a higher transvalvular gradient. In left ventricular failure, however, *parvus* and *tardus* may occur even with mild AS.

18. **How can you differentiate supravalvular from valvular aortic stenosis?**
Supravalvular AS is associated with right-to-left asymmetry of the arterial pulse: the right brachial is normal while the left resembles the pulse of *valvular* AS (*see* Fig. 10-3).This is akin to aortic coarctation and underscores the importance of examining both pulses.

19. **And what about *subvalvular* stenosis?**
In *subvalvular stenosis* of the hypertrophic variety (HOCM), the arterial pulse is usually brisk and with a double systolic impulse.

20. **What is the significance of a *brisk arterial upstroke*?**
It depends on whether it is associated with *normal* or *widened* pulse pressure. If associated with *normal pulse pressure,* a brisk upstroke usually indicates two conditions:
- The simultaneous emptying of the left ventricle into a high-pressure bed (the aorta) and a lower pressure bed. The latter can be the right ventricle (in patients with ventricular septal defect, VSD) or the left *atrium* (in patients with mitral regurgitation, MR). Both will allow a rapid left ventricular emptying, which, in turn, generates a brisk arterial upstroke. The pulse pressure, however, remains normal.

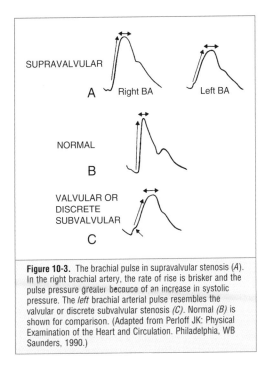

Figure 10-3. The brachial pulse in supravalvular stenosis (*A*). In the right brachial artery, the rate of rise is brisker and the pulse pressure greater because of an increase in systolic pressure. The *left* brachial arterial pulse resembles the valvular or discrete subvalvular stenosis *(C)*. Normal *(B)* is shown for comparison. (Adapted from Perloff JK: Physical Examination of the Heart and Circulation. Philadelphia, WB Saunders, 1990.)

- *Hypertrophic obstructive cardiomyopathy* (HOCM). Despite its association with left ventricular obstruction, this disease is characterized by a brisk and bifid pulse, due to the hypertrophic ventricle and its *delayed* obstruction.
  If associated with *widened pulse pressure,* a brisk upstroke indicates *aortic regurgitation (AR).* In contrast to MR, VSD, or HOCM, the AR pulse has rapid upstroke *and* collapse.

21. **In addition to AR, which other processes cause rapid upstroke and widened pulse pressure?**
    The most common are the *hyperkinetic heart syndromes* (high output states). These include anemia, fever, exercise, thyrotoxicosis, pregnancy, cirrhosis, beriberi, Paget's disease, arteriovenous fistulas, patent ductus arteriosus, aortic regurgitation, and anxiety—all typically associated with rapid ventricular contraction and low peripheral vascular resistance.

22. **What is *pulsus paradoxus*?**
    It is an exaggerated fall in systolic blood pressure during *quiet* inspiration. In contrast to evaluation of arterial contour and amplitude, pulsus paradoxus is best detected in a *peripheral* vessel, such as the radial. Although *palpable* at times, optimal detection of the pulsus paradoxus usually requires a sphygmomanometer (*see* Chapter 2, Vital Signs, questions 85–103).

23. **What is *pulsus alternans*?**
    It is the alternation of strong and weak arterial pulses, despite *regular rate and rhythm*. First described by Traube in 1872, *pulsus alternans* is often associated with alternation of strong and feeble heart sounds (*auscultatory alternans*). Both indicate severe left ventricular dysfunction (from ischemia, hypertension, or valvular cardiomyopathy), with worse ejection fraction and higher pulmonary capillary pressure. Hence, they are often associated with an S_3 gallop.

24. **What is *electrical* alternans?**

It's a beat-to-beat alternation of tall and small QRS complexes, still within the realm of a regular heart rate. It may also present as beat-to-beat variation in the direction, amplitude, and duration of *any other* component of the ECG waveform, although the QRS is usually the predominant one. Undetectable on physical exam, it may coexist with *mechanical alternans* (which manifests itself through pulsus alternans). The clinical significance of electrical alternans is its association with large pericardial effusions, seen in 5–10% of patients with tamponade.

25. **What is the best way to feel a pulsus alternans?**

Not on the carotids. Like *pulsus paradoxus,* pulsus alternans is best assessed in *peripheral* arteries because smaller vessels tend to magnify those variations in volume and amplitude that are crucial for the detection of both findings. To feel a pulsus alternans, either palpate the radial artery at the wrist or use the blood pressure cuff at the arm (beat-to-beat fluctuations in arterial pulse are paralleled by beat-to-beat fluctuations in systolic blood pressure). Slowly deflate the cuff until you hear the first Korotkoff sounds. Notice that only the stronger ejections do indeed produce a sound. After further deflating the cuff, notice that the weaker ejections become detectable, too, causing in fact a doubling of Korotkoff sounds. The difference in systolic blood pressure between stronger and weaker ejections is usually 15–20 mmHg, not too dissimilar from that of pulsus paradoxus. Finally, ask the patient to take a deep breath, or suddenly assume an upright position. This also may help elicit pulsus alternans.

26. **What is the mechanism of pulsus alternans?**

There are two schools of thought: one based on contractility and the other on hemodynamics. The *contractility* school attributes the pulse-to-pulse variation to a beat-to-beat change in left ventricular diameter, which, in turn, leads to a cycling of weaker and stronger ejections through swings in the Starling curve position. The *hemodynamic* school attributes, instead, the variation in left ventricular ejection to a relative change in systolic and diastolic duration. Whenever ejection lengthens (because of increased left ventricular filling), diastole is proportionally shortened. This, in turn, leads to a shorter (and weaker) ejection during the following cycle, with a subsequent proportional increase in diastolic filling. This will then trigger a new cycle of stronger ejection and shorter diastole, with reinitiation of the seesaw.

27. **Can pulsus alternans ever be normal?**

It may be encountered in very rapid heart rates (for example, paroxysmal tachycardia), where it does not carry the same ominous implications.

28. **What is *total* alternans?**

It's a *pulsus alternans* in which the weak pulse is too small to be detected so that the rate at the wrist is always half that at the apex.

29. **What is a *bigeminal pulse*?**

It is also a pulse in which beats occur in pairs (and with different strength), except that this time the rhythm is *irregular*, and the cause is a bigeminy.

30. **What is a *double-peaked pulse*?**

It is a pulse characterized by two palpable spikes per cycle (Fig. 10-4). The first peak always occurs in systole, whereas the second may instead occur during either systole (as part of the primary wave: *pulsus bisferiens* and *bifid pulse*) or diastole (as part of the secondary wave: *dicrotic pulse*).

31. **Define *pulsus bisferiens*.**

From the Latin *bis* (twice) and *ferio* (to strike [i.e., a "double-strike"]), *pulsus bisferiens* is an arterial pulse with two *palpable* systolic peaks of equal strength. First described by Galen, it has a large amplitude and quick upstroke/downstroke.

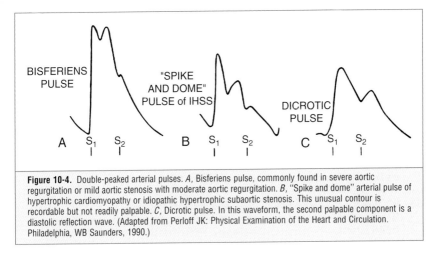

Figure 10-4. Double-peaked arterial pulses. *A*, Bisferiens pulse, commonly found in severe aortic regurgitation or mild aortic stenosis with moderate aortic regurgitation. *B*, "Spike and dome" arterial pulse of hypertrophic cardiomyopathy or idiopathic hypertrophic subaortic stenosis. This unusual contour is recordable but not readily palpable. *C*, Dicrotic pulse. In this waveform, the second palpable component is a diastolic reflection wave. (Adapted from Perloff JK: Physical Examination of the Heart and Circulation. Philadelphia, WB Saunders, 1990.)

32. What is the best way to detect a pulsus bisferiens?
Through *light* but firm compression of a large *central* artery, best if done by using the thumb and slightly elevating the patient's arm. Too strong of a compression may actually miss it. A pulsus bisferiens also can be detected by blood pressure cuff, as a closely split Korotkoff sound.

33. What is the diagnostic significance of a pulsus bisferiens?
It usually reflects *moderate to severe aortic regurgitation* (with or without aortic stenosis), but can also occur in other high output states. In aortic regurgitation, however, the double pulse is not only palpable, but sometimes is even *audible*. For example, it can be detected as:
- **Double Korotkoff sound:** This is heard during measurement of systolic blood pressure, with the cuff being slowly deflated. It coincides with the systolic arterial peak.
- **Traube's femoral sound(s):** Reported by Traube in 1867, this is a loud, explosive, and shot-like *systolic* sound heard over a large central artery (femoral usually, but also brachial or carotid) in synchrony with the arterial pulse. It is detected whenever *light* pressure is applied with the stethoscope's diaphragm over the artery, coupled with mild arterial compression distal to the stethoscope's head. Although more often single (and thus called *pistol shot sound*), it can also be *double* (hence, referred to as *Traube's femoral double sounds*) and sometimes even *triple*. It reflects the sudden systolic distention of the arterial wall—like a sail filling with wind. A single shot occurs in approximately one half of all AR patients, but may also take place in other high output states. Double sounds occur in one fourth of AR patients. Lack of arterial compression distal to the stethoscope's head sharply decreases the test's sensitivity, confining it to cases with severe left ventricular dilation. Like the water hammer pulse, Traube's sound(s) has 37–55% sensitivity for AR and 63–98% specificity.

34. What is Duroziez's double murmur?
It is a to-and-fro double murmur over a large central artery—usually the femoral, but also the brachial. It is elicited by applying gradual but *firm* compression with the stethoscope's diaphragm. This produces not only a systolic murmur (which is normal), but also a *diastolic* one (which is instead pathologic, and typical of AR). Duroziez's has 58–100% sensitivity *and* specificity for AR. False negatives may occur in mild disease, concomitant AS, inadequate ventricular *filling* (due to associated mitral stenosis), inadequate ventricular *emptying* (due to concomitant mitral regurgitation), or obstruction to waveform transmission (because of aortic coarctation). False positives may occur in all high-output conditions. In these disorders, the

murmur is not to and fro, but *continuous*, like that of an arteriovenous fistula. Moreover, the double murmur of high-output states is usually caused by *forward* flow, whereas in AR only one murmur is due to forward flow; the other is caused instead by *reverse* flow. The two can be easily separated by applying pressure first on the more cephalad edge of the diaphragm (which enhances the murmur of forward flow), and then on its more caudad end (which enhances the reverse flow murmur). This allows identification not only of AR but also of patent ductus arteriosus, the only other high-output state characterized by both forward and reverse flow.

35. **Who was Duroziez?**
A colleague and friend of Charcot. Paul L. Duroziez (1826–1897) had a general medical practice in Paris, but no official academic appointment. After serving as a surgeon during the Franco–Prussian war of 1870, he became president of the French Society of Medicine and Chevalier of the Legion of Honor. He described his homonymous finding at age 35, in 1861.

36. **What is the usefulness of all these auscultatory findings?**
More historical than clinical, although the intensity of femoral pistol shot sounds does indeed correlate with height of pulse pressure. Yet, neither Traube nor Duroziez predicts AR severity.

37. **What is the mechanism of pulsus bisferiens?**
Not clear. One theory explains the trough between the two peaks as a result of the Venturi effect caused by rapid blood flow. This would pull *inward* the aortic walls and trigger a transient arrest in flow—which, in turn, would stop the Bernoulli effect, restart the flow, and thus lead to the secondary peak.

38. **What is the prognostic value of a pulsus bisferiens?**
It indicates a very large stroke volume. Hence, it may disappear with left ventricular dysfunction.

39. **What is a *bifid pulse*?**
It is the classic pulse of HOCM. In contrast to bisferiens, the bifid pulse (from the Latin *bifidus*, cleft) is not detectable at the bedside, *unless there is severe outflow obstruction*. In fact, most HOCM patients have a *normal* carotid pulse, with its bifid nature only appearing on tracings (where it presents as a *spike and dome pattern*).

40. **What is the mechanism of the bifid pulse?**
It is a very rapid, early systolic emptying of the ventricle (causing the first brisk peak), followed by an obstruction, and then by another emptying (causing the second peak).

41. **What is a *dicrotic pulse*?**
It is also a double-peaked pulse (from the Greek *di*, two, and *krotos*, beat), except that in this case the additional impulse originates in *diastole,* as an accentuation of the secondary (or *dicrotic*) wave. Although the secondary wave is normally seen only on arterial recordings, the dicrotic pulse can actually be *felt*—usually over the carotids. It is probably due to a rebound of blood against the closed aortic valve, causing a secondary elastic wave. Since this "rebound" requires very elastic arteries, it can only be felt in young patients—and never above the age of 45. The dicrotic pulse is the least common of all the double-peaked pulses, easily separated from *bifid* and *bisferiens* because of its diastolic timing and longer interval between peaks.

42. **What is the clinical significance of a dicrotic pulse?**
It suggests low cardiac output and increased systemic vascular resistance, as in severe congestive cardiomyopathy or tamponade (especially during inspiration). Hence, it often coexists with pulsus alternans and gallop sounds. In these patients, the low cardiac output

reduces the primary wave, thus increasing the likelihood of feeling the secondary one. In addition, a dicrotic pulse also has been reported in *young* healthy individuals as a result of fever.

43. What is a *hypokinetic pulse*?
From the Greek *hypo* (diminished) and *kinesis* (movement), this is a pulse of *diminished amplitude*. Causes include:

- Obstruction to left ventricular outflow (aortic stenosis)
- Diminished left ventricular contraction (cardiomyopathy)
- Diminished left ventricular filling (mitral stenosis)

A small pulse is also called *parvus* ("small" in Latin), which usually presents as a slow upstroke (*tardus*, "delayed" in Latin). A reduced and delayed pulse (parvus and tardus) narrows significantly the differential diagnosis of a hypokinetic pulse, making AS more likely.

44. Is there any difference in sensitivity/specificify for tardus versus parvus?
A *pulsus tardus* is a better predictor of AS, with 30–90% sensitivity and even higher specificity. Instead, a pulse with small amplitude (*parvus*) but normal upstroke usually suggests decreased left ventricular contraction and/or filling. Hence, it argues for cardiomyopathy or mitral stenosis.

45. Can arterial characteristics modify a pulsus tardus?
Yes. The stiffer the vessel, the brisker the upstroke. That is why atherosclerosis may obliterate a pulsus tardus. And that is also why older AS patients may lack the typical arterial findings. This atherosclerosis-induced "acceleration" may even occur on *central* arteries.

46. Are there any other manifestations of arterial delay?
The *apical–carotid* and *brachio–radial delay* (respectively, a palpable delay between the apical and carotid impulse, and brachial and radial impulse). Both can occur in patients with valvular AS.

47. What is the carotid shudder?
It is a palpable thrill felt at the peak of the carotid pulse in patients with AS, AR, or both. It represents the transmission of the murmur to the artery and is a relatively specific but rather insensitive sign of aortic valvular disease (Fig. 10-5).

48. What is an *anacrotic* pulse?
Another sign of AS. The pulse is not only *small* (parvus) and *slow* (tardus), but also has an anacrotic notch on its ascending limb. This is visible on arterial tracings but *not palpable*. Hence, it has little clinical relevance. The name derives from the Greek *ana* (upwards) and *krotos* (impulse), and refers to the *upstroke (or ascending) limb* of the arterial tracing. It is an abbreviation for "*anadicrotic*" (*twice beating on the upstroke*).

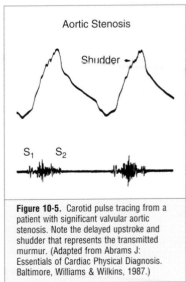

Figure 10-5. Carotid pulse tracing from a patient with significant valvular aortic stenosis. Note the delayed upstroke and shudder that represents the transmitted murmur. (Adapted from Abrams J: Essentials of Cardiac Physical Diagnosis. Baltimore, Williams & Wilkins, 1987.)

49. What is a *hyperkinetic* pulse?
A pulse with *large amplitude* and *rapid upstroke* (from the Greek *hyper*, large, and *kinesis*, motion). It is often referred to as *pulsus celer* (which is Latin for "fast"), to distinguish it from

the *slow* and *small* pulse (*tardus and parvus*) of AS. The large volume of a hyperkinetic pulse reflects increased stroke volume, whereas the quick rise reflects increased velocity of contraction.

50. **What are the causes of a hyperkinetic pulse?**
    Usually the *high-output states* (including AR), which are typically associated with a *widening pulse pressure*. Yet, a hyperkinetic pulse can also occur in mitral regurgitation or HOCM, but in this case the pulse pressure is normal. Finally, a hyperkinetic pulse may be felt in patients with decreased arterial compliance, like elderly individuals (especially if hypertensive).

51. **What is *Corrigan's pulse*?**
    It is one of the various names for the bounding and quickly collapsing pulse of aortic regurgitation. This is both visible *and* palpable. Another common term for it is *"water hammer,"* but also cannonball, collapsing, or pistol-shot pulse. Corrigan's may be so brisk as to cause other typical findings, such as De Musset's or Lincoln's signs (*see* Chapter 1, questions 53 and 54).

52. **Who was Corrigan?**
    Sir Dominic J. Corrigan (1802–1880) was an Irishman; in fact, the longest-serving president of the Irish College of Physicians, and a member of Parliament for the city of Dublin. He also was a personal physician to Queen Victoria. In 1832, he published a treatise titled "On Permanent Patency of the Mouth of the Aorta, or Inadequacy of the Aortic Valve," in which he reported a series of observations on AR. He also reported the visible (*not* palpable) characteristics of his famous pulse. Still, a brisk arterial pulse had been described by De Vieussens 100 years before, but Corrigan was the first to make the correlation between this pulse and aortic regurgitation.

53. **What is a water hammer?**
    A very popular Victorian toy. It consisted of a sealed test tube, partially filled with water or mercury, and all in a vacuum. Since solids and liquids fall at the same rate in a vacuum, the inversion of the tube caused the column of fluid to fall rather precipitously, hitting the glass with a brisk jolt. This made the Victorian children happy and the gadget almost as popular as today's electronic gizmos. The comparison between the slapping impact of a water hammer and the brisk bounding pulse of AR was first made in 1844 by the English physician Thomas Watson. It remains part of medical lore today, long after the demise of its homonymous toy.

54. **What is the best way to feel a Corrigan's pulse?**
    By elevating the patient's arm while at the same time feeling the radial artery at the *wrist*. Raising the arm higher than the heart reduces the intra-radial diastolic pressure, collapses the vessel, and thus facilitates the palpability of the subsequent systolic thrust.

55. **What is a pulsus *durus*?**
    A pulse so hardened that it is difficult to compress (*durus*, hard in Latin). This is usually a finding of arteriosclerosis, which may be associated with Osler's sign (*see* Chapter 2, questions 70–72).

56. **Can the compressibility of the arterial pulse predict the systolic blood pressure?**
    Yes. To do so, palpate the radial artery with the fingers of your *left* hand, while at the same time compressing the brachial artery with the thumb of your *right* hand. Push on the brachial until you have obliterated the radial pulse. If this requires *mild* force, the blood pressure is probably around 120 mmHg or less. If it requires *intermediate* force, the blood pressure is 120–160 mmHg. Finally, if it requires *high* force, the blood pressure is probably above 160 mmHg.

57. **How do you auscultate for carotid bruits?**
    By placing your bell on the neck in a quiet room and with a relaxed patient. Auscultate from just behind the upper end of the thyroid cartilage to immediately below the angle of the jaw.

58. **What other findings can mimic a carotid bruit?**
   - **Systolic heart murmurs:** These are only *transmitted* to the neck. Hence, in contrast to a bruit, they are louder over the precordium than the neck.
   - **Venous hums:** These are innocent murmurs caused by flow in the internal jugular vein. In contrast to carotid bruits, they are loudest in diastole (although, actually, *continuous*) and can only be heard in a sitting position (*see* questions 120–123).

   Most carotid bruits are heard in *systole*. Only a few are both systolic and diastolic. Why this is so is unclear. The major issue of a bruit, of course, is ruling out *carotid artery stenosis*.

59. **What is the interobserver agreement on carotid bruits?**
   Quite good for *detecting* bruits, but only fair for evaluating their intensity, pitch, or duration.

60. **Can carotid bruits occur in children?**
   Yes. In fact, they are present in 20% of children younger than 15 years of age.

61. **And what about adults?**
   They occur in 1% of *healthy* adults. Still, prevalence and incidence increase with age. For example, prevalence of *asymptomatic* bruits rises from 2.3% between 45 and 54 years, to 8.2% above age 75. In fact, incidence of new bruits is 1% per year in adults $\geq$ 65—twice the rate of people aged 45–54. Finally, bruits are very common in *high output states*. In hemodialysis patients, they are often louder on the side of the A-V fistula, frequently associated with a subclavian bruit.

62. **What is the significance of a carotid bruit in asymptomatic ambulatory patients?**
   It depends on the age. In a 50-year-old man, an asymptomatic carotid bruit is associated with increased incidence of both cerebrovascular and cardiovascular events, with average annual rates of stroke and transient ischemic attacks that are three times higher. This increased risk decreases sharply with age, becoming essentially nonexistent among people older than 75.

63. **What is the significance of a carotid bruit in an asymptomatic preoperative patient?**
   It depends on the surgery. Asymptomatic preoperative bruits are rather common in the surgical population (10% of patients), a prevalence much higher than in the general population (4.4%). Yet, they do not necessarily predict increased risk of perioperative stroke, although they do predict transient postoperative dysfunction and behavioral abnormalities. Still, in patients undergoing by-pass heart surgery, the incidence of hemodynamically significant carotid artery stenosis is high (2.8–11.8%, with no correlation in the asymptomatic patient between presence of a bruit and severity of carotid disease). Risk of perioperative stroke is age related (1–3% in patients of all ages, but 3.8 times higher in those older than 70). Hence, detecting a bruit prior to coronary revascularization is ominous, and it mandates further diagnostic studies.

64. **What is the correlation between symptomatic carotid bruit and high-grade stenosis?**
   It's high. In fact, bruits presenting with transient ischemic attacks (TIAs) or minor strokes in the anterior circulation should be evaluated aggressively for the presence of high-grade (70–99%) carotid stenosis, since endarterectomy markedly decreases mortality and stroke rates. Still, while presence of a bruit significantly increases the likelihood of high-grade carotid stenosis, its absence doesn't exclude disease. Moreover, a bruit heard over the bifurcation may reflect a narrowed *external* carotid artery and thus occur in angiographically normal or completely occluded *internal* carotids. Hence, surgical decisions should *not* be based on physical exam alone; imaging is mandatory.

D. CENTRAL VENOUS PRESSURE AND JUGULAR VENOUS PULSE (WAVEFORM)

"The visible oscillations in this region consist of a series of filling and collapses, sometimes prominent and easy to recognize ... There is found then, aside from the slow oscillations caused by the respiratory movements and simultaneous with them, the following sequence of movements which is repeated with constant and perfect regularity: at first a slow elevation, then two quick elevations, finally two deep depressions, after which the series begins again. Now each series of this kind corresponds to a cardiac cycle. These impulses sometimes have such force and amplitude that at first it might be believed that they represent pulsation of the carotid artery or of the subclavian. But after a little attention one is soon convinced that they actually take place in the internal jugular."
—Pierre Carl Potain: On the movements and sounds that take place in the jugular veins.
Bull Mem Soc Med Hop (Paris) 4:3, 1867.

"We come now to the study of a subject which gives us far more information of what is actually going on within the chambers of the heart. In the study of the venous pulse we have often the direct means of observing the effects of the systole and diastole of the right auricle, and of the systole and diastole of the right ventricle. The venous pulse represents therefore a greater variety of features, and is subject to influence so subtle that it may manifest variations due to the changing conditions of the patient, during which the arterial pulse reveals no appreciable alteration."
—James MacKenzie: The Study of the Pulse, Arterial, Venous and Hepatic, and
the Movements of the Heart. Edinburgh, Young J. Pentland, 1902.

"Clinical analysis of the venous pulse may not be easy, but there can be no question that five minutes spent observing the movements of neck veins may be as informative as auscultation."
—Paul Wood: Diseases of the Heart and Circulation. London, Eyre & Spottiswoode, 1950.

Observation of the *jugular venous pulse* and measurement of the *central venous pressure* are more recent acquisitions than the evaluation of the arterial pulse, yet they can still provide a wealth of valuable clinical information, especially when trying to assess intravascular volume, evaluate right ventricular function, test the integrity of the pulmonic and tricuspid valves, and investigate the status of the pericardium. Skills are difficult—at times even intimidating. Yet, they are worth the effort, even in our times of invasive hemodynamic monitoring.

65. **What is the history behind the examination of neck veins?**
The first report of venous pulsations goes back to the 17th century, when the Italian Giovanni Maria Lancisi (1654–1720) described a "systolic fluctuation of the external jugular vein" in a patient with tricuspid regurgitation (i.e., the large systolic jugular wave replacing the normal trough that is still referred to as the *Lancisi's sign*—in these patients, also watch for earlobe pulsations, especially on the right side). In 1867, Pierre Carl Potain carefully described the jugular waveform in a paper titled "Movements and Sounds that Take Place in The Jugular Veins." Forty years later, the Scottish Sir James MacKenzie published *The Study of the Pulse*, a seminal work, which summarized 20 years of clinical assessment of both venous and arterial pulsations, and established the jugular venous pulse as one of the essential elements of cardiovascular examination. It also contributed the standard waveform terminology (A, C, and V waves and X–Y descent) still used nowadays. Yet, it was only in the 1950s that the examination of the jugular venous pulse (and pressure) became a standard component of bedside assessment, thanks to the influence of the charismatic British physician Paul Wood.

66. **What is the role of physical exam in assessing neck veins?**
   - To estimate the central venous pressure
   - To evaluate the *venous pulse*

67. **What is the central venous pressure (CVP)?**
The pressure within the right atrium/superior vena cava system (*i.e., the right ventricular filling pressure*). As pulmonary capillary wedge pressure reflects left ventricular end-diastolic pressure (in the absence of *mitral* stenosis), so central venous pressure reflects *right* ventricular end-diastolic pressure (in the absence of *tricuspid* stenosis).

68. **Which veins should be evaluated for assessing venous pulse and CVP?**
Central veins, as much in direct communication with the right atrium as possible. The ideal one is therefore the *internal jugular*. Of course, as part of a comprehensive examination, all visible veins should be evaluated. Since this chapter focuses on the *cardiovascular exam*, we will limit our discussion to *jugular waveform* and *central venous pressure*. Evaluation of peripheral veins is covered in Chapter 22, The Extremities and Peripheral Vascular Exam, questions 41–62.

69. **What is the clinical value of jugular venous distention and pulse?**
It is a "poor man's" monitor of right heart hemodynamics. More specifically:
- Evaluation of *jugular venous distention* provides a noninvasive assessment of jugular venous *pressure*. This, in turn, provides an estimate of CVP and *intravascular volume*.
- Evaluation of *jugular waveform* provides instead additional information on right ventricular function, the status of the tricuspid and pulmonic valves, and the presence (or absence) of pericardial constriction.

70. **How difficult is it to evaluate the jugular veins?**
Quite difficult, especially in patients with very low CVP or short and fat necks. It is especially difficult during mechanical ventilation or situations characterized by wide respiratory swings in CVP (such as status asthmaticus, or respiratory distress of any etiology). In fact, critically ill patients offer the greatest challenge to the assessment of jugular venous *pulse* and *pressure*. In one intensive care unit study, *jugular venous pulsations* were adequate for examination in only 20% of the patients, and *central venous pressure* could be measured by physical exam in only one half of the cases. In another study, *central venous pressure* could be accurately determined in two thirds of critically ill patients. Thus, the more severe and acute the patient's condition, the more difficult and inaccurate is the bedside determination of jugular venous pulse and pressure.

71. **Should one inspect the right or the left internal jugular vein?**
Ideally the right, since it is in a more direct line with the right atrium and thus better suited to function as both a manometer for *venous pressure* and a conduit for atrial *pulsations*. Moreover, CVP may be spuriously higher on the left as compared to the right because of the left innominate vein's compression between the aortic arch and the sternum.

72. **Can the external jugulars be used for evaluating central venous pressure?**
Theoretically not, practically yes. "Not" because:
- While going through the various fascial planes of the neck, they often *become compressed*.
- In patients with increased sympathetic vascular tone, they may *become so constricted* as to be barely visible.
- They are farther away from the right atrium and thus in a less straight line with it. Yet, both internal *and* external jugular veins can actually be used for estimating CVP since they yield comparable estimates.
  Hence, if the only visible vein is the external jugular, do what Yogi Berra recommends you should do when coming to a fork on the road: take it.

73. **But don't external jugulars have valves?**
They do, but so do the *internal* jugulars. Yet, this doesn't interfere with estimation of CVP since the normal flow of blood is *toward the heart*, and not *from* it. It might interfere, though, with the evaluation of the venous pulse (*see* question 79).

74. Still, aren't the internal jugulars too deep for an accurate inspection?
They *are* quite deep and thus not as visible as the *external* jugular (in fact, if you see a plump subcutaneous neck vein, as turgid as the one on the dorsum of your hand, it is probably the *external* jugular) yet the pulsations of the internal can be transmitted quite well through the overlying sternocleidomastoids, making its waveform recognizable as a skin flickering.

75. What is the anatomy of internal and external jugular veins?
The *external* jugulars lie *above* the sternocleidomastoid muscles, coursing obliquely from behind and laterally toward the angle of the jaw (Fig. 10-6). The *internal* jugulars lie instead *below* the

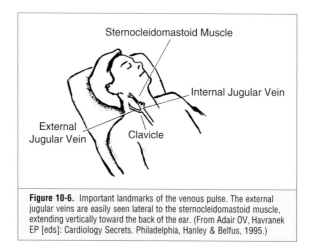

Figure 10-6. Important landmarks of the venous pulse. The external jugular veins are easily seen lateral to the sternocleidomastoid muscle, extending vertically toward the back of the ear. (From Adair OV, Havranek EP [eds]: Cardiology Secrets. Philadelphia, Hanley & Belfus, 1995.)

sternocleidomastoids, crossing them in a vertical straight line. At the junction with the subclavian veins, the internal jugulars create a dilation known as the *bulb*, which is often visible between the two heads of the sternocleidomastoid muscles.

76. How do you examine neck veins?
By carefully positioning the patient (so that the veins fill enough to become visible) and then by tangentially shining a light across the neck. The venous pulse will only be visible, *not* palpable.

77. How important is the patient's position during examination of the neck veins?
Of enormous importance:
- The *head* should be supported, so that the neck muscles are fully relaxed and not impinging on the jugular veins.
- The *trunk* should be inclined and raised. The angle of inclination must allow the top of the column of blood in the internal jugular to reach above the clavicle, but still to remain below the jaw. This inclination will vary depending on CVP:
- In patients with *normal CVP,* the required angle is usually 30–45 degrees above the horizontal.
- In patients with *elevated CVP*, the required angle is >45 degrees. In fact, patients with severe venous congestion may have to sit upright and take deep inspiration in order to lower the meniscus down into full view. In some of these patients, the level of venous pulsation may still remain behind the angle of the jaw, where it will appear to flicker the earlobes.

- In patients with *very high CVP*, the internal jugular will be so "full" that pulsations may not be visible even when the patient is fully upright. The risk in this case is to overlook the high venous pressure and call it normal.
- In patients with *low CVP,* the required angle is usually between 0 and 30 degrees.
- In patients with *very low CVP,* the neck veins will be so empty that pulsations may not be visible at all, even when the patient is fully horizontal.

Hence, to get a good look at venous pulsations, you may need to vary the patient's position based on *volume status*.

78. How do you tell apart the carotid pulse from the jugular venous pulse?
By the following differentiating features:

- **The waveform is different:** The venous pulsation is diffuse, at least *bifid*, and with a *slow* upward deflection. Conversely, the carotid pulse is well localized, *single*, and with a *fast* outward deflection. Also, the most striking event in the venous pulse is the troughs, whereas in the arterial pulse, it is the ascent.
- **The response to position is different:** The carotid pulse never varies with position. The venous pulsations classically do so. In fact, as the patient sits up or stands, they move down toward the clavicle and may even disappear below it. Conversely, as the patient reclines, venous pulsations gradually climb toward the angle of the jaw. They may even disappear behind the auricle.
- **The response to respiration is different:** In the absence of intrathoracic disease (and Kussmaul's sign—*see* questions 115–118), the top of the venous waveform descends toward the heart during inspiration (because of lower intrathoracic pressure and greater venous return). The carotid pulse, instead, remains unchanged. The only exception is pulsus paradoxus, and even in this case, the variation is rarely visible, at most palpable. Note that inspiration makes jugular "pulsations" *more visible* (by enhancing venous return), even though it also lowers the mean jugular "pressure."
- **The response to palpation is different:** The jugular venous pulse is too light to be palpable. Even gentle pressure will collapse the vein, engorge its more distal segment, and obliterate the pulse. Conversely, the carotid is not only palpable but quite forceful too.
- **The response to abdominal pressure is different:** Sustained pressure on the abdomen (the *abdominojugular reflux test, see* questions 106–114) will *not* change the carotid pulse, but will increase (at least momentarily) even the normal venous pulse (*see* Table 10-3).

79. How do you evaluate the jugular venous pulse?
With great difficulty and lots of practice.

- Examine the *right* internal jugular vein (which is in more direct line with the right atrium).
- Position the patient at such an angle that the jugular meniscus (i.e., the top of the venous *flickering*) is well seen. Shine a light tangentially to better visualize the flickering.
- Carefully inspect the level of the venous column and the timing and amplitude of the waveform and its components. Note respiratory variations (*see* questions 84 and 85).

If you still have difficulty in relating the various jugular ascents/descents to the cardiac cycle, either auscultate the heart or simultaneously palpate the *right* radial artery and *left* carotid.

Note that the external jugulars transmit the pulse poorly. So, while they are adequate for estimating *central venous pressure*, they are not well suited for *jugular pulse* evaluation.

80. What are the components of the jugular waveform?
It depends on whether you are looking at a patient or a tracing. Jugular vein undulations reflect phasic pressure changes in the right atrium. Yet, because the fluctuations in venous pressure are so mild (3–7 mmHg, or 4–11 cmH$_2$O), peaks and troughs of the venous pulse can be easily *recorded,* but remain difficult to appreciate at the bedside. As a result:

- *On venous tracing,* the jugular pulse consists of *three positive waves* (A, C, and V) and *three negative descents* (X, X$_1$, and Y). The A wave is followed by the X descent, the C wave by the X$_1$ descent, and the V wave by the Y descent.

TABLE 10-3.   DIFFERENTIATION BETWEEN JUGULAR AND CAROTID PULSES

Characteristic	Internal Jugular Vein and Jugular Venous Pulse	Carotid Artery and Carotid Pulse
Location	Low in neck and lateral	Deep in neck and medial
Contour	Double peaked and diffuse	Single peaked and sharp
Character	Undulant, not palpable	Forceful, brisk, easily felt
Response to position	Varies with position	No variation
Response to respiration	Mean pressure decreases on inspiration (height of column falls), but A and V waves become more visible	No variation
Response to abdominal pressure	Displaces pulse upward and induces transient increase in mean pressure	Pulse unchanged
Effect of palpation	Wave visible but nonpalpable	Pulse unchanged
	Gentle pressure 3–4 cm above the clavicle obliterates pulse and fills the vein	Vessel difficult to compress

(Adapted from Cook DJ, Simel N: Does this patient have abnormal central venous pressure? JAMA 275:630–634, 1996; and Abrams J: Essentials of Cardiac Physical Diagnosis. Philadelphia, Lea & Febiger, 1987.)

- At *the bedside*, the jugular venous pulse consists instead of *only two positive waves* (A and V—with A taller than V) and *two negative descents* (X_1 and Y—with X_1 steeper than Y). Neither the C wave nor the X descent is visible (C is usually lost in the A wave, and X is merged with X_1). Note that descents are easier to spot than ascents (*see* Fig. 10-7).

81. **What is the physiology of the jugular venous pulse?**
    The jugular venous pulse reflects the relationship between volume of blood in the venous system, venous vascular tone, and right heart hemodynamics. Hence, during *diastole* it reflects right *ventricular* filling pressure, whereas during *systole* it reflects right *atrial* pressure.

82. **What is the physiology of the various ascents and descents of the jugular venous pulse?**
    It is the physiology of right-sided chambers. Thus, assessing the jugular venous pulse is important, not only to visualize peaks and troughs, but also to relate these undulations to various physiologic and clinical events, such as the ECG, the carotid pulse, and the heart sounds. More specifically:
    - The **A wave** (the first and dominant positive wave) is produced by right atrial contraction. It follows the P wave on ECG, coincides with the fourth heart sound (if present), and slightly precedes both the first heart sound and carotid upstroke.

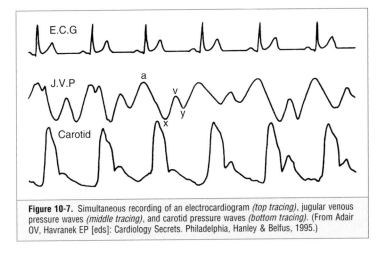

Figure 10-7. Simultaneous recording of an electrocardiogram *(top tracing)*, jugular venous pressure waves *(middle tracing)*, and carotid pressure waves *(bottom tracing)*. (From Adair OV, Havranek EP [eds]: Cardiology Secrets. Philadelphia, Hanley & Belfus, 1995.)

- The **C wave**, the second positive wave (only visible on recordings), is produced by the bulging of the tricuspid cusps into the right atrium and thus coincides with ventricular *isovolumetric* contraction. Note that a very small component of "C" is produced by the transmitted carotid pulsation—in fact, MacKenzie considered it an entirely carotid artifact; hence, the label "C"). Also, note that the interval between A and C corresponds to the P–R interval on ECG (this was one of the methods used by Wenckebach to describe the second-degree heart block that still carries his name). Yet, since the C wave is not visible at the bedside, it will be omitted from the remainder of our discussion.
- The **early X descent** (located between A and C) is produced by right atrial relaxation. The most dominant later trough *(X₁ [i.e., the "x-prime"])* is produced instead by the pulling of the valvular cusps into the right ventricle. This downward and forward movement of valve and atrium floor (*descent of the base*) coincides with right ventricular *isotonic* contraction and acts as a plunger, creating a sucking effect that draws blood from the great veins into the right atrium. The X_1 descent *occurs* during systole, *coincides* with ventricular ejection and the carotid pulse, *takes place* between S_1 and S_2, and *ends* just before S_2. Note that this discussion disregards the early X descent and uses instead this term to refer to the *combined* X and X_1 troughs—the only one visible at the bedside.
- The **V wave** (the third positive wave) occurs toward the end of ventricular systole and during the early phase of ventricular diastole. It coincides with the apex of the carotid pulse and peaks immediately after S_2. Because the ventricle relaxes while the tricuspid valve is still closed, blood flowing into the right atrium starts building up, generating a positive wave.
- The **Y descent** (the final negative trough) occurs during early ventricular diastole. It is due to the opening of the tricuspid valve and the emptying of the right atrium. It corresponds to S_3.

Clinically, the only visible peaks are A and V; the only visible troughs are a combination of X_1 and X (which we will herein refer to as "X") and Y; the A wave is usually more prominent than the V wave, whereas the X descent is usually more prominent than the Y descent. Overall, it is easier to time the pulse by using the X and Y *descents* than the A and V *waves*.

83. **Who was Wenckebach?**

Karel F. Wenckebach (1864–1940) was a Dutch physician. Building on an 1873 observation by the Italian physiologist Luigi Luciani, he reported in 1899 the phenomenon that still carries his name. He described it in a 40-year-old woman who had presented with an irregular pulse. Wenckebach based his conclusions on tracings of the patient's arterial pulse, observations of her venous pulse, and intra-atrial and intraventricular recordings in a frog. His insight preceded the invention of electrocardiography by 2 years, the discovery of the atrioventricular node by 7 years, and the description of the sinoatrial node by 8 years. Still, despite his genius he remained a simple and unassuming man who was full of charm, had a self-deprecating humor, and a life-long love for the arts and the English countryside. He was famous for quipping that he was not a great man, just a "happy man." His colleagues loved him and many affectionately referred to him as "Venky." His many friends included Sir William Osler and James MacKenzie (with whom he maintained a long correspondence, praising him for his 1902 book *The Study of the Pulse*). A master of physical diagnosis and a pioneer in arrhythmias, Wenckebach linked his name not only to the homonymous *phenomenon*, but also to one of the first reports on the beneficial use of quinine in atrial fibrillation. He taught at Utrecht, Groningen, Strasbourg, and, finally, Vienna, where he died of urosepsis just after the onset of World War II.

84. **What is the influence of respiration on the jugular venous pulse?**
Inspiration *increases* venous return. This, in turn, distends the right-sided chambers and, because of the Starling effect, makes right atrial and right ventricular contraction stronger. As a result, the *jugular venous pulse* becomes more *visible* in inspiration, with brisker X and Y descents (i.e., the troughs of the venous pulse). Even the positive waves become more accentuated. Conversely, exhalation *lessens the A wave*, so much so to make "V" dominant.

85. **What is the influence of respiration on the jugular venous *pressure*?**
The opposite. Inspiration *lowers* the mean jugular venous pressure, exhalation increases it.

86. **Which diseases can be diagnosed by jugular venous pulse?**
Quite a few. Some are both common and important, affecting either *waves* or *descents* (*see* Fig. 10-8).

87. **What are the most important abnormalities of jugular *waves*?**
For both this and the next question, *see* Fig. 10-9.
- **Giant A wave.** In addition to tricuspid stenosis, this also can occur in increased right ventricular end-diastolic pressure (from pulmonic stenosis, primary pulmonary hypertension, pulmonary emboli, or chronic pulmonary disease). In these patients, the large A wave reflects a strong atrial contraction against a stiffer ventricle presenting with a concomitantly blunted and small Y descent. The acoustic counterpart of a giant A wave is a right-sided S_4, and its electric equivalent is a P pulmonale. Giant A waves also may be seen in marked *left* ventricular hypertrophy (like AS, severe hypertension, or hypertrophic obstructive cardiomyopathy). In these patients, the ventricular septum bulges toward the *right*, making right ventricular filling more difficult (the Bernheim effect, from Hippolyte Bernheim, the French physician and hypnotist who described it in 1910).
- **"Cannon" A wave** is the hallmark of atrioventricular dissociation (i.e., the atrium contracts against a closed tricuspid valve). It is different from the other prominent outward wave (i.e., the presystolic giant A wave), insofar as it begins just after S_1, since it represents atrial contraction against a closed tricuspid valve. The giant A wave, on the other hand, begins just *before* S_1—like the large V wave of tricuspid regurgitation (*see* below). *Intermittent* cannon A waves reflect atrioventricular dissociation in a setting of ventricular tachycardia, whereas *regular* cannon A waves reflect atrioventricular dissociation in a setting of supraventricular tachycardia with retrograde atrial activation.
- The **V wave** is classically increased in tricuspid regurgitation (TR), during which it becomes the dominant wave, associated with a brisk Y collapse (a more gentle Y descent usually indicates concomitant regurgitation and stenosis). Abdominal compression may help to unmask more subtle and subclinical cases. Prominent V waves can become so large that they were dubbed

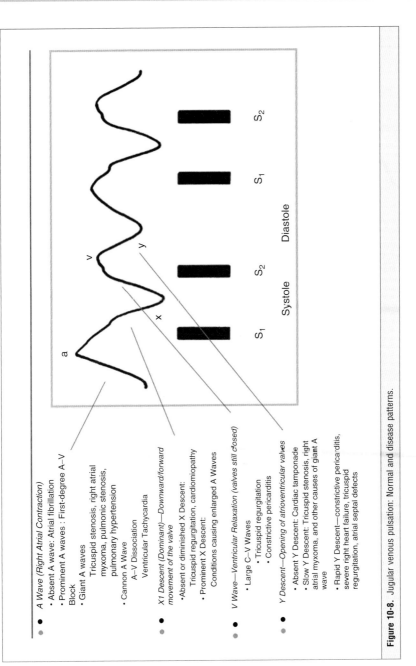

● *A Wave (Right Atrial Contraction)*
  • Absent A wave: Atrial fibrillation
  • Prominent A waves : First-degree A–V Block
  • Giant A waves
       Tricuspid stenosis, right atrial myxoma, pulmonic stenosis, pulmonary hypertension
  • Cannon A Wave
       A–V Dissociation
       Ventricular Tachycardia

● *X1 Descent (Dominant)—Downward/forward movement of the valve*
  • Absent or diminished X Descent:
       Tricuspid regurgitation, cardiomiopathy
  • Prominent X Descent:
       Conditions causing enlarged A Waves

● *V Wave—Ventricular Relaxation (valves still closed)*
  • Large C–V Waves
       • Tricuspid regurgitation
       • Constrictive pericarditis

● *Y Descent—Opening of atrioventricular valves*
  • Absent Y Descent: Cardiac tamponade
  • Slow Y Descent: Tricuspid stenosis, right atrial myxoma, and other causes of giant A wave
  • Rapid Y Descent—constrictive pericarditis, severe right heart failure, tricuspid regurgitation, atrial septal defects

Figure 10–8. Jugular venous pulsation: Normal and disease patterns.

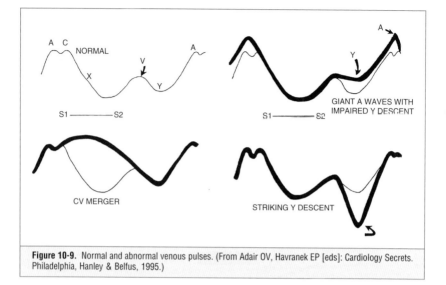

Figure 10-9. Normal and abnormal venous pulses. (From Adair OV, Havranek EP [eds]: Cardiology Secrets. Philadelphia, Hanley & Belfus, 1995.)

by Paul Wood "the venous Corrigan." In fact, they may even cause bobbing of the earlobes (the Lancisi's sign). Since the C and V merger responsible for the giant V wave entirely eliminates the X descent, a giant wave is easy to spot: it starts just after S_1 and leaves the patient with only one ascent (the V wave) and one descent (the Y descent). The giant V wave is not too sensitive for tricuspid regurgitation (TR), being present in only 40% of the cases.

- **Equally prominent A and V waves** can occur in atrial septal defect, wherein the V wave in the higher-pressure left atrium is transmitted through the perforated septum into the right atrium, and from there to the jugular veins. Still, equally prominent A and V waves are much more commonly suggestive of simple right ventricular failure.

88. **What are the most important abnormalities of jugular *descents*?**
    - A **prominent X descent** is seen in patients with vigorous ventricular contraction (and thus requiring strong atrial contractions), like *tamponade* or *right ventricular overload*.
    - A **diminished X descent** (to the point of becoming even less prominent than the Y descent) is seen in *atrial fibrillation* or *cardiomyopathy* (wherein right ventricular contraction is not forceful enough to "pull down" the atrial floor). TR, of course, would *obliterate* the X descent.
    - A **prominent Y descent** is seen in patients with increased venous pressure, regardless of etiology. A very brisk Y descent is often referred to as Friedreich's sign, from the German clinician and neurologist, Nikolaus Friedreich, who described it in 1864. In combination with the prominent X descent, it creates two steep troughs (the "W" sign). This occurs in one third of *constrictive pericarditis* cases, where it is often associated with an early diastolic extra sound (pericardial knock). Friedreich's sign is not too sensitive for constrictive pericarditis, but quite specific, with the only differential diagnosis being restrictive cardiomyopathy.
    - A **diminished-to-absent Y descent** is seen in patients with increased central venous pressure, like tamponade or tricuspid stenosis. Note that the Y descent is usually minimal in normal subjects, too; hence, an abnormally diminished Y descent has clinical significance *only if the patient has high central venous pressure*.

89. **How do you estimate the CVP?**
    - By *positioning the patient* so that you can get a good view of the internal jugular vein and its oscillations. Although it is wise to start at 45 degrees, it doesn't really matter which angle

you will eventually use to raise the patient's head, as long as it can adequately reveal the vein. In the absence of a visible internal jugular, the external jugular may suffice.

- By *identifying the highest point of jugular pulsation* that is transmitted to the skin (i.e., the meniscus). This usually occurs during exhalation and coincides with the peak of "A" or "V" waves. It serves as a bedside pulsation manometer.
- By *finding the sternal angle of Louis* (junction of the manubrium with the body of the sternum). This provides the standard zero for *jugular* venous pressure (the standard zero for the "central" venous pressure is instead the center of the right atrium).
- By *measuring in centimeters the vertical height from the sternal angle to the top of the jugular pulsation*. To do so, place two rulers at a 90-degree angle: one horizontal (and parallel to the meniscus) and the other vertical to it and touching the sternal angle (*see* Fig. 10-10). The extrapolated height between the sternal angle and meniscus represents the *jugular venous pressure* (JVP).
- By *adding five* to convert jugular venous pressure into *central* venous pressure.

This method relies on the fact that the *zero point* of the entire right-sided manometer (i.e., the point where central venous pressure is, by convention, zero) is the center of the right atrium. This is vertically situated at 5 cm below the sternal angle, a relationship that is present in subjects of normal size and shape, regardless of their body position. Thus, using the sternal angle as the *external reference point*, the vertical distance (in centimeters) to the top of the column of blood in the jugular vein will provide the *JVP*. Adding 5 to the JVP will yield the CVP.

90. **How is "Louis" pronounced?**
It depends. If you refer to the *sternal angle*, it should be "French-like," since it was indeed the French surgeon Antoine Louis who first described it (Dr. Louis is much more famous for having co-authored with the internist Joseph-Ignace Guillotin the homonymous capital punishment device, which presumably chopped aristocrats' heads just above the angle of Louis). If, on the other hand, you are referring to the *maneuver* that relies on the sternal angle for estimating central venous pressure, then you should pronounce it "English-like," since it was the British physician Sir Thomas Lewis (student of MacKenzie) who first realized that the normal jugular vein distention is never more than 2–3 cm above the angle of Louis. A subsequent variant of this observation (i.e., that central venous *pressure* can be estimated at the bedside by adding 5 to the vertical height of the internal jugular vein above the angle of Louis) is what we call today the "method of Lewis." Hence, it doesn't really matter how you pronounce it, since either will be correct.

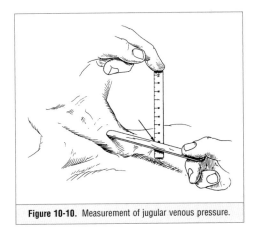

Figure 10-10. Measurement of jugular venous pressure.

91. What is the normal central venous pressure?

As estimated by the method of Lewis, a normal *central* venous pressure should be <7 cm H_2O (some authors have suggested 8 cm H_2O). This means that the *jugular* venous pressure (i.e., distention) should not be >2–3 cm (two fingerbreadths) above the angle of Louis.

92. Is there any faster way to assess central venous pressure?

Yes. A nice, quick and dirty method consists in having the patient sit up. Visible neck veins in the upright position indicate a central venous pressure >7 cm H_2O, which is *pathologic*. This is because the clavicles lie at a vertical distance of about 2 cm above the sternal angle. Hence, if central venous pressure is normal, the veins should *not* be visible).

93. Are there alternative methods to assess the CVP?

Yes, but they have not been validated:

- *Von Recklinghausen's maneuver* consists in asking the patient to lie supine, with the palm of one hand laid down over the thigh, and the other laid down over the bed (thereby 5–10 cm below the first hand). Patients have *high* CVP if the veins of both hands are engorged but *normal* CVP if only the lower hand veins are engorged.
- An alternative but similar maneuver consists of inspecting the veins of the back of the hand in a reclining patient as the arm is slowly and passively raised. The level at which the veins collapse can then be related to the angle of Louis and the CVP measured.

Both these methods may give falsely high readings because of local obstruction or peripheral venous constriction. Hence, they are not recommended for general use.

94. How precise is the clinical assessment of CVP?

When well performed (and in stable patients), it can be quite accurate, with bedside estimates of CVP within 4 cm H_2O of intravenous catheter measurement in almost 90% of the cases. Still, interobserver (and intraobserver) variability may be as high as 7 cm. This becomes especially problematic in the unstable patient, where expertise plays an important role. For instance:

- In a study of 50 intensive care unit patients, agreement on CVP values was substantial between students and residents, moderate between students and attending physicians, and modest between residents and staff. Factors that interfered with the precision of the estimate included variations in patients' positioning, poor ambient lighting, confusion between carotid and venous pulsations, and changes in CVP with respiration.
- In a second study, an attending physician, a critical care fellow, a medical resident, an intern, and a student were asked to predict whether the CVP of 62 patients was low, normal, high, or very high. Right heart catheterization provided the gold standard. The *sensitivity* of clinical examination was 0.33, 0.33, and 0.49, respectively for the identification of low (<0 mmHg), normal (0 to 7 mmHg), or high (>7 mmHg) CVP. The *specificity* of the exam was instead 0.73, 0.62, and 0.76, respectively. Accuracy was greater in patients with low cardiac indexes (<2.2 L/min) and high pulmonary artery wedge pressures (>18 mmHg). It was lower in comatose patients or patients on mechanical ventilation. A higher precision (i.e., interobserver agreement) did not translate into a greater accuracy.
- In a third study, Eisenberg and colleagues compared bedside assessment of 97 critically ill patients with pulmonary artery catheter readings. They compared various hemodynamic variables, including CVP. Based on clinical assessment, physicians were asked to predict whether the CVP was <2, 2–6, or >6 mmHg. Predictions were correct only 55% of the time. CVP was underestimated more frequently than *overestimated* (27% and 17% respectively).

95. So what conclusions can be drawn about the clinical use of CVP assessment?

When compared to the gold standard of a central venous catheter, clinical measurement of CVP is overall poor, especially in the acutely ill patient. In the aforementioned study of 50 critically ill patients, for example, the pooled accuracy of the test was 56%. All groups involved (students, residents, and attending physicians) tended to *underestimate* central venous pressure (*see* question 96), and level of expertise was not a guarantee of accuracy. In fact, the correlation coefficient between clinical assessment and central venous catheter recording was highest for medical students (0.74), a little lower for residents (0.71), and lowest for staff physicians (0.65). These correlations slightly improved after exclusion of patients on mechanical ventilation, suggesting that CVP assessment is more accurate in patients who breathe spontaneously. Hence, bedside assessment of CVP is only accurate at the extremes of presentation:

- A *low* CVP increases the likelihood by threefold that the measured CVP will also be low. It also makes it very unlikely that the measured CVP will be high.
- A *high* CVP at the bedside (because of neck veins distended more than 3 cm above the angle of Louis) increases the likelihood by about fourfold that the measured CVP will also be high. In fact, no patient with a clinically high CVP had a low measured CVP.
- Finally, a CVP assessed as *normal* at the bedside is truly indeterminate (with likelihood ratios approaching 1). Thus, clinical estimates of "normal" CVP provide no helpful information because they neither increase nor decrease the probability of an abnormal CVP.

96. **Why does bedside assessment tend to *underestimate* central venous pressure?**
Because the semi-erect (or erect) position required for the neck veins' visualization lengthens the distance between the angle of Louis and the zero reference point by as many as 3 cm. To reduce this underestimation, many physicians measure CVP in *exhalation*.

97. **What is the significance of a low jugular venous pressure?**
It reflects a low CVP, usually due to intravascular depletion from GI (vomiting, diarrhea), urinary (diuretics, uncontrolled diabetes mellitus, or diabetes insipidus), or third space losses.

98. **What is the significance of an *elevated* jugular venous pressure?**
It usually reflects a high CVP. This can be due to either *hypervolemia* or *impedements to right-sided filling*. Among the latter are (in a rostrocaudal fashion):

- **Superior vena cava obstruction** (in this case, there will be no jugular venous pulse and the abdominojugular reflux test will be negative).
- **Obstruction to right ventricular inflow** (such as tricuspid stenosis and right atrial myxoma, but also constrictive pericarditis or tamponade, where neck vein distention is a *sine qua non*)
- **Tricuspid regurgitation**
- **Decreased right ventricular compliance** with increased end-diastolic (and right atrial) pressure. Possible causes include right ventricular failure or infarction, pulmonic stenosis, and pulmonary hypertension.
- **Left ventricular failure.** This is a common cause of pulmonary hypertension. In fact, in patients presenting with either angina or dyspnea, a high CVP argues in favor of left ventricular failure. Conversely, normal neck veins are unhelpful in separating normal from increased left-atrial pressure.

Finally, CVP does *not* predict left-sided ejection fraction.

99. **What is the significance of neck vein distention in assessing chronic heart failure?**
In a prospective study of 52 patients undergoing in-hospital evaluation for heart transplantation, Butman et al. found that jugular venous distention, a positive abdominojugular test, pulmonary crackles, and a left-sided S_3 all independently predicted higher right-sided pressures and worse cardiac performance. Jugular venous distention (whether at rest or inducible) had the best sensitivity (81%), specificity (80%), and predictive accuracy (81%) for elevation of pulmonary capillary wedge pressure. In fact, the probability of an elevated "wedge" was 0.86 when either variable was present. Hence, the bedside cardiovascular examination of patients with chronic heart failure is quite useful for identifying increased right- *and* left-sided pressures. In this study, baseline or induced jugular venous distention was both sensitive and specific.

100. **What is the prognostic significance of abnormal jugular venous pressure in heart failure?**

Together with S_3, it represents an *ominous* prognostic variable, independently associated with adverse outcomes, including progression of heart failure. This was shown by Drazner et al. in a large study of 2569 patients with either symptomatic heart failure or a history of it. In multivariate analyses adjusted for other markers of heart failure severity, elevated jugular venous pressure was associated with a significant increase in the risk of death or hospitalization for heart failure. The presence of S_3 was similarly (and independently) associated with increased risk.

101. **How are the neck veins in tamponade?**

Distended. This is a *must*, together with dyspnea/tachypnea, tachycardia, and clear lungs. Given this constellation of four symptoms/findings, the differential diagnosis is narrowed to five major entities: right ventricular infarction, massive pulmonary embolism, constrictive pericarditis, tension pneumothorax, and tamponade. The first four present with a positive Kussmaul's sign in approximately one half of the cases, but never have a pulsus paradoxus >21 mmHg. Conversely, tamponade comes with no Kussmaul's, but does present with a *pulsus* of 20–50 mmHg (*see* Chapter 2, questions 92–95).

102. **What is the significance of leg swelling without increased central venous pressure?**

It reflects either bilateral venous insufficiency or noncardiac edema (usually hepatic or renal). This is because any cardiac (or pulmonary) disease resulting in right ventricular failure would manifest itself through an increase in central venous pressure.

103. **What is the significance of leg edema *plus ascites* in the absence of increased CVP?**

It also argues in favor of a hepatic or renal cause (cirrhotics do *not* have high CVP). Conversely, a high CVP in patients with ascites and edema argues in favor of an underlying cardiac etiology.

104. **What is the prognostic value of an increased CVP in preoperative patients?**

If untreated, it predicts postoperative pulmonary edema and/or infarction.

105. **What are the jugular findings of right ventricular infarction?**

- The right ventricular filling pressure is increased (as a result of an ischemic and less compliant chamber). Since the ventricle also becomes unable to handle incoming venous flow, the mean *jugular (and central) venous pressures* will be similarly increased. This has high specificity (96.8%) but low sensitivity (39%) for right ventricular infarction.
- The jugular venous pulse exhibits a prominent "A" wave. It also shows "X" and "Y" descents so steep as to almost mimic constrictive pericarditis. Still, despite its high specificity (100%), a rapid "Y" descent has low sensitivity (17.3%) for right ventricular infarction. Moreover, jugular venous pressure and waveform are both significantly affected by the concomitant magnitude of damage to the interventricular septum and *left* ventricular free wall.
- Positive Kussmaul's sign is as specific as a JVP increase, but less sensitive (26.1%).
- The abdominojugular reflux test can be positive.
- Finally, an associated tricuspid regurgitation (TR) will give additional findings, such as giant V waves, pulsatile liver, and right earlobe bobbing.

106. **What is the hepatojugular reflux?**

An old term for the *abdominojugular reflux*, a maneuver first described by the British William Pasteur in 1885 as a sign of *TR*, and then rekindled in 1898 by the French Edouard Rondot. Rondot also is the author of the unfortunate term "hepatojugular reflux" and the first to suggest that a positive response is *not* pathognomonic of TR, but can also occur in other disorders.

107. What is it used for?
To unmask *subclinical* right ventricular failure (and silent tricuspid regurgitation) but also to confirm *symptomatic* left ventricular failure (*see* question 113). Hence, the "Pasteur-Rondot maneuver" is a very helpful tool, albeit one that is often misused and misinterpreted.

108. What is the physiology of the abdominojugular reflux?
It is a cardiac stress test for patients whose jugular venous pressure is either normal or only borderline elevated (hence, no need to use it in patients who already have jugular venous distention). Steady pressure onto the abdomen increases venous return by shifting blood from the splanchnic bed into the thorax and right atrium, like a sort of "poor man's" *fluid challenge*. If the right ventricle cannot handle this extra load, there will be *sustained increase* in JVP.

109. Does abdominal pressure cause any change in cardiac output?
No. Moreover, the changes in central venous pressure that result from this maneuver cannot be attributed to variations in esophageal pressure or to a compression of the heart by elevation of the diaphragm. Instead, various observations are consistent with the overall hypothesis, that the increased right-sided filling pressure induced by abdominal compression does indeed reflect both *the volume of blood* in the abdominal veins and *the ability of the ventricles to respond to an increased venous return*. Hence, its value for unmasking congestive heart failure

110. Is compression of the *liver* necessary to elicit a response?
No. In fact, it can actually be detrimental in patients with passive hepatic congestion, since compression of the right upper quadrant (and a distended glissonian capsule) might indeed elicit pain and a Valsalva's response. As a result, pressure over the periumbilical area (or any other area of the abdomen) has become the method of choice. Hence, the more current term of *abdominojugular (reflux) test*.

111. How do you perform an abdominojugular test?
By observing the jugular venous pressure before, during, and after abdominal compression:
- Position the supine patient so that the jugular venous pulsations are properly monitored (an angle of 45 degrees will usually suffice). Then instruct the patient to relax and breathe normally through the open mouth. This will avoid the false positive increase in jugular venous pressure caused by a Valsalva's maneuver inadvertently triggered by abdominal discomfort.
- Apply your hand over the patient's mid abdomen (periumbilical area), with fingers widely spread and palm gently rested. Once the patient is well relaxed, apply gradual and progressive pressure for at least 15 seconds: firm, inward, cephalad, and soon reaching a steady level of 20–35 mmHg. This can be confirmed by placing an unrolled bladder of a standard adult blood pressure cuff between the examiner's hand and the patient's abdomen. The cuff should be partially inflated with six full-bulb compressions.
- Note that the precision of the test may vary, based on the force of abdominal compression. Different investigators have in fact suggested different force: Ducas recommended 35 mmHg (equivalent to a weight of approximately 8 kg), whereas Ewy used 20 mmHg.
- Throughout the maneuver (i.e., before, during, or after compression), observe the column of blood in the internal and external jugular veins.
- To avoid the risk of false positive neck vein distention from breath-holding or "bearing down," consider a trial run. This also can be used to demonstrate in advance the force that will be applied onto the abdomen.
- You might also look for a softening of the first heart sound during the application of abdominal pressure. This represents the auscultatory equivalent of a positive response.

112. **When is the abdominojugular test considered positive?**

When there is an *increase* in jugular venous pressure *of more than 3 cm in height* (which, according to Ducas, is the upper limit of normal) that remains *sustained* though all 15 seconds of compression. Conversely, the test is considered *negative* when any of the following occurs:

- No change in JVP
- Sustained change, but not large enough (i.e., <3 cm)
- *Enough change, but not sustained.* In this case, there may be an initial bulging of the external jugular vein at the beginning of abdominal compression (and also of the peaks and troughs of the internal jugular), and the JVP may even increase by more than 3 cm, but this is transient and returns to normal (or near normal) during the remainder of the compression.

A positive "reflux" is sometimes easier to observe as *an abrupt fall in JVP* when the pressure is being *released*. For the test to be positive, this drop should be at least *4 cm* (Ewy et al).

113. **What is the significance of a positive abdominojugular reflux?**

In patients presenting with dyspnea and/or angina, it argues in favor of *bi*-ventricular failure and suggests a *pulmonary capillary wedge pressure >15 mmHg*. This was confirmed at cardiac catheterization by Ewy et al. Patients with positive response also had lower left ventricular ejection fraction and stroke volume and higher mean pulmonary arterial and right atrial pressure, confirming biventricular failure. Conversely, a negative test in a patient with dyspnea would strongly argue *against* the presence of increased left atrial pressure.

In the absence of left ventricular failure, a positive test points instead to the *right chambers*, suggesting an inability of the atrium and ventricle to handle an increased venous return. This is particularly useful in subclinical cases, where a positive test has high sensitivity and specificity for predicting right atrial pressure >9 mmHg and right ventricular end-diastolic pressure >12 mmHg. Differential diagnosis includes impaired right ventricular preload (increased intravascular volume), decreased right ventricular compliance (right ventricular hypertrophy), decreased right ventricular systolic function (right ventricular infarction), or elevated right ventricular afterload (pulmonary hypertension).

Tricuspid regurgitation, tricuspid stenosis, restrictive cardiomyopathy, and constrictive pericarditis are also a common cause of a positive test. The only condition *not* presenting with a positive abdominojugular reflux is cardiac tamponade. Hence, the test is not specific to any one disorder, but is instead a reflection of either a right ventricle that cannot accommodate an increased return or a *left* ventricle that is dysfunctional.

Pearl:

Although recently shown to correlate with pulmonary capillary wedge pressure (and thus reflecting left ventricular function), the abdominojugular maneuver is traditionally used to either augment or unmask a murmur of tricuspid regurgitation. For this, it has a specificity of 100% and a sensitivity of 66%, whereas the Rivero-Carvallo maneuver (inspiratory increase in intensity of the tricuspid regurgitation murmur) has a specificity of 100% and a sensitivity of 80%. When combined, the two have sensitivity of 93% and a specificity of 100%.

---

114. **Shouldn't the abdominal pressure be applied for at least 1 minute?**

No. This was recommended in the past, but it is not the case anymore. In fact, Ewy used 10 seconds, and so did Ducas, who also showed that CVP stabilized by that point and did not change over the subsequent 60 seconds. Sochowski, on the other hand, showed that 62 of 65 patients stabilized their pressure by *15* seconds. Hence, the choice of 15 seconds.

115. **What is Kussmaul's sign?**
It is the paradoxical increase in JVP that occurs during inspiration. Jugular venous pressure normally *decreases* during inspiration because the inspiratory fall in intrathoracic pressure creates a "sucking effect" on venous return. Thus, Kussmaul's sign is a true physiologic paradox. This can be explained by the inability of the right heart to handle an increased venous return.

116. **Which disease processes are associated with a positive Kussmaul's?**
Those that interfere with venous return and right ventricular filling. The original description was in a patient with *constrictive pericarditis* (Kussmaul's is still seen in one third of severe and advanced cases, where it is often associated with a positive abdominojugular reflux). Nowadays, however, the most common cause is *severe heart failure*, independent of etiology. Working backwards from the heart to the superior vena cava, other causes of this sign include:
- Cor pulmonale (acute or chronic)
- Constrictive pericarditis
- Restrictive cardiomyopathy (such as sarcoidosis, hemochromatosis and amyloidosis)
- Tricuspid stenosis
Remember that Kussmaul's is also present in 33–100% of patients with right *ventricular infarction*. Thus, in a setting of acute myocardial infarction, Kussmaul's should *not* be interpreted as a sign of tamponade, but as a clue to concomitant right ventricular injury.

117. **What can be said about the association of pulsus paradoxus and Kussmaul's sign?**
Both were first described by Kussmaul, yet Kussmaul's *never* occurs in "pure" tamponade (if it does, concomitant epimyocardial fibrosis is present); however, it does occur in one third of patients with "pure" constrictive pericarditis. Pulsus paradoxus, on the other hand, *does not* occur in "pure," totally dry constrictive pericarditis (if it does, a concomitant amount of pericardial effusion is present). Still, it does occur in almost all patients with tamponade.
A small pulsus paradoxus (>10 but <21 mmHg) occurs in two thirds of patients with right ventricular infarction, whereas Kussmaul's occurs in 33–100% of right ventricular infarctions.
To avoid confusion, you should use a *high cutoff* for pulsus paradoxus (>21 mmHg). This will limit the positivity of the test to only tamponade, a condition where Kussmaul doesn't occur.

118. **What is the association between Kussmaul's sign and the abdominojugular reflux?**
They share the same pathophysiology. Both, for example, occur in situations of diffuse peripheral venous constriction with secondary increase in central venous pressure, such as severe heart failure and constrictive pericarditis. And both result from the inability of the heart to handle an increase in venous return, either because of pump failure or various mechanical impediments (constrictive pericarditis, tricuspid stenosis, and cor pulmonale—acute or chronic).

119. **How can you improve the clinical examination of the jugular veins?**
Blind examination of patients with indwelling central venous catheters may provide a valuable feedback. Pocket cards displaying the normal jugular pulse also may be helpful. Finally, evaluation of patients with tachycardia, irregular cardiac rhythms, rapid and deep respirations, or need for mechanical ventilation may provide very useful challenges and thus hone the skill.

120. **What is the "venous hum"?**
It is a *functional* murmur (*see* Chapter 12, questions 44 and 45) produced by turbulent flow in the internal jugular vein. It is *continuous* (albeit louder in diastole) and at times strong enough

to be associated with a palpable thrill. It is best heard on the right side of the neck, just above the clavicle, but sometimes it can become audible over the sternal/parasternal areas, both right and left. This may lead to misdiagnoses of carotid disease, patent ductus arteriosus, or AR/AS.

121. **What is the best way to elicit a venous hum?**
Have the patient sit up, with head turned away from the side of auscultation (i.e., rotated 30–60 degrees *leftward* if listening over the *right* supraclavicular area). The *hum* vanishes upon reclining and similarly fades (or altogether disappears) with other maneuvers that reduce venous return, such as pressing over the jugular vein distal to the hum (i.e., just above the stethoscope) or performing Valsalva.

122. **What is the mechanism of the venous hum?**
It is a mild compression of the internal jugular vein by the transverse process of the atlas, in subjects with strong cardiac output and increased venous flow. Hence, it is common in young adults or patients with a high output state.

123. **How prevalent is this finding?**
It can be heard in 31–66% of normal children and 25% of young adults. It also is encountered in 2.3–27% of adult outpatients. It is especially common in situations of arteriovenous fistula, being present in 56–88% of patients undergoing dialysis and 34% of those in *between* sessions.

124. **Can any other cardiac event be heard at the neck?**
Beside transmitted systolic ejection murmurs, right-sided S_3, and S_4 gallops also may be heard over the neck. These usually occur in patients with right-ventricular failure and elevated right-sided pressure. Similarly, the murmur of TR may at times be heard over the neck.

E. THE PRECORDIAL MOVEMENT AND IMPULSE

"In the first place, then, when the chest of a living animal is laid open and the capsule that immediately surrounds the heart is slit up or removed, the organ is seen now to move, now to be at rest; there is a time when it moves, and a time when it is motionless."
—William Harvey, Exercitatio Anatomica De Motu Cordis et Sanguinis in Animalibus (An Anatomical Exercise on the Motion of the Heart and Blood in Animals). Frankfurt: W. Fitzer, 1628.

"In the natural condition of the organ, the heart, examined between the cartilages of the fifth and sixth ribs, at the lower end of the sternum, communicates, by its motions, a sensation as if it corresponded evidently with a small point of the thoracic parietes, not larger than that occupied by the end of the stethoscope."
—René T.H. Laënnec, Treatise on Mediate Auscultation. Paris: Didot Jeune, 1819.

Inspection and palpation of *precordial impulse and movements* complete the preauscultatory evaluation of the cardiovascular system. In fact, *percussion* of the cardiac area (although still quite accurate when competently performed) has become more a memory of the past than a standard of today's practice. Conversely, evaluation of the precordial *impulse* remains a very important part of the exam. It can provide valuable information on intracardiac size and function and may even be the first clue of ventricular enlargement, well before any ECG or x-ray change.

125. **What is the history behind precordial palpation?**
It goes back 3500 years, to the Ebers Papyrus of 1550 B.C., which was the principal medical document of ancient Egypt. The papyrus covered 15 diseases of the abdomen, 29 of the eyes,

and 18 of the skin. It also listed no fewer than 21 cough treatments. In a section titled "Beginning of the Secret of the Physicians: Knowledge of Heart's Movement and Knowledge of the Heart," palpation of the cardiac impulse was clearly described. Following that initial information, chest palpation remained part of the medical armamentarium up to medieval times. Only with William Harvey, though, did the motions of the heart become again a specific topic of *scientific* discussion. In his 1628 book *De Motu Cordis*, Harvey wrote: "[T]he heart is erected and rises upward to a point so that at this time it strikes against the breast and the pulse is felt externally." Subsequently, important contributions to the art of precordial palpation came from Laënnec, his teacher Jean-Nicolas Corvisart, and Sir James MacKenzie.

126. **Which precordial impulse can be appreciated on physical exam?**
The only one that can be normally seen (and palpated) in healthy subjects is the *apical impulse*, also known as the PMI (point of maximal impulse)—a rather confusing term for what is nothing more than a brisk movement of left ventricle and septum against the chest wall. This is typically felt over the left fifth interspace midclavicular line, and can be absent in >50% of the cases. In disease states, additional precordial or chest wall impulses may occur, reflecting mechanical events of ventricles, atria, and large vessels. Hence, the need for a systematic search.

127. **What precordial areas should be examined?**
The same four used for cardiac auscultation. In addition to the *apex* per se (which reflects primarily the left ventricular impulse), you should palpate the *two basilar areas* (right and left parasternal interspaces, reflecting, respectively, the aortic and pulmonary outflow tracts) and the *left lower sternal area* (reflecting the right ventricular and atrial projection).

128. **Can the right ventricle be appreciated in a normal person?**
No. Right ventricular contraction produces neither visible nor palpable chest wall movements. Only occasionally (and usually in children or young people with narrow anteroposterior diameter) it may become possible to feel a gentle right ventricular activity. The same applies for the two basilar areas, which in the absence of pathology offer no palpable impulse.

129. **How do you assess the precordial impulse(s)?**
- First *inspect,* since this may prove even more valuable than palpation. Shine a tangential light across the chest, which can help you visualize retractions and outward motions.
- Then *palpate* the precordium, thoroughly assessing all major areas. With the patient in the supine position, *localize* impulses and evaluate their *force*. Then assess the impulse *size* by asking the patient to lie in left lateral decubitus. This also might help you elicit an otherwise undetectable apical impulse, as well as other impulses, such as a palpable S_3 or S_4. Use your palm to detect *heaves or lifts* (i.e., *sustained* precordial movements*)*, the proximal metacarpals to identify *thrills*, and the finger pads to localize the various abnormalities. To clarify semantics, note that a *heave/lift* is a forceful and sustained systolic *thrust* that raises the palpating hand a little. The three terms are often used interchangeably.

130. **How do you time precordial events?**
By simultaneously palpating the carotid, or by concomitantly auscultating for S_1 and S_2.

131. **Which characteristics of the apical impulse should be analyzed?**
- **Location:** Normally over the fifth left interspace midclavicular line, which usually (but not always) corresponds to the area just below the nipple. *Volume loads* to the left ventricle (such as aortic or mitral regurgitation) tend to displace the apical impulse downward and laterally. Conversely, *pressure loads* (such as aortic stenosis or hypertension) tend to displace the impulse more upward and medially—at least initially. Still, *a failing and decompensated ventricle*, independent of its etiology, will typically present with a downward and lateral shift in PMI. Although not too sensitive, this finding is very specific for cardiomegaly, low ejection fraction, and high pulmonary capillary wedge pressure.

Correlation of the PMI with anatomic landmarks (such as the left anterior axillary line) can be used to better characterize the displaced impulse.

- **Size:** As measured in left lateral decubitus, the normal apical impulse is the size of a dime. Anything larger (nickel, quarter, or an old Eisenhower silver dollar) should be considered pathologic. A diameter >4 cm is quite specific for cardiomegaly.
- **Duration and timing:** This is probably one of the most important characteristics. A normal apical duration is brief and never passes midsystole. Thus, a *sustained impulse* (i.e., one that continues into S_2 and beyond—often referred to as a "heave") should be considered pathologic until proven otherwise, and is usually indicative of pressure load, volume load, or cardiomyopathy. For separating these conditions, use the overall clinical picture:
  - In patients with no murmurs, consider cardiomyopathy and a low ejection fraction.
  - In patients with a systolic ejection murmur, consider instead severe pressure load from AS.
  - In patients with a diastolic murmur of aortic regurgitation (which causes a *volume* load), consider the disease to be mild if the apical impulse is nonsustained.
- **Amplitude:** This is not the length of the impulse, but its *force*. A *hyperdynamic* impulse (often referred to as a "thrust") that is forceful enough to lift the examiner's finger can be encountered in situations of volume overload and increased output (such as aortic regurgitation and ventricular septal defect), but may also be felt in normal subjects with very thin chests. Similarly, a *hypodynamic* impulse can be due to simple obesity, but also to congestive cardiomyopathy. In addition to being hypodynamic, the precordial impulse of these patients is large, somewhat sustained, and displaced downward/laterally.
- **Contour:** A normal apical impulse is single. Double or triple impulses are clearly pathologic. Hence, a normal apical impulse consists of a single, dime-sized, brief (barely beyond S1), early systolic, and nonsustained impulse, localized over the fifth interspace midclavicular line.

132. **What are the most common abnormal apical movements?**
- A **double systolic apical impulse** can be seen in patients with *hypertrophic obstructive cardiomyopathy* (HOCM). This may even present as a *triple* apical impulse (*triple ripple*), with one impulse being presystolic (and corresponding to a strong atrial contraction) and the other two being instead systolic (corresponding to the initial ventricular contraction, and a delayed one necessary to overcome the outflow obstruction by the septum). A thrill is often present. Note that a double systolic impulse also may be encountered in patients with left ventricular dyskinesia due to either ischemia or aneurysm of the wall (*see* question 138). In fact, one third of patients with ventricular aneurysm present with abnormal precordial findings.
- A **presystolic apical impulse** represents the palpable equivalent of a fourth heart sound. It is an important finding because it provides a clue to reduced left ventricular compliance, as in the case of either ischemia or pressure load (such as aortic stenosis or hypertension). In aortic stenosis, a palpable S_4 usually correlates with a significant gradient between the left ventricle and aorta. It is often associated with a palpable thrill over the second right interspace.
- An **early diastolic apical impulse** represents the palpable equivalent of S_3. It is more difficult to palpate than the presystolic impulse and usually indicates a dilated left ventricle. This can be the result of either volume load (i.e., mitral regurgitation) and/or left ventricular failure. In the latter, there may be an associated *sustained* apical impulse.

133. **What is the significance of a precordial movement in the left lower sternal area?**
- A **sustained** movement *that begins immediately after S_1* usually reflects a pressure (or volume) load to the right ventricle.
- A **sustained** movement *that begins late in systole* reflects instead severe mitral regurgitation with dilation of the left atrium.
- A **hyperdynamic** movement can be a sign of atrial septal defect, but is much more common in situations of high output, thin chests, or sternal malformations.

134. **What is a retracting impulse?**
One that moves *inward* in systole and *outward* in diastole. This is the opposite of the normal apical impulse, which has instead an early systolic outward movement followed by a mid to late systolic retraction. Timing of the events by either auscultation or carotid palpation is therefore key to separating the two.

135. **What are the causes of a retracting impulse?**
Constrictive pericarditis (where up to 90% of patients may present with the finding) and *severe tricuspid regurgitation*. In the latter condition, patients usually exhibit a peculiar rocking motion of the chest in systole, with a retraction at the apex (now occupied by the enlarged right ventricle) and a bulge over the epigastric and tricuspid areas (now occupied by the enlarged right atrium).

136. **What are the precordial findings of tricuspid regurgitation?**
In addition to those previously listed, adult patients with TR almost always have precordial evidence of pulmonary hypertension and right ventricular hypertrophy, such as a palpable P_2 over the pulmonic area and a right ventricular parasternal impulse. At times, the right ventricular impulse may even be palpable over the epigastric or subxiphoid area. A pulsatile liver in synchrony with each systole also is appreciated.

137. **What precordial evidence suggests mitral stenosis?**
Palpability of both first and second heart sounds. S_1 becomes palpable because of the sharp loudness characteristic of this disease, and S_2 (primarily its P_2 component) because of the concomitant pulmonary hypertension. Thus, the absence of a palpable P_2 argues strongly against the presence of pulmonary hypertension. Note that the opening snap can become palpable, too, and an apical diastolic thrill may at times be felt in left lateral decubitus. Since the apical impulse of mitral stenosis is usually hypodynamic (as a result of impaired left ventricular filling), the presence of a hyperkinetic impulse argues strongly against the purity of the disease and suggests instead the possibility of concomitant aortic or mitral regurgitation.

138. **What precordial evidence suggests angina? Previous infarction?**
In angina, the apical impulse is usually normal, but there may be a transiently palpable S_4 (presystolic impulse) or a dyskinetic apical area. Conversely, in cases of a preexisting infarction, the apical impulse may at times be just superior and medial to the normal apical location. Such an ectopic impulse usually suggests left ventricular aneurysm or dyskinesia.

139. **What are the precordial findings of a dilated aorta or pulmonary artery?**
A dilated pulmonary artery (as in patients with pulmonary hypertension) may often be felt at the upper left parasternal area. Conversely, a dilated aorta (as, for example, in patients with aortic aneurysm) may often be felt at the *right* parasternal area.

140. **What is a thrill?**
A palpable vibration associated with an audible murmur (*see* Chapter 12, question 7). A thrill automatically qualifies the murmur as being >4/6 in intensity and thus pathologic.

141. **What is the value of precordial percussion?**
When properly carried out, precordial percussion retains some clinical value. It can even outline the cardiac area with errors of only 1 cm. But given the difficulty in mastering this skill (and today's ubiquity of sophisticated imaging), cardiac percussion has become one of those areas of physical examination that have clearly yielded to technology-based diagnosis.

SELECTED BIBLIOGRAPHY

1. Amoroso T, Greenwood RN: Posture and central venous pressure measurement in circulatory volume depletion. Lancet 2:258–260, 1989.
2. Basta LL, Bettinger JJ: The cardiac impulse. Am Heart J 197:96–111, 1979.
3. Benchimol A, Tippit HC: The clinical value of the jugular and hepatic pulses. Prog Cardiovasc Dis 10:159–186, 1967.
4. Boicourt OW, Nagle RE, Mounsey JPD: The clinical significance of systolic retraction of the apical impulse. Br Heart J 127:379–391, 1965.
5. Borst JGG, Molhuysen A: Exact determination of the central venous pressure by a simple clinical method. Lancet 2:304–309, 1952.
6. Bude RO, Rubin JM, Platt JF, et al: Pulsus tardus: Its cause and potential limitations in detection of arterial stenosis. Radiology 190:779–784, 1994.
7. Butman SM, Ewy GA, Standen JR, et al: Bedside cardiovascular examination in patients with severe chronic heart failure: Importance of rest or inducible jugular venous distension. J Am Coll Cardiol 22:968–974, 1993.
8. Cintron GB, Hernandez E, Linares E, et al: Bedside recognition of right ventricular infarction. Am J Cardiol 47:224–227, 1981.
9. Constant J: Using internal jugular pulsations as a manometer for right atrial pressure measurements. Cardiology 93:26–30, 2000.
10. Cook DJ, Simel N: Does this patient have abnormal central venous pressure? JAMA 275:630–634, 1996.
11. Davison R, Cannon R: Estimation of central venous pressure by examination of the jugular veins. Am Heart J 87:279–282, 1974.
12. Dell'Italia J, Starling MR, O'Rourke RA: Physical examination for exclusion of hemodynamically important right ventricular infarction. Ann Intern Med 99:608–611, 1983.
13. Drazner MH, Rame JE, Stevenson LW, et al: Prognostic importance of elevated jugular venous pressure and a third heart sound in patients with heart failure. N Engl J Med 345:574–581, 200.
14. Ducas J, Magder S, McGregor M: Validity of the hepatojugular reflux as a clinical test for congestive heart failure. Am J Cardiol 52:1299–1303, 1983.
15. Eddleman EE, Langley JO: Paradoxical pulsation of the precordium in myocardial infarction and angina pectoris. Am Heart J 63:579–581, 1962.
16. Ellen SD, Crawford MH, O'Rourke RA: Accuracy of precordial palpation for detecting increased left ventricular volume. Ann Intern Med 99:628–630, 1983.
17. Ewy GA: The abdominojugular test. Ann Intern Med 109:456–460, 1988.
18. Forssell G, Jonasson R, Orinius E: Identifying severe aortic valvular stenosis by bedside examination. Acta Med Scand 218:397–400, 1985.
19. Ikram H, Nixon PGF, Fox JA, et al: The hemodynamic implications of bisferiens pulse. Br Heart J 26:452–459, 1964.
20. Lange RL, Boticelli JT, Tsagaris TJ, et al: Diagnostic signs in compressive cardiac disorders: Constrictive pericarditis, pericardial effusion, and tamponade. Circulation 33:763–777, 1966.
21. Lorell B, Leinbach RC, Pohost GM, et al: Right ventricular infarction: Clinical diagnosis and differentiation from cardiac tamponade and pericardial constriction. Am J Cardiol 43:465–471, 1979.
22. McGee SR: Physical examination of venous pressure: A critical review. Am Heart J 136:10–18, 1998.
23. O'Neill TW, Barry M, Smith M, et al: Diagnostic value of the apex beat. Lancet 1:410–411, 1989.
24. Sauve JS, Laupacis A, Ostbye T, et al: The rational clinical examination. Does this patient have a clinically important carotid bruit? JAMA 270:2843–2845, 1993.
25. Smith D, Craige E: Mechanisms of the dicrotic pulse. Br Heart J 156:531–534, 1986.
26. Sochowski RA, Dubbin JD, Naqvi SZ: Clinical and hemodynamic assessment of the hepatojugular reflux. Am J Cardiol 66:1002–1006, 1990.
27. Surawicz B, Fisch C: Cardiac alternans: Diverse mechanisms and clinical manifestations. J Am Coll Cardiol 20:483–499, 1992.
28. Wiese J: The abdominojugular reflux sign. Am J Med 109:59–61, 2000.

CHAPTER 11

HEART SOUNDS AND EXTRA SOUNDS

Salvatore Mangione, MD

". . . the gallop stroke is diastolic and is due to the beginning of sudden tension in the ventricular wall as a result of blood flowing into the cavity. It is more pronounced if the wall is not distensible and the failure of distensibility may depend on either a sclerotic thickening of the heart wall (hypertrophy) or to a decrease in muscular tonicity . . . the sound is dull, much more so than the normal sound. It affects the tactile sensation, more perhaps than the auditory sense. If one attempts to hear it with a flexible stethoscope, it lacks only a little, almost always, of disappearing completely."

—Potain PC: Note sur les dedoublements normaux des bruits du coeur.
Bull Mem Soc Med Hop Paris 3:138, 1866.

A. GENERALITIES

Conventional teaching has long recognized auscultation of the heart as the centerpiece of physical diagnosis. Indeed, proper identification of the various findings can still allow the prompt recognition of many important cardiac diseases. This is particularly true in the area of sounds and extra sounds, a field that has fascinated physicians since the introduction of stethoscopy. A plethora of *gallops, clicks, snaps, knocks,* and *plops* has since entered our everyday vocabulary. Accordingly, we have granted all but a few of these sounds a "high pass" in our conventional teaching test. The few that failed did so, not because of the paucity of information they deliver, but because of the rarity of the disease processes they represent.

B. CARDIAC AUSCULTATION: SOME SUGGESTIONS

1. **Why is cardiac auscultation so difficult?**
   - **Cardiac sounds are often at the threshold of audibility.** The human ear can only perceive sounds between 20 and 20,000 Hz: it can neither reach *beyond* (as dolphins and whales do) nor go *below* it (as elephants often do). Yet, in this range, it has a preferential bandwidth of 1000–5000 Hz, corresponding to that of the human voice. Yet, most cardiac sounds are <500 Hz. In fact, many are so low pitched to be almost inaudible (S_3 or S_4 can be <100 Hz).
   - **Cardiac sounds are crammed in a very little time interval.** At a rate of 70/minute, a cycle of 0.8 seconds can easily harbor four to five sounds, many barely detectable.
   - **Hospital rooms are noisy.**
   - **Patients' hair and respiration create misleading artifacts.**
   - **The obesity epidemic** has given many patients a much fattier chest muffler.
   - **Pathology has shifted from rheumatic to coronary,** thus reducing the pool of teaching patients.
   - **Our ever-increasing fascination with the inanimate and the machine** (and the sophistication of technology), compounded by:
     - **Medicolegal issues** (which have made imaging a self-protecting necessity)
     - **Patients' demands and expectations**
     - **Reduced emphasis on bedside skills during training and reduced availability of teachers**
     - **Time constraints** (which make resorting to technology an ever-increasing need)

2. **How can you make auscultation a little easier?**
   - Take your time.
   - Be thorough.
   - Control noise in the room.
   - Separate systole from diastole (easily done in normal rates by recognizing the acoustic differences of S_1 and S_2 plus the long and short intervals; in faster hearts, it may require simultaneous assessment of the arterial pulse or precordial impulse).
   - "Inch" (move your stethoscope inch by inch, from auscultatory area to auscultatory area).
   - Know how to use your tool: (1) bell versus diaphragm; (2) patient's position (supine, seated, and left lateral decubitus); (3) changes with respiration; and (4) dynamic bedside maneuvers (straight-leg raising, squatting-standing, Valsalva, hand-gripping, exercise).
   - When challenged by feeble and crammed signals, focus on one sound at a time.
   - Develop *pattern recognition*. This means practice, practice, practice.... In fact, you may need to hear an individual acoustic event as many as 500 times before you can master it.

C. NORMAL HEART SOUNDS

3. **What are the normal heart sounds?**
   They are the first (S_1) and second (S_2) heart sounds.

4. **What are the hemodynamic and acoustic characteristics of the cardiac cycle?**
   The cardiac cycle starts with contraction of the atria (S_4), which completes the ventricular diastolic filling and results in electrical activation (and contraction) of the ventricles themselves. This, in turn, closes the atrioventricular valves (S_1) and starts the *isometric* phase of systole. Opening of the semilunar valves (which may cause ejection sounds/clicks) signals the beginning of *isotonic* contraction, with expulsion of ventricular content into the great vessels. Closure of the semilunar valves (S_2), and subsequent reopening of the atrioventricular valves, restarts diastole, and the cycle begins anew. Note that diastole is always longer than systole, unless the heart rate exceeds 120/minute. Knowledge of the interrelationship between intracardiac pressure and valve motions is crucial for understanding heart sounds and murmurs.

5. **What are the cardiac areas?**
   They are areas of chest wall projection that correspond to the four cardiac valves (*see* Chapter 12, questions 1 and 2). In a clockwise fashion:
   - **Aortic area:** Second right parasternal interspace
   - **Pulmonic area:** Second left parasternal interspace
   - **Erb's point:** Third left parasternal interspace (area of left ventricular outflow)
   - **Mitral area:** Apex (fifth interspace left midclavicular line)
   - **Tricuspid area:** Fourth to fifth left parasternal space, at times extending into the epigastrium/subxiphoid

(1) FIRST HEART SOUND (S_1)

6. **Where is S_1 best heard?**
   At the apex (for its mitral component) and over the subxiphoid/epigastrium (for the tricuspid).

7. **How is S_1 generated?**
   By the vibration of valves, ventricles, and blood that coincides with:
   1. **Closure** of the atrioventricular (A-V) valves
   2. **Opening** of the semilunar valves. This in turn leads to two separate sounds, caused by:

- Opening of the semilunar valves per se
- Blood being ejected into the large vessels

In the absence of pathology, only A-V closure is responsible for S_1. Semilunar opening is silent.

8. **Which characteristics of S_1 are clinically valuable and should therefore be identified?**
The most valuable is *intensity* (and variations thereof). The next most valuable is *splitting*.

9. **How do you tell S_1 from S_2?**
The *area of greatest intensity* is different (apical for S_1 and basilar for S_2), and so is the *timing* (beginning of the short interval for S_1 versus beginning of the long interval for S_2). Finally, S_1 is lower pitched and longer than S_2, but still high pitched enough to require the diaphragm.

10. **What is the significance of S_2 being *louder than S_1 at the apex*?**
It suggests two possible explanations:
- S_2 is indeed louder than S_1 (usually as a result of either pulmonary or systemic hypertension).
- S_2 is normal, whereas S1 is *softer*.

11. **Which factors are responsible for the loudness of S_1?**
In addition to *shape* and *thickness* of the chest wall, three major factors play a role:
1. **The rate of rise in left ventricular pressure:** This is a function of *ventricular contractility*, with stronger contractions causing a faster rise in left ventricular pressure and thus brisker and more forceful A-V closure. Hence, a loud S_1 is typical of the *hyperkinetic heart syndrome*, whereas a soft (muffled) S_1 is instead common in congestive heart failure, whose failing ventricles can only generate a *slow* rise in systolic pressure.
2. **The separation between atrioventricular leaflets at the onset of ventricular systole:** The closer the leaflets, the softer S_1 is; conversely, the wider apart the leaflets, the louder S_1 is. This mechanism feeds into two other important variables:
   - *The duration of the P-R interval:* A short P-R forces the ventricles to contract while the leaflets are still widely separated, so that their closure occurs on a steeper part of the left ventricular pressure curve. This, in turn, means a more forceful and louder closure. Conversely, a long P-R provides enough time for the leaflets to come close to each other, thus softening S_1. A muffled S_1 used to be quite common in rheumatic fever with first degree A-V block. The progressive P-R lengthening of the Wenckebach phenomenon may also gradually (and increasingly) soften S_1.
   - *The atrioventricular pressure gradient:* A large A-V pressure gradient keeps the leaflets widely separated until ventricular pressure rises high enough to shut them close. Since the closure takes place on a steeper part of the left ventricular pressure curve, it will be forceful and loud. Hence, the longer the ventricle has to contract in order to close the A-V valve, the louder S_1 will be. This is quite common in mitral stenosis, where it contributes to the loudness of S_1.
3. **The thickness of the atrioventricular leaflet:** The thicker the leaflets, the louder S_1 is (banging hardbacks against each other generates more noise than banging paperbacks). Still, a soft S_1 may indicate leaflets that are too rigid. Hence, a thickened and stenotic mitral valve may generate a booming S_1 *early on* in the disease, but a softer (or absent) S_1 when the leaflets get eventually *calcified* and *fixed*.

12. **What factors can affect the rate of rise of ventricular pressure?**
The most important is *contractility*. An increase in left ventricular contractility (because of exogenous or endogenous inotropics) will *intensify* the mitral component of S_1. Conversely, a *decrease in* contractility (because of congestive heart failure) will *soften* it.

13. **Which diseases present with a *variable intensity* of S_1?**
Heart blocks, such as *second degree* (i.e., Mobitz I or Wenckebach) and *third degree*:

TABLE 11-1. INTENSITY OF S_1

Loud	Variable	Soft
Short P-R interval (<160 msec)	Atrial fibrillation	Long P-R interval (>200 msec)
Increased contractility (hyperkinetic states)	Atrioventricular block (Wenckebach and third degree)	Decreased contractility (left ventricular dysfunction)
Thickening of mitral (or tricuspid) leaflets	Ventricular tachycardia (due to atrioventricular dissociation)	Left bundle branch block
Increased atrioventricular pressure gradient (stenosis of the A-V valves)	Pulsus alternans	Calcification of A-V valve(s)
		Premature closure of mitral valve (acute aortic regurgitation)
		Mitral (or tricuspid) regurgitation

- In second-degree A-V block, there is *progressive softening of S_1*, while S_2 remains constant. This is due to the increasing P-R lengthening, until a beat is eventually dropped. It is so typical of Mobitz I that Wenckebach could describe it even before electrocardiogram (ECG) availability.
- In third-degree A-V block (typical of Morgagni-Adams-Stokes syndrome), the change in S_1 intensity is instead *random and chaotic* because the atrium and ventricle march to the beat of a different drummer, with rates that are totally independent—when ventricular contraction catches the A-V valves wide apart, S_1 booms; when it catches them partially closed, S_1 softens. The varying S_1 intensity is so typically random to allow the recognition of complete block just on the basis of auscultation (Table 11-1).

14. **What was the role of Morgagni in describing complete heart block?**
He had actually reported it almost 100 years before Adams and Stokes, in a merchant from Padua whom he had evaluated: "When visiting by way of consultation, I found with such a rarity of the pulse that within the 60th part of an hour the pulsations were only 22. And this rareness, which was perpetual, was perceived to be even more considerable, as often as many as two (epileptic) attacks were at hand. So that the physicians were never deceived from the increase of the rareness they foretold a paroxysm to be coming on."

15. **Who was Mobitz?**
Woldemar Mobitz was a German cardiologist who during the first half of the 20th century linked his name to various arrhythmias and to the eponymous second-degree A-V block.

16. **What is the intensity of S_1 in atrial fibrillation?**
Variable. This is due to the irregular ventricular rate, which may catch the A-V valves widely open, partially closed, or in between.

17. **How can you separate the variable S_1 of atrial fibrillation from that of complete A-V block?**
In atrial fibrillation, the rhythm is irregularly irregular, whereas in third degree, A-V block is a *regular bradycardia* (due to either nodal or ventricular "escape").

18. **How is S_1 in mitral stenosis (MS)?**
    Booming (in 90% of the patients). A loud S_1 should always alert the clinician to the possibility of MS and thus prompt a search for its associated diastolic rumble. Conversely, a soft S_1 argues *against* the presence of *uncomplicated* MS (i.e., one where the valve is still relatively pliable). The loud S_1 is usually the result of:
    - **Thickening of the mitral leaflets:** In the late stages of MS, however, leaflets can become stiff and poorly mobile, which, in turn, softens S_1 and eventually eliminates it.
    - **High atrioventricular pressure gradient:** This is produced by the stenotic valve and keeps the A-V leaflets maximally separated at the onset of ventricular contraction.

19. **What other conditions can be associated with a *loud* S_1?**
    In addition to *mitral stenosis* and the *hyperkinetic heart syndrome*, a loud S_1 is often encountered in:
    - Hypertrophic ventricles
    - Holosystolic mitral valve prolapse with regurgitation (where the prolapse delays the tension of the redundant mitral leaflet, thus allowing it to occur at peak of ventricular contraction, which makes it louder). A similar mechanism takes place in:
      - A left-atrial myxoma. Here it is the tumor that delays the closure of the mitral valve, thus allowing it to occur at peak of ventricular contraction and making it, therefore, louder. As a result, 80% of patients with this condition will have a loud S_1.
      - Short P-R interval, as in the pre-excitation syndromes of Wolff-Parkinson-White and Ganong-Levine syndromes.

20. **Which conditions can be associated with a *soft* S_1?**
    Other than *calcific mitral stenosis*, a soft S_1 is usually heard in either *early* closure of the mitral valve (aortic regurgitation) or *late* closure (prolonged P-R interval). Alternatively, a soft or absent S_1 can result from inadequate left ventricular contraction because of *congestive heart failure*, *myocardial infarction*, or *left bundle branch block* (where the left ventricle not only contracts ineffectively, but also late, with M_1 *following* T_1; "M" for mitral and "T" for tricuspid).

21. **Which atrioventricular valve closes first?**
    The mitral, followed by the tricuspid (high pressure beds always *close* earlier). Since mitral closure is much louder than tricuspid, the first component of S_1 is usually referred to as M_1 and predominates in the formation of the sound.

22. **Which semilunar valve opens first?**
    The pulmonic, followed by the aortic (low pressure beds always *open* earlier). As for the intensity, the aortic ejection sound is usually louder than the pulmonic, but still not enough to become audible in the normal patient.

23. **What is the sequence of closure and opening of the various valves at the time of S_1?**
    In sequence:
    - Mitral closure (M_1)
    - Tricuspid closure (T_1)
    - Pulmonic opening
    - Aortic opening
    The first two events are the only real contributors to S_1, whereas the last two may become audible (as *ejection* clicks/sounds) in case of disease.

24. **What is the significance of a *narrowly split* S_1?**
    It reflects the audible separation of M_1 and T_1, a normal phenomenon that may at times be detected by listening over the lower left sternal border/epigastric area (where the tricuspid component is louder and thus easier to separate from its mitral counterpart).

25. **Is the tricuspid component of S_1 (T_1) audible at the apex?**
No. It *is* only audible over the lower left sternal border (LLSB). T_1, however, may become audible at the apex in case of (1) *thickening of the tricuspid valve leaflets* (i.e., early tricuspid stenosis) or (2) *right ventricular pressure overload* (such as pulmonary hypertension or atrial septal defect).

26. **What is the significance of a split S_1 at the *base*?**
It does *not* indicate the audible separation of M_1 and T_1, but instead the presence of an *early ejection sound*. This can be of either pulmonic or aortic origin.

27. **What is the significance of a *widely split* S_1 at the LLSB?**
It usually indicates a delayed closure of the *tricuspid valve*, most commonly because of a right bundle branch block. Note that a bundle branch block is also a cause of split S_2.

28. **What is the significance of an *apparently split* S_1 at the *apex*?**
It may represent a *normal* S_1 that is either *preceded* by an S_4 or *followed* by an early systolic (ejection) sound. This is an important differential diagnosis to keep in mind.

29. **How can one separate a truly split S_1 from a "pseudo-split" S_1?**
A truly split S_1 is usually heard over the *lower left sternal border*. Conversely, an S_4 of left atrial origin is only audible at the *apex*, whereas an early systolic click is usually louder over the *base*. To separate S_4 from an early systolic click, keep in mind that S_4 is lower pitched, best heard with the bell, softer, located *before* the true S_1, and only heard at the *apex*. An early ejection click is instead higher pitched, best heard with the diaphragm, louder, located *after* the true S_1, and best heard at the *base* (although it can also radiate down to the apex).

(2) SECOND HEART SOUND (S_2)

30. **Where is S_2 best heard?**
At the base. More specifically, over the second/third *left* parasternal interspace for its pulmonic component and over the second or third *right* parasternal interspace for the aortic one. Because of its medium to high frequency, S_2 requires the diaphragm of the stethoscope.

31. **How is S_2 generated?**
By *sudden deceleration of blood* following the closure of aortic (A_2) and pulmonic (P_2) valves.

32. **Which of the two semilunar valve closes earlier?**
The aortic, due to systemic pressure being normally higher than pulmonic pressure.

33. **How clinically useful is S_2?**
Very useful. In fact, it has been suggested that careful evaluation of S_2 ranks with electrocardiography and radiology as one of the most valuable routine screening tests for heart disease. (Leatham used to call it "the key to auscultation of the heart".)

34. **Which S_2 characteristics are more valuable clinically?**
Sound *intensity* and sound *splitting*. Of these, splitting (and variations thereof) is the most informative. This is in contrast to S_1, where *intensity* (and variations) are the most important.

35. **What is a *physiologic splitting* of S_2?**
It is the *inspiratory* widening of the normal interval between A_2 and P_2. This is triggered by:
- Increased venous return to the *right* ventricle (due to negative intrathoracic pressure). This delays P_2.
- Decreased venous return to the *left* ventricle (due to pooling of blood in the lungs). This anticipates A_2.

Although there is always a small interval between A_2 and P_2, only in inspiration does this get large enough to become audible (i.e., 30–40 msec.)

36. What is the effect of exhalation on semilunar valve closure?
The opposite. It delays A_2 (more venous return to the *left* side) and anticipates P_2 (less venous return to the *right* side), so that the interval between the two components becomes too narrow for being appreciated by the human ear.

37. How common is a physiologic splitting of S_2?
Not very common. In a study of 196 normal adults examined in the supine position, only 52.1% had an audible inspiratory split of S_2. Physiologic splitting was much more common in younger individuals (60% of those between ages 21 to 30, and 34% of those older than 50). Indeed, after age 50, S_2 appeared single in more than 60% of subjects, as opposed to 36% for all ages. Hence, in older patients a single S_2 should not be considered evidence for a delayed A_2 (and therefore it should *not* suggest underlying aortic stenosis [AS] or a left bundle branch block) (*see* Fig. 11-1).

> **Pearl:**
> A physiologic S_2 split occurs in 60% of subjects younger than 30 and 30% of those older than 60.

38. Why does S_2 splitting disappear with aging?
Because of *senile emphysema*, with greater air muffling of the pulmonic component of S_2.

39. How important is a patient's position on S_2 splitting?
Very important. A supine position increases venous return, lengthens right ventricular systole, and thus widens the physiologic splitting of S_2. Conversely, a sitting (or standing) position decreases venous return, shortens right ventricular systole, and narrows the physiologic split (Fig. 11-2). This is especially important when analyzing an *expiratory* splitting of S_2. In a study by Adolph and Fowler, 22/200 (11%) normal subjects had an expiratory split while supine, but only 1/22 maintained it upon sitting or standing. Hence, a true *expiratory splitting of S_2* is one that is present *both* in a recumbent *and* upright position.

40. What is the significance of a true expiratory splitting of S_2?
It indicates one of three conditions:
- A wide (physiologic) splitting of S_2
- A fixed splitting of S_2
- A paradoxical splitting of S_2

With the exception of the *wide (physiologic) splitting* (that may be normal in the young, but *abnormal* in those older than 50), both the *fixed* and the *paradoxical splitting* reflect cardiovascular pathology.

41. What is a wide (physiologic) splitting of S_2? What causes it?
It is a splitting so wide as to present *throughout respiration*, albeit still more marked in *inspiration*. It occurs in (1) delayed closure of the *pulmonic* valve (delayed P_2), (2) premature closure of the *aortic* valve (premature A_2), or (3) a combination thereof.

42. What are the causes of delayed closure of the pulmonic valve?
The classic one is a complete right bundle branch block, which delays both the depolarization of the right ventricle and the closure of the pulmonic valve, making the physiologic splitting of S_2 audible both in inspiration *and* expiration. Loss of pulmonary recoil (because of *idiopathic dilation*) or severe impedance to right ventricular emptying also can delay the pulmonic closure. The latter can occur in (1) pulmonic stenosis (where the interval between A_2 and P_2

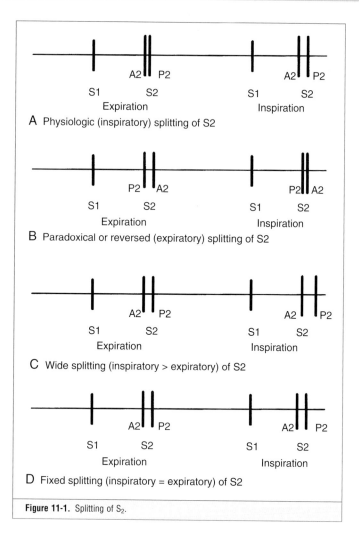

Figure 11-1. Splitting of S_2.

correlates with the severity of stenosis), (2) massive pulmonary embolism, (3) cor pulmonale with right ventricular failure, and (4) atrial septal defect. In pulmonary embolism, an audible expiratory splitting of S_2 (with a loud and palpable P_2) has both diagnostic and prognostic significance, reflecting acute cor pulmonale and usually resolving in hours or days.

43. **What are the causes of premature closure of the aortic valve?**
The most common is a rapid emptying of the left ventricle, as in severe mitral regurgitation or ventricular septal defect. A premature closure of the aortic valve also can occur in severe congestive heart failure, usually because of a reduction in left ventricular stroke volume. Finally, a widely split S_2 also may occur in tamponade, where expansion of the two ventricles is limited and fixed. During inspiration, the *right ventricle* fills relatively more, pushing the septum leftward and thus further impairing *left* ventricular filling. This reduces left ventricular stroke volume, anticipates A_2, and makes S_2 widely split. The opposite occurs in exhalation.

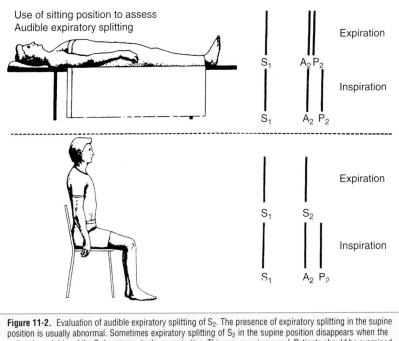

Figure 11-2. Evaluation of audible expiratory splitting of S_2. The presence of expiratory splitting in the supine position is usually abnormal. Sometimes expiratory splitting of S_2 in the supine position disappears when the patient is upright and the S_2 becomes single on expiration. This response is normal. Patients should be examined carefully in the sitting and standing positions whenever S_2 appears to be abnormally split during expiration. (Adapted from Abrams J: Essentials of Cardiac Physical Diagnosis. Philadelphia, Lea & Febiger, 1987.)

44. What is a *fixed splitting* of S_2? What does it mean?

It is an S_2 that remains audibly split *throughout respiration,* both in the supine and upright positions, and with a *consistent interval between its two components.* Although encountered in severe ventricular failure, a fixed splitting of S_2 should suggest a *septal defect* (most often *atrial* but occasionally *ventricular*), especially if associated with pulmonary hypertension. The defect (and its shunt) eliminate the respiratory changes in right and left ventricular stroke volume, thus *fixing* the S_2 splitting (more rarely, a fixed S_2 split will occur in severe impedance to right ventricular emptying, such as that of pulmonary stenosis, pulmonary hypertension, or massive pulmonary embolism—with or without bundle branch block). These patients cannot cope with the increased venous return of inspiration by increasing right ventricular stroke volume. Hence, they maintain their S_2 widely and persistently split *throughout* respiration (*see* Fig. 11-3).

45. What is the differential diagnosis of a fixed splitting of S_2?

A late-systolic click (which *precedes* S_2) and an early diastolic extra sound (which *follows* S_2):

- **The late-systolic click** varies with bedside maneuvers and is loudest at the apex (conversely, the split S_2 is unchanged with maneuvers and only heard at the base).
- The two most **common early diastolic extra sounds** are the *S_3* and the *opening snap* (OS) of mitral (or tricuspid) stenosis (for a discussion of how to differentiate an opening snap from a widely split S_2 or an S_3, *see* questions 103, 104, and 130). OS is primarily apical, whereas the split S_2 is basilar. Still, OS can be loud enough to transmit to the base, thus producing a triple lilt in inspiration (OS + split S_2, with a loud P_2 because of pulmonary hypertension). Note that the interval between S_2 and OS is wider than that between the two components of S_2. Finally, an OS is usually (but not necessarily) associated with a diastolic rumble.

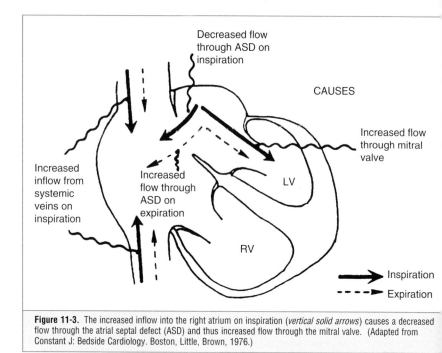

Figure 11-3. The increased inflow into the right atrium on inspiration (*vertical solid arrows*) causes a decreased flow through the atrial septal defect (ASD) and thus increased flow through the mitral valve. (Adapted from Constant J: Bedside Cardiology. Boston, Little, Brown, 1976.)

46. **What about *tumor plop* and *pericardial knock*?**

    They are two other (albeit less common) early diastolic sounds that should be included in the differential diagnosis of a fixed splitting of S_2. The *tumor plop* is the opening sound of an atrial myxoma. It typically varies with the patient's position and from cycle to cycle. The *pericardial knock* is instead a loud apical sound that is widely separated from S_2 (and thus easily differentiated from a fixed splitting of S_2, which is more basilar and closely separated). The knock also comes with signs of constrictive pericarditis, like distended neck veins, hepatomegaly, and leg edema in the absence of crackles.

47. **What is a *paradoxical splitting* of S_2? What does it mean?**

    A paradoxical (or reversed) splitting indicates a second sound that becomes audibly split only in *exhalation*, while remaining single in *inspiration*. It means pathology until proven otherwise. The behavior (opposite to the physiologic inspiratory split of normal subjects—hence, the paradox) usually results from a delay in aortic closure, so that A_2 now *follows* P_2. Since the respiratory changes of the two valves remain the same, inspiration will *narrow* their closure, whereas exhalation will widen it. Hence, the expiratory (or paradoxical) splitting.

48. **What are the causes of paradoxical S_2 splitting?**

    - **Delayed aortic closure.** This is indeed the most common reason, usually due to a complete left bundle branch block (where reversed S_2 splitting can occur in 84% of the cases). Other causes include increased impedance to left ventricular emptying (hypertension, AS, coarctation) or left ventricular dysfunction. The latter can occur in acute ischemia and various cardiomyopathies.
    - **Early pulmonic closure.** This is a much less common cause of paradoxical splitting, usually due to decreased right ventricular filling—from either tricuspid regurgitation or right atrial myxoma.

49. Is paradoxical S_2 splitting a sign of myocardial ischemia?
Yes. Even though paradoxical splitting of S_2 rarely occurs with *stable* coronary artery disease, it may often be heard during acute decompensation, such as after exercise or during angina. It also may be heard during the first three days following an acute myocardial infarction (in as many as 15% of patients). Finally, it is commonly heard in elderly hypertensive patients with underlying coronary artery disease and evidence of heart failure.

50. What is the significance of a "single splitting" of S_2?
It refers to either a single S_2 or to an S_2 so narrowly split in inspiration as to be inaudible in its two separate components. A single S_2 is usually due to:
- **Aging:** The audible splitting of S_2 decreases in prevalence with age, to the point of becoming absent in most subjects older than 60. This is probably due to the muffling of P_2 by the "physiologic" senile emphysema.
- **Emphysema:** The hyperinflated lungs will muffle P_2 during inspiration, thus making A_2 the only audible sound. Because this phenomenon is less pronounced in exhalation, these patients may be misdiagnosed as having *paradoxical splitting of S_2* (while, in fact, they have a *pseudo-paradoxical splitting* that becomes evident only in expiration).
- **Reversed (or paradoxical) splitting:** In this case, the split will indeed occur only in exhalation.
- **Pulmonary hypertension:** Increased impedance on right ventricular emptying makes the ventricle unable to cope with the increased venous return of inspiration. Hence, there will be no inspiratory lengthening of right ventricular systole and no inspiratory splitting of S_2.
- **Semilunar valvular disease:** Stiffening and reduced mobility of semilunar valves may also lead to the disappearance of either A_2 or P_2, thus making S_2 "single."

51. Which is louder: A_2 or P_2?
A_2. This is consistent throughout the precordium. In fact, there is *only one site* where P_2 is loud enough to become audible: the *pulmonic area* (second or third left parasternal interspace). This is also the only site where physiologic splitting of S_2 can be heard.

52. How can you differentiate the two components of S_2?
By remembering that only A_2 is heard at the apex (in the absence of pulmonary hypertension, P_2 is too soft to be transmitted there). Hence, to tell A_2 from P_2, move the stethoscope from the base to the apex, and then pay attention to which component of S_2 gets softer: if it is the first component, then P_2 precedes A_2; if it is the second component, then A_2 precedes P_2. This maneuver may help differentiate a right bundle branch block (where A_2 precedes P_2) from a left bundle branch block (where P_2 precedes A_2).

53. What is the significance of S_2 physiologically split at the apex?
It suggests pulmonary hypertension, with P_2 so loud to transmit downward. This is common in *primary* pulmonary hypertension and atrial septal defect, but less common in other conditions.

54. What is the significance of a loud P_2 or A_2?
It suggests increased pressure in the pulmonic or systemic circulation. In fact, S_2 *louder than S_1 at the apex* also suggests *pulmonary* or *systemic* hypertension. Note that high output states may also be associated with a loud S_2, very much like they are associated with a loud S_1. These include aortic regurgitation and atrial or ventricular septal defects.

55. What is the significance of S_2 softer than S_1 at the base?
It depends on which basilar area is involved (and thus on which of the S_2 components is softer). If S_2 is softer than S_1 over the *aortic* area, then A_2 is diminished, suggesting fibrosis or calcification of the aortic valve (i.e., aortic stenosis). Conversely, if S_2 is softer than S_1 over the *pulmonic* area, then P_2 is decreased, and the most likely explanation is pulmonic stenosis.

56. **What is a "Tambour" S_2?**
It is a loud and ringing S_2, very rich in overtones. *Tambour* ("drum" in French) conveys the peculiar character of this sound, which usually indicates a dilation of the aortic root. In patients with an aortic regurgitation murmur, it suggests Marfan's syndrome, syphilis (Potain's sign), or a dissecting aneurysm of the ascending aorta (Harvey's sign).

57. **What makes P_2 louder than A_2?**
Pulmonary hypertension. Alternatively, aortic stenosis with reduced valve mobility can make A_2 *softer* than P_2. Note that, despite conventional teaching, a loud P_2 has not been validated as a clue to pulmonary hypertension. This is in contrast to a *palpable* P_2 over the pulmonic area, which is indeed a strong predictor of pulmonary systolic pressure >50 mmHg.

58. **What are the other precordial findings of pulmonary hypertension?**
A right-sided S_4, a pulmonic ejection sound, murmurs of tricuspid and/or pulmonic regurgitation, an audible splitting of S_2 at the apex, and, of course, a palpable P_2.

59. **What can soften A_2 or P_2?**
In addition to emphysema, the most common cause is reduced pulmonic or systemic pressure. Soft A_2 or P_2 also can be due to reduced mobility of the semilunar valves, from either calcification or sclerosis, an important marker of severe stenosis.

D. EXTRA SOUNDS

60. **What are extra heart sounds?**
They are *pathologic* sounds that may occur *in addition to* the normal sounds (S_1 and S_2). Based on location within the cardiac cycle, extra sounds are classified into *systolic* (usually referred to as *clicks:* early systolic, mid systolic, and late systolic) or *diastolic* (usually referred to as *snaps, knocks, or plops*) (*see* Table 11-2 and Fig. 11-4). For each of them, we shall review acoustic characteristics, pathogenesis, and clinical significance.

61. **Are S_3 and S_4 extra sounds?**
They are more *heart sounds* than *extra sounds*. Still, they reflect pathology (S_4 always and S_3 most of the times), and thus their significance is closer to that of extra sounds.

TABLE 11-2. EXTRA SOUNDS

Systolic		Diastolic	
Timing	Sound	Timing	Name
Early systolic	Ejection sounds (aortic or pulmonary) Click (mitral or tricuspid) Aortic prosthetic valve sounds	Early diastolic	Opening snap (mitral or tricuspid) Early S_3 Pericardial knock Tumor "plop"
Mid-to-late systolic	Click (mitral or tricuspid)	Mid-diastolic	S_3 Summations sound ($S_3 + S_4$)
		Late diastolic (presystolic)	S_4 Pacemaker sound

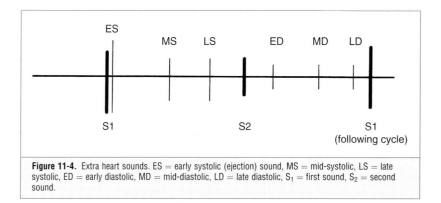

Figure 11-4. Extra heart sounds. ES = early systolic (ejection) sound, MS = mid-systolic, LS = late systolic, ED = early diastolic, MD = mid-diastolic, LD = late diastolic, S_1 = first sound, S_2 = second sound.

62. **Where are these extra sounds best heard?**
    It depends. Snaps, knocks, and "plops" are best heard at the apex, whereas clicks (especially *ejection* clicks) can be heard at both the base and the apex.

63. **Where are S_3 and S_4 best heard?**
    At the apex, but barely, since their low frequency (20–50 Hz) puts them at the threshold of audibility. Hence, use the bell and remember to *palpate*: in thin patients they may be more palpable than audible (especially the S_4).

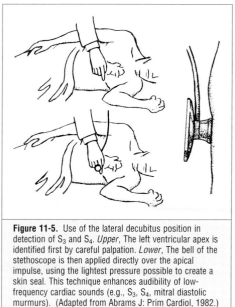

Figure 11-5. Use of the lateral decubitus position in detection of S_3 and S_4. *Upper*, The left ventricular apex is identified first by careful palpation. *Lower*, The bell of the stethoscope is then applied directly over the apical impulse, using the lightest pressure possible to create a skin seal. This technique enhances audibility of low-frequency cardiac sounds (e.g., S_3, S_4, mitral diastolic murmurs). (Adapted from Abrams J: Prim Cardiol, 1982.)

64. **Which bedside maneuvers can intensify S_3 and S_4?**
    Maneuvers that *increase venous return, intracardiac blood volume,* and *flow across the atrioventricular valves* (Fig. 11-5). These include (1) leg raising, (2) mild exercise (such as assuming the left lateral decubitus—or even coughing a few times may unmask a gallop), (3) abdominal compression, (4) the release phase of Valsalva, and (5) respiration. Held-*exhalation* tends to intensify the *left*-sided S_3 and S_4 (with S_4 increasing in *early* exhalation and S_3 in end-exhalation), whereas held-*inspiration* tends to intensify the *right*-sided S_3 and S_4. Conversely, maneuvers that *decrease* venous return, intracardiac blood volume, and transvalvular flow (such as sitting, standing, and the strain phase of Valsalva) will soften a pathologic S_3 or S_4 and totally eliminate a physiologic S_3. Note that all these maneuvers increase (or decrease) the intensity of both S_4 and S_3, but they will do so much more dramatically with S_3.

(1) Diastolic Extra Sounds

65. How many diastolic extra sounds can be encountered?
Five. Of these, two are common (S_4 and S_3); one less common (the opening snap of mitral or tricuspid stenosis); and two very uncommon (the opening "plop" of atrioventricular myxoma and the pericardial knock). Only the S_4 occurs late in diastole (or *pre-systole*); all others are early diastolic. Two are low pitched and soft (S_3 and S_4); two high pitched and loud (opening snap and pericardial knock); and one medium pitched and of varying intensity (tumor "plop").

Third Heart Sound (S_3)

66. What is an S_3?
It is a low-pitched, soft, *early* diastolic extra sound of great value. First described by Potain in the second half of the 19th century, S_3 is an important clue to ventricular dysfunction. In a nationwide survey of primary care directors, it was ranked as the most useful extra sound.

67. How easy is it to detect an S_3?
Not easy at all, since the sound is low pitched and often of such a varying intensity to be fleeting. Not surprisingly, variability in detection can be quite wide, with individual skills and experience playing a major role. Among four trained observers examining 81 hospitalized patients, agreement was only 48–73% for pairs of observers. Hence, S_3 is valuable but frustrating. Still, it should be sought aggressively in any patient suspected of congestive failure.

68. How is S_3 best detected?
In left-lateral decubitus and by holding the bell very gently over the apex. This will bring the ventricle closer to the chest wall, thus improving sound transmission. Of course, asking the patient to turn on the side after a negative supine exam requires a high index of suspicion. A high index of suspicion also is needed for other "bedside maneuvers" that may elicit the S_3.

69. Why the bell?
Because it filters out all the extraneous high frequencies, thus making the feeble S_3 more easily detectable. Given its low pitch, S_3 may be inaudible through the diaphragm. In fact, it may be inaudible even through the bell when *too much pressure* is applied (thus transforming it into a diaphragm). This little trick can be used to confirm that the sound in question is indeed an S_3, and not, for example, a higher-pitched extra sound—like an opening snap.

70. How is S_3 after an extra systole?
Louder. The mechanism is the same: increased ventricular filling following the premature beat.

71. Should S_3 be pursued over the point of maximal apical impulse (PMI)?
Yes. In fact, at times S_3 is too soft to be heard anywhere else. That the PMI is the best area of auscultation derives directly from the site of origin of S_3, the left ventricular wall.

72. Can S_3 be palpable?
Yes. In thin patients with left ventricular hypertrophy, S_3 may be more palpable than audible—especially in left-lateral decubitus.

73. Can S_3 be transmitted to the supraclavicular fossa?
This has indeed been reported, usually on the right side, and occasionally all the way up into the right internal jugular vein. The same transmission has been reported for S_4.

74. **Which is easier to detect: S_3 or S_4?**
S_4. It is higher pitched and louder, even though not quite as long (the S_3 is often prolonged by a series of low-pitched and humming vibrations, rumble-like—*see* question 90).

75. **How is S_3 produced?**
Not by the left ventricle *hitting* against the chest wall, but instead by the sudden and abnormal *deceleration in left ventricular flow* that coincides with the end of rapid filling. This occurs in patients with *abnormal left ventricular compliance* or *increased left ventricular preload* (the latter can be physiologic in young and bradycardic athletes, and pathologic in atrioventricular regurgitation or left-to-right shunt). Either mechanism will make S_3 more detectable, through greater *intensity* (higher preload) or higher *frequency* (abnormal compliance).

76. **Why does S_3 occur in early diastole?**
Because it coincides with the *rapid (and passive) phase of ventricular filling,* which occurs in early diastole just after the opening of the A-V valves. This normally accounts for 80% of ventricular filling, with the other 20% taking place *much later* in diastole, and at the time of atrial contraction (*active* filling). This late phase coincides with the atrial *kick,* and is heralded not by S_3 but by S_4. Hence, S_3 signals the phase of early (or passive) ventricular filling, whereas S_4 indicates the phase of late (or active) ventricular filling. Both sounds occur within the ventricle.

77. **Is S_3 always a *gallop*?**
No. A *gallop* is any triple lilt whose cadence resembles the canter of a horse. Accordingly, a *ventricular* gallop (i.e., a gallop produced by S_3) is only one of *three* forms of gallop (*see* also S_4 and *summation gallop*). The *sine qua non* for a gallop is its *lilt,* which usually requires S_1 and S_2 to be almost as soft as the pathologic extra sound. It also requires a relatively *fast heart rate,* even though gallops can at times be rather slow, as long as they maintain the necessary *cadence.* Still, tachycardia remains the prerequisite for the *summation* gallop (*see* questions 81–84).

78. **Can a gallop be physiologic?**
No, a gallop is always pathologic. Hence, S_3 can be physiologic and yet not be a gallop, whereas the S_3 "gallop" is always pathologic. Whether due to S_3 or S_4, a gallop is *usually ominous.*

79. **Who first used the term *gallop*?**
Pierre Carl Potain, who in the second half of the 19th century wrote about the "triple bruit du coeur" and the "bruit de galop"—an expression of his teacher, Jean-Baptiste Bouillard (in addition to describing both S_3 and S_4, Potain also contributed to the measurement of blood pressure).

80. **What are the most important gallops?**
The **ventricular** gallop (where the lilt is due to a *third* heart sound, together with a soft S_1 and S_2) and the **atrial** gallop (where the lilt is instead due to a *fourth* heart sound, together with S_1 and S_2). Traditionally, we try to mimic these rhythms by saying in a cadenced fashion: *Ken-tù-cky* (for an early diastolic, or S_3, gallop) and *Tèn-ne-ssee* (for a late diastolic, or S_4, gallop). Finally, there is a third and less common gallop, called **summation**.

81. **What is a *summation* gallop?**
It is the peculiar lilt of very tachycardic patients, who have both atrial *and* ventricular gallops. Often referred to as "S_7" ($S_3 + S_4$), the summation gallop owes its genesis to a *tachycardia*-induced shortening of diastole, causing the merge of S_3 and S_4 into a single extra sound (S_7).

82. **What are the causes of a summation gallop?**
Diseases causing both a stiff *and* a failing ventricle, like hypertensive congestive heart failure. A summation gallop also may occur in *hypertrophic cardiomyopathy* and in first-degree A-V block (where the prolonged P-R moves the S_4 *backward* in diastole, thus merging it with S_3).

83. **What are the acoustic characteristics of a summation gallop?**
    It is higher pitched, longer, and louder than either S_3 or S_4 (in fact, often louder than S_1 and S_2). It also is easily palpable. Given its longer duration (and its location in early/mid-diastole), S_7 can often be misinterpreted as a mid-diastolic rumble. It can, however, be easily recognized as a combination of two separate acoustic events by simply slowing the heart rate. This can be done with a cautious carotid massage (beware of elderly and possibly atherosclerotic patients).

84. **Is a *quadruple rhythm* the same as a summation gallop?**
    No. A quadruple rhythm is a gallop lilt characterized by both S_3 *and* S_4, each *separately* audible. This is usually caused by a rate not fast enough to produce summation. More than the galloping of a horse, a quadruple rhythm resembles the steel-rail humming of a passing train.

85. **What is a *physiologic* S_3?**
    It is the sound often heard in healthy children and young adults, usually in association with a venous hum or an innocent systolic murmur. A physiologic S_3 occurs in 20–90% of young volunteers, usually thin and with more rapid early diastolic left ventricular inflow. It also can occur in athletes, especially if *bradycardic*. It is due to a more energetic expansion and filling of the left ventricle, probably caused by higher cardiac output (and lower heart rate). It typically softens (or disappears) upon assuming an upright position (because of the decreased venous return). Given the slowing of ventricular relaxation associated with aging (which delays diastolic filling), S_3 *in those older than 40* should be considered pathologic until proven otherwise.

86. **Can a physiologic S_3 occur in any other situation?**
    Yes. It can occur in patients with increased sympathetic tone or higher catecholaminemia, causing rapid circulation time and tachycardia (*hyperkinetic heart syndrome*).This, for example, affects 80% of pregnant women. An S_3 of this type often coexists with a cervical *venous hum*.

87. **What is the clinical significance of a *pathologic* S_3?**
    It reflects either (1) *increased ventricular preload* (i.e., diastolic overload) or (2) *reduced ventricular function* (i.e., systolic impairment, with decreased myocardial contractility and low ejection fraction). The first (and less common) mechanism plays a role in *high output failure*; the second (and more common) plays instead a role in the *low output failure of dilated* cardiomyopathy (conversely, *hypertrophic* cardiomyopathy is more often associated with $\underline{S_4}$).

88. **How does a pathologic S_3 differ from a physiologic S_3?**
    A pathologic S_3 is softer, lower pitched, and more likely associated with a gallop. It also is longer. At times, however, the two may be indistinguishable. Hence, the best differentiating feature is "the company it keeps": a pathologic S_3 comes with symptoms or abnormal signs.

89. **Why is the pathologic S_3 softer and lower pitched?**
    Because of reduced ventricular contractility. This also causes the tachycardia and softer S_1/S_2 of these patients. Altogether, these findings make the pathologic S_3 more subtle and elusive.

90. **What is the low-pitched diastolic murmur that often follows a pathologic S_3?**
    It is the sound produced by the sudden rush of blood across the A-V valve. This low-pitched, short, early diastolic rumble often occurs in situations of ventricular dysfunction or increased transmitral flow, as in cases of regurgitation. It may even present in patients who lack an S_3. It is, however, rarely encountered in association with a *physiologic* S_3. Hence, the presence of an early diastolic rumble *and* an S_3 should be considered pathologic until proven otherwise.

91. **What are the hemodynamic implications of an S_3?**
    They depend on the mechanism responsible for its generation.
    - In patients with **increased left ventricular preload** (diastolic overload), the atrial pressure is not necessarily elevated, while cardiac index and ejection fraction may even be increased.

- In patients with **systolic dysfunction** (and abnormal *ventricular compliance*), the cardiac index and ejection fraction are instead both decreased, whereas left atrial, pulmonary diastolic, pulmonary capillary wedge, and left ventricular pressures are all increased. Hence, the left ventricle is dilated and the end-diastolic volume increased. S_3 in ventricular dysfunction reflects ejection fraction <30% and filling pressure >25 mmHg. That the sound is partly due to an increased atrial pressure is demonstrated by its disappearance after diuresis.

92. **Does the presence of S_3 predict higher levels of B-type natriuretic peptide (BNP)?**
    Yes, and intuitively so, considering that both findings originate from increased left ventricular end-diastolic pressure. In a study of 100 consecutive adults presenting to a cardiology clinic, Marcus et al. noted that BNP levels were significantly higher in patients with S_3 as compared to those *without* S_3 (476 ± 290 pg/mL versus 175 ± 198 pg/mL, p <.0005). Overall, presence of S_3 had 41% sensitivity and 97% specificity for detecting elevated BNP levels (with a positive predictive value of 96% and a negative predictive value of 49%). Only one patient with S_3 had a BNP level <100 pg/mL (which in this study was the cut-off for congestive heart failure).

93. **So what are the clinical implications of S_3?**
    Quite a few. S_3 is such an accurate predictor of poor systolic function (and elevated atrial pressure) that its absence argues in favor of an ejection fraction >30%. In patients with congestive heart failure, S_3 is the best predictor for response to digitalis and overall mortality. If associated with elevated jugular venous pressure, it predicts more frequent hospitalizations and worse outcome. S_3 also is the most significant predictor of cardiac risk during noncardiac surgery. Even in the absence of other signs of decompensation, it can identify patients at risk of perioperative or postoperative failure and infarction. If preoperative diuresis is *not* instituted, it also can predict mortality. Finally, presence of S_3 in mitral regurgitation reflects worse disease (i.e., higher filling pressure, lower ejection fraction, and more severe regurgitation).

> **Pearl:**
> You diagnose mitral regurgitation in systole, but you assess its severity in diastole.

94. **Which conditions are responsible for an S_3 of diastolic overload?**
    - **Intracardiac or intravascular shunts,** such as a ventricular septal defect (VSD) or a patent ductus arteriosus (PDA). Note that an *atrial* septal defect is *not* responsible for diastolic overload of the left ventricle because the right-to-left atrial shunt actually *decreases* the transmitral flow (while the increased *tricuspid* flow is much less likely to cause a *right*-sided S_3).
    - **Mitral regurgitation (MR)** with increased diastolic flow across the mitral valve. Here, S_3 is louder and higher pitched than the more typical S_3, almost resembling an opening snap. S_3 in MR does not necessarily indicate heart failure, but it *does* indicate a severe regurgitation.

95. **What about the diastolic overload of aortic regurgitation (AR)?**
    In contrast to mitral regurgitation, presence of S_3 in chronic *AR does* indicate left ventricular dysfunction. In fact, it may help with selecting patients for catheterization and valve replacement.

96. **What is the effect of pulmonary hypertension on the S_3 due to diastolic overload?**
    It depends. If the diastolic overload is caused by a left-to-right shunt (such as VSD or PDA), the development of *pulmonary hypertension* will gradually decrease the shunt and thus reduce the transmitral flow across. This will progressively soften S_3 and eventually eliminate it—an important clue to the development of Eisenmenger's syndrome. In these patients, the return of an audible S_3 usually indicates development of a new *right*-sided (and *not* left-sided) failure.

97. **What is Eisenmenger's syndrome?**

It is any left-to-right shunt complicated by pulmonary hypertension, shunt reversal, and cyanosis. This is usually more common with patent ductus arteriosus or ventricular septal defects, and less with atrial septal defects. The syndrome was first described by the German physician Victor Eisenmenger (1864–1932).

98. **Is S_3 common in *aortic stenosis* (AS)?**

No, it's actually *uncommon*. When present, it indicates ventricular decompensation and elevated filling pressure. Aortic stenosis is otherwise more frequently associated with S_4.

99. **How common is S_3 during a *myocardial infarction*?**

Not uncommon in the early stages, but resolving in matter of days or weeks. In fact, a persistent post infarction S_3 has ominous implications, predicting greater myocardial damage, higher likelihood of congestive heart failure, and worse mortality.

100. **Is S_3 always generated by the left ventricle?**

No. It also can be generated by the *right* ventricle, through the same mechanisms of either ventricular dysfunction/flaccidity or increased transvalvular flow.

101. **Which disease processes are associated with a *right*-sided S_3?**

Processes characterized by either increased blood flow across the tricuspid valve (because of severe TR) or increased impedance to right ventricular emptying (because of cor pulmonale or massive pulmonary embolism).

102. **How can you differentiate right from left ventricular S_3?**

Mostly through the different location (the *right-sided S_3* is best heard over the left lower sternal border/epigastric area, and not at the apex). Response to respiration also will be different (Fig. 11-6): the right-sided S_3 gets louder with *inspiration*, whereas the left-sided gets louder with *exhalation* (Carvallo maneuver). Finally, a right-sided S_3 is often associated with a parasternal "lift" (*see* Chapter 10, Cardiovascular Exam, question 129).

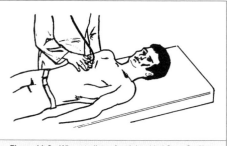

Figure 11-6. Where to listen for right-sided S_3 or S_4. Note the use of the bell of the stethoscope. (Adapted from Tilkian AG, Conover MB: Understanding Heart Sounds, 3rd ed. Philadelphia, WB Saunders, 1993.)

103. **What is the differential diagnosis of S_3?**

- **A split S_2:** In contrast to S_3, a split S_2 is higher pitched (and thus best heard through the diaphragm) and "basilar." It also has respiratory variations, but does *not* soften with either a sitting or standing position.
- **Tumor (plop):** The hallmark of this sound is its cycle-to-cycle variability, which is *not* a feature of S_3.
- **Pericardial knock and opening snap:** In contrast to S_3, both the knock and the snap (OS) are medium- to high-frequency sounds—thus best detected through the diaphragm.

104. How can S_3 be further differentiated from an opening snap (OS)?

S_3 occurs a little later in diastole than OS (and much later than the split S_2): 120 msec after A_2 (and often even later), as opposed to 100 msec for OS. Although this may seem trifling to the untrained ear, it can actually help differentiate the two sounds. In addition, S_3 is softer, lower pitched, and heard through the bell. Finally, because the left ventricle is usually small in mitral stenosis, OS tends to be a little closer to the *left sternal border* than S_3 (which is instead loudest at the apex).

105. How common is S_3 in mitral stenosis (MS)?

Very *uncommon*. In fact, *presence* of S_3 argues strongly against significant stenosis because the valvular obstruction of MS prevents the rapid left ventricular early diastolic filling that is so crucial for the genesis of S_3.

Fourth Heart Sound (S_4)

106. What is an S_4?

It is a low-pitched, soft, *late* diastolic (and thus, *pre*systolic) extra sound. It is much more common than S_3, but never physiologic. Still, some authors consider it a "normal" sound of aging, due to the reduction in ventricular compliance that results from either hypertrophy (i.e., hypertension) or fibrosis (i.e., ischemia)—two time-honored companions of old age.

107. How is S_4 best detected?

Very much like the S_3: over the apex, through the bell, and in left lateral decubitus. Note that S_4 (and S_3) are often inaudible in a supine position and become transiently more evident *only upon assuming a left-lateral decubitus* position. As in the case of S_3, a firm pressure on the bell will usually soften or eliminate S_4.

108. Can S_4 be palpable?

Yes, as a presystolic movement. This is best detected in the left-lateral decubitus position and over many cardiac cycles (because of its respiratory variation). In fact, S_4 is often easier to palpate than S_3, thus allowing for a bedside differentiation between these two diastolic extra sounds. A palpable S_4 should always be considered pathologic (conversely, an S_4 that is *only audible* can often be a simple by-product of aging).

109. How common is S_4? Can it be normal?

It depends on the method used to detect it. By phonocardiography, it is so common that it may indeed reflect no true pathology. In fact, S_4 can be *recorded* in 75% of normal middle-aged subjects, as a response to the effects of aging on ventricular compliance. Still, an *audible*, *loud*, and even *palpable* S_4 reflects almost always an underlying pathology—independent of the patient's age. Even in older adults (where it may be common even in the absence of clear-cut pathology), the presence of a *distinctly audible S_4* should suggest underlying disease. Indeed, follow-up of these "normal" patients usually reveals coronary artery pathology.

110. Can S_4 occur in younger individuals?

Yes. It has been recorded in younger subjects with no clear underlying pathology, but just an increase in blood flow.

111. What are the auscultatory differences between S_3 and S_4?

S_4 is higher pitched, louder, shorter, and, of course, differently timed, since it is late diastolic and thus *preceding S_1* (which serves as an important reference point). S_3 is instead early diastolic and thus *following S_2*. Both vary with respiration (S_3 more prominently than S_4).

112. **Why is S$_4$ late diastolic?**

Because it is generated immediately *before ventricular systole*. Hence, it is *pre*systolic.

113. **How is S$_4$ produced?**

By atrial contraction, primarily left sided, but at times right sided, too. Yet, it is *not* generated by atrial systole per se, but by the resulting forceful tension of the *ventricle/A-V valve apparatus*. Hence, S$_4$ is often more persistent than S$_3$, since its reason (strong atrial contraction) is usually chronic.

114. **What is the hemodynamic significance of an S$_4$?**

Not as ominous as that of S$_3$. S$_4$ corresponds to an increase in *late* ventricular diastolic pressure, but in contrast to S$_3$, it reflects normal atrial pressure, normal cardiac output, and normal ventricular diameter. It also is associated with loud S$_1$ and S$_2$, since ventricular systole is usually adequate, and many patients are even hypertensive.

115. **What are the clinical implications of S$_4$?**

More benign that those of S$_3$, insofar as S$_4$ has no adverse postoperative implications. It is even questionable whether it predicts severity of AS. It simply indicates a hypertrophic but *compensated* ventricle, with reduced ventricular distensibility and decreased *passive* filling in early to mid-diastole. This places greater demand on the atria, which now have to handle 30–40% of the entire ventricular filling (instead of the usual 20%). The resulting stronger atrial *kick* will rush blood into the noncompliant ventricle and thus produce S$_4$, which in tachycardic patients may assume a gallop cadence. Hence, S$_4$ indicates *diastolic* rather than systolic dysfunction.

116. **Which disease processes can cause an S$_4$?**

Diseases with ventricles so thick to require a strong atrial contraction (in fact, P waves may also become prominent). Among these are:

- **Hypertension,** either systemic or pulmonary (note that S$_4$ may precede the electrocardiographic signs of ventricular hypertrophy)
- **Aortic stenosis** (where S$_4$ is usually associated with a gradient >70 mmHg)
- **Coarctation of the aorta**
- **Hypertrophic cardiomyopathy** (an audible, and palpable, S$_4$ is almost a *sine qua non* for this condition)
- **Coronary artery disease** (S$_4$ can be heard in as many as 90% of patients with myocardial infarction)
- **Prolonged P-R interval**

117. **What happens when these hypertrophic ventricles fail?**

Once ventricular *hypertrophy* evolves into ventricular *failure* (with a dilated and flaccid ventricle), the S$_4$ gradually softens and eventually disappears, leaving in its place an S$_3$. Hence, S$_4$ implies an earlier, more compensated (and less severe) ventricular dysfunction.

118. **How common is S$_4$ in *myocardial infarction* (MI)?**

Very common early on, and overall benign, given the ventricular stiffness of ischemia. Yet the presence of S$_4$ at more than 1 month after MI does predict higher 5-year mortality.

119. **Can S$_4$ occur in *mitral regurgitation*?**

Only if acute. Otherwise, mitral regurgitation is typically associated with an *S$_3$*.

120. **Can a right-sided S$_4$ be differentiated from a *left*-sided one?**

Yes. Like the right-sided S$_3$, a right-sided S$_4$ is best heard over the lower-left sternal border or subxiphoid areas. At times, it may even be heard over the neck veins. Also, a right-sided S$_4$ is commonly associated with other signs of right ventricular strain, like distended neck veins with large A or V waves, a loud P_2, and a right ventricular heave. Finally, as with all right-sided findings, a right-sided S_4 is usually louder in *inspiration*.

121. Can patients with atrial fibrillation have an S_4?
No, since they cannot muster an adequate atrial contraction. The same applies to atrial flutter.

122. What is the differential diagnosis of an S_4?
- A **split S_1**: In contrast to S_4, a split S_1 (1) widens (or shortens) with respiration in one third of patients, (2) does not soften upon standing or sitting, (3) is best heard with the diaphragm, and (4) presents all the way up to the upper left sternal border (the S_4, instead, is mostly localized over the apex or lower sternal border).
- **S_1-ejection click (sound) complex:** This may easily simulate an S_4–S_1 complex and thus be difficult to separate. In contrast to S_4, both S_1 and ES are medium to high pitched and thus best heard with the diaphragm. They also do not soften when the patient assumes an upright position (as does the S_4). Finally, ES is usually audible all the way up to the base, intensifying with *exhalation* when pulmonic in origin. Note that although S_4 can be palpable (as a presystolic impulse), a split S_1 and the ES can only be audible.

Opening Snap

123. What is an opening snap?
It is a pathologic, loud, snapping, short, high-pitched, and early diastolic extra sound of patients with mitral (or tricuspid) stenosis. It is loudest over the lower left sternal border (a little less at the apex), and is best heard by either using the diaphragm or by applying firm pressure on the bell (thus converting it into a diaphragm). It is produced by the tensing and deceleration of a stenotic but still mobile A-V valve (Fig. 11-7). In this, it resembles the snapping of a sail that is filling with wind. Note that in *mitral* stenosis, much of the snapping is produced by the filling of the *anterior* leaflet, which is larger and more mobile than the posterior.

124. Why are these sounds called "snaps"?
Because of convention. Extra sounds produced by the atrioventricular valves are

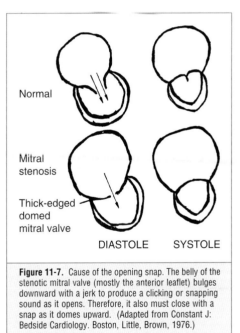

Figure 11-7. Cause of the opening snap. The belly of the stenotic mitral valve (mostly the anterior leaflet) bulges downward with a jerk to produce a clicking or snapping sound as it opens. Therefore, it also must close with a snap as it domes upward. (Adapted from Constant J: Bedside Cardiology. Boston, Little, Brown, 1976.)

normally referred to as *snaps* (if occurring in *diastole* and caused by the abnormal opening of the leaflets) and *clicks* (if occurring in *systole* and caused by the prolapse and backward ballooning of the leaflets). Clicks of A-V prolapse are usually mid- to late-systolic, although they also can be early systolic, but in this case, they are more commonly due to abnormal *semilunar* ejection and thus referred to as ejection *sounds*.

125. **Is the opening of a normal atrioventricular valve audible?**
No. Only in patients with hyperkinetic heart syndrome, the increase in blood flow may render it audible. This, however, represents more the exception than the rule. In all other cases, an audible sound of A-V opening indicates thickening and stiffening of leaflets, making them behave like a sail that suddenly fills under wind—with ballooning, billowing, and a final snap caused by the tight grip of the chordae.

126. **How can one distinguish an opening snap from the closing of S_2?**
By their different timing. There is usually enough separation between the closing of the aortic valve (A_2) and the opening of the mitral valve to make them perceived as two separate acoustic events. This interval is around 100 ms and is commonly referred to as the A_2–OS.

127. **Does the *timing* of OS (i.e., the length of A_2–OS) reflect the severity of stenosis?**
Yes: the earlier the snap, the worse the stenosis. OS timing is controlled by:
- The pressure in the left atrium at the time of mitral opening (the greater the pressure, the earlier the snap)
- The heart rate (bradycardia delays the snap, whereas tachycardia anticipates it)
- The stiffness of the mitral valve (the stiffer the valve, the longer the A_2–OS and thus the later the snap)
- Myocardial contractility (ventricular dysfunction lengthens the A_2–OS and *delays* the snap)
- The closing pressure for the aortic valve (the higher the aortic pressure, the later the snap)

128. **Does the intensity of OS reflect the severity of stenosis?**
Yes. A soft (or absent) snap suggests a stiff and poorly mobile mitral valve, usually *calcific* (although it also might reflect the thickness of the chest wall, or the degree of emphysema). Other conditions that also may *soften* OS include *heart failure, a very large right ventricle* (which pushes the *left* ventricular wall away from the chest surface), and *pulmonary hypertension* (that reduces flow at both the mitral and pulmonic levels). Conversely, increased venous return (and raised left atrial pressure) *increases the intensity* of the snap. This can occur after leg raising or mild exercise, like turning from supine to the left decubitus position.

129. **How common is an opening snap in patients with mitral stenosis?**
Common. In the absence of calcification, it occurs in 75–90% of all patients. It usually reflects a milder form of the disease and thus is absent in more advanced (and calcific) cases.

130. **How can one distinguish the pulmonary sound of a split S_2 from an opening snap?**
With difficulty. Both P_2 and OS are high pitched and short. And the time interval between A_2 and P_2 is similar to that between A_2 and OS (both are 30–100 msec). Hence, to separate P_2 from OS, you should rely on (1) *the area of maximum intensity* (OS is louder at the lower left sternal border/apex, whereas P_2 is louder at the base); (2) *the respiratory variations* (in the absence of left bundle branch block, the *expiratory* widening of a "split S_2" is more likely to represent an opening snap than an A_2–P_2 complex); and (3) *the intensity of S_1* (a soft S_1 tends to exclude an opening snap). In case of pulmonary hypertension, the best way to differentiate P_2 from OS is *not* the apical intensity of the sound (which can be quite loud), but its respiratory variations.

131. **What is a *tricuspid* opening snap?**
It is the opening sound of a stenotic tricuspid valve. This may occur in 5% of MS patients.

132. **How can one differentiate a mitral from a tricuspid opening snap?**
By respiration. Like all right-sided findings, the tricuspid opening snap is louder in *inspiration*. The OS of mitral stenosis is instead louder in *exhalation*.

Pericardial Knock

133. **What is a pericardial knock?**
It is a sharp, loud, and high-pitched early diastolic sound that coincides with initial ventricular filling. Hence, it represents a special form of S_3, even though louder, earlier, and higher pitched. It is best detected by placing the diaphragm between the apex and left sternal border.

134. **How is the pericardial knock produced?**
By sudden deceleration of the left ventricle, as it encounters a thick and calcific pericardium. This is a mechanism similar to that of S_3, even though the deceleration of the knock is even more abrupt—hence, its loudness.

135. **Is the pericardial knock common in acute pericarditis?**
No. It is always absent in acute/subacute pericarditis (where, instead, the *rub* is a more typical finding). Even in tamponade, knocks are absent. Conversely, they are encountered in 30–90% of patients with *chronic calcific and constrictive pericarditis*. This used to be the sequela of an old tuberculous process, but nowadays is usually the result of coronary artery bypass surgery.

136. **What other physical findings may accompany constrictive pericarditis?**
- **Findings of right-sided heart failure:** Hepatomegaly (90–100%), ascites (50–90%), leg edema (60%), and often anasarca. The key feature, however, is distention of neck veins (present in 98% of cases), with typically deep X and Y descents that mimic on tracing an "M" or "W." The deep "Y" (Friedreich's sign present in 60–90% of cases) is due to the fact that ventricular filling is only impaired at the very end of diastole.
- **Kussmaul's sign:** Inspiratory *distention* (and not collapse) of the neck veins. This is present in one half of patients with constriction.
- **Pulsus paradoxus:** This can be present in up to 40% of the cases, but *only* in the low range of 10–20 mmHg (*see* Chapter 2, question 92).
- **Systolic retraction of the apical impulse** (*see* Chapter 10, questions 134 and 135): This occurs in 90% of cases.

137. **What is the differential diagnosis of a pericardial knock?**
S_3 and *opening snap (OS)*. The knock occurs later than OS and is much louder and higher pitched than S_3. Since it can be well heard over the pulmonic area, it also may need to be differentiated from a split S_2, which has respiratory variations, lack of transmission to the apex, and shorter interval.

Mitral (or Tricuspid) Valve Myxoma

138. **What is a tumor plop?**
It is a sound produced by the diastolic prolapse of a pedunculated left (or right) atrial myxoma, billowing back through either the mitral or tricuspid orifice. It is rare (being present in only 10% of myxoma patients), but does go into the differential diagnosis of an early diastolic extra sound, together with S_3, the opening snap, the pericardial knock, and the split S_2. Its hallmark is *variability*, insofar as it is intermittent and varying in *intensity, timing,* and *quality*. Changes in body posture may occasionally induce a sudden drop in blood pressure (with or without syncope). This is due to a transient obstruction by the tumor of the diastolic ventricular flow.

(2) Systolic Extra Sounds

Early Systolic Click (i.e., Ejection Sound)

139. **What is an ejection sound (ES)?**
It is a high-pitched and clicky early systolic sound that is often louder than S_1 and always best heard through the diaphragm. It used to be referred to as *ejection "click"* (*or early systolic click*), but nowadays is most commonly called the *ejection "sound,"* since this avoids confusion with the mid/late systolic *click* of atrioventricular prolapse.

140. **What is the mechanism of production?**
Ejection sounds are produced by blood flowing across the semilunar valves and into the large vessels (Fig. 11-8). Thus, they are normal, but usually inaudible, components of S_1. Only in disease, however, they become loud enough to be identifiable as separate *acoustic events*. In patients with *no* cardiovascular pathology, *ejection sounds* are usually the result of a *hyperkinetic heart syndrome*. In patients *with* cardiovascular pathology, they reflect instead one of two processes:

- The opening (or doming) of a congenitally bicuspid semilunar valve with/without stenosis
- A dilatation of the aortic (or pulmonic) root. The enlarged trunk creates the sound through its sudden tensing in early systole. This is invariably associated with arterial stiffening or high pressure in the corresponding vascular bed (i.e., pulmonary or systemic hypertension).

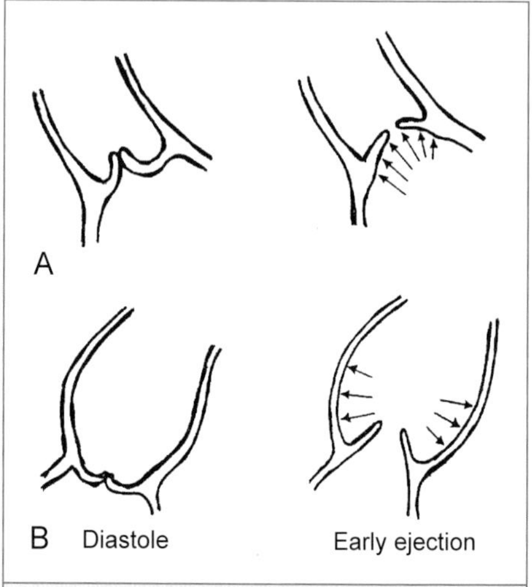

Figure 11-8. Origin of ejection sounds. *A,* Ejection sound or click produced by the opening motion of a thickened, often stenotic aortic or pulmonary valve. *B,* Ejection sound produced by the sudden tensing of the proximal aorta or pulmonary artery during early ejection. This is usually associated with a dilated and/or hypertensive great vessel. (Adapted from Abrams J: Essentials of Cardiac Physical Diagnosis. Philadelphia, Lea & Febiger, 1987.)

141. **How do you distinguish an aortic from a pulmonic ejection sound?**
- By their different **location** (left upper parasternal border for the pulmonic, apex for the aortic—even though the latter also can be heard over the aortic area).
- By their different **response to respiration:** The aortic ES has constant intensity throughout respiration, whereas the pulmonic gets louder in exhalation and softer in inspiration because the ballooning of the pulmonic valve (which causes the sound) tends to be less in inspiration, due to the increase in venous return that, in turn, causes a stronger right atrial contraction. The inspiratory softening (and even disappearing) of the pulmonary ES is very much in contrast to the respiratory behavior of *all* other right-sided findings, whose intensity *increases* during inspiration, while *decreasing* during exhalation (Rivero-Carvallo maneuver).

142. **Can an ejection sound be accompanied by a systolic *murmur*?**
Yes. In fact, ejection *sounds* due to a bicuspid valve are often immediately followed by an ejection *murmur*. This is caused by a relative stenosis of the bicuspid valve, leading, in turn, to a post-stenotic dilation of the aortic (or pulmonic) root. The dilation further enhances the ejection sound, thus perpetuating the cycle. Hence, an ejection sound identifies a concomitant systolic murmur as *pathologic* and places the cause of the stenosis at the valvular level.

143. **And so, what causes an aortic ES?**
   - **Forceful ejection** of blood into a *normal* aortic root (as it may occur in high output states, like AR) or *normal* ejection of blood into a *stiffened and dilated* aortic root (as may occur in patients with hypertension, atherosclerosis, aortic aneurysm, or aortic regurgitation)
   - **Normal ejection** of blood through an *abnormal aortic valve*. This is either a native trileaflet valve that has been stiffened and fused by a rheumatic process or (more commonly) a congenital bicuspid valve.

144. **Where is the aortic ES best heard?**
It depends. In patients with semilunar valve disease, it is well heard at the base, but even better at the *apex*. In some cases, the apex may actually be the only area where the ES is detectable. This is also true in patients with emphysema. When the ES originates from the aortic *root*, it is best heard throughout the *sash* area of aortic projection (from the apex to the right shoulder), with highest intensity at the base. The aortic ejection sound is also best heard with the patient sitting up and in held exhalation.

145. **What is the significance of an aortic ejection sound in *aortic stenosis*?**
It argues in favor of *valvular* AS (ejection sounds are absent in both *subvalvular* and *supravalvular* AS). More importantly, an ejection sound argues in favor of a *bicuspid* aortic valve.

146. **What is the clinical significance of the *intensity* of an aortic ES?**
It reflects the *mobility* of the valve; therefore, ES will soften with fibrosis and disappear with calcification (usually indicating a transvalvular gradient >50 mmHg)—hence, the higher prevalence of ejection sounds in young individuals, whose stenotic valves tend to be more pliable and mobile than those of the elderly.

147. **Can the opening of a *pulmonary* bicuspid valve be responsible for an ejection sound?**
Yes. In patients with valvular pulmonic stenosis, the sudden opening and upward movement of a dome-shaped valve will generate an ejection sound.

148. **Does a pulmonic ejection sound indicate severity of pulmonary stenosis (PS)?**
To the contrary. It indicates mild to moderate disease (which is intuitive, since *ejection sounds* reflect mobility of the valve). Only rarely does it correlate with right ventricular pressure >70 mmHg. In more severe PS cases, the ES tends to occur earlier, either merging with S_1 or preceding it.

149. **What is the significance baseline of the *intensity* of a pulmonic ES?**
Not as valuable as that of an *aortic* ES. In fact, a softer click may occur in both mild and severe forms of valvular PS. Still, given the baseline intensity of the click, *this* will vary with respiration (louder in exhalation and softer in inspiration), as does the intensity of the systolic ejection murmur that may accompany it.

150. **What causes a nonvalvular pulmonic ejection sound?**
Two possible mechanisms, both taking place in the pulmonary *artery*.

- **Pulmonary hypertension:** The ES is caused by ejection of blood into a stiffened pulmonary trunk. The timing of the sound correlates with pulmonary artery diastolic pressure—the higher the pressure, the later the systolic occurrence of ES.
- **Dilation of the pulmonary artery:** Contrary to the *valvular* pulmonic ejection sound, these two *arterial* ES remain constant throughout respiration.

151. **What is the differential diagnosis of an ejection click?**
The most difficult is its differentiation from a split S_1. Less difficult is the separation from either S_4 (softer, lower pitched, *preceding* S_1, and best detected through the bell) or a mid/late systolic click (high pitched and loud as the ejection sound, but timed a bit later in systole).

152. **What is the Means-Lerman scratch of hyperthyroidism?**
It is a raspy and scratchy systolic sound heard over the pulmonary artery of patients with hyperthyroidism. Described in 1932 by the American physicians J. Lerman and J.H. Means, it resembles a combination ejection murmur/ejection sound. It also can resemble a pericardial friction rub, since it has similar grating qualities and an increase in exhalation. In fact, the Means-Lerman scratch *is* caused by the rubbing of a hyperdynamic pericardium against the pleura. It is less common than the other cardiovascular findings of hyperthyroidism, such as *tachycardia* (with 90% of patients having a resting heart rate >90 beats/minute); *bounding peripheral pulses*; *wide pulse pressure*; *active precordium*; *louder heart sounds*; and a *systolic ejection murmur* (in up to 50% of cases). Moreover, *Means-Lerman* is not exclusive of thyrotoxicosis, having been described in other hyperdynamic conditions, such as anemia or fever.

Mid- to Late-Systolic Click

153. **What are mid- to late-systolic click(s)?**
They are short, high-pitched, and clicky extra sounds that are best heard over the apex and left-lower parasternal area. The diaphragm of the stethoscope, various bedside maneuvers, and a left-lateral decubitus position may all be necessary to bring them out.

154. **What is the clinical significance of a single (or multiple) mid- to late-systolic click(s)?**
It indicates the presence of mitral (or tricuspid) valve prolapse (MVP). In fact, simple identification of a typical click and/or murmur complex suffices—no further testing is needed.

155. **What are the auscultatory characteristics of a systolic click due to MVP?**
The major one is *variability* from cycle to cycle: in intensity, number, and timing. Clicks also may acquire association with late-systolic murmur and even fade enough to elude unskilled clinicians. At times, they may be multiple, further confusing the inexperienced observer.

156. **Why do clicks of mitral valve prolapse not occur in early systole?**
Because they have different modes of generation:
- **Early systolic clicks** are *ejection* sounds due to blood flowing across the semilunar valves and into the arterial root (aortic or pulmonic). Hence, they occur at the beginning of ventricular ejection (i.e., early systole).
- **Mid- to late-systolic clicks,** on the other hand, are *regurgitant* sounds caused by the posterior *billowing* of a mitral leaflet. Since this requires a significant decrease in left ventricular size, mid-systolic clicks *usually* take place during mid to late systole.
Yet, as always in medicine, there are exceptions that confirm the rule. Some clicks of prolapse, for example, may either follow or overlap with S_1 (thus creating a loud summation sound). These are usually caused by a billowing so severe to occur even in the large and distended ventricle of early systole.

157. How can one recognize MVP when the click coincides with S_1?

By the combination of a holosystolic murmur of regurgitation *plus* a loud "S_1" (which is actually the summation of S_1 *and* click). A loud S_1 is otherwise uncommon in patients with simple MR.

158. What are the acoustic characteristics of the click(s)?

The click(s) is mid to late systolic, loudest over the apex or left sternal border, and at times multiple. In two thirds of the cases, it precedes the murmur; in one third, it immediately follows it.

159. How are these clicks generated?

By the combined backward snapping of a prolapsing mitral leaflet and the sudden stretch of its chordal apparatus (*chordal snap*). This would also explain the occasional multiple clicks. Yet, some authors have argued that the contraction of the papillary muscles may actually *prevent* the leaflet from prolapsing directly back into the atrium. In this case, the click might be due to the *ballooning* of the leaflet itself, very much like the sound of a sail suddenly filled by wind.

160. Which bedside maneuvers can change the timing of an MVP click/murmur?

Maneuvers that modify left ventricular *diameter* (Fig. 11-9). For a more detailed discussion, please refer to Chapter 12, questions 22, 24, 178, and 179.

161. Are mid- to late-systolic clicks always associated with a late systolic murmur?

Not at all. If associated, however, they suggest the presence of mitral valve prolapse *with* regurgitation. Yet, many MVP patients have only the click (or clicks). Since presence of a murmur (and thus *regurgitation*) may vary from day to day and cycle to cycle, this affects the issue of prophylaxis. Many cases of endocarditis have been documented in patients with only a mid-systolic click, suggesting that regurgitation may only occur at times. Yet, the general consensus is that clickers stay clickers and murmurers stay murmurers.

162. Can patients with MVP present with a diastolic click?

Yes. 5–15% of all MVP patients have indeed an *early diastolic* click. This is still caused by the ballooning of the mitral leaflet, albeit *in a reversed* direction.

163. What is the differential diagnosis of a mid-systolic click?

It depends on timing. Earlier clicks tend to be confused with *ejection* sounds, split S_1, or even S_4 (which, however, is softer and lower pitched). Mid to late clicks, on the other hand, can be confused for a split S_2 or, even for an S_2/opening snap complex. Presence of a late-systolic murmur following the click may further confuse, suggesting an opening snap/diastolic rumble complex. Finally, multiple systolic clicks also may be confused for pericardial friction rubs.

E. PERICARDIAL FRICTION RUB

164. What are the auscultatory characteristics of a pericardial friction rub?

It is a scratching, scraping, grating, crackling, crunchy, squeaky, creaking, and typically fleeting *noise,* heard in patients with inflammation of the pericardial layers. It is very different from a murmur or an extra sound. In fact, it was first described by Collin in 1820 as the "crackling of new leather." Because of its high frequency, it is best heard by applying firm pressure on the diaphragm of the stethoscope, so that the tensing of the skin may further help transmission.

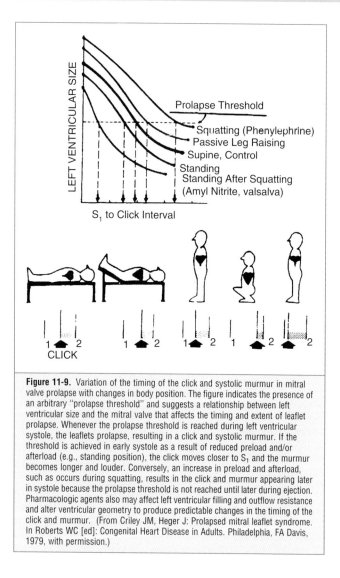

Figure 11-9. Variation of the timing of the click and systolic murmur in mitral valve prolapse with changes in body position. The figure indicates the presence of an arbitrary "prolapse threshold" and suggests a relationship between left ventricular size and the mitral valve that affects the timing and extent of leaflet prolapse. Whenever the prolapse threshold is reached during left ventricular systole, the leaflets prolapse, resulting in a click and systolic murmur. If the threshold is achieved in early systole as a result of reduced preload and/or afterload (e.g., standing position), the click moves closer to S_1 and the murmur becomes longer and louder. Conversely, an increase in preload and afterload, such as occurs during squatting, results in the click and murmur appearing later in systole because the prolapse threshold is not reached until later during ejection. Pharmacologic agents also may affect left ventricular filling and outflow resistance and alter ventricular geometry to produce predictable changes in the timing of the click and murmur. (From Criley JM, Heger J: Prolapsed mitral leaflet syndrome. In Roberts WC [ed]: Congenital Heart Disease in Adults. Philadelphia, FA Davis, 1979, with permission.)

165. **How many components are in a rub?**
    As many as three: (1) one occurring anywhere in systole, although most commonly in mid-systole (and thus corresponding to ventricular contraction) and (2) two occurring instead in *early* and *late* diastole (and thus corresponding respectively to early ventricular filling and atrial contraction). These may give the rub a peculiar lilt, almost gallop-like.

166. **Do rubs always present with three components?**
    No. The systolic component is always present, but the diastolic ones may be absent, especially the *atrial*. In a review of 100 patients with pericardial friction rubs, Spodick found that around 50% had three components, 30% had two components, and only 15% had just one.

167. **Where are rubs best heard?**

    Throughout the precordium, although more than 80% tend to be louder along the left parasternal area and lower-left sternal border (third and fourth interspaces). Note that rubs vary tremendously from site to site, often being audible in only a very circumscribed area.

168. **Can rubs be palpable?**

    Yes. Very loud rubs *can* be palpable (the same is true for *pleural* friction rubs). One fourth of all rubs are, in fact, palpable.

169. **What bedside maneuvers can intensify a pericardial friction rub?**

    The most common is *inspiration*: in approximately one third of the patients, rubs become louder in *deep and held inspiration* because the inspiratory descent of the diaphragm stretches the pericardium, thus making the rubbing of the two layers more likely to occur and more intense. Note, however, that rubs also may be enhanced by held *exhalation*. This brings the heart closer to the chest wall but also increases venous return to the left ventricle, thus better stretching the pericardial layers onto each other. Finally, having the patient sit up, lean forward, and rest on elbows and knees also may increase contact between the visceral and parietal pericardium and thus their rubbing (Fig. 11-10).

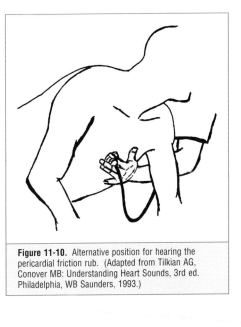

Figure 11-10. Alternative position for hearing the pericardial friction rub. (Adapted from Tilkian AG, Conover MB: Understanding Heart Sounds, 3rd ed. Philadelphia, WB Saunders, 1993.)

170. **How can one separate a pericardial from a pleural rub?**

    By asking patients to hold their breath, first in inspiration and then in exhalation. A pericardial rub will persist in at least one of the two (and usually in both), whereas a pleural rub will disappear. Remember, however, that patients with viral pleuropericarditis or Dressler's syndrome may actually have both a pleural *and* a pericardial friction rub.

171. **Which disease processes are associated with rubs?**

    - **Pericarditis**, usually acute or subacute. This can be *localized* (as in case of trauma or myocardial ischemia) or *diffuse* (viral or bacterial infections, radiation changes, uremia, and collagen vascular diseases like rheumatoid arthritis and systemic lupus erythematosus). Prevalence of rubs varies from condition to condition. In uremic pericarditis, for example, they can be heard in 14–83% of patients. Still, a rub is only one of the three diagnostic features of acute pericarditis (the others being chest pain and ECG changes).
    - **Acute myocardial infarction.** Rubs occur in 20% of cases, usually a few days into the course (they are typically absent in the first 24 hours). Rubs carry a worse prognosis, reflecting larger infarcts, more extensive coronary disease, lower ejection fractions, and a greater number of complications—including arrhythmias and pump failure (but not

tamponade). Although fleeting in simple post infarction pericarditis, rubs can last much longer in *post–myocardial infarction (Dressler's) syndrome*.

- A pericardial rub also can occur (albeit rarely) in patients with **pulmonary embolism**.
- Finally, a localized rub is often heard in patients with **metastatic involvement of the pericardium,** even though only 7% of all neoplastic effusions are associated with a rub. Curiously, in patients with known cancer who develop a rub, the finding argues against a neoplastic etiology, predicting instead either an idiopathic or a radiation-induced process.

172. **Does the presence of a rub exclude a pericardial effusion?**
    No. One tenth of all rubs will be associated with a pericardial effusion. In fact, rubs can occur in up to one fourth of *tamponade* cases. Although this is counterintuitive, it reflects a loculated process, capable of compromising ventricular filling (the *sine qua non* of tamponade) while simultaneously allowing parts of the pericardium to rub against each other. Hence, never exclude tamponade because of a rub. Instead, measure pulsus paradoxus— especially in patients with tachycardia, tachypnea, distended neck veins, and clear lungs (*see* Chapter 2, questions 93–97).

173. **What is the differential diagnosis of a pericardial friction rub?**
    A three-component rub must be differentiated from the to-and-fro murmur of *aortic regurgitation* and the continuous murmur of *patent ductus arteriosus,* and the systo-diastolic murmur of severe mitral regurgitation (*see* "lots of noise," Chapter 12, question 263). The scratching and creaking qualities of the rub will usually help recognize it. A three-component rub also may resemble a ventricular gallop (because its early diastolic component coincides with the S_3 timing), especially in tachycardic patients, who, after all, represent the majority of pericarditis cases. To identify the rub, rely on its loudness, high frequency, and typical scratchy quality. A one-component (systolic) rub may pose the greatest diagnostic challenge, since it is often misdiagnosed as a *systolic ejection murmur.* To sort it out, monitor the sound over time: a rub will usually change in quality and intensity, often acquiring one or two diastolic components.

174. **How about constrictive pericarditis?**
    It presents with a constellation of typical findings (discussed in question 136) that often include a knock, but *rarely* a rub (present in <5% of the cases).

SELECTED BIBLIOGRAPHY

1. Benchimol A, Desser KB: The fourth heart sound in patients without demonstrable heart disease. Chest 93:298–301, 1977.
2. Breen WJ, Rekate AG: Effect of posture on splitting of the second heart sound. JAMA 173:1326–1328, 1960.
3. Constant J.: Bedside Cardiology. Boston, Little, Brown & Co, 1985.
4. Evans W, Jackson F: Constrictive pericarditis. Br Heart J 14:53–69, 1952.
5. Folland ED, Kriegel BJ, Henderson WG, et al: Implications of third heart sounds in patients with valvular heart disease. N Engl J Med 327:458–462, 1992.
6. Fontana ME, Wooley CF, Leighton RF, et al: Postural changes in left ventricular and mitral valvular dynamics in systolic click—Late systolic murmur syndrome. Circulation 51:165–173, 1975.
7. Fowler NO, Adolph RJ, et al: Fourth sound gallop or split first sound. Am J Cardiol 30:441–444, 1972.
8. Hancock EW: The ejection sound in aortic stenosis. Am J Med 40:569–577, 1966.
9. Ishikawa M, Sakata K, Maki A, et al: Prognostic significance of a clearly audible fourth heart sound detected a month after an acute myocardial infarction. Am J Cardiol 80:619–621, 1997.
10. Ishmail AA, Wing S, Ferguson J, et al: Interobserver agreement by auscultation in the presence of a third heart sound in patients with congestive heart failure. Chest 91:870–873, 1987.

11. Leatham A: The second heart sound: Key to heart auscultation. Acta Cardiol 19:395, 1964.

12. Leech G, Brooks N, Green-Wilkinson A, et al: Mechanism of influence of PR interval on loudness of first heart sound. Br Heart J 43:138–142, 1980.

13. Marcus GM, Michaels AD, De Marco T, et al: Usefulness of the third heart sound in predicting an elevated level of B-type natriuretic peptide. Am J Cardiol 93:1312–1313, 2004.

14. McGee S: Evidence-based Physical Diagnosis. Philadelphia, Saunders, 2001.

15. Nelson WP, North RL, et al: Splitting of the second heart sound in adults forty years and older. Am J Med Sci 254:805–80, 1967.

16. Patel R, Bushnell DJ, Sobotka PA: Implications of an audible third heart sound in evaluating cardiac function. West J Med 158:606–609, 1993.

17. Perloff JK, Harvey WP: Mechanisms of fixed splitting of the second heart sound. Circulation 18:998–1009, 1958.

18. Pitt A, Pitt B, Schaefer J, et al: Myxoma of the left atrium: Hemodynamic and phonocardiographic consequences of sudden tumor movement. Circulation 36:408–416, 1967.

19. Posner MR, Cohen GI, Skarin AT, et al: Pericardial disease in patients with cancer: The differentiation of malignant from idiopathic and radiation-induced pericarditis. Am J Med 71:407–413, 1981.

20. Ronan JA: Cardiac auscultation: Opening snaps, systolic clicks, and ejection sounds. Heart Dis Stroke 2:188–191, 1993.

21. Ronan JA: Cardiac auscultation: The first and second heart sounds. Heart Dis Stroke 1:113–116, 1992.

22. Ronan JA: Cardiac auscultation: The third and fourth heart sounds. Heart Dis Stroke 1:267–270, 1992.

23. Shaver JA, O'Toole JD: The second heart sound: Newer concepts. Part 2: Paradoxical splitting and narrow physiological splitting. Mod Concept Cardiovasc Dis 46:13–16, 1977.

24. Spodick DH: Pericardial rub: Prospective, multiple-observer investigation of pericardial friction in 100 patients. Am J Cardiol 35:357–362, 1975.

25. Sutton G, Harris A, Leatham A: Second heart sound in pulmonary hypertension. Br Heart J 30:743–756, 1968.

26. Van de Werf F, Geboers J, Kesteloot H, et al: The mechanisms of disappearance of the physiologic third heart sound with age. Circulation 73:877–884, 1986.

CHAPTER 12

HEART MURMURS

Salvatore Mangione, MD

> *"That the stethoscope will come in general use notwithstanding its value I am extremely doubtful, because its beneficial application requires much time and gives a great deal of trouble both to the patient and the practitioner, and because its whole hue and character is foreign and opposed to our habits and associations. It must be confessed that there is something even ludicrous in the picture of a grave physician actually listening through a long tube to the patient's thorax as if the disease within were a living being that could communicate its conditions to the sense without. Besides, there is in this method a sort of bold claim and pretension to certainty, which cannot, at first sight, but be somewhat startling to a mind deeply versed in the knowledge and uncertainties of our art, and to the calm and cautious habits of philosophizing to which the physician is accustomed. On all these accounts and others that might be mentioned, I conclude that the new method will only in a few cases be speedily adopted, and never generally."*
> —John Forbes, preface to his translation of R.T.H. Laënnec, *De L'Auscultatione Mediate*. London, T. & J. Underwood, 1821.

INTRODUCTION AND BASIC ISSUES

Cardiac auscultation is the centerpiece of physical diagnosis, and recognizing murmurs is its most challenging aspect. It requires the identification of sounds jam-packed in less than 0.8 second, often overlapping, and not infrequently at the threshold of audibility. Stethoscopy is like learning a musical instrument and similarly rewarding. Hence, despite being as old as the battle of Waterloo, this little tool and its skillful use still occupy an important role in 21st-century medicine.

1. **What are the auscultatory areas of murmurs?**
   The classic ones are shown in Fig. 12-1 and Table 12-1. Auscultation typically starts in the aortic area, continuing in clockwise fashion: first over the pulmonic, then the mitral (or apical), and finally the tricuspid areas. Since murmurs may radiate widely, they often become audible in areas *outside* those historically assigned to them. Hence, "inching" the stethoscope (i.e., slowly dragging it from site to site) can be the best way not to miss important findings.

2. **What is Erb's point?**
   It is an additional and important area, located over the third/fourth interspace—just left of the sternum. It is named after the German neurologist (and pathologist) Wilhelm Heinrich Erb (1840–1921), who is otherwise more famous for his contributions in the field of neuromuscular dystrophies (Erb was to Germany what Charcot was to France, and Gowers to England. In fact, he was the first clinician to routinely use the reflex hammer in bedside examinations.) His homonymous point is an important site for the detection of aortic sounds and murmurs.

3. **How accurate is physical examination in detecting asymptomatic valvular disease?**
   Quite accurate: in fact, highly specific (98%), fairly sensitive (70%), and with positive and negative predictive values of 92%. Still, accuracy depends on the valve. For example, sensitivity

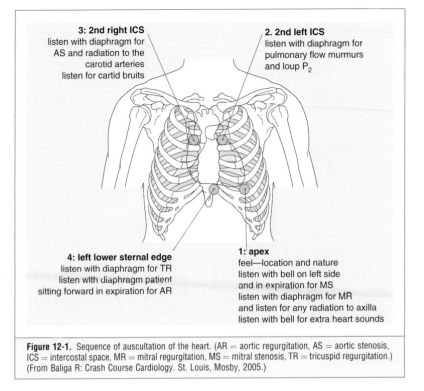

3: 2nd right ICS
listen with diaphragm for
AS and radiation to the
carotid arteries
listen for cartid bruits

2. 2nd left ICS
listen with diaphragm for
pulmonary flow murmurs
and loup P_2

4: left lower sternal edge
listen with diaphragm for TR
listen with diaphragm patient
sitting forward in expiration for AR

1: apex
feel—location and nature
listen with bell on left side
and in expiration for MS
listen with diaphragm for MR
and listen for any radiation to axilla
listen with bell for extra heart sounds

Figure 12-1. Sequence of auscultation of the heart. (AR = aortic regurgitation, AS = aortic stenosis, ICS = intercostal space, MR = mitral regurgitation, MS = mitral stenosis, TR = tricuspid regurgitation.) (From Baliga R: Crash Course Cardiology. St. Louis, Mosby, 2005.)

of exam for detecting the typical murmur of *aortic stenosis* (AS) is quite high (close to 100%), but specificity is much lower (70%) since other diseases (and many functional states) may present with a similar systolic murmur. The detection of moderate to severe mitral regurgitation (MR) has similar accuracy, very much for the same reason. Conversely, detecting moderate to severe *tricuspid* regurgitation (TR) has much higher specificity (close to 100%) since this murmur benefits from the Rivero-Carvallo confirmation. Specificity is also high for semilunar diastolic murmurs, although *sensitivity* for pulmonic regurgitation (PR) is only 15% (it is instead much higher for *aortic* regurgitation, especially if moderate to severe: close to 100%). Hence, detecting the typical murmurs of TR or PR argues very strongly for the presence of the disease. The same can be said of aortic regurgitation (AR). Conversely, absence of a typical murmur argues very strongly *against* the presence of significant AS or MR, but does *not* exclude PR or TR since these murmurs are usually very soft. Of course, *trivial regurgitation*s remain findings that are detectable by echo only.

4. **What is the clinical significance of murmurs?**
It depends on the murmur. For example, even though (almost) all diastolic and continuous findings are *pathologic* (and thus caused by *structural* abnormalities of valves, chambers, or great vessels), many systolic murmurs are *benign*.

5. **What, then, should be the approach to a newly detected murmur?**
The first step should be to use the cardiovascular exam to separate *pathologic* from *functional* murmurs (*see* below, questions 28–33). This is essential to avoid expensive and possibly

TABLE 12-1. LOCATIONS OF AUSCULTATORY SITES

Area	Prior Designation	Location	Murmurs Heard Best	Sounds Heard
Left ventricular	Mitral area	At apex impulse: extends to 3–5 LICS, 2 cm medially and laterally to left anterior axillary line. Isolated LVE: extends medially; isolated RVE may be displaced to left axila	Mitral stenosis Mitral regurgitation Aortic stenosis Aortic insufficiency IHSS Functional mid-diastolic rumble	LV S_3–LV S_4 A_2 Aortic ejection click Pericardial knock Opening snap of mitral stenosis Austin flint murmur
Right ventricular	Tricuspid area	Lower sternum and 3–5 LICS 2 cm to left and right. Isolated RVE: can extend laterally and occupy the apex	Tricuspid stenosis Tricuspid regurgitation Pulmonary regurgitation Ventricular septal defect	RV S_3 RV S_4 TV opening snap
Left atrial		Left posterior thorax between axillary line and spine at level of scapular tip	Mitral regurgitation	
Right atrial		Lower sternum and 4–5 RICS, 2 cm to right of sternum	Tricuspid regurgitation	
Aortic area	Erb's point (third left interspace)	3 LICS near sternal edge across manubrium to 1–3 RICS, may include 2 LICS, suprasternal notch, right sternoclavicular joint	Aortic stenosis Aortic insufficiency Aortic flow murmurs	A_2 Aortic ejection click
Pulmonary area		1–3 LICS adjacent to sternum, medial left intraclavicular area; posterior thorax: T4, 5 2–3 cm to either side of spine	Pulmonary stenosis Pulmonary regurgitation Pulmonary flow murmurs PDA murmur	P_2 Pulmonary ejection click
Descending thoracic area		Posterior thorax: T2–T16, 2–3 cm to either side of spine	Coarctation of aorta Aortic aneurysms Aortic stenosis Arotic stenosis	

LICS = left intercostal space, LVE = left ventricular enlargement, RVE = right ventricular enlargement, RICS = right intercostal space, IHSS = idiopathic hypertrophic subaortic stenosis, PDA = patent ductus arteriosus. LV = left ventricular, RV = right ventricular, TV = tricuspid valve. (Adapted from Abrams J: Essentials of Cardiac Physical Diagnosis. Baltimore, Williams & Wilkins, 1987.)

dangerous laboratory tests. Then, if the murmur is identified as *organic*, the physical examination should provide clues to its *site of origin*, its *hemodynamic cause*, and, possibly, its *severity*.

6. **Do the acoustic characteristics of the murmur help separate benign from pathologic?**
No. Acoustic characteristics *per se* (like *frequency* or *shape*) and even the *radiation pattern* are usually nonspecific and thus clinically unhelpful. There is only one valuable feature: the *intensity* of the murmur. Overall, benign murmurs are *softer* than pathologic ones and never louder than 3/6. Hence, they are never associated with a *palpable thrill* (which indicates grade 4 or higher).

7. **What is a thrill?**
It is a palpable vibratory sensation, often compared to the purring of a cat, and typical of murmurs caused by very high pressure gradients. These, in turn, lead to great turbulence and loudness. Hence, thrills are only present in pathologic murmurs whose intensity is >4/6.

MECHANISMS OF PRODUCTION

8. **How are murmurs produced?**
All murmurs (whether *functional* or *pathologic*) are produced by flow that becomes *turbulent enough* to cause audible vibrations in the various cardiac structures. Turbulence depends on flow *velocity*, which, in turn, depends on (1) local or concentric *narrowing* of vessels or valves (causing a pressure gradient) and (2) a sudden *change in vessel diameter*.

9. **What are the structural abnormalities that produce local narrowing and turbulent flow?**
Any of the following abnormalities in the orifice through which blood flows:
- Abnormal *size* (the smaller the orifice, the greater the turbulence; the greater the turbulence, the louder the murmur). This phenomenon also may occur when blood moves from a small into a large space, such as a dilated aortic root.
- Irregular *shape* (for example, an irregular valve opening)
- Irregular *edge* (the sharper the edge of the orifice, the higher the turbulence)

In addition to *structural* abnormalities, abnormal *blood viscosity* also can cause turbulence and murmurs (the lower the viscosity, the higher the turbulence, and thus the louder the murmur).

CLASSIFICATION

10. **How are murmurs classified?**
The first (and most important) separation is purely clinical: *pathologic* versus *functional*. The real classification, however, is based on the *phase* of the cardiac cycle where the murmur is located. Accordingly, murmurs are divided into *systolic, diastolic,* and *continuous*. This is clinically relevant, since diastolic and continuous murmurs are (almost) always pathologic, whereas systolic murmurs are often functional (Fig. 12-2).

Systolic murmurs are then further classified into *ejection* and *regurgitant*. This division, first proposed by Leatham in 1958, is based on the murmur's length and relationship to S_2. It defines *ejection* murmurs as forward flowing, crescendo-decrescendo, early to mid systolic, and ending always before S_2. Conversely, it defines *regurgitant* murmurs as backward flowing, plateau shaped, spanning *throughout* systole, and always incorporating S_2. Still, regurgitant murmurs also may be limited to late systole. In fact, they may even last *beyond* S_2. Yet, their hallmark remains the *extension into the S_2*. Although clinically valuable (regurgitant murmurs tend to be

Phonocardiogram (inspiration unless noted)	Description

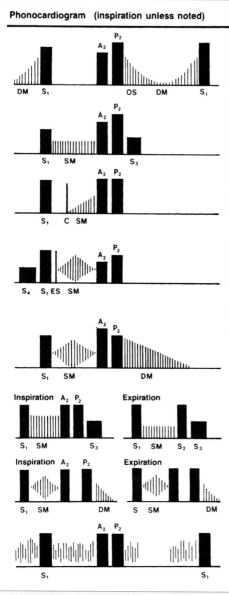

Mitral Stenosis

Precordium—Tapping apex beat; diastolic thrill at apex; parasternal lift. Auscultation—Loud S_1, P_2; diastolic opening snap followed by rumble with presystolic accentuation. Atrial fibrillation may be pulse pattern. Cold extremities.

Mitral Regurgitation

Precordium—Apical systolic thrill; apex displaced to left
Auscultation—Apical systolic regurgitant murmur following a decreased s_1; radiating to axilla; often hear S_3 due to increased left ventricular end diastolic volume.

Mitral Valve Prolapse

Most common in women younger than 30
Auscultation—A mid or late systolic click 0.14 seconds or more after S_1. Often followed by a high pitched systolic murmur; squatting may cause murmur to decrease.

Aortic Stenosis

Precordium—Basal systolic thrill; apex displaced anteriorly and laterally.
Carotids—Slow upstroke to a delayed peak.
Auscultation—A_2 diminished or paradoxically ejection systolic murmur radiating to carotids. Cold extremities.

Aortic Regurgitation

Often associated with Marfan's syndrome, rheumatoid spondylitis.
Precordium—Apex displaced laterally and anteriorly; thrill often palpable along left sternal border and in the jugular notch.
Carotids—Double systolic wave.
Auscultation—Decrescendo diastolic murmur along left sternal border; M_1 and A_2 are increased.

Tricuspid Regurgitation

Usually secondary to pathology elsewhere in heart.
Precordium—Right ventricular parasternal lift; systolic thrill at tricuspid area.
Auscultation—Holosystolic murmur increasing with inspiration; other: V wave in jugular venous pulse; systolic liver pulsation.

Atrial Septal Defect

Normal pulse; break parasternal life; lift over pulmonary artery; normal jugular pulse; systolic ejection murmur in pulmonic area; low pitched diastolic rumble over tricuspid area (at times); persistent wide splitting of S_2.

Pericarditis

Tachycardia; friction rub; diminished heart sounds and enlarged heart to percussin (with effusion); pulsus paradoxicus; neck vein distention, narrow pulse pressure and hypotension (with tamponade).

Figure 12-2. Phonocardiographic description of pathologic cardiac murmurs. (From James EC, Corry RJ, Perry JF: Principles of Basic Surgical Practice. Philadelphia, Hanley & Belfus, 1987.)

pathologic, whereas ejection murmurs are often *functional*), Leatham's classification is impractical since some regurgitant murmurs may have an ejection quality. Moreover, it relies on the bedside identification of S_2, which is not always easy. Hence, today's preference is for separating murmurs only on the basis of systolic timing (early, mid, late, and holo) and by using as reference points *both* S_1 and S_2. Accordingly:

- **Early systolic** murmurs would cluster around (and obscure) S_1.
- **Late systolic** murmurs would cluster around (and obscure) S_2.
- **Holosystolic** murmurs would obliterate both S_1 and S_2.
- **Mid-systolic** murmurs would spare them both.

11. **What are continuous murmurs?**
   They are sounds that originate outside the heart chambers and thus do not respect the systolic and diastolic boundaries of the cardiac cycle. Hence, they are driven by pressure gradients that persist *throughout* systole and diastole. This is what differentiates them from murmurs that occur *both* in systole and diastole (such as the to-and-fro of combined aortic stenosis and regurgitation) and what makes them resemble the noise of a *train in tunnel* or a *machine*.

12. **Why are systolic murmurs much more common than diastolic ones?**
   Because gradients generated in systole are much higher than those generated in diastole. Hence, systolic murmurs are more *hemodynamically likely* to occur. This is also why *diastolic* events (whether at rest or after exercise) should always be considered pathologic. Unless pathology is present, diastolic pressure gradients are too small to generate sound.

13. **Can exercise increase the intensity of a diastolic murmur?**
   Yes and no. Any increase in cardiac output (like the one of exercise, fever, or anemia) may enhance the *hemodynamic likelihood* of *any* murmur. Yet, this phenomenon still plays a greater role in systole rather than diastole.

14. **Once the phase of the cardiac cycle has been identified, which other characteristics of a murmur should be analyzed and described?**
   1. **The timing:** Murmurs can span throughout systole (*holo*systolic) or diastole (*holo*diastolic), or they may occur only in the early, mid, or late phases of each interval:
      - **Systolic murmurs:** *Holosystolic and late systolic murmurs* are clinically more important than early or mid-systolic murmurs because they are usually *pathologic*. Since benign systolic murmurs are *flow generated*, and since flow is maximal during the early part of systole, all benign systolic murmurs tend to be *short* and *early peaking*. They are never beyond S_2. In fact, a murmur that touches S_2 (whether holosystolic or late systolic) is pathologic and reflective of atrioventricular (A-V) regurgitation. Conversely, a murmur that occurs during the first half of systole (whether early or mid-systolic) is often benign and reflective of semilunar ejection. Hence, the longer the murmur, the worse the disease.
      - **Diastolic murmurs:** *Early diastolic murmurs* (starting immediately after S_2) reflect semilunar regurgitation, whereas *mid- to late-diastolic murmurs* (starting slightly after S_2) reflect A-V stenosis. Mid- to late-diastolic murmurs may extend into S_1 as a result of presystolic accentuation (due to strong atrial contraction), but are never truly *holodiastolic*. Conversely, murmurs of severe semilunar regurgitation may cover the entire length of diastole. This may provide useful clues to differential diagnosis. Note, however, that holodiastolic murmurs can be so faint in late diastole to become almost inaudible.
   2. The **intensity (or loudness):** Traditionally graded by the Levine system from 1/6 to 6/6:
      - 1/6: A murmur so soft as to be heard only intermittently and always with concentration and effort. Never immediately.
      - 2/6: A murmur that is soft but nonetheless audible immediately, and on every beat.
      - 3/6: A murmur easily audible and relatively loud
      - 4/6: A murmur relatively loud *and* associated with a palpable thrill (always pathologic)
      - 5/6: A murmur loud enough that it can be heard even by placing the edge of the stethoscope's diaphragm over the patient's chest
      - 6/6: A murmur so loud that it can be heard even when the stethoscope is not in contact with the chest, but held slightly above its surface

> **Pearl:**
> Everything else being equal, increased intensity usually reflects increased flow turbulence. Thus, a louder murmur is more likely to be pathologic and severe.

15. **Are *shape* and *frequency* of a murmur clinically useful?**

Not much. Although ejection murmurs tend to be typically crescendo-decrescendo (i.e., *diamond-shaped*), even regurgitant murmurs (such as the plateau of mitral regurgitation) may at times exhibit a late systolic accentuation. *Frequency* is instead more useful since it tends to correlate with flow velocity, which, in turn, correlates with pressure gradient. Hence, murmurs generated by high pressure gradients (such as AR) tend to be higher pitched (>300 Hz) than murmurs generated by low pressure gradients (such as MS), which are instead just 30–100 Hz. Because the human ear does not perceive well frequencies that are low, murmurs in this range are faint and subtle.

16. **What about *location* and *radiation* of a murmur?**

They are both important in differentiating systolic murmurs. For example, the *MR murmur* has an apical location and radiation to the axilla, whereas the AS murmur has a basilar location and radiation to the neck. Still, murmurs do not necessarily present with consistent location and radiation. For example, a TR murmur can at times be louder at the apex rather than the tricuspid area, especially when an enlarged right ventricle has posteriorly displaced the left ventricle.

17. **And what about the "quality" of a murmur?**

This also might help. For example, a *rough* and *harsh* systolic murmur would argue in favor of aortic stenosis, whereas a *blowing* and *musical* murmur would suggest instead mitral regurgitation. These characterizations may at times get carried away, leading to colorful descriptions—like the occasional *seagull murmur* of aortic regurgitation, a raucous sound resembling the call of a seagull that is produced by the eversion (or retroversion) of the right anterior aortic cusp.

18. **Which interventions and maneuvers can be used at the bedside to modify the intensity and characteristics of murmurs and make them more easily recognizable?**

Quite a few, all time honored and often linked to the name of the physician who first described them. They are primarily aimed at modifying *preload* (Valsalva and Rivero-Carvallo), *afterload* (handgrip), or both (squatting and standing). In addition, *variations* in length of cardiac cycle can affect not only preload and afterload, but also *contractility*.

19. **What is the effect of respiration on murmurs?**

It depends. Initially noted by Pierre Potain in 1866 (and then rediscovered by Carvallo in 1946 and Leatham in 1954), respiration has important effects on murmurs' *intensity* (not to mention on the splitting of S_2) because of its associated swings in intrathoracic pressure and venous return. As a result, all right-sided findings (*with the exception of the pulmonic ejection sound*) get louder on *inspiration* (because of greater venous return to the right ventricle). Conversely, all left-sided findings either soften or stay the same (because of decreased left-sided venous return, caused by lung pooling—or, alternatively, because of the inspiratory interposition of the pulmonary appendage between the cardiac apex and chest wall). This physiologic principle provides the basis for the Rivero-Carvallo sign/maneuver: an increase in intensity of the holosystolic murmur of TR during (or at the end of) a deep inspiration—a highly specific (100%) but not too sensitive (60%) tool for the bedside separation of TR from MR. In a study by Cha et al. of 35 patients with valvular disease, all 19 *with* Rivero-Carvallo had TR on ventriculography. Yet, of the 16 *without* Rivero-Carvallo, only five had normal ventriculography; five had 1+ regurgitation, and six had 3+/4+ regurgitation. Hence, Rivero-Carvallo is a reliable indicator of TR, but its absence does not exclude it. Since it may be difficult to hear the changes in murmur intensity *during* normal respiration, auscultation should always be carried out in two phases: first *at the end of a deep inspiration* (while the patient is in post inspiratory apnea [i.e., *holding breath* for 3 to 5 seconds]) and then *at the end of a deep expiration* (while the patient is in post expiratory apnea for 3–5 seconds). The loudness of the systolic murmur should then be compared between the two phases, remembering that *TR* will get louder in held-inspiration (and, possibly, higher pitched, too), whereas *MR* will remain unchanged or soften. Held exhalation is also useful when searching for either a pericardial rub, the soft murmur of aortic regurgitation, or the faint pulmonic mid-systolic murmur of a patient with loss of thoracic kyphosis (i.e., straight back syndrome murmur).

20. **What is the reversed Rivero-Carvallo sign?**
It is an inspiratory *reduction* in murmur intensity—reported in patients with hypertrophic obstructive cardiomyopathy (HOCM).

21. **Who was Carvallo?**
José Manuel Rivero Carvallo was a staff physician at the *Instituto Nacional De Cardiologia "Ignacio Chavez"* of Mexico City. Born in 1905, he reported his sign in 1946 as a way to separate tricuspid from mitral regurgitation. In medical folklore, he subsequently acquired a partner (Dr. Rivero, at times cited also as Rivera), who was actually just one of Carvallo's middle names. As a result, his sign/maneuver is often referred to as the Rivero-Carvallo sign.

22. **What is the effect of Valsalva on sounds and murmurs?**
Valsalva not only has important *hemodynamic* effects (that can be used for the recognition of congestive heart failure—*see* Chapter 2, questions 121–127), but may also elicit a diagnostic *auscultatory response* in patients with HOCM or mitral valve prolapse (MVP). This is mediated by a reduction in left ventricular diameter (caused by the strain), which in turn increases the left ventricular *gradient* of HOCM, thus intensifying its subvalvular systolic ejection murmur. This is the opposite of what happens to other murmurs of left ventricular outflow obstruction (such as, for example, *valvular* AS or PS), which instead *soften* with Valsalva (because of decreased venous return, with a resulting decrease in transvalvular gradients). The strain phase of Valsalva also anticipates the prolapse of a floppy mitral valve (by making the ventricle smaller, and thus "loosening up" the chordae tendineae). As a result, the click will occur earlier, and the murmur will lengthen. Hence, only two murmurs get *enhanced* by the straining phase of Valsalva: HOCM and MVP. In HOCM, the murmur gets louder, whereas in MVP it gets longer. Note that the *release period* of Valsalva may have opposite effects, based on the site of origin of the acoustic event being examined: *right*-sided murmurs will generally revert to their baseline intensity within 2–3 cardiac cycles, whereas *left*-sided murmurs will instead take a little longer (up to 5–10 cardiac cycles).

23. **Does S_2 change with Valsava?**
Yes, a widely split (but nonetheless normal) S_2 will be eliminated by the straining phase of Valsalva, whereas the fixed S_2 splitting of *atrial septal defect* will remain unchanged.

24. **What are the effects of posture on murmurs?**
Sitting, squatting, and *standing* all have profound effects on murmur characteristics. Many flow-related functional murmurs, for example, disappear upon sitting or standing (because of decreased venous return). The same occurs to the pseudo-fixed S_2 splitting of youth—separating it from the truly fixed split of atrial septal defect. Squatting/standing also can modify the findings of MVP and HOCM because squatting increases both *afterload* (by compressing femoral and iliac arteries) and *preload* (by squeezing abdominal venous content into the chest). This causes an increase in left ventricular diameter, which in turn *softens* the murmur of HOCM (less outflow obstruction) and *shortens* the one of MVP (more traction on the prolapsing valve through the tense chordae tendineae). Leg-raising in supine patients would do very much the same: *increased* venous return (and left ventricular volume/diameter) would *soften* HOCM and *shorten* MVP. Conversely, rapidly standing after 30 seconds of squatting would elicit a sudden drop in both afterload *and* preload, which, in turn, would decrease left

ventricular diameter and thus intensify the murmur of HOCM and lengthen the one of MVP (anticipating its associated click).

25. **What is isometric hand grip? What does it do to the murmur?**
Isometric hand grip is carried out by asking the patient to lock the cupped fingers of both hands into a grip, and then trying to pull them apart. The resulting increase in peripheral vascular resistance intensifies MR (and ventricular septal defect) while softening instead AS (and aortic *sclerosis*). Hence, a positive hand grip argues strongly in favor of MR. The same effect can be achieved by inflating above systolic levels two blood pressure cuffs around the patient's arms. The resulting increase in murmur intensity is even more specific for MR.

26. **What about variations in cardiac cycle?**
They also modify murmur intensity. For example, a longer diastolic pause (such as that following a premature beat) intensifies the murmur of *AS* because of lower systemic vascular resistances (due to the longer time available for aortic run-off into peripheral arteries) and higher left ventricular volume. This, in turn, increases contractility through Starling physiology, eventually resulting in higher transvalvular pressure gradients and thus a louder murmur. This triple phenomenon (lower afterload, higher preload, and increased contractility) also can be observed in situations of atrial fibrillation, where long and short cardiac cycles alternate randomly. Conversely, a murmur of *atrioventricular regurgitation* (like MR) tends to remain constant after a premature beat because the ejecting chamber has two available outlets: a normal forward/ejection one (large vessel) and an abnormal backwards/regurgitant one (atrium). This offsets the increase in ventricular contractility induced by a long diastole and thus keeps unchanged the intensity of a regurgitant murmur—even after a long diastolic phase. For instance, in the case of *MR*, the left ventricle can discharge into the left atrium (low pressure bed) or the aorta (high pressure bed). The percentage of blood ejected into each of these outlets depends on their relative resistance. After a long diastole (such as that following a premature beat), aortic resistance is decreased proportionally more than the atrial one (because even though the left atrium keeps filling during a long diastole, the aorta keeps *emptying*). As a result, although left ventricular volume is indeed higher after a premature beat (and so is contractility), proportionally more blood will be ejected into the aorta than into the atrium. This means that the regurgitant volume (and the intensity of the accompanying mitral murmur) will stay the same.

TABLE 12-2. CLASSIFICATION OF MURMURS DESCRIBED IN THIS CHAPTER*		
A. FUNCTIONAL (27–65)	**B. SYSTOLIC (66–194)**	**C. DIASTOLIC (197–258)**
Systolic	*Semilunar Ejection*	*Atrioventricular Stenosis*
• Still's murmur (46–50)	• Aortic stenosis	• Mitral stenosis (197–209)
	• Valvular (82–115)	
	• Subvalvular hypertrophic (116–128)	
	• Subvalvular "fixed" (129)	
	• Supravalvular (130)	
• Pulmonary systolic ejection murmur (51)	• Pulmonic stenosis (132–133)	• Mitral diastolic flow murmur (210)

Continued

TABLE 12-2. CLASSIFICATION OF MURMURS DESCRIBED IN THIS CHAPTER*— CONT'D

A. FUNCTIONAL (27–65)	B. SYSTOLIC (66–194)	C. DIASTOLIC (197–258)
• Supraclavicular arterial bruit (52) • Aortic sclerosis (56–65)	• Ventricular septal defect (134–138)	• Tricuspid stenosis (211–212) • Tricuspid diastolic flow murmur (213–215)
Continuous • Venous hum (53) • Mammary soufflé (54)	*AV Regurgitation* • Mitral regurgitation (142–170) • Mitral valve prolapse (171–184) • Tricuspid regurgitation (185–194)	*Semilunar Regurgitation* • Aortic regurgitation (216–251) • Pulmonic regurgitation (252–258)
Diastolic • Very rare, and always associated with either S3 or a diastolic rumble (33–34)		

*Not including continuous extracardiac murmurs like that of patent ductus arteriosus. The numbers in parentheses refer to the pertinent questions.

A. FUNCTIONAL MURMURS

27. **What are functional murmurs?**
They are *benign* findings caused by turbulent ejection into the great vessels. Functional murmurs have no clinical relevance, other than getting into the differential diagnosis of a systolic murmur.

28. **How can physical examination help differentiate functional from pathologic murmurs?**
There are two *golden* and three *silver* rules.
1. The **first golden rule** is to always judge (systolic) murmurs like people: by the company they keep. Hence, murmurs that keep *bad company* (like symptoms; extra sounds; thrill; abnormal arterial or venous pulse, ECG, or chest x-ray) should be considered pathologic until proven otherwise. These murmurs should receive lots of evaluation, technology-based included.
2. The **second golden rule** is that a diminished or absent S_2 usually indicates a poorly moving and abnormal semilunar valve. This is the hallmark of *pathology*. As a flip side, *functional* systolic murmurs are always accompanied by a well-preserved S_2, with *normal split*.
3. The **three silver rules** are:
   ■ All holosystolic (or late systolic) murmurs are pathologic.

- All diastolic murmurs are pathologic.
- All continuous murmurs are pathologic.

These silver rules are rooted in the pathogenesis of cardiac murmurs, which, in turn, relates to *intracardiac pressure gradients* and *blood flow velocity*. These are both maximal in early systole while tapering off during late systole and diastole. Hence, murmurs should never be generated during late systole or diastole. *In fact, they should never touch the S_2.* If so, they reflect a high pressure gradient and thus a *structural cardiac abnormality*. This is also why *benign systolic murmurs* should always be "ejection" (i.e., with a crescendo-decrescendo shape) and not holosystolic (i.e., starting with S_1 and ending with S_2—in plateau fashion). Hence, pay close attention to S_2, both in regard to intensity (with soft or absent S_2 arguing in favor of pathology) *and* in regard to its relation of the murmur (with murmurs that incorporate S_2 being more likely pathologic).

29. **Are these rules written in stone?**
Of course not. Yet, they remain useful for the practicing physician—simple but not simplistic. As such, keep them in mind at the bedside.

30. **So what should functional murmurs be like?**
They should be *systolic*, *short*, *soft* (typically <3/6), early peaking (never passing mid-systole), predominantly *circumscribed* to the base, and associated with a well-preserved and normally split-second sound. They should have an otherwise normal cardiovascular exam and often disappear with sitting, standing, or straining (as, for example, following a Valsalva maneuver).

31. **What should be the characteristics of "bad" systolic murmurs?**
They should be long, loud (and in fact, pathologic by definition if loud enough to generate a thrill—*see* below), late peaking, nonlocalized, and associated with a soft-to-absent S_2 that does not normally split. They also should be accompanied by other abnormal findings/symptoms.

32. **What are the synonyms for functional murmurs?**
Innocent, physiologic, benign, and systolic flow related.

33. **Can functional murmurs occur outside systole?**
Very rarely. Some innocent murmurs *may* indeed be *continuous*, and a few can even be *diastolic* (in a survey of 12,000 South African children, innocent mid-diastolic murmurs had an 0.3% prevalence). Yet, these are the exceptions that confirm the basic rule: murmurs that are either continuous or diastolic should be considered pathologic until proven otherwise.

34. **What are the causes of *benign diastolic* murmurs?**
Rapid ventricular filling—very much like the physiologic S_3. In fact, these benign diastolic murmurs are always associated with either a physiologic S_3 or some other type of benign rumbling murmur of filling (like Still's—*see* below, questions 46–50). *They never occur in isolation.*

35. **What are the clinical implications of functional murmurs?**
They are five:
- Functional murmurs are *not* caused by structural abnormalities.
- Functional murmurs do *not* have hemodynamic repercussions.
- Functional murmurs do *not* require endocarditis or antistreptococcal prophylaxis.
- Functional murmurs do *not* need any further work-up.
- Functional murmurs have an excellent long-term prognosis.

36. **How common are these functional murmurs?**
Extremely common. In young adults, systolic murmurs have a 5–52% prevalence, with echocardiography being normal in 86–100%. They also are extremely commonly in *pregnant* women, with as many as 80% having a benign ejection murmur during gestation. Finally, systolic murmurs are present in 29–60% of elderly medical outpatients or nursing home residents (*see* aortic *sclerosis*, questions 56–65), with echocardiography being normal in

44–100% of cases. *Hence, functional murmurs are the most common heart murmurs encountered by the generalist.* Indeed, each of us probably had a functional murmur at some point in life.

37. **Why are these murmurs better heard in children than adults?**
Because they are soft enough to be more easily detectable in thin subjects. Moreover, children have higher flow velocity, faster circulatory time, and more angulated great vessels—all facilitating the production of these findings. Hence, functional murmurs can be encountered in 40–50% of *children* between the ages of 2 and 14. In fact, in a study of more than 12,000 South African schoolchildren, functional murmurs had an astounding prevalence of 72%.

38. **Can functional murmurs occur immediately after birth?**
Not really. Functional murmurs are very rare *up to 2 years of age.* Hence, a murmur in a very small child should be considered pathologic until proven otherwise.

39. **Is high flow velocity present in nonpediatric patients?**
Yes. For example, in tachycardia, anemia, fever, or, quite simply, during and after exercise.

40. **How significant is a murmur that appears only after exercise, anemia, or fever?**
It might still be quite significant because:
- **Exercise** increases flow velocity and thus may elicit not only a functional but also a pathologic murmur that would be otherwise inaudible. Hence, mild exercise (such as going from supine to sitting or left lateral decubitus) can be quite helpful in unmasking subtle findings.
- **Anemia** accelerates circulatory time, which in turn elicits *innocent* findings (such as the *hemic murmur* of patients with normal valves and no pressure gradient) or possibly *pathologic ones*.
- **Fever** behaves very much like exercise and anemia.

41. **Are there other conditions where a higher stroke volume causes an ejection murmur?**
Yes. Patients with shunts, for example (due to atrial septal defect, ventricular septal defect, or patent ductus arteriosus), often present with *benign systolic ejection murmurs over the base,* all caused by an increase in pulmonary flow and stroke volume. Similarly, a bicuspid aortic valve (one of the most common congenital valvular abnormalities) also may be responsible for a benign ejection murmur. This is usually best heard over the second right interspace and is due to "doming" of the valve from an increased flow—not necessarily to an abnormal pressure gradient.

42. **Is a functional murmur always caused by an increase in flow velocity?**
Not necessarily. Although benign flow murmurs are much more likely in situations of *increased* flow velocity, they also may occur when flow *decreases*—for example, in patients with a dilated aortic or pulmonic root, which decelerates ventricular ejection. Hence, it is the rapid *change* in flow velocity (whether an increase or a *decrease*) that produces the murmur.

43. **What are the functional murmurs caused by reduced flow velocity?**
The most common is aortic *sclerosis,* wherein the aorta is dilated and tortuous.

44. **How many types of functional murmurs are known?**
There are four *systolic* murmurs and two *continuous* murmurs. There also is a *very rare* functional *diastolic* murmur of children, always associated with either Still's or a physiologic S_3.
In order of frequency, the four *systolic* murmurs are:
- Precordial vibratory murmur (Still's)
- Pulmonary ejection systolic murmur
- Supraclavicular (carotid) arterial bruit
- Aortic sclerosis murmur

The first three occur in children and adolescents, whereas the fourth one is typical of the elderly.

The two functional *continuous* murmurs are:

- Venous hum
- Mammary soufflé

45. What is the mechanism responsible for the generation of these functional murmurs?

It depends of the phase of the cardiac cycle:

- Functional **systolic** murmurs are due to rapid and vigorous ejection, across normal semilunar valves and into the large vessels. Because their site of origin is probably the large vessels themselves, these findings are loudest at the cardiac base (i.e., over the pulmonic [second to third left interspace] or aortic area [second to third right interspace]). Since the left ventricle generates higher pressures than the right, most functional systolic murmurs tend to occur over the *aortic* area.
- Functional **continuous** murmurs (like the venous hum and the mammary soufflé) are caused instead by turbulent flow in either the great veins or the great arteries.
- Finally, functional **diastolic** murmurs reflect a rapid and vigorous ventricular filling, with no intracardiac pressure gradient and no structural abnormalities. Hence, they have the same hemodynamic basis of a physiologic S_3, which they often accompany as a sort of extension. In fact, they are never an isolated finding. And yet, they are so rare as to validate the rule that *every diastolic murmur should be considered pathologic until proven otherwise.*

46. What is *Still's murmur*?

It is the quintessential innocent murmur, a mid-systolic ejection finding caused by flow across the aortic valve. It is best heard over the middle or lower left sternal border, although it often spills to the right upper sternal edge. It is soft and low pitched, with a somewhat musical quality—like plucking a rubber band or a string. In fact, it has been variously described as vibratory, twanging string, and fiddle-like. It is up to grade 3 in intensity (usually less), becomes louder with fever and increased cardiac output, and may be absent at times, usually when the child sits up or lies down. It was first described in 1909 by Dr. Still, who wrote in his pediatric textbook *Common Disorders and Diseases of Childhood*: "I should like to draw attention to a particular bruit which has somewhat of a musical character, but is neither of sinister omen nor does it indicate endocarditis of any sort. Its characteristic feature is a twangy sound, very like that made by twanging a piece of tense string. Whenever may be its origin, I think it is clearly functional, that is to say, not due to any organic disease of the heart either congenital or acquired."

47. Who has it?

One third of all children between 2 and 5. In fact, Still's is the most common innocent murmur of preschool-aged children. It also can be heard in young adults, even though it usually disappears at puberty.

48. What causes it?

No one knows for sure. Echo has failed to show anatomic differences between children *with* and children *without* the murmur, except for a recent report by Schwartz et al., who *did* find a smaller mean ascending aorta (relative to body surface area) in Still's. These children also had higher peak *ascending* and *descending* aortic velocity, suggesting that the smaller aorta may cause faster blood flow, and thus the murmur. Whatever its origin, Still's remains entirely benign.

49. What does it mean prognostically?

It means nothing. Children with Still's are normal and thus should be neither restricted in their physical activity, nor should they require endocarditis prophylaxis. Even more importantly, Still's should never be mentioned on insurance forms, school sports clearances, and dental visits.

50. **Who was Still?**

Sir Frederick George Still (1868–1941) was England's first professor of childhood medicine. A good-looking and shy man, who loved children but could not stand their mothers, Dr. Still received a solidly humanistic education, graduated from Guy's Hospital in London, and then became house physician at the Hospital for Sick Children, where he remained for the rest of his career. It was during medical school that he compiled 22 cases of children with rheumatoid arthritis, lymphadenopathy, and hepatosplenomegaly, which eventually became his doctor of medicine thesis (thus giving him, with Raynaud and Tooth, the distinction of an eponym after a medical school thesis). Dr. Still was a workaholic with a penchant for the classics, who never married but lived with his widowed mother until she died, taking her religiously to church every Sunday morning. Famous among London children for his waiting room full of toys, he retired in 1937—knighted by George VI for having been the personal physician to princesses Elizabeth and Margaret. He spent the last 4 years of his life in Salisbury, Rhodesia, where he fly fished a lot and taught English at the local church. He also wrote poetry, and the year he died he published a volume titled *Childhood and Other Poems,* which included the following lines:

For my garden is the garden of children / Cometh naught there but golden hours, / for the children are its joy and its sunshine, / and they are its Heaven-sent flowers.

51. **What is a *pulmonary* systolic ejection murmur?**

It is Still's right-sided counterpart: a systolic ejection murmur caused by flow across the *pulmonic* valve. It is heard over the mid to upper *left* sternal border, using the diaphragm due to its high frequency. P_2 is well preserved and normally split. Very common in thin adolescents, a variety of this murmur can be heard in patients with thoracic malformations that bring the pulmonary artery closer to the chest wall, such as pectus excavatum or straight back. Louder in the supine position, the pulmonary systolic ejection murmur fades upon sitting or standing.

52. **What is the *supraclavicular arterial bruit*?**

It is a murmur caused by ejection into the large vessels of the aortic arch and is best heard *above* (and not below) the clavicles, louder on the right because of the brachiocephalic arteries' branching.

53. **What is a *venous hum*?**

It is a continuous and physiologic *venous* sound—not uncommon in children, but rare in adults. For a more extensive description, refer to Chapter 10, questions 120–123.

54. **What is a *mammary souffle*?**

Not a fancy French dish, but a systolic-diastolic murmur heard over one or both breasts in late pregnancy, and typically disappearing at end of lactation. It is caused by increased flow along the mammary arteries, which explains why its systolic component starts just a little after S_1. It can be obliterated by pressing (with finger or stethoscope) over the area of maximal intensity.

55. **What can one do to sort out functional murmurs from pathologic ones?**

1. Start with **history**, specifically:
   - **Family history** (i.e., does any other family member have heart disease?)
   - **Past medical history** (antenatal and perinatal, postnatal, infancy, and childhood history)
   - **Personal history** (age murmur first heard, history of central cyanosis, feeding difficulties, poor weight gain). Also, benign murmurs should *never* present with cardiac symptoms, such as dyspnea, angina, lightheadedness, fatigue, failure to thrive, and cyanosis.
2. Then continue with the **physical examination**, looking for clubbing and cyanosis and any abnormalities in the following areas of the *cardiovascular exam*:
   - Respiratory pattern
   - Blood pressure
   - Peripheral pulses

- Neck veins exam
- Palpation of the precordium
- Palpation of the liver edge (look for hepatomegaly and a positive abdominojugular reflux)
- Auscultation of heart sounds
- Assessment of second heart sound (intensity, splitting, relation to the murmur)

3. Then carefully evaluate the murmur in its main *characteristics*, especially:
- Area of maximum intensity
- Timing and peak
- Intensity
- Quality and shape
- Transmission
- Variations with respiration
- Variations with exercise
- Variations with Valsalva maneuver (remember that the pulmonary ejection, the Still's murmur, and the venous hum all disappear with the onset of Valsalva, whereas the murmurs of HOCM and MVP increase—*see* question 22)
- Postural changes (supine position increases preload and thus exaggerates flow murmurs; squatting/standing enhances HOCM and MVP)
- Response to pharmacologic agents (nowadays this is rapidly fading)

4. Finally, **gather simple laboratory tests** (such as an electrocardiogram or a chest x-ray), and look for any associated "bad company."

56. **What is the most common systolic ejection murmur of the elderly?**
The murmur of *aortic sclerosis*. This is an early peaking systolic murmur that is so age related as to affect 21–26% of persons older than 65, and 55–75% of octogenarians (conversely, the prevalence of aortic *stenosis* is 2% and 2.6%, respectively).

57. **Why does the murmur of aortic sclerosis peak early?**
Because it is due to *flow* and *velocity* and *not* to a transvalvular pressure gradient. And since the greatest fraction of ventricular ejection occurs in the first half of systole, flow, velocity, and intensity of the murmur also will peak in early systole. Moreover, since the integrity of the valve is maintained in aortic sclerosis, the intensity of S_2 also will be preserved.

58. **What are the risk factors for aortic sclerosis?**
Age (twofold higher risk for each 10-year increase in age), *male gender* (twofold excess risk), *current smoking* (35% increase in risk), and a *history of hypertension* (20% increase in risk). Other significant factors include height and hypercholesterolemia. In fact, risk factors associated with aortic sclerosis (and stenosis) are quite similar to risk factors associated with *atherosclerosis*.

59. **What causes the murmur of aortic sclerosis?**
Either a degenerative change of the aortic valve or abnormalities of the aortic root. The latter may be *diffuse* (such as a tortuous and dilated aorta) or *localized* (like a calcific spur or an atherosclerotic plaque that protrudes into the lumen, creating a turbulent bloodstream).

60. **What are the degenerative changes of the aortic valve that can cause aortic sclerosis?**
Mostly a senile degeneration of the leaflets, with thickening, fibrosis, and occasionally calcification. This can stiffen the valve, and yet not cause a transvalvular pressure gradient. In fact, commissural fusion is typically absent in aortic sclerosis.

61. **What are the prognostic implications of aortic valve sclerosis?**
Serious. In a study of more than 5000 adults followed for approximately 5 years, aortic sclerosis carried a 40% increased risk of myocardial infarction and a trend toward an increased risk of

angina, heart failure, and stroke. Note that other "benign" conditions similarly devoid of hemodynamic consequences, such as mitral annular calcification (MAC) and aortic root sclerosis (ARS), also carry a higher risk of aortic atheromatous disease.

62. How frequent are MAC and ARS?

Quite frequent, at least when sought by transesophageal echocardiography. Prevalence of MAC and ARS beyond the fifth decade is 30% and 48%, respectively.

63. What is the reason for the worse clinical outcome of patients with aortic sclerosis?

It is neither hemodynamic instability (in fact, the valve abnormality is relatively benign) nor a progression to true AS (in a study of more than 2000 patients, progression occurred in only 16%—with most stenoses being mild). Instead, it is a concomitant and subclinical coronary artery disease (CAD). In fact, aortic sclerosis serves as a marker not only for the presence of CAD, but also of *systemic inflammation*. And since inflammation may stiffen valvular leaflets but also cause atheromatosis, aortic sclerosis identifies subjects at risk of adverse cardiovascular events.

64. Is there any evidence for this "inflammatory" theory?

Aortic sclerosis patients indeed have higher inflammatory markers, such as increased serum levels of C-reactive protein and fibrinogen. In fact, their risk of cardiovascular death increases with each tertile of C-reactive protein.

65. What should one do in clinical practice?

One should identify aortic sclerosis (by looking for its normal carotid pulse and typical soft and early peaking systolic ejection murmur). Once this has been confirmed, CAD should be ruled out and risk factor modification implemented, like smoking cessation and hypertension/hypercholesterolemia control. It is humbling to think that a new screening procedure for coronary risk in asymptomatic patients may now simply rely on the effective use of good old stethoscopy.

B. SYSTOLIC MURMURS

66. How common are systolic murmurs?

Extremely common, especially if ejection. Hence, the need to separate functional from pathologic.

67. What are the causes of a systolic murmur?

1. **Ejection** (i.e., increased "forward" flow over a semilunar valve). This can be:
   - *Physiologic:* Normal valve, but flow high enough to cause *turbulence* (anemia, exercise, fever, and other hyperkinetic heart syndromes)
   - *Pathologic:* Abnormal valve, with or without outflow obstruction (i.e., aortic stenosis versus aortic *sclerosis*)
2. **Regurgitation:** "Backward" flow from a high- into a low-pressure bed. Although this is usually due to incompetent A-V valves (mitral/tricuspid), it also can be due to ventricular septal defect.

68. What characteristics of a systolic murmur help differentiate ejection from regurgitation?

- The **relationship of the murmur to S_2**. Regurgitant systolic murmurs typically extend into S_2 (and sometimes even beyond it), whereas ejection murmurs always end before it. This may be difficult to detect, since S_2 is often soft (and even absent in severe semilunar stenosis).
- The **change of the murmur after a longer diastole**. This is especially evident after a premature beat (*see* question 26), with ejection murmurs of semilunar stenosis becoming *louder,* and regurgitant murmurs of atrioventricular insufficiency remaining constant.

- The **response of the murmur to bedside maneuvers** (previously discussed)
- The **musical quality of the murmur**. This is only present in situations of regurgitation.

69. **What is the precision of physical examination for the evaluation of systolic murmurs?**
    Precision (i.e., interobserver agreement) varies depending on finding and observer (most studies have evaluated cardiologists). Overall, precision of examination for *any* systolic murmur is only fair in the clinical setting (kappa, 0.30). Precision for a *loud* systolic murmur (grade 2 or louder) also is only fair in the clinical setting (kappa, 0.29). Precision for a *late peaking* systolic murmur is instead excellent (kappa, 0.74). Finally, precision for a systolic *click* is good (agreement of 85%).

(1) SYSTOLIC *EJECTION* MURMURS

70. **What is the definition of an ejection murmur?**
    It is a *systolic* murmur that is produced by *forward* blood flow—usually across the semilunar valves and into one of the large vessels.

71. **What are the characteristics of an ejection murmur?**
    - It starts immediately after S_1 (or after an ejection sound associated with S_1).
    - It has a crescendo-decrescendo pattern (hence, it is shaped like a diamond or a *kite*).
    - It ends before the ipsilateral component of the second sound.

72. **Are all ejection murmurs crescendo-decrescendo?**
    They *tend* to be because murmur intensity is regulated by the transvalvular *pressure gradient*, which, in turn, depends on *velocity* and *acceleration* of flow. Whenever these increase, the pressure gradient also increases, and so does the intensity of the murmur. For instance, in the ejection murmur of AS, the pressure gradient (and loudness) builds up during the very first part of ventricular contraction and peaks around *mid*-systole. By then the ventricle starts losing contractility; flow *velocity* and *acceleration* decrease; the *pressure gradient* diminishes, and the intensity of the murmur abates. This is reflected by the *decrescendo* pattern of the murmur's second half.

73. **What is the pitch of a systolic ejection murmur?**
    Low to medium. This can help differentiate ejection from *regurgitant* murmurs, which tend instead to be higher pitched.

74. **In addition to pitch, are there other differences between ejection and regurgitant murmurs?**
    - Clearly **location**. Ejection murmurs (such as AS) are loudest over the base, whereas regurgitant murmurs (such as MR) are most intense at the apex. The only exception is the Gallavardin phenomenon (*see* questions 92 and 93).
    - **Transmission** also is different (to the neck for an ejection murmur and to the axilla for a regurgitant one).
    - **Changes after a long diastole**. AS (but *not* MR) is louder after a long pause, like that following a premature ventricular contraction (or the long cardiac cycle of atrial fibrillation).
    - **Handgrip** intensifies regurgitant murmurs, but softens ejection ones.
    - **Duration**. Regurgitant murmurs audibly extend all the way into S_2, whereas ejection murmurs end before it.
    - **Shape**. Although *systolic regurgitant murmurs* may at times have a crescendo-decrescendo pattern, this is rather uncommon, and typically associated with higher frequency components than systolic *ejection* murmurs. Yet, despite all of these differentiating features, bedside separation can at times be very difficult.

75. **Everything else being equal, is the intensity of an ejection murmur related to its severity?**
    Yes. The louder the murmur, the higher the transvalvular pressure gradient. This rule of thumb requires, of course, that other parameters of murmur intensity (such as thickness of chest wall, degree of emphysema) remain constant. When this is the case, a softer murmur (such as a grade 2 or less) argues in favor of a lower pressure gradient than a louder murmur (grade 4 or higher). *The only exception is congestive heart failure,* where reduction in contractility softens ejection murmurs without necessarily indicating a lower transvalvular pressure gradient.

76. **Does loudness of an ejection murmur always predict severity of disease?**
    No. Many factors may *intensify* an ejection murmur *without* necessarily reflecting worse disease. In addition to obvious conditions (such as a thin chest wall or a dilated aortic/pulmonic root), all *high-output states* tend to cause *louder* ejection murmurs that do not necessarily reflect higher pressure gradients. Instead, they indicate high flow velocity, as in the *hyperkinetic heart syndrome.*

77. **What are the effects of respiration on left-sided ejection murmurs?**
    Inspiration decreases flow into the left-sided chambers. Hence, in AS it will decrease transvalvular flow, pressure gradient, and murmur intensity. Exhalation does instead the opposite.

78. **What is the effect of inspiration on *right*-sided ejection murmurs like pulmonic stenosis?**
    It intensifies it because of increased right-sided venous return. Yet, this may be counterbalanced by lung expansion, which interposes a larger cushion of air between the heart and stethoscope. Since this is usually more an issue in the *upper half* of the chest (where the *base* of the heart is located), the inspiratory intensification of PS may be best heard in the *lower* chest.

79. **What is the effect of *standing* on the intensity of a PS murmur?**
    It magnifies the respiratory variations. This is counterintuitive, considering that standing *decreases* right ventricular stroke volume (due to reduced venous return). Still, the inspiratory *increase* in return (and pulmonary blood flow) tends to be proportionally higher while standing. Hence, the right-sided ejection murmur of PS will be *proportionally* louder in inspiration than expiration.

80. **What is the effect of *Valsalva* on systolic ejection murmurs?**
    It depends on the phase (*straining* or *releasing*). Overall, all ejection murmurs (except HOCM) fade during *straining*, due to decreased venous return. Yet, as soon as straining is released, *all* ejection murmurs intensify, peaking within 2–3 beats (for the pulmonic ejection murmur) or 6–8 beats (for the aortic ejection murmur). The delayed peak of AS is due to the longer time needed for the blood that had been pooled during straining to finally reach the left ventricle and the aorta.

I. AORTIC STENOSIS

81. **What are the three main types of aortic stenosis?**
    Supravalvular, valvular, and subvalvular. These can be easily separated by evaluating the central arterial pulse (*see* Chapter 10, questions 18 and 19 and Fig. 10-3). In addition, *subvalvular stenosis* is further divided into (1) *hypertrophic subaortic stenosis* (also called HOCM [i.e., hypertrophic obstructive cardiomyopathy]) and (2) *fixed, fibrotic subvalvular stenosis.*

Valvular Aortic Stenosis

82. **What are the causes of valvular AS?**
    - Congenital
    - Degenerative
    - Inflammatory (i.e., rheumatic)

Congenital AS occurs predominantly in patients younger than 50, whereas *degenerative* AS is more common in the elderly, usually as a result of age-related thickening and calcification of a normal (or bicuspid) semilunar valve. In fact, nowadays calcific valvular disease is the most common cause of aortic stenosis in the Western world. Inflammatory (or *rheumatic*) AS, while still very common worldwide, has instead become increasingly rare both in the United States and Europe. It should still be suspected in anyone presenting with *multivalvular* disease, such as combined mitral *and* aortic regurgitation.

83. **What is the most common *congenital* cause of valvular AS?**
A bicuspid semilunar valve. This is one of the most frequent congenital heart abnormalities, present in around 2% of the general population. A bicuspid valve may remain completely silent throughout the patient's life, or simply present as an early systolic (ejection) click. In most cases, however, bicuspid valves stiffen over time, eventually calcifying and stenosing—a not uncommon reason for AS in the elderly. Alternatively, they may fail—usually at an earlier stage in life.

84. **What is the progression of valvular changes in aortic stenosis?**
Calcific stenosis represents the final stage of an *active process* that starts with (1) focal thickening of the valvular subendothelium; progresses to (2) mild, irregular thickening of the leaflets, without any outflow obstruction (*aortic sclerosis*); and eventually results in (3) greater stiffening and calcification, with a reduced valvular area and clinically significant outflow obstruction.

85. **Is aortic root dilation a common feature of valvular AS?**
Yes. Postobstructive dilation occurs in approximately 25% of patients with AS. Yet, root diameter does not reflect degree of stenosis and does not necessarily result in concomitant *regurgitation*.

86. **What is the link between AS and coronary artery disease (CAD)?**
A link almost as strong as the one between aortic *sclerosis* and CAD—especially in symptomatic patients. CAD occurs in one half of those patients with AS who end up dying or requiring valvular surgery, but only in one fourth of those without adverse outcome. Event-free survival at 3 years is 63% in CAD patients, as opposed to 86% in those without it, confirming its ominous prognosis.

87. **How much reduction in valvular area is necessary for the AS murmur to become audible?**
At least 50% (the minimum for creating a pressure gradient at rest). Mild disease may produce loud murmurs, too, but usually significant hemodynamic compromise (and symptoms) do not occur until there is a 60–70% reduction in valvular area. This means that early to mild AS may be subtle at rest. Exercise, however, may intensify the murmur by increasing the output and gradient.

88. **What is the normal aortic area?**
3 cm². A valvular area >1.5 cm² reflects mild disease, 1–1.5 cm² moderate disease, <1.0 cm² severe disease, and <0.7 cm² *critical* disease. Symptoms usually occur with an orifice <1 cm².

89. **What is the frequency of clinically significant outflow obstruction?**
1–2% of adults older than 65, with most patients eventually requiring valve replacement.

90. **What is the pathophysiology of left ventricular outflow obstruction?**
It is a physiology of *pressure* load, with compensatory hypertrophy and typically well-preserved systolic function—at least initially. This is in contrast to aortic *regurgitation* (AR), wherein *volume* load causes instead progressive left ventricular *dilation* and dysfunction—even in the

absence of symptoms. This is why AR with severe ventricular dysfunction may often be asymptomatic, whereas AS with ventricular dysfunction is *always* symptomatic. Hence, in contrast to AR, the clinical outcome of AS is *very closely related to* the *presence or absence of symptoms*: once these occur, outcome is poor, with 2-year survival below 50%. Yet, even advanced and symptomatic AS may greatly benefit from valvular replacement, since the resulting relief in afterload increases systolic function, improves ejection fraction, and dramatically reduces symptoms.

91. Where is the murmur of aortic stenosis louder?

Over the second right parasternal interspace, but also all the way down to the *apex*. This area of surface projection is referred to as the "sash," and is much wider than the traditional aortic area.

92. What is the Gallavardin phenomenon?

One noticed in some patients with AS, who may exhibit a dissociation of their systolic murmur into two components:

- A **typical AS-like murmur** (medium to low pitched, harsh, right parasternal, typically radiated to the neck, and caused by high velocity jets into the ascending aorta)
- A **murmur that instead mimics MR** (high pitched, musical, and best heard at the apex)

This phenomenon reflects the different transmission of AS: its medium frequencies to the base, and its higher frequencies to the apex. The latter may become so prominent as to be misinterpreted as a separate apical "cooing" of MR. Gallavardin attributed this finding to solid tissue transmission of the musical components of AS; although more recently, Burch suggested that a concomitant papillary muscle dysfunction might produce *real* mitral regurgitation.

93. Who was Gallavardin?

One of the premier European cardiologists of his times, but also a refined aesthete and humanist. The son of a homeopathic physician, Louis Gallavardin (1875–1957) was a consummate bedside diagnostician, who contributed enormously to the understanding of hypertension, cardiomyopathy, and coronary artery disease (he antedated Attilio Maseri's description of vasospasm as one of the causes of myocardial infarction). In this regard, he described a painless variant of exertional angina called "blockpnea" (a term he coined in 1933), a condition characterized by an agonizing feeling of blocked respiration, almost apnea-like, which slows the patient to a standstill. He also reported on valvulopathies, like the pulmonary edema of MS (still called the "reticissimente de Gallavardin"), and the transformation of the harsh murmur of AS into a higher-pitched apical sound (the Gallavardin's phenomenon, 1925). A modest man with an interest in the humanities, a prodigious memory, and an impressive knowledge of art and books, Gallavardin mustered such a strong respect among peers that he often overrode everybody else's opinion. This is why it took three decades before Reid and Barlow were eventually able to delineate the true nature of the mid-systolic click, which Gallavardin had erroneously attributed to pleuropericardial lesions.

94. What are the characteristics of the AS murmur?

It is typically crescendo-decrescendo, mid-systolic, medium pitched, harsh, and with a rasping or coarse quality. Note that although absence of a murmur argues strongly *against* AS, its presence is less of a positive predictor, given the wide differential diagnosis of a systolic murmur.

95. How can one separate the murmur of AS from that of aortic sclerosis?

By the same rules previously outlined for separating pathologic from functional murmurs:

- **"The company it keeps":** A systolic ejection murmur associated with a reduced and delayed arterial pulse, a sustained apical impulse, a palpable precordial thrill, electrocardiographic evidence of left ventricular hypertrophy, and symptoms of outflow obstruction (exertional dizziness/syncope, chest pain, and dyspnea) is much more likely due to aortic *stenosis* than a similar murmur with none of the associations.

- **Auscultatory characteristics:** AS is more likely to be *long*, late peaking, associated with a soft to absent S_2 (at least in its aortic component), and radiated to the right carotid. It may even have the ejection sound of a bicuspid valve. Conversely, aortic *sclerosis* is *short*, *early peaking*, and with a well-preserved (and even loud) S_2, since many patients have in fact hypertension. Ejection sounds are uncommon in this condition, and so is radiation to the neck.
- Finally, all things being equal, **murmur intensity** may help. A murmur of aortic *sclerosis* is softer. In fact, less than grade 4 in 98% of the cases (and thus never accompanied by a palpable *thrill*).

96. **Of all these characteristics, which are the most useful for ruling in (or ruling out) aortic stenosis?**
The ones arguing most strongly in favor of AS are a reduced/delayed carotid upstroke, a mid to late peak, a soft to absent A_2, a palpable precordial thrill, and an apical–carotid (or brachioradial) delay. Except for the thrill, all other features also have significant likelihood ratios in separating *severe* AS from mild to moderate disease or from aortic sclerosis. Conversely, lack of radiation to the right carotid artery argues most strongly *against* AS.

97. **What is the *apical–carotid* and *brachioradial* delay?**
It is a palpable delay between the apical and carotid impulse and between the brachial and radial impulse. Patients with valvular AS may have both.

98. **How valuable is a pulse that is parvus and tardus?**
Valuable, but mostly in younger subjects because various factors in the elderly may result in a misleadingly *brisk* carotid upstroke, with early peak and normal amplitude in spite of severe stenosis. Among these are changes in arterial compliance, impedance, concomitant aortic regurgitation, and, more importantly, increased wall stiffness due to coexisting hypertension or atherosclerosis. Hence, the frequent lack of *parvus* and *tardus* in older patients.

99. **Is the timing of peak intensity always reflective of severity of disease?**
No. Although this finding *does* correspond to the time course of the transvalvular pressure gradient (with progressive delaying in peak corresponding to more severe obstruction), it also is true that early peaks can simply be the result of an increased transvalvular *flow rate*—as seen, for example, in patients with coexisting aortic regurgitation, a not uncommon event in AS. Peripheral vascular impedance wave reflections (and compliance) also may affect the timing of peak intensity, thus making this finding a less specific predictor of severity in the elderly.

100. **And how can one differentiate AS from the other systolic murmurs?**
Mitral regurgitation, tricuspid regurgitation, hypertrophic cardiomyopathy, and mitral valve prolapse also can be ruled in (and ruled out) through physical exam—at least by cardiologists, even though the studies supporting this conclusion tend to be smaller and of lower quality. Still, it appears that in the hands (and ears) of specialists, the clinical examination can accurately detect various causes of abnormal systolic murmurs. It also can exclude *pathology*. In fact, one could state with Etchells that a cardiologist's assessment of a murmur as "normal" significantly reduces the likelihood of disease, whereas its assessment as being "abnormal" significantly increases it. Whether this conclusion also applies to noncardiologists needs to be determined.

101. **Are there any other murmur characteristics that can predict the severity of AS?**
Intensity, but only in younger individuals. In older patients, various other factors (such as concomitant obstructive lung disease or obesity) may in fact soften even the most severe of murmurs. Since the bone is a good sound conductor, auscultation over the neck (or right clavicle) may help to restore adequate murmur intensity in these patients. Note that the murmur may soften considerably (and almost disappear) when the failing ventricle becomes unable to overcome a high pressure gradient and thus generate enough turbulence. Hence, soft

AS murmurs may paradoxically indicate advanced disease. Still, in *asymptomatic* patients, absence of a murmur (or a 1/6 grade) argues strongly against the presence of significant obstruction.

102. **And what about the intensity of S_2?**
Also very important. Although a small number of AS patients may have loud murmurs in spite of mild to moderate disease, loudness together with a *soft or absent aortic component of S_2 (A_2)* almost always reflects severe obstruction. Conversely, a well-preserved (and physiologically split) S_2 argues strongly against the presence of severe AS. The only exceptions are concomitant mitral regurgitation, pulmonary hypertension, or right ventricular conduction delay.

103. **What are the reasons for a soft S_2 in AS?**
Either calcification of the aortic cusps (which renders closure inaudible) or a prolongation of left ventricular ejection time (which delays A_2 and thus renders its interval from P_2 too narrowed to be audible). The latter is indeed common in patients with reduced left ventricular function and thus provides an important predictor of disease severity.

104. **What about the transmission of the murmur?**
Toward the neck and right carotid. Although traditionally linked to AS (and in fact, arguing *against it* if lacking), this type of transmission does *not* reflect disease severity.

105. **Is there any other acoustic event that may suggest severe AS?**
Intuitively, one could think of the S_4 and the early systolic click. And yet:
- Presence of an audible S_4 *does* reflect severe left ventricular hypertrophy (with a transvalvular pressure gradient >70 mmHg), but *only* in younger patients. Older subjects may already have a "normal" S_4. Conversely, a *palpable* S_4 always reflects severe disease.
- An early systolic (ejection) click usually indicates a *valvular* AS, typically due to a congenitally bicuspid aortic valve. Still, *presence of a click does not correlate with severity of obstruction*. Moreover, an early systolic click tends to be more frequent in younger patients, since AS in the elderly is usually due to calcification of a normal trileaflet valve.

106. **Are there any other findings that do not predict severity of AS?**
Narrow pulse pressure, *paradoxical splitting of S_2*, and *third heart sound*. Although traditionally linked to AS, these do *not* correlate with AS severity.

107. **How is the point of maximal impulse (PMI) in AS?**
There are two major characteristics:
- **Location of PMI:** In the typical patient with concentric left ventricular hypertrophy, the PMI is usually well *sustained,* but only mildly displaced to the left. An increased displacement usually indicates the development of left ventricular failure or concomitant aortic regurgitation.
- **Apical thrill:** A palpable thrill is common in AS and does not reflect disease severity. To detect it, have the patient sit up, lean forward, and hold his or her breath in forced exhalation.

108. **How are the neck veins in patients with AS?**
They may have a prominent "A" wave, as a result of the "Bernheim phenomenon."

109. **What is the "Bernheim phenomenon"?**
It is a phenomenon first described in 1910 by the French physiologist P.I. Bernheim. It consists of an interaction between the left and right ventricle, such that a change in the function of one leads inevitably to an alteration in the function of the other. In other words, a dilation/hypertrophy of the left ventricle would compress the *right* ventricle, resulting in its impaired filling. This is in part due to the restraining influence of the pericardium (which ensures

that any increase in *left* ventricular volume occurs at the expense of the *right* ventricle, as a result of leftward shift in the septum), and in part due to the secondary pulmonary hypertension caused by increased left ventricular filling pressure. Hence the prominent "A" wave of patients with AS.

110. **What is the "reverse Bernheim phenomenon"?**

It is a *leftward* shift of the interventricular septum, secondary to pressure or volume load of the *right* ventricle. This causes a decrease in left ventricular size, contractility, compliance, and ejection fraction, as well as an increase in diastolic pressure of the left ventricle—hence, a left ventricular *diastolic* dysfunction. Although never actually suggested by Bernheim, this phenomenon is noticed in a wide array of pulmonary diseases with right ventricular hypertrophy.

111. **What then are the valuable clinical predictors of severe AS?**

Clearly, ECG presence of left ventricular hypertrophy or radiologic evidence of valvular calcification. As for the bedside, Otto et al. found the three most useful predictors to be:
- Murmur **intensity** and **timing** (the louder and later peaking the murmur, the worse the disease)
- A **single S_2**
- **Delayed upstroke/reduced amplitude of the carotid pulse** (pulsus parvus and tardus)

Still, no single physical finding has both high sensitivity *and* specificity for detecting *severe* valvular obstruction. Some findings (such as murmur grade = 3 or decreased carotid upstroke) have high *specificity* but lack sensitivity. Others (like murmur peak in mid-to-late systole, or murmur intensity = 2) have high *sensitivity* but low specificity. Hoagland et al. found predictive value in combining five bedside findings: (1 and 2) reduced and delayed carotid upstroke (2 and 3 points, respectively); (3) murmur loudest over the aortic area (2 points); (4) reduced A_2 (3 points); and (5) radiologic calcification of the valve (4 points). Scores >10 identified severe obstruction, whereas scores <6 identified mild obstruction. Intermediate scores were not helpful.

112. **And what about bedside predictors of clinical outcome?**

In the same aforementioned study, Otto et al. found the *intensity* of the systolic murmur, the *timing* of its peak, the presence of a *single S_2*, and *delayed/reduced carotid amplitude* to be all significant univariate predictors of clinical outcome. On multivariate analysis, however, only the *carotid upstroke amplitude* remained predictive. Hence, physical examination appears to correlate with disease *severity* and *prognosis,* but this correlation is not too close. Echocardiography remains, therefore, essential to reliably exclude severe obstruction and to predict clinical outcome.

113. **Why is physical examination inadequate in predicting disease severity?**

Not because of interobserver variability or examiners' expertise, but because of the pathophysiology of AS, and its modulating coexisting conditions: old age, emphysema, atherosclerotic changes of the arterial wall, or concomitant AR. As a result, bedside exam has low *specificity* for detecting severity (due to the many false positives of moderate disease) and occasionally low *sensitivity*. Yet, it can accurately separate *mild* from moderate to severe AS.

114. **In summary, what is the role of physical examination in valvular AS?**

It varies, depending on the clinical situation. In patients with cardiac symptoms, a loud (grade 3 or 4) and late peaking systolic murmur associated with a significantly reduced (and delayed) carotid upstroke strongly argues in favor of severe AS and thus prompts treatment. In this case, bedside findings can be quite specific. In other situations, however (like preoperative evaluation for noncardiac surgery), the goal of the exam may simply be the exclusion of severe disease. In this setting, an early peaking and soft *murmur* (grade 2 or less) with a normal carotid upstroke and a physiologically split S_2 all argues against significant disease. They are, in fact, very sensitive—yet not 100%. Hence, echocardiography may still be necessary to completely exclude AS.

115. **What are the clinical implications for a primary care physician?**
First of all, that it is crucial to consider AS in any adult presenting with a systolic murmur *and* symptoms of outflow obstruction (*judge murmurs like people, by the company they keep*). Hence, listen (with both the stethoscope *and* your ears) to what your patients are trying to tell you. Still, beware that early symptoms may be subtle (a mild exercise intolerance, for example, usually ascribed to "getting old") and that the classic triad of angina, dyspnea, and syncope is usually limited to the most advanced cases. Secondly, keep in mind that it is very difficult to *rule out* AS only on the basis of auscultation—the major exceptions being a very soft (grade 1/6) systolic murmur or a physiologically split S_2. Hence, rely on ultrasonography to evaluate all symptomatic adults with a systolic murmur. Echo can visualize anatomy, estimate severity of obstruction, and provide crucial monitoring of disease progression.

Aortic *Subvalvular* Stenosis

Subvalvular "Hypertrophic"

116. **What is the pathophysiology of HOCM?**
It Is a disproportionate (and asymmetric) thickening of the interventricular septum. As this bulges in systole, it draws medially the anterior mitral leaflet, thus causing a dynamic systolic obstruction to left ventricular outflow.

117. **Where is this murmur best heard?**
It depends. When septal hypertrophy obstructs not only left but also *right* ventricular outflow, the murmur may be louder at the left lower sternal border. More commonly, however, the HOCM murmur is louder at the *apex*. This may often cause a differential diagnosis dilemma with the murmur of MR.

118. **How can one differentiate the systolic ejection murmur of valvular AS from that of HOCM?**
   - **Location:** HOCM is subvalvular—and, hence, louder over Erb's point, or even the apex whereas typical AS is loudest over the aortic area.
   - **Timing of onset** is also different: The murmur of valvular AS starts immediately after S_1, whereas HOCM starts a little later—usually in mid-systole (since the obstruction is dynamic and, hence, more likely to occur when the ventricular lumen is reduced—as during systole).
   - **Arterial pulse** is delayed and reduced in AS, but brisk and bifid in HOCM.

119. **Does timing of onset of the HOCM murmur reflect severity of disease?**
Yes and no. In *moderate to severe* HOCM, the onset of the murmur is often anticipated, suggesting a severe subaortic pressure gradient. Conversely, early murmurs also may be due to very rapid ejection (in HOCM, 80% of the left ventricular volume is usually ejected during the first half of systole, as compared to only 50% in the normal patient). Rapid ejection can manifest itself with a short and early systolic sound (ejection click) immediately following S_1.

120. **What bedside maneuvers can modify the murmur of HOCM?**
Maneuvers/factors that change left ventricular (LV) volume: a smaller volume brings the septum closer to the anterior mitral leaflet, thus causing a greater obstruction and a *louder* murmur. Conversely, a larger LV volume separates the upper septum from the anterior mitral leaflet, thus causing less obstruction and a *softer* murmur. *Note that these are the same maneuvers that can respectively lengthen or soften the findings of mitral valve prolapse* (*see* below, questions 178 and 179).

121. **Which factors _increase_ left ventricular volume?**
    - Exhalation
    - Bradycardia
    - Volume infusion
    - Passive leg raising for 20 seconds (which can easily be carried out in most patients, even frail ones)
    - Squatting after standing—the latter increases both _preload_ (by "milking" blood out of leg veins and abdomen) and _afterload_ (by compressing femoral and iliac arteries)

    Passive leg raising and standing-to-squatting have excellent sensitivity and specificity for _softening_ the murmur of HOCM (both close to 90%). Hence, absence of softening strongly argues against presence of the disease.

122. **Which factors _reduce_ left ventricular volume?**
    - Inspiration
    - Tachycardia
    - Volume depletion
    - Administration of vasodilators, such as sniffing amyl nitrate
    - Valsalva maneuver (which during its "strain" phase lowers preload—_see_ question 22)
    - Standing after squatting (which lowers both preload and afterload)

    Both Valsalva and squatting-to-standing have excellent specificity for _intensifying_ the murmur of HOCM (both close to 90%, with Valsalva having an even higher positive likelihood ratio). Hence, if positive, both maneuvers argue strongly for the presence of the disease.

123. **How accurate are these maneuvers in recognizing HOCM?**
    Quite accurate. Studies of cardiologists have indeed shown that passive leg raising and squatting-to-standing both have a good likelihood ratio in predicting the presence or absence of the murmur.

124. **How does _valvular_ AS respond to these maneuvers?**
    Very differently. For example, squatting _softens_ HOCM (because it increases left ventricular diameter), whereas it _intensifies_ valvular AS (because it increases both venous return and contractility due to the larger left ventricular diameter). Standing reduces venous return and thus intensifies HOCM (smaller ventricular diameter), whereas it softens valvular AS (through a decreased stroke volume).

125. **How does a long diastolic pause after a premature beat affect the murmur of HOCM?**
    Not in the same way as it affects the murmurs of valvular or subvalvular "fixed" AS. In a study of 14 patients with HOCM, 40 with valvular AS and four with discrete subaortic AS, _all_ experienced increases in left ventricular outflow gradient following a post extrasystolic beat. And yet, while 42 of the 44 (95%) with either valvular AS or discrete subaortic stenosis had increases in murmur intensity, only nine of 14 (64%) with HOCM did. In fact, only two (29%) of seven patients with HOCM and resting gradients of more than 25 mmHg had murmur increases. Hence, the murmur of HOCM does _not_ increase consistently with the magnitude of the outflow tract gradient.

126. **Can the murmur of HOCM be partially related to a murmur of mitral regurgitation?**
    Yes. In fact, HOCM is often associated with an apical murmur of MR. This is due to the pull-down on the mitral valve (especially its anterior leaflet) by the thickened and hypertrophic left ventricle, which not only causes outlet obstruction but also A-V regurgitation. Evidence of MR is encountered in 75% of all HOCM cases. In these patients, the murmur behaves like the HOCM murmur, insofar as it is delayed in onset and ends before A_2. Hence, if MR spans _throughout_ systole, it is much more likely to be due to _primary_ mitral regurgitation.

127. **Are there any other associated physical findings in HOCM?**
   - **Brisk arterial pulse:** This may be bifid on tracing (spike-and-dome waveform). Yet, in contrast to the *pulsus bisferiens* of AR, the bifid of HOCM is usually undetectable at the bedside (unless the obstruction is very severe).
   - **Double or *triple* apical impulse:** The "triple-ripple" reflects a *strong atrial contraction* (which, in turn, can cause an S_4) and a *double ventricular contraction* (early rapid ejection, followed by obstruction, and subsequent late slow ejection. This is also the mechanism for the bifid pulse).
   - **S_3:** This is rare in HOCM, unless the degree of associated MR is severe.
   - **Single split S_2** (due to delayed closure of the aortic component, from increased impedance to left ventricular emptying): In severe HOCM, S_2 can become paradoxically split (10% of cases).
   - **Nonejection systolic click:** The likely explanation is inequality of the functional length of the mitral chordae tendineae, secondary to asymmetric myocardial hypertrophy.

128. **In summary, how accurate is physical exam for the diagnosis of HOCM?**
   Quite accurate, at least in the hands of cardiologists and when supported by bedside maneuvers such as passive leg raising or squatting-to-standing.

Subvalvular "Fixed"

129. **What is the cause of a "fixed" subvalvular aortic stenosis?**
   Usually, some sort of discrete obstructive fibrosis. This may be either *below* the valve (as a thin membrane) or *on the ventricular septum*. In other patients, the obstruction is produced instead by a concentric fibrous ring and some muscular hypertrophy, just 2 cm below the aortic valve.

Aortic *Supravalvular* Stenosis

130. **What are the characteristics of supravalvular aortic stenosis?**
   Supravalvular AS is usually produced by a localized discrete narrowing above the sinuses of Valsalva. The area of highest intensity for this murmur is either the suprasternal notch or the first right interspace (as opposed to the *second* right interspace for the murmur of *valvular* AS, and the *Erb's point* for the murmur[s] of *subvalvular* stenosis). Radiation is more toward the *right* carotid than the left (as is in patients with *valvular* AS).

131. **What are the other characteristics of supravalvular AS?**
   Male gender plus a number of congenital abnormalities, like hypercalcemia and a peculiar "elfin" facies, with wide-set eyes, upturned nose, patulous lips, baggy cheeks, small chin, and a peculiarly deep, husky voice. These patients also tend to have a stronger pulse (and a higher blood pressure) in the *right* arm and carotid as compared to the left. Although the ejection murmur may be occasionally accompanied by an aortic regurgitant one, it is almost never associated with an aortic ejection click.

II. AORTIC VERSUS PULMONIC STENOSIS

132. **How does the murmur of pulmonic stenosis (PS) differ from that of aortic stenosis (AS)?**
   - **Location:** The area of maximum intensity for AS is the second right interspace or the apex, whereas that of PS is the *left sternal border*.
   - **Respiration:** AS is louder in exhalation, whereas PS is *louder in inspiration*.
   - **Standing:** It makes the PS murmur proportionally louder in inspiration.
   - **Valsalva maneuver:** Straining softens both murmurs. Still, immediately after release, the PS murmur reaches its highest intensity after only two to three beats, whereas AS takes much longer.

133. **What other auscultatory features can help differentiate pulmonic from aortic stenosis?**
- An ejection click can occur in both PS and AS. Yet, only the one of PS fades or disappears with inspiration (which represents the only exception to the Rivero-Carvallo's rule that *all* right-sided findings get louder in inspiration).
- A widening of the normal and physiologic splitting of S_2 argues in favor of PS. A *paradoxical* splitting of S_2, on the other hand, argues in favor of AS.
- Finally, the presence of an S_4 gallop during inspiration is more likely to be associated with PS, whereas presence of an S_4 gallop during *exhalation* is more likely to be associated with AS.

III. MISCELLANEOUS EJECTION MURMURS

Ventricular Septal Defect (VSD)

134. **What are the characteristics of a VSD murmur?**
They are similar to those of both *regurgitant* and *ejection* murmurs. Indeed, a VSD may cover the entire systole with a plateau, crescendo-decrescendo, decrescendo, or crescendo murmur.

135. **Can the shape of a VSD murmur help identify the type of defect?**
Yes. A crescendo-decrescendo murmur usually indicates a defect in the *muscular part of the septum*. Ventricular contraction closes the hole toward the end of systole, thus causing the decrescendo phase of the murmur. Conversely, a defect in the *membranous septum* will enjoy no systolic reduction in flow and thus produce a murmur that remains constant and holosystolic.

136. **Is there any relationship between the intensity of the murmur and the size of the defect?**
No. Murmurs of varying intensity may occur with either small or large defects. Yet, whenever the defect is very large, the intensity of the murmur is usually very loud. Note, however, that a soft murmur may actually occur when very large defects are associated with severe pulmonary hypertension. In this case, the murmur usually follows an *ejection sound* (which is the hallmark of high pulmonary pressures) and ends with a very loud single S_2, continuing into an early diastolic murmur of pulmonary regurgitation (the Graham Steell murmur).

137. **Where is the VSD murmur best heard?**
Along the left lower sternal border, often radiating left to right across the chest.

138. **How can one differentiate MR from VSD?**
The MR murmur can be delayed in onset and exhibit a crescendo pattern toward S_2. This never occurs in a ventricular septal defect: even though some VSD murmurs may exhibit a crescendo pattern, they *always start immediately after S_1*. Finally, an early crescendo-decrescendo shape is *not* typical of MR, but is frequently seen in very small congenital muscular VSDs. *Hence, the key to the recognition of a VSD murmur is that, in contrast to MR, it <u>always</u> starts immediately after the mitral component of S_1.*

(2) SYSTOLIC *REGURGITANT* MURMURS

139. **What is a systolic regurgitant murmur?**
One characterized by a pressure gradient that causes a *retrograde* blood flow across an abnormal opening. This can be (1) a ventricular septal defect, (2) an incompetent mitral valve, (3) an incompetent tricuspid valve, or (4) fistulous communication between a high-pressure and a low-pressure vascular bed (such as a patent ductus arteriosus).

140. Is "regurgitation" the same as "insufficiency"?

Yes and no. All these acoustic events should be called murmurs of *regurgitation*, since insufficiency (or incompetence) solely defines the anatomic (and functional) features of the valve, and not the blood flow derangement that is the hallmark of true regurgitation: a backflow from a high- to a low-pressure chamber.

141. What are the auscultatory characteristics of systolic regurgitant murmurs?

They tend to start immediately after S_1, often extending into S_2. They also may have a musical quality, variously described as "honk" or "whoop." This is usually caused by vibrating vegetations (endocarditis) or chordae tendineae (mitral valve prolapse, dilated cardiomyopathy) and may help separate the more musical murmurs of A-V regurgitation from the *harsher* sounds of semilunar stenosis. Note that in contrast to systolic ejection murmurs like AS or VSD, systolic *regurgitant* murmurs do not increase in intensity after a long diastole (*see* questions 26 and 68). In fact, if the intensity of a systolic murmur *does* increase, but only at the base, then it usually reflects the presence of *two* murmurs: one of *ejection* (becoming louder at the base) and one of *regurgitation* (remaining instead unchanged at the apex). Still, in mitral valve prolapse this rule does not hold, since the regurgitation of MVP is dictated by left ventricular volume: with larger volumes (such as those following a long diastole) causing instead *reduced* regurgitation, and thus a *softer* murmur.

I. Mitral Regurgitation

142. How prevalent is mitral valve regurgitation (MR)?

Very prevalent: 500,000 discharge diagnoses annually in the United States, making it the most common nonfunctional murmur. Echocardiographically, it can be detected in 80% of adults, even though very few of these require surgical attention (only 18,000 a year), suggesting that most cases are technological incidentalomas. Hence, the need to identify patients with *clinically significant disease* and provide them with appropriate care and follow-up.

143. What is the pathophysiology of MR?

It is a backflow into the atrium, leading eventually to the most pronounced *left atrial enlargement* of *all* valvular diseases. This typically comes with atrial fibrillation and increased pulmonary pressure. It also causes chronic *volume load* to the left ventricle, which, in turn, leads to its compensatory *dilatation*. Although this manages, at least initially, to maintain cardiac output, it eventually results in electrical irritability (sudden death) and myocardial decompensation.

144. What are the causes of MR?

They vary, depending on patient's *age* and *acuteness* of condition. Overall, MR may be due to diseases of the *valve per se* (annulus, leaflets, chordae, and papillary muscles) or to *alterations in left ventricular function/structure* (from ischemic disease or dilated cardiomyopathy). Identification of the mechanism *is* crucial, since it determines (together with severity) clinical outcome, medical therapy, and the potential need for surgical intervention.

145. What are the most common "valvular" causes of MR in adults?

There are four:

- Myxomatous degeneration of the valve (mitral valve prolapse)
- Dysfunction of the papillary muscle(s), usually on an ischemic basis. This occurs in 10–20% of acute myocardial infarction cases, usually transiently, but still predicting a less favorable outcome.
- Rheumatic valvular damage (rare in the United States and typically associated with some degree of mitral stenosis)
- Rupture of the chordae, usually infectious

In surgical series, the most common causes of *severe* MR are (in increasing frequency): endocarditis (10–12%), rheumatic heart disease (3–40%), ischemia (13–30%), and mitral valve prolapse (20–70%). Although the latter is common in surgical series, most patients with MVP only have mild disease, and thus never require surgery.

146. What are the most common "valvular" causes of MR in *children*?

In *infants,* the most common is a *dysfunction of the papillary muscles,* associated with either an anomalous left coronary (arising from the pulmonary artery) or endocardial fibroelastosis. Other congenital abnormalities that can lead to MR are endocardial cushion defect (with a cleft mitral leaflet) and myxomatous degeneration (often associated with Marfan's; approximately 50% of Marfan patients may have MR). Finally, myocarditis also may cause regurgitation in infants.

147. Can left ventricular dilation and systolic dysfunction cause MR?

Yes. In fact, *it is the most common cause of adult MR.* Ventricular dilation may be due to cardiomyopathy, or MR *per se,* since dilation of the atrioventricular ring from MR renders the valve even more incompetent (hence, the dictum: *mitral regurgitation begets regurgitation*). This, however, usually causes *mild* regurgitation since the valvular orifice remains otherwise constant. Moreover, systolic contraction of the *muscular ring in the annulus* behaves like a sphincter, further minimizing regurgitation. That is why *annulus calcification* in the elderly is such an ominous event: it disables the sphincter and renders the valve *truly* incompetent. Yet, even this form of MR is only mild to moderate, mostly because the decreased left ventricular function cannot generate massive regurgitation. Hence, the murmur is usually soft. Moreover, patients with MR from cardiomyopathy often have such a low ejection fraction that they cannot *afford* surgical repair, since the failing valve provides a much-needed low-pressure escape to ventricular emptying.

148. Once the typical murmur is detected and recognized, what is the prognosis of MR?

It depends on the *etiology* and *severity*. MR may remain asymptomatic for a long time, with average interval from diagnosis to symptoms of approximately 16 years. This may be even longer in mild to moderate disease since most series are indeed restricted to *severe* disease. Yet, once symptomatic, *severe* MR without surgery has poor prognosis, with survival rates of 33% at 8 years, and average mortality of approximately 5% per year. Most deaths are due to pump failure, but sudden death plays a role, too. Other comorbid conditions (such as atrial fibrillation, cerebral ischemic events, and endocarditis) also may worsen outcome.

149. How is MR detected in adults?

It depends:

- **Asymptomatic patients** *with primary valve disease* (i.e., mitral valve prolapse or a rheumatic sequela) get diagnosed by either detecting the typical systolic murmur or performing an echo for some other reasons.
- **Symptomatic patients** *with primary disease* instead come to attention because of heart failure, atrial fibrillation, or endocarditis—often precipitated by some hemodynamic stress, like pregnancy, anemia, or infection.
- Finally, **patients with secondary MR** (i.e., ischemia or endocarditis) get recognized during evaluation of the underlying process.

150. What is the significance of detecting a typical MR murmur?

It strongly argues in favor of MR, with sensitivity and specificity of 80%. Conversely, absence of a murmur does argue *against* moderate to severe disease.

151. What are the characteristics of the MR murmur?

It is loudest at the apex, radiated to the left axilla or interscapular area, high pitched, plateau, and extending all the way into S_2 (holosystolic). S_2 is normal in intensity, but often widely split.

152. **Can the "pitch" identify gradient?**

Yes. Pitch depends on *pressure gradient* and *flow*. If the gradient is high (and the flow is low), the MR murmur is high pitched. Conversely, if the gradient is low (and the flow is high) the murmur is low pitched. Cases in between tend to have mixed frequency.

153. **Can the murmur of MR radiate medially?**

Yes. Rupture of the *posterior* chordae may redirect the regurgitant stream toward the atrial septum and aorta, thus producing a murmur that not only radiates into the neck like AS, but also has its crescendo pattern. Conversely, rupture of the *anterior* chordae may push the stream posteriorly into the mid-thoracic spine, or even toward the top of the head. At times, it may even direct flow *across the chest*, resembling a ventricular septal defect, and thus creating issues of differential diagnosis in post infarction patients.

154. **Are all MR murmurs plateau?**

No. Shape depends on where the murmur starts in systole. Late starters usually extend into S_2; conversely, early starters immediately follow S_1. Hence, the shape of MR can be *plateau, crescendo-decrescendo, crescendo* (starting at mid-systole), and even *decrescendo* (starting after S_1 and ending toward mid-systole). Usually, the loudest MR murmurs are holosystolic and crescendo-decrescendo (yet not as pronounced as the crescendo-decrescendo pattern of AS).

155. **Can the MR murmur extend beyond S_2?**

Yes. This occurs when left ventricular pressure remains higher than left atrial pressure, even after aortic closure, thus leading to a post-S_2 ongoing regurgitation.

156. **What are the best bedside predictors of MR severity?**

The same predictors of murmur severity in general: *intensity and length*. Hence, the louder (and longer) the MR murmur, the worse the regurgitation. Intensity is a particularly strong predictor of severity, especially in MR due to neither ischemia nor dilated cardiomyopathy. In a study of 170 consecutive patients, none of those with silent disease had a regurgitant volume >50 mL, and only one had a regurgitant fraction >40% (similar data were found for AR patients—*see* below, questions 236 and 237). Yet, since murmur grading is rather subjective, interobserver variability may be an issue, as can be obesity and emphysema.

157. **What is the implication for the clinician?**

That one should pay closer attention to murmur intensity: a murmur grade 4 or louder has a positive predictive value of 91% for severe MR. Conversely, a murmur grade <2 argues so strongly *against* significant regurgitation (predictive value of 97%) to make unnecessary any repeat confirmatory testing. Finally, a grade 3 murmur (which occurs in more than one third of MR patients) may reflect any degree of regurgitation, prompting a search for other signs of severity.

158. **What are the other bedside signs of severe MR?**

- **Left ventricular enlargement:** This can be determined by palpation, as a downward and lateral displacement (and enlargement) of the apical impulse. A *left-lower parasternal* impulse also argues strongly in favor of severe disease, usually reflecting a dilated left atrium.
- **Widened S_2 splitting:** This is typical of severe MR and due to early closure of its aortic component. In time, it may become offset by the development of pulmonary hypertension, which, in turn, narrows S_2 splitting.
- **Concomitant S_3:** This occurs in 90% of severe MR cases, with S_3 loudness being directly related to severity of regurgitation. A third sound has 77% specificity for severe MR, but only 41% sensitivity. Note that S_4 is rare in MR, unless there is *acute* regurgitation.

- **Diastolic flow murmur:** In addition to S_3, severe MR is often accompanied by an early diastolic rumble that follows S_3 like an extension. The longer and louder the rumble, the worse the MR.

> **Pearl:**
> Hence, MR is diagnosed in systole, but its severity is assessed in diastole, by the presence of S_3, and/or an early diastolic rumble.

159. **So what is the role of echocardiography in MR?**
It allows an accurate evaluation of the presence, severity, and cause of MR. Hence, it should be obtained in all suspicious systolic murmurs, either because of their intermediate or high *intensity* (i.e., >3/6) or because of concomitant symptoms and findings.

160. **Since both MR and AR cause similar peripheral findings, how can you separate the two?**
Both conditions cause left ventricular *volume load* and thus resemble each other peripherally. Yet, the *arterial pulse* is brisk and *single* in MR, but often bisferiens in AR. The *PMI* is enlarged, sustained, and downward/laterally displaced in both processes; yet only in MR does it often present with an early diastolic extra impulse (S_3-like). Finally, *neck veins* are usually normal in both.

161. **Can a murmur of severe regurgitation be nonetheless soft and almost silent?**
Yes. In addition to obesity or emphysema, its most common reason is *acute* MR from transient papillary muscle ischemia. Most of these patients have *silent but severe* regurgitation, manifesting itself as either paroxysmal nocturnal dyspnea or "flash pulmonary edema" (conversely, transient ischemia in chronic MR presents as a *new, loud, and symptomatic murmur*). In addition to the dramatic presentation, the only other clues to diagnosis are a large left ventricle and a widely split S_2.

162. **Can the shape of the murmur differentiate the various causes of regurgitation?**
Yes. *Plateau* murmurs are more likely to be *rheumatic*, whereas murmurs that start in mid-systole and "grow" into S_2 are more likely to be due to either *mitral valve prolapse* or *papillary muscle dysfunction*. Because in this case the papillary muscle is not contracting well, its chordae become progressively longer as the ventricle gets smaller. This causes a murmur that grows louder throughout systole, is crescendo-like, and often has a *cooing* character—like the cry of a *seagull*.

163. **Is there any bedside maneuver that can help identify papillary muscle dysfunction?**
Passive leg raising for 20 seconds. This increases left ventricular volume and thus may elicit the murmur of *papillary muscle dysfunction*. Passive leg raising comes in handy in patients with angina and left ventricular failure who have transient and subtle MR.

164. **Can you separate MR of ruptured chordae from MR of dysfunctional papillary muscles?**
Yes. *Dysfunctional* papillary muscle(s) are either asymptomatic or presenting with mild congestive failure. *Ruptured* chordae (or papillary muscles) present instead *much* more dramatically, with an intense MR murmur (3/6 or greater), a loud S_3, and a *flash pulmonary edema*. In fact, the large amount of backflow in these patients may even increase atrial pressure so rapidly to eventually slow regurgitation early on in systole. Hence, the MR murmur typically starts immediately after S_1 and then softens (and even disappears) at mid-systole.

This is the opposite of the murmur of *dysfunctional* papillary muscle, which starts instead at mid-systole, has a crescendo pattern, and usually ends at S_2 (although it also may last into mid-systole or even stay holosystolic). Patterns of radiation also may be unusual in ruptured chordae tendineae (*see* question 153). Finally, the MR of ruptured chordae is often associated with an S_4. This is due to the Starling's effect of a dilated atrium, which results in greater contractility and thus a stronger (and louder) systole. S_4 is instead rare in MR from dysfunctional papillary muscles, and is almost absent in rheumatic disease.

165. What is the cause of ruptured chordae tendineae?
Usually, infective endocarditis. Very often, however, the rupture is *idiopathic*. In this case, the valve (or chordae) has a congenital myxomatous degeneration that makes it more prone to spontaneous rupture, especially during unusual strains. This is especially common in MVP.

166. What are the characteristics of the acute MR murmur?
The foremost is the patient's instability due to incapacity of the normal-sized left atrium to accommodate the regurgitating stream. As a result, acute MR patients are often in florid pulmonary edema, with pulmonary hypertension and distended neck veins. In addition, the acute MR murmur tends to be very short, and even absent, since the left atrium and ventricle often behave like a common chamber, with no pressure gradient between them. Hence, in contrast to that of chronic MR (which is either holosystolic or late systolic) the *acute* MR murmur is often early systolic (exclusively so in 40% of cases) and is associated with an S_4 in 80% of the patients.

167. Is the murmur of MR increased or softened by respiration?
It depends on the *phase* of respiration, and its effect on right- and left-sided venous return. Usually, MR is *softened* by inhalation, whereas TR is heightened. The opposite occurs in exhalation.

168. What are the effects of other bedside maneuvers/vasoactive drugs on the intensity of MR?
To understand these effects, one has to remember that in MR the left ventricle has two possible discharge outlets: a high resistance bed (the aorta) and a low resistance bed (the left atrium). *Increases* in peripheral vascular resistance (by vasopressors, but also handgrip or squatting) will increase regurgitation and heighten the murmur. Conversely, they will soften AS.

169. What is the effect on MR of standing?
It increases peripheral vascular resistance, but its effect on the murmur depends on the etiology of MR. If primarily due to a *dilated left ventricle,* the murmur will get *softer* during standing (because *decreased venous return* causes a reduction in ventricular size). If, on the other hand, MR is due to other reasons, then the murmur will get *louder* during standing (because the increased peripheral vascular resistance increases the degree of regurgitation). This effect may nonetheless be upset by the drop in venous return caused by standing, and thus the intensity of the murmur may stay unchanged. Finally, if MR is due to *MVP,* a smaller left ventricle (as in standing) will cause *more* prolapse. Hence, standing may prolong and intensify the MVP murmur.

170. In summary, how accurate is physical examination for diagnosing MR?
It depends. In the ears of cardiologists, the absence of an apical late systolic/holosystolic murmur strongly argues against the presence of MR (except in acute MI). Cardiologists also can accurately distinguish left-sided regurgitant murmurs (like MR and VSD) by using transient arterial occlusion. Noncardiologists (especially house officers) are instead much less accurate.

II. Mitral Valve Prolapse

171. What is mitral valve prolapse (MVP)?

An entity that throughout its history has received many names, with the most current being *mitral valve prolapse syndrome,* since this is indeed a syndrome, characterized not only by auscultatory findings, but also arrhythmias, atypical chest pain, abnormal ECG, panic attacks, and, possibly, valve infection. MVP is the most common congenital valvular disease, with a prevalence of 1–2%. In this section, we will focus on its murmur. For the click, refer to Chapter 11, questions 153–163.

172. What is the underlying abnormality of MVP?

A redundancy of one or both mitral leaflets, causing a systolic ballooning (and posterosuperior prolapsing) into the left atrium. This may present with a sharp mid- (or late) systolic *click,* possibly followed by a regurgitant murmur. Women are twice as often affected by MVP, which may even be familial (with autosomal dominant inheritance). Although systolic clicks had been known for decades, they were incorrectly given an extracardiac origin—mostly through the influence of Gallavardin. It was Reid and Barlow who first correctly interpreted them as due to MVP.

173. Which leaflet is most commonly involved?

Usually the posterior, which often has a myxomatous degeneration. This is commonly seen in Marfan patients, who indeed often have MVP. Yet, most MVP patients have no features of Marfan's, although 20–30% *do* have some of its minor traits, such as tall stature, low body mass index, straight backs, pectus excavatum, scoliosis, greater arm span than height, and unusual joint flexibility.

174. Is myxomatous degeneration limited to the mitral valve?

No, it often extends to the *tricuspid* valve.

175. Who was Barlow?

John Brereton Barlow was chief of cardiology at Witwatersrand University in South Africa (Witwatersrand is Afrikaans for "white water reef"—*under which the gold lies,* since the homonymous and nearby mountain range is the source of 40% of all the *gold* ever mined on *earth*). Born in Cape Town in 1924, Barlow became well known because of his rugby skills, which eventually gained him a university admission to Johannesburg. As a med student, he became known for his frequent reference to rare and bizarre syndromes, which eventually earned him the nickname of "canary" (the South African equivalent of our "zebra," since over there zebras are not a rarity, whereas canaries are. In a tribute to his reputation as eccentric, Barlow later on kept canaries outside his office). After serving in the British Army during World War II, he graduated from medical school and then trained for 3 years in Soweto, and 3 more years in London, under Sir John McMichael. It was there that he learned to challenge conventional wisdom (*holy cows make great burgers*), a penchant that eventually helped him make his most iconoclastic observation: that the mid- and late systolic click(s) were *not* extracardiac in origin (as Gallavardin had suggested), but due instead to "billowing" (and regurgitation) of the mitral leaflet. Although this had already been suggested by John Reid in the 1950s, it was so controversial that Barlow's initial paper was rejected by *Circulation,* and eventually printed in short form in the *Maryland State Medical Journal* and the *American Heart Journal* (1963). The term mitral valve "prolapse," however, was introduced by John Michael Criley during Barlow's 1964 visit to Johns Hopkins. Criley also was the one to point out that the phenomenon was *not* due to filling of a subvalvular ventricular aneurysm (as Barlow had initially thought), but to a prolapsing of the mitral leaflet. Barlow accepted this observation and always credited Criley. Still, he never liked the term *prolapse,* preferring instead "billowing." As a physician, he was the ultimate clinical cardiologist, in the classical and bedside-oriented

British style. He practiced in Johannesburg for over 40 years, caring for underprivileged Soweto children and influential politicians like 1993 Nobel laureate Nelson Mandela. His passion for auscultation (and the bedside) was reflected in the Oslerian dedication of his textbook, *Perspectives on the Mitral Valve:* "To all students of medicine who listen, look, touch, and reflect; may they hear, see, feel, and comprehend."

176. What are the characteristics of the mitral valve prolapse murmur?
It is a mitral *regurgitant* murmur—hence, loudest at the apex, mid to late systolic in onset (immediately following the click), and usually extending all the way into the second sound (A_2). In fact, it often has a *crescendo* shape that *peaks* at S_2. It is usually not too loud (never greater than 3/6), with some musical features that have been variously described as *whoops* or *honks* (as in the honking of a goose). Indeed, musical murmurs of this kind are almost always due to MVP.

177. Can mitral valve prolapse be silent? Can anything make it louder?
Click and murmur may often be absent. Bedside maneuvers, such as mild exercise, may, however, bring them back—either together or separately. Various positions and different phases of respiration can do the same—mostly by changing left ventricular *size*, since a *larger* ventricle pulls down on the ballooning valve, thus delaying/preventing its prolapse. This "trimming of the sail" through tense chordae can postpone (and possibly eliminate) the click. It also can shorten the murmur. Conversely, a *smaller* ventricle facilitates the posterior ballooning of the valve, thus causing earlier and more severe regurgitation. Hence, an *earlier* click and a *longer* murmur.

178. Which bedside maneuvers can *reduce* left ventricular size?
Inspiration, tachycardia (from mild exercise), *standing* (after squatting), and the straining phase of *Valsalva*. In other words, the same maneuvers previously described for HOCM. These reduce left ventricular size through a decrease in *preload*, thus *anticipating* click, *lengthening* murmur, and making both more audible. Squatting-to-standing also makes the murmur *louder*.

179. Which bedside maneuvers can *increase* left ventricular size?
Exhalation, bradycardia, passive leg raising, and *squatting.* These all delay the click, shorten the murmur, and lessen the severity of regurgitation. Drugs that slow heart rate (and thus enlarge the left ventricle) also will do the same. Hence, the common use of beta blockers in MVP.

180. In summary, how accurate is physical examination for the diagnosis of MVP?
It depends on the examiner. If a cardiologist hears a systolic click (with or without a murmur), then the likelihood of echocardiographic MVP is very high. Conversely, absence of both click *and* murmur strongly argues *against* MVP. Finally, presence of a holosystolic murmur *without a click* significantly increases the likelihood of long-term complications from MVP, such as cardiac death, progressive regurgitation requiring surgery, endocarditis, and systemic embolism; absence of both click *and* murmur makes instead these complications much less likely.

181. Do patients with an isolated click necessarily develop regurgitation?
No. When followed for as long as 8 years, they do not develop significant regurgitation. Hence, clickers tend to stay clickers, which may have importance for prophylaxis (*see* Chapter 11).

182. And what about the need for valvular replacement in patients with a murmur?
Still relatively low. Overall, MVP is associated with mild to moderate regurgitation, as indicated by the mid to late onset of the murmur. With time, regurgitation may worsen, but this is still rare, with only 3% of patients eventually requiring valve replacement. Severe but initially

asymptomatic MVP also has a favorable 5-year outlook, with only one third of patients becoming symptomatic enough to require surgery. In fact, a much more common cause of *severe* regurgitation is rupture of malformed chordae, resulting in a flail leaflet. This has a poor 10-year outcome, independent of symptoms (90% of patients die or undergo surgery). Finally, an even more frequent reason for surgery is infective endocarditis, often the presenting manifestation of a previously silent MVP.

183. What is the differential diagnosis of MVP?
The most important is *papillary muscle dysfunction* from infarction/ischemia, since this, too, can cause "prolapse." These patients are usually older (and more symptomatic) than those with MVP. *HOCM* also may prolapse the mitral valve, usually because of the unequal length of the chordae tendineae. Finally, a split S_1 or ejection sounds (early systolic clicks) may need to be differentiated from the click of MVP, which is later in systole and changed by maneuvers.

184. Can bedside maneuvers identify a murmur of papillary muscle dysfunction?
Yes, since this neither lengthens nor intensifies with sitting, standing, or Valsalva.

III. Tricuspid Regurgitant (TR) Murmur

185. What are the most common causes of tricuspid regurgitation?
- **Primary TR** is usually the result of direct valvular damage, without any preexistent pulmonary hypertension. This is typically *acute* and due to either endocarditis (almost always from drug abuse) or trauma. Primary TR also can be a congenital anomaly, as in Epstein's disease.
- **Secondary TR** requires instead either a *pressure* load to the right ventricle (i.e., pulmonary hypertension) or a *volume* load (as in atrial septal defect). This is often *chronic,* eventually causing right ventricular dilation, pulling apart of leaflets, and valvular incompetence.

186. What is the most common cause of pulmonary hypertension in the United States?
Left ventricular failure. Think of pulmonary hypertension in terms of (1) *post capillary etiologies* (left ventricular failure, mitral stenosis, cor triatriatum, veno-occlusive pulmonary disease); (2) *capillary etiologies* (pulmonary obstructive, restrictive, and vascular diseases); and (3) *pre-capillary etiologies* (pulmonary emboli and primary pulmonary hypertension).

187. Where is the TR murmur best heard?
Over the left lower sternal border or the epigastric/subxiphoid area. At times, however, it may be best heard over the apex—especially when the right ventricle has become large enough to displace the *left* ventricle laterally and posteriorly. Occasionally, a TR murmur can be heard only over the free edge of the liver—especially in patients with "muffling" by chronic obstructive pulmonary disease (COPD) and air trapping.

188. What are the diagnostic features of a TR murmur?
It depends. If caused by *pulmonary hypertension,* it has a typical holosystolic duration with inspiratory accentuation (Rivero-Carvallo sign, positive in 2/3 of patients). Often, there is a whooping or *honking* quality. Note that the murmur remains intensified *as long as* inspiration is held, since right ventricular return is indeed increased *throughout* inspiration. The murmur may also intensify in response to *other* maneuvers that increase right-sided venous return, like having the patient bend the knees toward the chest, passively elevate the legs, or engage in mild exercise. Finally, presence of a typical murmur argues strongly in favor of TR, whereas its absence does not exclude it.

189. **How can one differentiate TR from MR?**

By their different area of maximal intensity. Still, a very enlarged right ventricle may at times expand leftwards and thus replace the left ventricle in its apical location. Conversely, a very enlarged *left* ventricle (as often seen in *MR*) may expand rightwards and thus confuse the listener. Hence, the easiest way to separate these two murmurs is indeed the inspiratory maneuver of Rivero-Carvallo, which intensifies only TR. Other useful findings are *hepatic pulsatility* (30–91% of TR patients—usually arguing in favor of moderate-to-severe disease with specificity >90%) and *response to the abdominojugular reflux* (MR elicits no response, whereas TR induces a positive reflux with concomitant increase in murmur intensity—Vitum sign, 60% sensitivity and 100% specificity). *Neck vein examination* can be helpful, too, since 70–85% of TR patients will have typical giant V waves with deep Y descents (i.e., the *Lancisi sign*, from Giovanni Lancisi, physician to three popes). This is often associated with the *flickering* of *earlobes* from regurgitating blood (80% sensitivity). MR patients have neither of these findings. Finally, TR gets louder within 1 second into the *release* phase of Valsalva, whereas MR takes longer (3 seconds).

190. **Does the Lancisi sign predict severity?**

No. A giant systolic "V" wave may be absent in regurgitations so severe to prevent the diastolic collapse of the vein (i.e., in patients with persistently high central venous pressure [CVP]). It may instead be very prominent in patients whose regurgitation is too mild to cause high CVP.

191. **How can one measure central venous pressure (CVP) in TR?**

With great difficulty. Estimation of CVP in TR can be misleading because of the interference by the large systolic regurgitant wave, which makes reading venous diastolic pressure much more complicated. To overcome this problem, you should rely on *mean* venous pressure. This is determined by identifying the patient's position in which the systolic regurgitant wave becomes visible: the more upright this position is, the higher the diastolic central venous pressure will be.

192. **What are the other bedside findings of chronic TR?**

90% of patients have distended neck veins, plus peripheral edema and/or ascites.

193. **In summary, how accurate is physical examination for the diagnosis of TR?**

Once again, it depends on the examiner. Overall, cardiologists can accurately detect the murmur of moderate to severe TR, especially if using quiet inspiration and sustained abdominal pressure.

194. **How does *acute* TR differ from its chronic counterpart?**

In many ways. Whenever regurgitation is sudden, its murmur is typically limited to early systole, and often decrescendo because right atrial pressure rises so rapidly to eventually stop backflow at mid-systole—a phenomenon similar to that behind acute *MR* (*see* question 166). In fact, whenever regurgitation is so severe that the *atrium and ventricle become a single chamber*, the murmur of TR (and MR) is absent. This may occur in patients whose chordae rupture. Finally, many of the peripheral manifestations of TR (leg edema, ascites, pulsatile liver), and even some of its jugular findings, may be absent acutely, since pulmonary pressure remains low and TR less prominent.

C. DIASTOLIC MURMURS

195. **What are the causes of a diastolic murmur?**

Primarily two, both pathologic:

- **Forward flow** through a narrowed A-V valve (i.e., mitral or tricuspid stenosis). This also can occur with increased transvalvular flow due to either atrial septal defect or MR/TR.
- **Backward flow** through an incompetent semilunar valve (i.e., pulmonic or aortic regurgitation).

196. **How are diastolic murmurs classified?**
By their timing. Hence, the most important division is between murmurs that start *just after S_2* (i.e., *early* diastolic—reflecting semilunar regurgitation) versus those that start *a little later* (i.e., mid to late diastolic, often with a presystolic accentuation—reflecting atrioventricular stenosis).

(1) DIASTOLIC ATRIOVENTRICULAR VALVE MURMURS

I. Mitral Stenosis

197. **What are the most common causes of mitral stenosis (MS)?**
The most common is rheumatic fever, causing inflammation, fibrosis, and fusion of the leaflets, often with superimposed calcification. A less-common reason is a congenital anomaly of one papillary muscle, which renders it linked by chordae tendineae to *both* mitral leaflets (*parachute mitral valve*). An even less-frequent cause is a left atrial myxoma (often presenting with a tumor "plop" and a syncope triggered by change in position) or a calcified bacterial vegetation that obstructs the inlet. Note that MS may be mimicked by various conditions, including (1) *mitral annular calcification* (in fact, detecting an apical diastolic rumble in elderly patients has specificity close to 100% for this condition) and (2) the early diastolic murmur of a large mitral flow, as seen in severe MR or VSD. These are neither MS nor Austin Flint murmurs (see under aortic regurgitation).

198. **Where is the murmur of MS best heard?**
At the apex, but a bit more medially than normal, since the left ventricle of MS is smaller. Hence, before listening to the apex with your bell, carefully palpate the PMI with the patient in left-lateral decubitus position.

199. **What is the timing of the diastolic murmur of MS? What is its relationship to S_2?**
The MS murmur is mid to late diastolic, insofar as it does *not* immediately follow S_2 (like the murmur of semilunar regurgitation), but is instead separated by a little pause. In fact, it often follows the *opening snap* (which may or may not be audible) and then rumbles through diastole.

200. **What is the shape of the diastolic rumble of MS?**
It has an initial *crescendo* pattern with a mid-diastolic peak (since the most rapid phase of ventricular filling occurs in early diastole), followed by a *decrescendo* phase and a final *presystolic accentuation*. This late diastolic "crescendo" has been traditionally attributed to a forceful left atrial contraction, but probably has a different mechanism, since it also can be heard in patients without a valid atrial contraction (like those in atrial fibrillation). Hence, it is probably due to a further increase in mitral narrowing caused by the onset of ventricular systole.

201. **What is the pitch of the MS rumble?**
Very low. The MS murmur is so low pitched to be detectable only in left lateral decubitus, by the bell, and after paying extraordinary attention because the *rumble* is more the result of *flow* than of a true atrioventricular pressure gradient. In fact, even in severe MS the maximum gradient is only 30 mmHg at the *beginning* of diastole and 10 mmHg at the *end* of it. This is definitely much lower than the peak gradient encountered in significant *systolic* obstruction, such as that of AS (where it may easily reach 50 mmHg). Since murmurs produced by *flow* tend to be lower pitched than those produced by gradient, the MS murmur has typical low frequencies. This has led to many adjectives, such as *rumbling* and *laboring,* first used by Austin Flint in 1884.

202. Is a very intense murmur reflective of more severe stenosis?

It depends. If the patient does not have concomitant mitral regurgitation, a loud murmur (usually accompanied by a thrill [i.e., >4/6]) does indeed reflect severe stenosis. Conversely, a loud murmur also indicates absence of significant pulmonary hypertension—which is a good prognostic sign because a reduction of flow from the right into the left chambers (as the result of severe pulmonary hypertension) would actually *decrease* the intensity of the MS rumble.

203. What are the other physical findings of mitral stenosis?

- **Loudness of S_1:** This is a very important feature, so much so that traditional teaching considers MS unlikely in patients lacking it. The reasons for the increased intensity are primarily two: a higher A-V pressure gradient (which prevents the slow juxtaposition of leaflets) and thickening of the leaflets themselves. Note that patients whose valve becomes calcified, or otherwise less mobile, may paradoxically *soften* S_1—even though their MS is quite severe.
- **Small apical impulse:** This is due to the reduced ventricular filling of MS and is also the reason why the *arterial pulse* may be small in MS patients (and often irregularly irregular, given the predisposition to atrial fibrillation). Hence, a hyperkinetic or downward/laterally displaced PMI argues in favor of a concomitant regurgitant disease (aortic or mitral).
- **Increased central venous pressure and prominent "A" wave:** This is common in MS patients with pulmonary hypertension. By the time pulmonary hypertension causes pulmonic and tricuspid regurgitation, other physical findings appear (a giant venous "V" wave, pulsatile liver, right ventricular heave, palpable P_2, Graham Steell murmur, and a holosystolic TR murmur).

204. Which maneuvers can be used to intensify the MS rumble?

First of all, maneuvers that can bring the left ventricle closer to the chest wall, and thus to the stethoscope. The most common is the *left-lateral decubitus*. Maneuvers that increase cardiac output (and thus flow across the stenotic valve) also can intensify the murmur. For example, asking the patient to engage in brief exercise (such as getting up from bed) immediately before auscultation. Or listening while the patient is squatting during a hand-grip maneuver. Finally, listening while the patient is raising the straightened legs also may enhance the murmur. If this is too cumbersome, one may simply ask the patient to raise his or her legs while keeping the knees bent toward the chest. At times, even a few bouts of coughing or the completion of a Valsalva straining maneuver (with auscultation carried out during the *release* phase) may do the trick.

205. And what about respiration?

Exhalation also can increase murmur intensity because it not only causes the heart to get closer to the stethoscope (due to diminished lung aeration), but it also squeezes blood from the lungs into the left chambers, thus increasing flow across the stenotic valve. Overall, left-sided findings intensify in *expiration*, whereas right-sided findings intensify in *inspiration*. The reasons are physiologically different, but grounded on the same principle: increased venous return.

206. What is then the best strategy to detect the MS murmur?

The best strategy consists of listening over the *apex*, with the patient in the *left lateral decubitus* position, at *the end of exhalation*, and after a *short exercise*. Finally, applying the bell with very light pressure also may help (strong pressure will instead completely eliminate the low frequencies of MS).

207. And what about the concomitant presence of mitral regurgitation?

If the patient also were to have MR, the MS murmur would be louder *independent of the pressure gradient* because MR increases not only left ventricular size (thereby bringing the left ventricle *closer* to the stethoscope), but also left atrial volume (due to the regurgitation). This, in turn, increases diastolic flow through the stenotic mitral valve, and thus the MS rumble.

208. Which conditions are instead associated with a softer murmur of MS?

The most common is emphysema. Low transvalvular flow also may soften the murmur. Though severe MS is typically the reason for this, severe pulmonary hypertension, cardiomyopathy, and concomitant tricuspid stenosis may do it, too. Finally, a large right ventricle (which is the end result of pulmonary hypertension) may displace posteriorly its left-sided counterpart, thus pushing it away from the anterior wall—and the stethoscope. This, in turn, will make the MS murmur softer.

209. What is the effect of atrial fibrillation on the intensity of MS?

It softens the murmur. This is due to its tachycardia and also to the absence of a valid atrial contraction (which can increase cardiac output by about 25% in patients with significant MS).

II. Mitral Diastolic Flow Murmur

210. What are "mitral diastolic flow murmurs"?

They are murmurs produced by excessive flow across a normal mitral valve. These "flow murmurs" can be encountered in moderate to severe MR, a high *alpha state* (like thyrotoxicosis), or even situations of left-to-right shunt at either the ventricular or arterial level (such as VSD or PDA). In all these conditions, the large amount of blood reaching the left atrium creates a characteristic early diastolic flow rumble that may be easily confused for MS. A similar murmur also can be heard in pronounced bradycardia, which also causes an early diastolic transvalvular rush. All these murmurs are similar to that of MS, insofar as they are low pitched, rumbling, and separated from S_2 by a little delay. They also are heard at the apex, in left lateral decubitus, and with the bell. In contrast to MS, however, they occur at the same time as the S_3, thus remaining primarily limited to *early* diastole (whereas the MS murmur tends instead to rumble *throughout* diastole, often with a presystolic accentuation). A diastolic flow murmur can at times be heard in *acute rheumatic fever,* presenting with mitral regurgitation and cardiomegaly. It is preceded by S_3 and is called the Carey Coombs murmur (from the English physician who described it in 1924). Finally, early to mid-diastolic murmurs should be differentiated from a *summation gallop* (i.e., the louder sound of merged S_3 and S_4 in patients with tachycardia).

III. Tricuspid Diastolic Murmurs

211. What is the mechanism of a tricuspid diastolic murmur?

It is very much the same as that of a *mitral* diastolic flow murmur: the valve may either be the site of *stenosis*, or of a diastolic *flow* murmur unrelated to any narrowing.

212. Where are these murmurs mostly heard?

Over the right ventricular area (i.e., the epigastrium/subxiphoid site), but also over the lower parasternal areas (left and right). Note that whenever the right ventricle is very dilated, it may actually displace backwards the left ventricle and position itself over the true apex.

213. What are the most common causes of a tricuspid diastolic flow murmur?

It depends. Increased flow through the tricuspid valve may occur in *atrial septal defects*, and thus produce a diastolic flow rumble. A similar rumble also may occur in situations of *TR*, also as a result of increased diastolic flow. Both these murmurs can be intensified by minimal exercise, like holding up the patient's legs, bending them backwards, or simply having the patient take deep inspirations (panting). Still, the major differential diagnosis for a diastolic *flow* murmur is *stenosis* of the corresponding valve (i.e., tricuspid stenosis [TS]). The hallmark of TS is its very accentuated presystolic component, which is typical of it, and absent in tricuspid diastolic flow murmurs. Also, TS tends to occur *without* S_3, whereas the tricuspid diastolic flow murmur is often accompanied by it.

214. How frequently does tricuspid stenosis occur in patients with MS?
In as many as 5%. It is usually detected over the same area of tricuspid diastolic flow murmurs.

215. How can one differentiate TS from MS?
In addition to having different locations, the TS murmur increases with inspiration, whereas the one of MS softens (Rivero-Carvallo phenomenon). The murmur of TS also is louder in the right-lateral decubitus position, whereas that of MS is louder in the *left*-lateral decubitus position. Finally, the MS murmur tends to have a low-pitched quality, whereas the one of TS has instead a more *scratchy* quality.

(2) DIASTOLIC SEMILUNAR VALVE MURMURS

I. Aortic Regurgitation (AR)

216. How frequent is AR?
It accounts for approximately 10% of all cases of valvular heart disease.

217. What are its causes?
Primarily two: (1) aortic *cusp* disease and (2) aortic *root* dilation. Before antibiotics, the two most common forms of adult AR were rheumatic fever (through its direct *cusps'* involvement) and syphilis (through its *root* dilation). Although they both remain leading causes of AR worldwide, nowadays the most common mechanism in the West is a "leaky" *bicuspid* valve. This usually starts to fail in the fourth or fifth decade of life and eventually progresses to full-blown AR over a few years. A failed bicuspid valve was rumored to be behind Arnold Schwarzenegger's 1997 surgery.

218. How does rheumatic fever cause aortic regurgitation?
By an inflammatory shrinkage/retraction of the cusps, which prevents the leaflets from fully juxtaposing. Inflammation also may *fuse the commissures,* resulting in combined AS *and* AR.

219. What are the other "valvular" causes of AR?
The major ones are:
- **Calcific aortic degeneration:** This is an age-related process that may affect a congenitally bicuspid valve and result in AR, with or without stenosis. Still, only 5% of bicuspid valves develop AR. Moreover, calcific degeneration also can occur with a normal trileaflet valve.
- **Myxomatous degeneration:** This may involve either the aortic or mitral valve, where it presents as mitral valve prolapse. Unrelated to Marfan's, it may occur in up to 15% of patients with chronic and progressive AR.
- **Infective endocarditis**
- **Aging tissue prosthesis:** This is usually the result of an age-related structural deterioration of a bioprosthetic valve.
- **Trauma**
- **Ventricular septal defect (VSD):** This is due to leaflet prolapse into a large VSD.

220. What are the "root" causes of aortic regurgitation?
Several—all related to an enlarged ascending aorta. The most common are degenerative aortic dilation of the elderly, cystic medial necrosis of Marfan's, syphilitic aortitis, and dissection of the ascending aorta. Root diseases have recently become more frequent than cusps diseases.

221. What about hypertension?
Severe hypertension also may cause aortic regurgitation (in as many as 60% of patients), usually because of either a bicuspid aortic valve or a dilation of the aortic ring. Most of the time, however, the leakage is minimal and mostly limited to an echocardiographic finding.

222. **Is there any way to separate at the bedside "valvular" AR from "root" AR?**
Location. Proctor Harvey proposed in 1963 that *valvular* AR tends to be loudest over the Erb's point (left parasternal area), whereas "root" AR over the aortic area (right parasternal area). This is intuitive if one considers the anatomy. Note that a *tambour* S_2 (loud and ringing sound, with rich aortic overtones) suggests the presence of a dilated aortic root, serving as a drum-like ("tambour" in French) echoing chamber for the vibration of the regurgitating flow. Indeed, a *bruit de tambour* ("sound of drum") used to be a typical 19th-century finding of syphilitic aortitis.

223. **What is the pathophysiology of chronic AR?**
In chronic AR, the left ventricle (LV) receives blood from both the atrium and aorta. This results in a *volume load* that, over time, leads to *the greatest ventricular enlargement of any heart disease* (which, in the past, led to the creation of the colorful term "ox-like heart"—"cor bovinum"). Although the LV end-diastolic volume becomes quite large, LV compliance also increases. As a result, LV end-diastolic pressure remains near normal, and LV hypertrophy is in fact minimal. Regurgitant flow, however, may be huge. In severe cases, regurgitant flow may exceed 20 L/min, with total LV output of almost 30 L/min. Eventually, a persistent rise in preload and afterload leads to myocardial dysfunction and a drop in cardiac output. This process of decompensation, however, is gradual and always precedes the onset of symptoms. Ultimately, the rise in left-ventricular end-diastolic pressure causes an increase in left-atrial, pulmonic, right-ventricular, and right-atrial pressures. Detection of the onset of LV dysfunction is crucial for timing surgery. Note that the *cor bovinum* (i.e., a heart of >500 g) was a common outcome of aortic regurgitation only historically. In fact, recent data from Germany (Fluri et al.) suggest that not only this condition is decreasing in frequency (from one in four to one in five of all "cardiac" autopsies), but it is also becoming increasingly associated with nonvalvular risk factors, such as coronary atherosclerosis, hypertension, COPD, and male gender. It is also being found at a more advanced age, suggesting the beneficial impact of recent therapeutic interventions (like ACE-inhibitors, beta blockers, statins, PTCA, and cardiac surgery).

224. **What are the symptoms of AR?**
Most patients are asymptomatic, and the diagnosis is usually established through detection of the typical diastolic murmur during a routine physical exam. In fact, in contrast to *acute* AR, chronic AR may be present for years before its initial symptom (*exertional dyspnea*) develops. This will then evolve into *orthopnea* and *paroxysmal nocturnal dyspnea*. The patient's awareness of the heartbeat (due to left ventricular enlargement, heart pounding, and palpitations) is also a frequent AR symptom, whereas *chest pain* tends to be much less common than in AS: only 20% of patients experience it (with evidence of coronary artery disease in 10% of these cases). Still, nocturnal *angina* (often accompanied by diaphoresis) is not uncommon and usually due to diastolic hypotension triggered by sleep-related bradycardia. Some patients with AR also may report abdominal pain, presumably due to splanchnic ischemia.

225. **What are the "central" signs of chronic AR?**
- **Blood pressure:** The hallmark of severe, chronic AR is a marked reduction in diastolic pressure, along with some increase in *systolic* values due to higher stroke volume. Hence, *pulse pressure* widens, often exceeding 80 mmHg. At times, determination of diastolic blood pressure may be especially difficult, since Korotkoff sounds can remain audible all the way to 0. Thus, diastolic pressure should be established at *point of muffling,* and *not* of disappearance.
- **Arterial pulse:** Typical, with brisk upstroke and downstroke, tall amplitude, and prominent carotid pulsations ("dance of the carotids"). These, in turn, may cause a pulsatile movement of head, larynx, and uvula. Abdominal pulsations may be visible in the suprarenal region.

- **Precordial impulse:** Enlarged, sustained, and downwards/laterally displaced. This is due to the enormous left ventricular dilation that is so typical of regurgitant diseases like AR and MR (volume load). In contrast to MR, AR rarely presents with a palpable S_3 (*see* question 245).

226. What are the typical auscultatory findings of AR?

Depending on severity, there may be up to three murmurs (one in systole and two in diastole) plus an ejection click. Of course, the typical auscultatory finding is the *diastolic tapering murmur,* which, together with the brisk pulse and the enlarged/displaced PMI, constitutes the bedside diagnostic triad of AR. A characteristic early diastolic murmur argues very strongly in favor of the disease.

227. What is the *click* of AR?

It is an early systolic *ejection* sound caused by one of three mechanisms: (1) a bicuspid semilunar valve, (2) a brisk and turbulent ejection (usually indicative of a large regurgitation), or (3) a dilated aortic root. The latter is not uncommon in severe AR and leads to further regurgitation.

228. What about the systolic murmur?

It may be caused by concomitant AS, but most commonly indicates *severe regurgitation*, followed by an increased systolic flow across the valve. Hence, it is often referred to as "comitans" (Latin for *companion*). It provides an important clue to the severity of regurgitation. Hence, semilunar regurgitation is diagnosed in *diastole* (by the presence of an early diastolic and tapering murmur), but its severity is assessed in *systole* (by the presence of a concomitant ejection flow murmur and, possibly, of an early systolic click).

229. Is there any way to separate the comitans murmur of AR from the systolic murmur of AS?

The flow murmur of AR tends to be shorter than that of AS, with louder S_2 and brisker pulse.

230. What about the two diastolic murmurs?

They are (1) the tapering diastolic murmur of aortic regurgitation per se and (2) the rumbling diastolic murmur of *Austin Flint* (i.e., functional mitral stenosis).

231. What are the characteristics of the decrescendo murmur of AR?

The major one is that it starts *immediately after* the aortic component of S_2 (i.e., in early diastole) and that it *tapers*. If AR is trivial, the murmur may be short enough to be only early diastolic. At times, just an echo finding. Hence, absence of a murmur excludes moderate to severe disease.

232. Where is it best heard?

Usually over Erb's point (third or fourth interspace, left parasternal line), but at times also over the aortic area, especially when a tortuous and dilated root pushes the ascending aorta anteriorly and to the right. This is common in case of ascending aortic aneurysm or severe atherosclerotic disease. Occasionally, the murmur is best heard at the apex, and at times even near the axilla or mid-left thorax (Cole-Cecil murmur). In fact, the surface projection of the AR murmur is the famous "sash" (i.e., an oblique line that goes from the aortic area to the apex).

233. What is the typical pitch of the AR murmur?

Variable and depending on the severity of regurgitation. *Mild* disease has a high-pitched, blowing, and musical murmur. *Severe* AR, on the other hand, has only a few medium- to high-pitched components. Occasionally, the diastolic murmur acquires a very musical quality, like a seagull cry or "dove-coo" murmur. This has been shown by echo to coincide with the coarse fluttering of the aortic posterior wall during the opening of the mitral valve—which explains why a triphasic dove-coo murmur is rare in patients with AR of rheumatic origin, who often have concomitant mitral involvement, hampering its diastolic opening and thus limiting aortic root vibrations.

234. **What maneuvers can increase the loudness of a soft AR murmur?**
Positional maneuvers. The decrescendo diastolic murmur of AR is best heard by having the patient sit up and lean forward while holding breath in exhalation. Using the diaphragm and pressing hard on the stethoscope also may help since this murmur is rich in high frequencies. Finally, increasing peripheral vascular resistances (by having the patient squat) will also intensify the murmur.

235. **How do you differentiate the MS murmur from that of AR?**
AR starts immediately after the aortic component of S_2, whereas MS is always delayed a little, often heralded by an opening snap. In addition, MS has a presystolic accentuation that AR lacks.

236. **What auscultatory characteristics of AR correlate with severity of regurgitation?**
The major ones are *length* (the longer the diastolic murmur, the worse the AR) and *intensity*.

237. **How does intensity of AR predict severity?**
The louder the murmur, the worse the regurgitation. In fact, this is a characteristic that AR shares with MR: a murmur grade of 3 or louder carries a high probability of severe regurgitation, with a positive predictive value of 79%. Conversely, a murmur grade <1 argues so strongly against significant regurgitation that confirmatory testing may not even be required. Finally, a grade 2 murmur (which is quite frequent, occurring in more than one third of all AR patients) may reflect *any* degree of regurgitation. In this case, other signs of severity should be pursued, such as *length* of the diastolic murmur, concomitant systolic flow murmur/ejection sound, and presence of Austin Flint. Still, the longer and the louder the murmur of AR, the worse the disease.

238. **What is Austin Flint (A-F)?**
It is a mitral stenosis–like diastolic rumble, best heard at the apex, and due to the regurgitant aortic stream preventing full opening of the anterior mitral leaflet. It was first described by the homonymous cardiologist during the height of the American Civil War.

239. **How common is this finding?**
Rare in mild disease, but it can occur in more than 50% of moderate to severe AR cases.

240. **Is the presence of an Austin Flint murmur an indication of severe regurgitation?**
Yes, but not necessarily. Although A-F usually requires an aortic regurgitant volume of at least 50 mL, it also has been reported in patients with moderate regurgitation. Still, its presence *does* indicate a high left ventricular end-diastolic pressure and a high left atrial mean pressure.

241. **How can one differentiate the A-F murmur from one of mitral stenosis?**
Whereas the murmur of MS is mid-diastolic with a presystolic accentuation, the A-F murmur is presystolic in only half of the cases (the other half has both the mid-diastolic and presystolic components). In addition, A-F usually lacks the opening snap (which is instead common in MS), while it may have instead an S_3 (which is extremely rare in MS). Finally, reducing aortic pressure (and thus AR) tends to attenuate (or eliminate) the Austin Flint murmur, while instead intensifying the rumble of MS. Of course, an echo of the mitral valve would definitively differentiate the two.

242. **Who was Austin Flint?**
He was a Massachusetts cardiologist, who was greatly influenced at Harvard by one of the first American followers of Laënnec. A superb clinician and teacher, Flint taught in Buffalo (where he helped create the local medical college), Chicago, New Orleans, and finally New York, where

he was professor of medicine at Bellevue before moving to Long Island Hospital, where he died of a stroke in 1886, at age 74. A proponent of European diagnostic methods (who wrote that "the diagnosis of cardiac disease is for the most part based on physical signs"), Flint popularized the binaural stethoscope and became so well respected as to eventually be referred to as "the American Laënnec." His many contributions were mostly in cardiology, but he also forayed into pulmonary medicine, authoring the (in)famous term of "bronchovesicular breath sounds." Eventually, he ascended to the presidency of the American Medical Association. He had a son (whom in a fit of creativity he named Austin) who graduated from Jefferson Medical College of Philadelphia and became a well-respected physiologist and cofounder of New York University.

243. Which other bedside findings correlate with severity of regurgitation?
Hill's sign. If >60 mmHg, it argues very strongly in favor of severe regurgitation (*see* Chapter 2, questions 110–115). So does a diastolic blood pressure <50 mmHg and a pulse pressure >80 mmHg. Conversely, a diastolic blood pressure >70 and a pulse pressure <60 argue strongly *against* severe disease. Finally, absence of an enlarged or sustained apical impulse also argues against severe disease. Yet, these predictors of severity only apply to patients with *chronic* AR. Acute AR is *very* different.

244. What are the other auscultatory findings of AR?
Softness of S_1 and loudness of S_2 (due to increased elastic aortic recoil). S_2 also is single in AR. Note that in more severe AR, S_2 tends to become muffled.

245. And how about the presence of S_3 in AR?
S_3 gallops *may* occur in patients with pure AR, although they usually are much more common in patients with multivalvular disease. In isolated AR, S_3 reflects left ventricular dysfunction rather than more severe regurgitation. Hence, it may help in selecting patients for catheterization and surgery.

246. What are the "peripheral" signs of AR?
They are a plethora of eponyms, many going back more than 150 years, and most being just curious observations that, with a few exceptions, do not correlate with disease severity. Instead, they correlate with the wide pulse pressure of AR and its brisk arterial rise that can cause visible (and palpable) jolts. In fact, jolts of this sort have been reported even for the cervix and spleen. We reviewed some of these findings in the Vital Signs and Arterial Pulse sections of Chapters 2 and 10. Here are some more:
- Increased **pulse pressure** with systolic hypertension
- **Hill's sign:** Exaggerated difference in systolic pressure between the upper and lower extremities
- **Pulsus bisferiens**
- **Water hammer pulse:** Visible, forceful, and bounding peripheral pulses
- **Corrigan's pulse:** Quickly collapsing pulse, both *visible* and palpable
- **De Musset's sign:** Bobbing of the head. Lincoln's sign is a variant (*see* Chapter 1, questions 53 and 54).
- **Müller's sign:** Systolic pulsations of the uvula, accompanied by redness and swelling of the velum palati and tonsils. First described in 1889 by the German laryngologist Friedrich von Müller, who, together with Hamman, is actually more famous for his homonymous auscultatory sign: the crunching and rasping precordial sound that occurs in synchrony with each heartbeat in patients with spontaneous mediastinal emphysema (and that was first described by Laënnec).
- **Landolfi's sign:** Systolic contraction and diastolic dilation of the pupil. Named after the Italian Michele Landolfi (1878–1959), professor of semiology at the University of Naples.
- **Becker's sign:** Retinal arteries' pulsation; also described in Graves' disease

- **Oliver-Cardarelli sign:** Pulsation of the larynx synchronous with ventricular systole. It is elicited by grasping the *cricoid cartilage* between index finger and thumb while the patient is sitting up with the chin fully uplifted. By applying a *gentle upward pressure on* the larynx, one would feel a tracheal tug in cases of brisk aortic ejection—as, for example, in patients with AR. More typically, however, the tracheal tug would suggest an aneurysm of the aortic arch—also possibly associated with aortic regurgitation. Yet, the finding also can be due to a mediastinal tumor or simple chronic obstructive lung disease (*see* Chapter 13, questions 141–144).

All these *visible* (and *palpable)* signs are enhanced by exercise, as a result of increased pulse pressure. In addition, there are two more peripheral findings that are instead exclusively *auscultatory* (*see* Chapter 10, questions 33–36): (1) *Traube pistol shot sound(s)* and (2) *Duroziez double murmur*. Both have sensitivity of 37–55% and specificity of 63–98% for AR. Neither predicts severity.

247. **What is Quincke's pulse (sign)?**
It is another peripheral AR sign, albeit a vastly discredited one, since it is totally nonspecific. It consists of alternate reddening and blanching of the fingernails, coinciding with each cardiac cycle, and is easily visualized by lightly compressing the nail bed with a glass slide. It can occur in anyone with a hyperkinetic heart. In fact, even the ingestion of a few strong espressos might do it. An equivalent of this is the so-called *lighthouse sign* (flushing and blanching of the forehead and face). Similarly nonspecific is the lip pulsation of AR patients.

248. **Who was Quincke?**
Heinrich Irenaeus Quincke (1842–1922) was the son of a prominent German physician, who studied under Virchow and Helmholtz and went on to become a rather fussy gentleman with a penchant for horseback riding and argumentative conversations. Quincke taught in Vienna, Berlin, and Bern, until eventually taking the chair of internal medicine at the University of Kiel. He remained there until he retired as emeritus in 1908. His most notable contribution is neither the description of capillary pulsations in aortic regurgitation nor the description of angioneurotic edema (none of which was a *first*), but his introduction of the lumbar puncture as a diagnostic and therapeutic technique. Quincke also was the first to advocate surgical drainage of lung abscesses and better positioning of bronchiectatic patients for easier expectoration.

249. **What are the signs of acute and severe AR?**
Sudden and severe AR does not allow time for ventricular adaptation and enlargement. Hence, LV diameter remains small, and *pulse pressure actually narrows*. As a result, stroke volume cannot increase adequately and thus forward cardiac output declines. To compensate for the reduced stroke volume, the heart rate increases sharply. Eventually, rising LV end-diastolic pressure leads to early closure of the mitral valve. Hence, the murmur of acute AR is almost never holodiastolic, but instead early to mid-diastolic and thus more difficult to recognize. In fact, the most typical auscultatory sign of sudden and severe AR is a soft or absent S_1, due to premature mitral closure. Still, the hallmark is *clinical instability*. Patients are typically tachycardic, orthopneic, cyanotic, clammy, vasoconstricted, and gravely ill—often in overt failure or shock.

250. **What are the causes of "acute" AR?**
- Aortic dissection
- Bacterial endocarditis
- Trauma (either penetrating or blunt)

251. **What are the morbidity and mortality of AR ?**
It varies. *Acute AR* carries a grave prognosis unless promptly corrected. *Chronic AR* is instead well tolerated, with less than 4% of patients per year requiring surgical replacement.

The 10-year survival rates are 85–95% in mild disease, and 50% in *moderate* disease. But average survival decreases to less than 2 years after onset of congestive heart failure.

II. Pulmonary Regurgitation

252. What is the differential diagnosis of an AR murmur?
It has to be differentiated from the Graham Steell murmur, especially in patients with MS and pulmonary hypertension (who could be easily misdiagnosed as having AR with an Austin Flint).

253. What is the Graham Steell murmur?
It is an early diastolic, tapering, high-pitched, and blowing murmur of pulmonic regurgitation (PR). It is due to pulmonary hypertension, which, in the 1888 description by Graham Steell, was the result of *mitral stenosis*. It is best heard over the second left interspace and thus may be confused for the murmur of *AR*—except that PR typically intensifies with held inspiration (Rivero-Carvallo).

254. Who was Graham Steell?
A Scottish physician and the author of a 1906 cardiology textbook that won the praise of Sir James MacKenzie. The son of a sculptor and the nephew of the Scottish National Gallery curator, Steell grew up in Edinburgh, where he also attended medical school. He subsequently transferred to Manchester, where he became the leading cardiologist of Northern England. A charismatic bedside teacher, but a boring lecturer whose classes often went unattended, Steell was a champion boxer as a youth, an animal lover, and one of the first promoters of physical exercise as the key to a long and productive life. His commitment served him well, since he lived into his 90s.

255. What are the other findings of a PR murmur?
They are the typical findings of pulmonary hypertension: loud P_2, a pulmonic ejection sound, distended neck veins, and a possible murmur of tricuspid regurgitation. In fact, a PR murmur occurs in 12% of patients with tricuspid regurgitation. Note that a PR murmur also can be heard in fluid-overloaded renal patients, just before their dialysis session.

256. How sensitive is this murmur for pulmonic regurgitation?
Not much, only 10% because the lower pressures of the pulmonary circuit make this murmur much softer than the one of AR and thus harder to detect. This is especially true in PR from endocarditis, which has lower pulmonary pressures and thus a murmur that is even softer and later starting. Hence, absence of a PR murmur does *not* exclude PR.

257. Is a PR murmur common in pulmonary embolism (PE)?
Usually not. In fact, findings of pulmonary hypertension are not too common in pulmonary embolism: distended neck veins (3%), loud pulmonary component of S_2 (19–57%), S_4 or S_3 (6–34%) are overall rare. Similarly rare are the findings of *thrombotic disease*, such as a swollen and tender calf (15–52%) or unilateral leg swelling (16%), although their specificity is usually much higher than the sensitivity, so that they achieve a positive likelihood ratio of 2.6.

258. What about the other findings of PE?
The only one that is common is tachycardia (81%), which has low specificity but a positive likelihood ratio (2.5). Everything else is much less frequent: respiratory rate >25 (48%), pleural rub (4–18%), use of accessory respiratory muscles (17%), cyanosis (3–19%), fever (7%), and diaphoresis (11–36%). Note that some misleading findings (like chest wall tenderness) can be present in up to one tenth of patients with PE, thus contributing to the difficulty of the diagnosis.

D. CONTINUOUS MURMURS

259. What are continuous murmurs?

They are systolic murmurs that *go beyond* S$_2$, thus extending into diastole. This is due to their *extracardiac origin,* usually from an abnormal communication between high- and low-pressure beds (which explains their ongoing gradient and *sound*). Although not really "murmurs that never end," they *are* present throughout systole *and* diastole—as high-pitched noises that peak late in systole (around S$_2$) and then soften immediately afterwards, ending before the next S$_1$. Note that murmurs that cover systole *and* diastole but are *not* continuous are called instead "to-and-fro"—as, for example, the murmur of *aortic stenosis and regurgitation*, or the murmur of aortic regurgitation with its concomitant systolic ejection flow. They are so-called because their flow goes in opposite direction during systole as compared to diastole.

260. If continous murmurs are extracardiac, what conditions are responsible for them?

Conditions of:

- Abnormal communication between high-pressure and low-pressure vascular beds. Hence, the continuous flow, such as in *patent ductus arteriosus* (PDA) or in simple *arteriovenous fistulas*.
- Abnormally increased vascular flow. The latter can occur in either *veins* (venous hum) or *arteries* (like the mammaries of breast-feeding women or the intercostals of coarctation).

261. Why are these murmurs continuous?

Because their pressure gradient persists throughout systole and diastole, thus causing a *no-stop flow* that is always turbulent and noisy. In PDA, this never-ending stream of high-pressure/high-oxygen blood between the aorta and pulmonary artery eventually leads to pulmonary hypertension. This, in turn, gradually decreases the pressure gradient between the two vessels, eventually fading the diastolic component of the murmur. After reversal of the shunt, the murmur will cease altogether, while the patient becomes cyanotic and findings of severe pulmonary hypertension ensue. This is the *Eisenmenger's syndrome* (i.e., pulmonary hypertension from an initial left-to-right shunt that has evolved into shunt reversal and cyanosis). First described by the homonymous Austrian physician (1864–1932), Eisenmenger's from PDA is often associated with clubbing, which, like cyanosis, involves the feet but not the hands since the reversed shunt only affects the dependent portion of the aorta (*see* "differential clubbing," question 105 in Chapter 13).

262. What is the Nicoladoni-Israel-Branham sign?

It is a circulatory phenomenon initially observed in angioma racemosum of the extremities, but it is present in *all* arteriovenous fistulas, whether pathological or surgical: compression of the fistula causes a reflex bradycardia *whenever there is significant flow through the fistula.* First described by Nicoladoni in 1875 (and then by Israel in 1877 and Branham in 1890), it was subsequently rediscovered by Wigdorowitsch in 1915.

E. SYSTOLIC-DIASTOLIC MURMURS/SOUNDS

263. What is the differential diagnosis of "lots of noise" throughout the cardiac cycle?

"Noise" throughout systole and diastole usually reflects four possible processes (*see* Fig. 12-3):

- The to-and-fro murmur of AR with its companion systolic flow murmur (or, alternatively, a combined murmur of aortic regurgitation *and* stenosis)
- A PDA murmur
- A three-component pericardial friction rub (*see* Chapter 11, questions 164–174)
- Less commonly, "lots of noise" may indicate a holosystolic murmur of severe MR accompanied by its high-flow diastolic rumble.

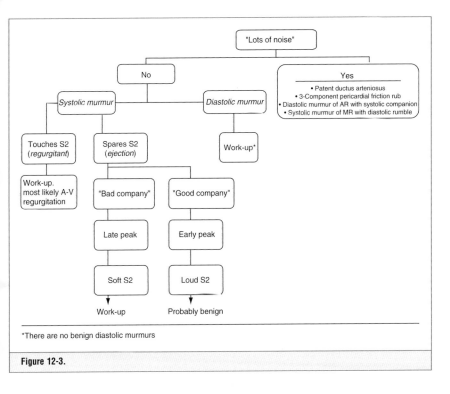

Figure 12-3.

*There are no benign diastolic murmurs

SELECTED BIBLIOGRAPHY

1. Aronow WS, Kronzon I: Correlation of prevalence and severity of aortic regurgitation detected by pulsed Doppler echocardiography with the murmur of aortic regurgitation in elderly patients in a long-term health care facility. Am J Cardiol 63:128–129, 1989.

2. Barlow JB, Bosman CK, Pocock WA, et al: Late systolic murmurs and nonejection ("mid-late") systolic clicks: An analysis of 90 patients. Br Heart J 30:203–218, 1968.

3. Burch GE, Phillips JH: Murmurs of aortic stenosis and mitral insufficiency masquerading as one another. Am Heart J 66:439–442, 1963.

4. Cha SD, Gooch AS: Diagnosis of tricuspid regurgitation. Arch Intern Med 143:1763–1768, 1983.

5. Cha SD, Gooch AS, Maranhao V: Intracardiac phonocardiography in tricuspid regurgitation: Relation to clinical and angiographic findings. Am J Cardiol 48:578–583, 1981.

6. Chun PKC, Dunn BE: Clinical clue of severe aortic stenosis: Simultaneous palpation of the carotid and apical impulses. Arch Intern Med 142:2284–2288, 1982.

7. Cohn KE, Hultgren HN: The Graham Steell murmur re-evaluated. N Engl J Med 274:486–489, 1966.

8. Constant J, Lippschutz EJ: Diagramming and grading heart sounds and murmurs. Am Heart J 70:326–332, 1965.

9. Danielsen R, Nordrehaug JE, Vik-Mo H: Clinical and haemodynamic features in relation to severity of aortic stenosis in adults. Eur Heart J 12:791–795, 1991.

10. Dennison AD: Aortic regurgitation: Multiple eponyms, physical signs and etiologies. J Ind State Med Assoc 52:1283–1289, 1959.

11. DePace NL, Nestico PF, Morganroth J: Acute severe mitral regurgitation: Pathophysiology, clinical recognition, and management. Am J Med 78:293–306, 1985.

12. Desjardins VA, Enriquez-Sarano M, Tajik AJ, et al: Intensity of murmurs correlates with severity of valvular regurgitation. Am J Med 100:149–156, 1996.

13. Devereux RB, Perloff JK, Reichek R, et al: Mitral valve prolapse. Circulation 54:3–14, 1976.

14. Emi S, Fukuda N, Oki T, et al: Genesis of the Austin Flint murmur: Relation to mitral inflow and aortic regurgitant flow dynamics. J Am Coll Cardiol 21:1399–1405, 1993.

15. Etchells E, Glenns V, Shadowitz S, et al: A bedside clinical prediction rule for detecting moderate or severe aortic stenosis. J Gen Intern Med 13:699–704, 1998.

16. Etchells E, Bell C, Robb K: Does this patient have an abnormal systolic murmur? JAMA 277:564–571, 1997.

17. Folland ED, Kriegel BJ, Henderson WG, et al: Implications of third heart sounds in patients with valvular heart disease. The Veterans Affairs Cooperative Study on Valvular Heart Disease. N Engl J Med 327:458–462, 1992.

18. Fontana ME, Wooley CF, Leighton RF, et al: Postural changes in left ventricular and mitral valvular dynamics in systolic click-late systolic murmur syndrome. Circulation 51:165–173, 1975.

19. Forssell G, Jonasson R, Orinius E: Identifying severe aortic valvular stenosis by bedside examination. Acta Med Scand 218:397–400, 1985.

20. Frank S, Braunwald E: Idiopathic hypertrophic subaortic stenosis: Clinical analysis of 126 patients with emphasis on the natural history. Circulation 37:759–788, 1968.

21. Freeman AR, Levine SA: The clinical significance of the systolic murmur: A study of 1000 consecutive "noncardiac" cases. Ann Intern Med 6:1371–1385, 1933.

22. Grayburn PA, Smith MD, Handshoe R, et al: Detection of aortic insufficiency by standard echocardiography, pulsed Doppler echocardiography, and auscultation: A comparison of accuracies. Ann Intern Med 104:599–605, 1986.

23. Henein MY, Xiao HB, Brecker SJ, et al: Bernheim "a" wave: Obstructed right ventricular inflow or atrial cross talk? Br Heart J 69:409–413, 1993.

24. Leach RM, McBrien DJ: Brachioradial delay: A new clinical indicator of the severity of aortic stenosis. Lancet 335:1199–1201, 1990.

25. Lembo NJ, Dell'Italia LJ, Crawford MH, et al: Bedside diagnosis of systolic murmurs. N Engl J Med 318:1572–1578, 1988.

26. McCraw DB, Siegel W, Stonecipher HK, et al: Response of heart murmur intensity to isometric (handgrip) exercise. Br Heart J 34:605–610, 1972.

27. McGee S: Evidence-Based Physical Diagnosis. Philadelphia, WB Saunders, 2001.

28. Nellen M, Gotsman MS, Vogelpoel L, et al: Effects of prompt squatting on the systolic murmur in idiopathic hypertrophic obstructive cardiomyopathy. Br Med J 3:140–143, 1967.

29. Otto CM, Lind BK, Kitzman DW, et al: Association of aortic-valve sclerosis with cardiovascular mortality and morbidity in the elderly. N Engl J Med 341:142–147, 1999.

30. Otto CM: Clinical practice: Evaluation and management of chronic mitral regurgitation. N Engl J Med 345:740–746, 2001.

31. Otto CM: Valvular aortic stenosis: Which measure of severity is best? Am Heart J 136:940–942, 1998.

32. Perloff JK: Auscultatory and phonocardiographic manifestations of pulmonary hypertension. Prog Cardiovasc Dis 9:303–340, 1967.

33. Perloff JK: Clinical recognition of aortic stenosis: The physical signs and differential diagnosis of the various forms of obstruction to left ventricular outflow. Prog Cardiovasc Dis 10:323–352, 1968.

34. Roldan CA, Shively BK, Crawford MH: Value of the cardiovascular physical examination for detecting valvular heart disease in asymptomatic subjects. Am J Cardiol 77:1327–1331, 1996.

35. Sutton GC, Craige E: Clinical signs of severe acute mitral regurgitation. Am J Cardiol 20:141–144, 1967.

CHEST INSPECTION, PALPATION, AND PERCUSSION

CHAPTER 13

Salvatore Mangione, MD

> *"According to a German physician, if the chest covered with a simple shirt is struck with the hand, it gives back a dull sound on the side where vomica is, as if one was striking a flesh piece, whereas if the chest opposite side is struck, it gives back a resonant sound, as if one was striking a drum. However, I still doubt that this information is generally correct."*
>
> –Tissot SAAD: Avis au peuple sur sa santé. Paris, 1782.

> *"A most violent and startling knocking was heard at the door.... The object that presented itself to the eyes of the astonished clerk was a boy—a wonderfully fat boy—standing upright at the mat, with his eyes closed as if in sleep. He had never seen such a fat boy..., and this, coupled with the utter calmness and repose of his appearance, so very different from what was reasonably to have been expected of the inflictor of such knocks, smote him with wonder.... The extraordinary buy spoke not a word; but he nodded once and seemed to the clerk's imagination to snore feebly."*
>
> –Charles Dickens, Pickwick Papers

GENERALITIES

Chest inspection, palpation, and percussion are the foundations of physical exam. Percussion is 15 years older than the United States, the brainchild of an Austrian innkeeper's son who figured out that patients' chests could behave like barrels of wine. Although rather "ancient," these maneuvers retain considerable value. Their skilled use may in fact still provide key pieces to our diagnostic mosaic. Indeed, bedside diagnosis of lung diseases requires *all* these maneuvers to yield useful information.

> **Pearl:**
>
> In contrast to cardiac diseases, where a bedside diagnosis can often be achieved by auscultation alone, a pulmonary diagnosis usually requires a comprehensive and competent performance of all parts of the exam, starting with inspection, palpation, and percussion.

1. **What are the main components of the chest exam?**
They are the same as for any other section of the exam: inspection, palpation, percussion, auscultation, and ... *contemplation*. This last (but not least) component was added by William Osler, as the necessary pondering of information garnered through the four preceding stages. Pondering was so important for Sir William that several portraits actually depict him at the bedside, deeply engrossed in his own contemplative thoughts. Yet, with the fading of bedside rounds, contemplation took a hit, becoming the latest casualty in the never-ending feud between science and art for the soul of medicine.

2. **What is the usual sequence in a typical pulmonary exam?**
The patient usually remains seated, with the physician moving from front to back and sides. Initial assessment includes an evaluation of *effort, rate, and depth of respiration*. It also should

identify any wheeze, or grunt, or noisy sound that might be audible *without the need of a stethoscope*. Sequential inspection of the anterior, posterior, and lateral chest should then be carried out. Finally, palpation, percussion, and auscultation complete the exam. The examination should be thorough and go from the chest surface toward the inner structures (Fig. 13-1).

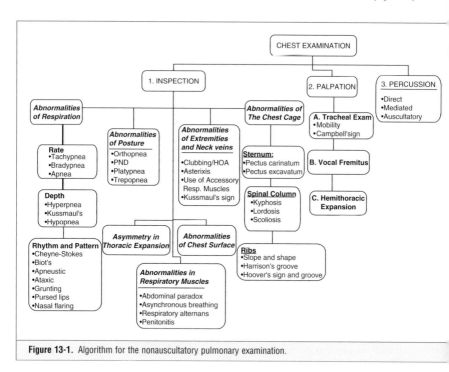

Figure 13-1. Algorithm for the nonauscultatory pulmonary examination.

A. CHEST INSPECTION

3. **What kind of information can be gathered through inspection?**

   In addition to gross abnormalities of body habitus (such as the Pickwickian type of obesity-hypoventilation or sleep apnea), an astute examiner also should look for seven important areas of anomaly:

   - Abnormalities of respiration
   - Abnormalities of posture
   - Abnormalities in the use of respiratory muscles
   - Asymmetry in thoracic expansion
   - Abnormalities of the chest cage
   - Abnormalities of the chest surface
   - Assessment of extremities and neck veins

4. **What are the most common abnormalities of *respiration*?**

   Mostly the ones related to the *vital signs* of the respiratory pump, such as pattern of breathing and its three main components: (1) *rate*, (2) *depth*, and (3) *rhythm*. Each of them may be abnormal, and all may be evaluated by simply observing the patient during the interview. In addition, *grunting, nasal flaring,* and *pursed-lip respiration* also can be detected through bedside observation (see later).

5. **What are the abnormalities of *posture*?**
These, too, can be detected by simple observation, even before the patient undresses. They are mostly related to *compensatory postures,* designed to improve the efficiency of the respiratory "pump." Patients with chronic obstructive pulmonary disease (COPD), for example, usually sit up and lean forward, so that they can better tense the accessory respiratory muscles and improve their contractility. Patients may lean so much forward to eventually have to prop themselves up by their resting elbows against the thighs. With time, the protracted pressure on the thighs leads to hyperpigmented calluses immediately above the knees (Dahl's sign).

6. **What are the main abnormalities in the *use of respiratory muscles*?**
In addition to recruitment of accessory muscles of respiration, the main abnormality is an asynchronous contraction of the diaphragm and intercostals (*paradoxical respiration*), an important sign of impending respiratory failure.

7. **What about *asymmetry in thoracic expansion*?**
This, too, can be detected by simple inspection, even though it is usually best evaluated by palpation.

8. **What *abnormalities of the chest cage* can be detected by inspection?**
Abnormalities of the spine, ribs, and sternum. All may adversely affect *lung mechanics* and thus lead to compensatory postures.

9. **And what about *abnormalities of the chest surface*?**
They are pallor or cyanosis, hyperpigmentation or hypopigmentation, expiratory bulges, collateral circulations, dermatomic lesions, and chest wall fistulas. All are detectable by astute observation.

10. **What about *assessment of extremities and neck veins*?**
Although often carried out separately, examination of neck veins and extremities is an important aspect of respiratory evaluation. Finding *clubbing,* for example, or *asterixis* may provide valuable information toward the recognition of an underlying respiratory disease. The same can be said for the detection of either nicotine stains (usually on fingers) or a smoker's face (deep and premature wrinkles coupled with skin coarsening), both indications of unrepentant smoking even before a social history is obtained. Finally, distended neck veins in patients with either cor pulmonale or pulmonary embolism also can be a very important diagnostic sign.

(1) Abnormalities of Respiration

Abnormalities in the *Rate* of Inspiration

11. **What are the main abnormalities in respiratory rate?**
The major ones are an *increase* and a *decrease*. The normal respiratory rate in an adult should be around 20 ± 5 breaths a minute. Hence, *tachypnea* indicates a rate faster than 25/minute, whereas *bradypnea* usually indicates a rate slower than 8/minute, as observed in narcotic-induced respiratory depression.

12. **Can *tachypnea* be considered normal?**
Probably not. Still, a respiratory rate >20 breaths/minute is often seen in elderly nursing home residents with chronic medical conditions but no active disease.

13. **What is the clinical significance of true tachypnea?**

It usually indicates moderate to severe *cardiorespiratory disease*, requiring a compensatory increase in the work of breathing. In hospitalized patients, it carries a bad prognosis. In fact, on internal medicine wards, it predicts cardiorespiratory arrest. It also argues in favor of *pneumonia*, both in the inpatient and outpatient settings. In hospitalized pneumonia patients, it can even predict death, thus providing a far more accurate prognostic indicator than either tachycardia or abnormal blood pressure. It also predicts *failure to wean* from mechanical ventilation.

14. **Can absence of tachypnea be helpful?**

Yes, because tachypnea is so common in chest diseases that its presence adds relatively little, whereas its absence challenges a cardiac or respiratory diagnosis. For example, tachypnea is so frequent in pulmonary emboli (92% of patients) that a normal respiratory rate argues strongly against the diagnosis. The same can be said for tamponade, where tachypnea is a *must*. Conversely, in an acute abdomen, tachypnea directs attention to a *supra*diaphragmatic rather than subdiaphragmatic process.

15. **Does tachypnea predict *hypoxemia*?**

Not necessarily. In fact, some patients might actually be hypoxic as a result of *hypo*ventilation (and therefore of *bradypnea*). Others might use instead tachypnea to fully compensate for hypoxemia. Hence, the need for monitoring not only the respiratory rate, but also oxygen saturation.

16. **What is the clinical significance of *bradypnea*?**

It should prompt consideration of *hypothyroidism*, but it also may suggest a central nervous system disease, or, as indicated before, the use of narcotics and sedatives.

17. **What is *apnea*?**

It is the absence of respiration for at least 20 seconds while awake or 30 seconds while asleep. It is often seen in patients with either neuromuscular dysfunction (central apnea) or airway obstruction induced by rapid eye movement (REM) sleep (obstructive sleep apnea). Note that apnea also remains the final event of *all* respiratory failures, whether due to pulmonary or neuromuscular disease.

Abnormalities in the *Depth* of Respiration

18. **What are the main abnormalities in the depth of respiration?**

Hyperpnea and hypopnea (Fig. 13-2).

19. **What is *hyperpnea*?**

It is an increase in tidal volume, usually accompanied (but not necessarily) by an increase in rate. In other words, hyperpnea is a rapid *and deep* respiration. The classic form was first described by Kussmaul in patients with diabetic ketoacidosis, who attempt to compensate by hyperventilating. This compensation also can be observed in any of the other anion gap metabolic acidoses, which can be recalled with the mnemonic **make up** a list: **m**ethanol poisoning, **a**spirin intoxication, **k**etoacidosis, **e**thylene glycol ingestion, **u**remia, **p**araldehyde administration, and **l**actic acidosis.

20. **Is there a difference between hyperpnea and the hyperventilation of cardiorespiratory disease?**

Yes. In cardiorespiratory disease, vital capacity is typically compromised, and thus breaths are *shallow*, with the increase in ventilation due primarily to a faster rate. In contrast, true hyperpnea relies more on increased *tidal volume*. Since this does not rebreathe dead space as much, it is a better CO_2 controller. Hence, *hyperpnea* rather than *tachypnea* is the compensation of choice in metabolic acidosis.

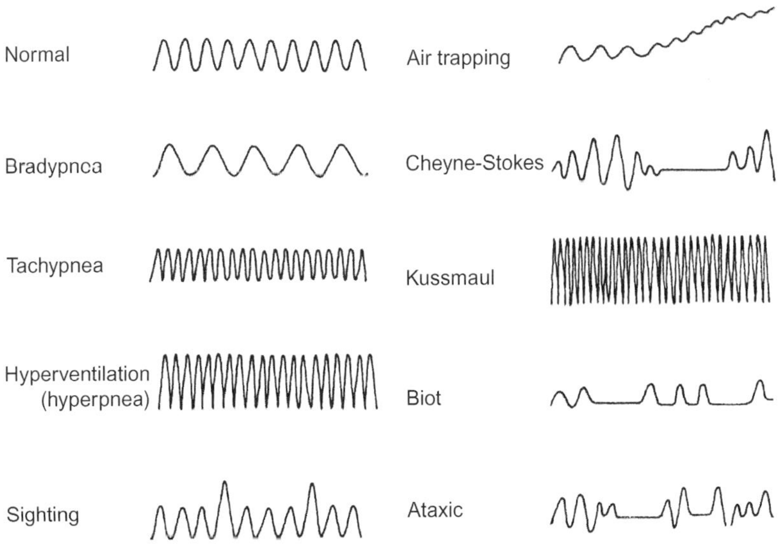

Figure 13-2. Patterns of respiration. The horizontal axis indicates the relative rates of these patterns. The vertical swings of the lines indicate the relative depth of inspiration. (Adapted from Seidel HM, Ball JW, Dains JE, Benedict GW: Mosby's Guide to Physical Examination, 3rd ed. St. Louis, Mosby, 1995.)

21. **Who was Kussmaul?**
Adolf Kussmaul (1822–1902) was a graduate of Heidelberg and Würzburg (where he studied under Virchow) and a part-time German Army surgeon. He was the first to describe periarteritis nodosa and progressive bulbar paralysis. He also was the first to attempt gastroesophagoscopy, pleural tapping, and peritoneal lavage. His name is linked to the respiration of patients with metabolic acidosis, the clinical description of pericarditis, pulsus paradoxus, aphasia, and, of course, *Kussmaul's sign,* the inspiratory increase in jugular venous pressure (and distention) seen in patients with obstruction to right-sided venous return (*see* Chapter 10, questions 115–118). A meticulous and precise man famous for complaining that none of his colleagues could write good German, Kussmaul contributed satirical poems to a weekly magazine under the pseudonym of Gottlieb Biedermeier, an imaginary and unsophisticated poet who eventually came to symbolize the values and tastes of the early 19th-century German bourgeois: reliable, hard-working, but boringly unimaginative (like in the Biedermeier style of furniture. *"Bieder"* is German for "everyday, plain" while *"Meier,"* or Meyer, is a common German last name).

22. **What is *hypopnea*?**
It is shallow respiration, usually indicative of impending respiratory failure or obesity-hypoventilation (Pickwickian syndrome). In this regard, hypopnea is often associated with periods of apnea (*see* question 17).

Abnormalities in *Rhythm* and *Pattern* of Respiration

23. **What are the main abnormalities in respiratory rhythm?**
They are many, and usually the result of disruption in the neurogenic control of the respiratory pump. Hence, they are often seen in *comatose patients.* Thus, they are valuable to recognize because they may help localizing the site of the neurologic lesion (*see* Fig. 13-2). Moving

downward in a rostrocaudal fashion, from the uppermost to the lowermost neurologic center, the most common abnormalities of respiratory rhythm are (1) Cheyne-Stokes respiration, (2) Biot's respiration, (3) apneustic breathing, (4) central hyperventilation, and (5) ataxic (agonal) respiration.

24. **What is Cheyne-Stokes respiration?**
It is a form of *periodic* breathing (i.e., a regularly irregular pattern consisting of a series of cycles). Each "cycle" has a constant respiratory *rate* but variable *depth,* insofar as it progressively increases in amplitude (crescendo), eventually culminating in a peak followed by a decrescendo period. This fades into complete *apnea,* from which another cycle restarts. The crescendo-decrescendo phase lasts approximately 30 seconds, whereas the apneic period is usually just a little shorter.

25. **What is the physiologic repercussion of Cheyne-Stokes?**
Mostly a swing in cerebral blood flow, caused by alternating *hyperpnea* (higher cerebral flow) and *hypopnea* (lower cerebral flow). These are probably responsible for some of the mental status changes described in these patients, such as alertness, agitation, and increased muscle tone during *hyperpnea,* followed by sleepiness, motionlessness, and decreased tone during *apnea.*

26. **What is the clinical significance of Cheyne-Stokes?**
   - It may be encountered in normal people as a result of *aging* or simply sleep.
   - It also can be seen in normal individuals who recently moved to high altitudes, where environmental hypoxia leads to a heightened CO_2 response of the respiratory centers.
   - The classic association, however, is with *congestive heart failure,* where Cheyne-Stokes is found in as many as one third of cases, reflecting worse function and prognosis. The reduced cardiac output of these patients leads to a lag between alveolar CO_2 and the *arterial* CO_2 delivered to the medulla. Hence, low alveolar CO_2 is reflected *much later* in the blood that bathes the medulla. This asynchrony between alveoli and medulla, coupled to higher sensitivity of the respiratory centers to CO_2, eventually leads to the hyperpnea-hypopnea-apnea cycle.
   - Cheyne-Stokes also can be seen in various *neurologic disorders* (such as meningitis, bilateral or unilateral cerebral infarctions/hemorrhage, and traumatic brain stem or supratentorial damage) in which the underlying mechanism is heightened sensitivity of the respiratory centers to carbon dioxide stimulations. As a result, any increase in CO_2 blood levels leads to excessive hyperventilation, until the CO_2 bottoms out and respiration ceases completely. Eventually, the apnea-induced increase in CO_2 leads to another phase of hyperpnea, and the cycle starts anew.

27. **What are the therapeutic implications of Cheyne-Stokes?**
Given its major swings in ventilation (and O_2 blood levels), patients with Cheyne-Stokes respiration may require administration of supplemental oxygen and, overall, have a worse prognosis.

28. **Who were Cheyne and Stokes?**
John Cheyne (1777–1836) was a Scot and himself the son of a surgeon, often helping his father to care for patients by bleeding and dressing them. After graduating at age 18 from the University of Edinburgh, he served in the army for 4 years. During this time, he took part in the battle of Vinegar Hill, which broke Irish resistance to British rule. In 1809, he went to Dublin, where he was eventually appointed Physician-in-General for Ireland, becoming the founder of modern Irish medicine.

William Stokes (1804–1878) was instead a bona-fide Irishman and the son of the anatomy professor who had succeeded John Cheyne at the College of Surgeons School in Ireland. Although lacking in formal education (his father wanted to protect him from a society that did not abide by the scriptures), Stokes eventually went to Edinburgh, where he received his doctor of medicine in 1825. In Scotland, he learned of Laënnec and his recent invention, the "cylinder." He soon became so enamored of this little tool that he even wrote an introductory book about it, the first of its kind in the English language. In fact, Stokes was such a vocal advocate for the use of stethoscopy that he provoked quite a few reactions (and even some sarcasm) among his colleagues. Still, he was a well-liked physician, who worked among the poor during the Dublin typhus epidemic in 1826 (he even contracted the disease but survived) and then again during the subsequent cholera epidemic. His name is linked not only to the eponymous pattern of respiration but also to Stokes-Adams syncope, which the Irish surgeon Robert Adams had described in 1827 and which Stokes included in his 1854 book, *Diseases of the Heart and Aorta*. Of course, the Italian Morgagni had preceded them both by describing the condition almost 100 years before (*see* Chapter 11, question 14).

29. **What other abnormalities in rhythm are worthy of recognition? What is their significance?**
    - **Biot's respiration** is a variant of Cheyne-Stokes, insofar as it is a succession of hyperpneas/hyperventilations and apneas, but *without* the typical crescendo-decrescendo pattern, the abrupt beginning, and the regularity. It is also less common than Cheyne-Stokes. Biot's is usually observed in patients with either meningitis or medullary compression. Hence, it carries a worse prognosis, usually resulting in complete apnea and cardiac arrest.
    - **Apneustic breathing** is a peculiar pattern of respiration, characterized by a deep inspiratory phase followed by a breath-holding period and a rapid exhalation. It is typical of brain stem (pons) lesions.
    - **Central hyperventilation** is often encountered in patients with midbrain/upper pontine lesions. It is an ongoing pattern of hyperpnea *and* tachypnea (i.e., deep *and* rapid respirations), which tends to be different from Kussmaul's respiration, insofar as it is not as fast, but usually deeper.
    - **Ataxic ventilation:** From the Greek *a-* (lack of) and *taxis* (order), this is a totally anarchic respiratory rhythm—a sort of fibrillation of the respiratory centers, with back-and-forth shifts from hyper- to hypo-ventilation, and from hyperpnea to hypopnea, all intermingled with periods of apnea. It is seen in patients with damage to the medulla, typically preceding death. Hence the term, *agonal respiration*.

30. **What is a grunting respiration?**
    It is another abnormal respiratory pattern. A typical grunting respiration is the *râle de la mort,* a pre-terminal gurgling-and-grunting sound produced by patients too ill to clear secretions. The expression translates as "death rattle" (*râle* is rattle in French), and in the olden days, it used to be a sign of severe pneumonia with impending respiratory muscle fatigue and death. The *râle de la mort* also is the main cause of Laënnec's botched nomenclature, insofar as the inventor of the stethoscope became so sensitive to the emotional overtones of the term râle to eventually prefer at the bedside its Latin equivalent *rhonchus*. This triggered a tremendous (and ongoing) confusion in lung sound terminology.

31. **What is the clinical significance of a grunting respiration?**
    Very much the same as in Laënnec's days. It can still be heard in adults with respiratory muscle fatigue (and impending arrest), but nowadays it is much more frequent in children, where it usually presents as a short and low-pitched noise produced by forced expiration against a closed glottis. The "grunt" is due to the sudden opening of the glottis and the loud rush of air from the larynx. Its physiology (and significance) is akin to pursed-lip respiration (*see* below, questions 32 and 33), insofar as it leads to an increase in expiratory airway pressure, which then acts as a mechanical splint against alveolar collapse, increasing tidal volume and oxygenation while decreasing respiratory rate and CO_2. An increased intra-alveolar pressure also has a positive effect against transudation of fluid in patients with pulmonary edema, and thus it is often observed during acute episodes of left ventricular failure.

32. What is *pursed-lip respiration*?

Another respiratory pattern, typically seen in *obstructive lung disease*—usually *emphysema* (Fig. 13-3). Given the alveolar hyperinflation (and reduced lung elasticity) of COPD, patients are at risk for expiratory airway closure and air-trapping. Hence, they resort to pursed lip exhalation, as if they were inflating a balloon. This increases intra-airway pressure, thus inducing auto-PEEP (positive end-expiratory pressure). It is often accompanied by an expiratory wheeze or *grunt*.

33. What is the physiologic impact of pursed-lip respiration?

It increases arterial O_2 while decreasing CO_2. It does so by behaving as an E-PAP in a Bi-PAP machine (i.e., by providing an *expiratory* positive airway pressure). It also slows respiratory rate (by as much as 40%), improves tidal volume, and decreases dyspnea. The mechanism for the latter is unclear, although it probably involves an effect on interstitial J-receptors as well as an overall reduction in the work of breathing.

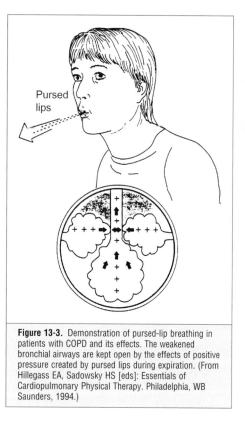

Figure 13-3. Demonstration of pursed-lip breathing in patients with COPD and its effects. The weakened bronchial airways are kept open by the effects of positive pressure created by pursed lips during expiration. (From Hillegass EA, Sadowsky HS [eds]: Essentials of Cardiopulmonary Physical Therapy. Philadelphia, WB Saunders, 1994.)

34. What is *nasal flaring*?

It is the outward inspiratory motion of the nostrils—a valuable sign of respiratory distress. Often associated with the use of accessory muscles.

(2) Abnormalities of Posture

35. What are the most common compensatory postures for improving oxygenation and ventilation?

Orthopnea, platypnea, and *trepopnea*—which indicate, respectively, easier breathing while upright, supine, or lying on one side. Also important is *paroxysmal nocturnal dyspnea* (PND).

36. What is *orthopnea*?

It is a dyspnea that is aggravated by lying flat. Conversely, it is relieved by sitting upright. It comes from the Greek *orthos* (upright) and *pneo* (breathing)—(i.e., *upright respiration*).

37. What is the clinical and physiologic significance of orthopnea?

Usually indicates *congestive heart failure,* where it can help identify patients with low ejection fraction. Conventional wisdom has traditionally interpreted orthopnea as a "poor man's" phlebotomy, pooling blood in the dependent areas of the body and thereby decreasing venous return and ventricular preload. Yet, in patients with congestive heart failure, orthopnea and pulmonary capillary wedge pressure correlate very little. Still, the need for orthopnea is often relieved whenever left ventricular failure degenerates into *bi*-ventricular failure, suggesting that failure of the right ventricle may indeed provide a useful "unloading" to left ventricular filling and pulmonary congestion.

38. Can orthopnea also occur in patients with lung disease?
Yes. Although more common in *heart* disease (in as many as 95% of cases), orthopnea also may be observed in *lung* disease, since sitting upright improves both vital capacity and lung compliance. Hence, orthopnea can occur in many pulmonary conditions, such as pneumonia, bilateral diaphragmatic paralysis, and pleural effusion. It also can occur in bilateral *apical* lung diseases, usually bullous. Whenever these patients sit up, they increase perfusion to the lower lung fields (as a result of gravity). Since these areas also are the best ventilated (because of bilateral apical disease), orthopnea improves ventilation/perfusion matching and gas exchange and thus relieves dyspnea.

39. And what about patients with COPD?
In COPD (which often presents with apical bullae), an upright position improves not only gas exchange but also *lung mechanics* (because of the increased stretch of accessory respiratory muscles). Hence, COPD patients often tend to prop themselves up, so that they can better use their respiratory muscles. They do so by clasping the side of the bed or pushing with the elbows over the thighs (*see* question 5, Dahl's sign).

40. What about asthma?
Orthopnea also is an important sign of asthma, especially *severe* asthma. In fact, when present at the time of initial emergency evaluation, it is a good predictor of poor outcome. Patients who cannot lie flat have a worse pulmonary function and a greater need for admission. The same is true for diaphoresis. Both findings were reported by Brenner in acute asthmatics and represent the scientific validation of the time-honored dictum that patients who "do not look good" (because they are sweaty and in an obligatory upright position) usually do poorly.

41. So, is orthopnea a cardiac or a pulmonary sign?
It is both. Because of all the above reasons, orthopnea should *not* be interpreted as a sign of a cardiac rather than respiratory etiology. The contrary is actually the case. Yet, *absence* of orthopnea in *pulmonary* patients *does* argue against concomitant presence of left ventricular failure.

42. Can orthopnea be encountered in patients with neither cardiac nor pulmonary disease?
Yes. For instance, it can be seen in patients with massive ascites, obesity, or bilateral phrenic nerve paralysis. In both cases, an upright position helps relieve the intra-abdominal pressure on the lungs.

43. What is *PND*?
It is a very common and dramatic presentation, characterized by a nocturnal spell (paroxysm) of acute dyspnea (air hunger). After 1–2 hours of sleep, the patient suddenly awakens, sits upright, lowers the legs down the side of the bed, opens the window to catch some fresh air, and after a few minutes feels better enough to go back to sleep.

44. What is the mechanism of relief in PND?
It is the upright posture, of course, and not the fresh air (although cold air blown into the face of patients has been shown to give a refreshing feeling in both cardiac and pulmonary diseases). The peripheral blood-pooling caused by sitting upright effectively decreases venous return, thereby reducing pulmonary capillary pressure and lung congestion. PND is, therefore, a frequent sign of left ventricular failure.

45. **Can PND be seen in pulmonary patients, too?**
Yes. Like orthopnea, it can be seen in bullous and bilateral apical disease. Both basilar perfusion and lung mechanics are improved when the patient sits upright and leans forward.

46. **What is *platypnea*?**
From the Greek *platus* (flat) and *pneo* (respiration), platypnea is an obligatory *supine respiration*. In other words, patients with platypnea breathe better when they lie flat. Hence, it is the opposite of orthopnea: it is a *dyspnea in the erect position,* promptly relieved by recumbency. Platypnea is often associated with *orthodeoxia,* which is a hemoglobin oxygen desaturation upon sitting upright.

47. **What is the clinical significance of platypnea?**
Unlike orthopnea, platypnea is usually due to a right-to-left shunt, which can be either intracardiac or intrapulmonary. In *intrapulmonary* shunts, platypnea requires a *bibasilar* process (and not biapical, like orthopnea). In this case, an upright posture increases perfusion to the lower lobes, worsens ventilation/perfusion (V/Q) matching, and leads to oxygen desaturation and dyspnea. Conversely, a supine position improves V/Q matching and relieves dyspnea. Given its physiology, platypnea occurs in:
   - **Multiple recurrent pulmonary emboli** (which, because of gravity, tend to involve primarily the bases)
   - **Pleural effusion** (which can cause bibasilar atelectasis) or *bibasilar pneumonia*
   - **Cirrhosis** (which often has arteriovenous shunting at the lung bases)
   - **Intrapulmonary right-to-left shunt**, such as an arteriovenous malformation, often basilar in location
   - **Intracardiac right-to-left shunt,** usually due to an atrial septal defect. This produces platypnea only when associated with an increase in pulmonary resistances, as in cases of pleurocardial/pericardial effusion or status post lobectomy/pneumonectomy. An upright position will reduce the shunt by redirecting blood toward the atrial septum and by possibly increasing pressure over the right atrium. A supine posture will have instead the opposite effect.

48. **What is *trepopnea*?**
From the Greek *trepo* (twisted) and *pneo* (breathing), this is a "twisted respiration" characterized by the patient's inability to lie supine (or prone), and instead by preference for the *lateral decubitus* position. Trepopnea is often referred to as "down with the good lung," meaning that in cases of *unilateral lung disease,* the patient can breathe better when placed on a side, typically with the good lung down.

49. **What is the physiology behind trepopnea?**
It is an increased perfusion to the dependent lung, which happens to be the good one, thus causing better (V/Q) matching, better oxygenation, and more comfortable respiration.

50. **What are some of the disease processes associated with trepopnea?**
The classic one is a *unilateral lung collapse,* from an endobronchial obstructing lesion or a massive effusion. In both situations, the patient feels better (and has improved oxygenation) whenever the *good* lung is "dependent." A similar mechanism also can explain the preferential right lateral decubitus position of patients with congestive heart failure from dilated cardiomyopathy (since this relieves the pressure applied on the left lung by the enlarged heart), or the preferential lateral decubitus position of patients with a mediastinal or endobronchial tumor that compresses the airways only in a particular position.

51. **Are there any contraindications to lying with the "good" lung down?**
Any unilateral lung disease due to "spillable" material, like pneumonia (intra-alveolar *pus*) or hemorrhage (intra-alveolar *blood*). In this case, intrabronchial spread into the dependent good

lung would only make things worse. Hence, patients with "spillable" unilateral disease should always lie with the *bad* lung down, since protecting the good lung is more important than improving oxygenation. Finally, lying with the good lung down is physiologically *detrimental* in small children with unilateral lung disease.

(3) Abnormalities in the Use of Respiratory Muscles

52. What are these?

These are abnormalities in the respiratory muscle "pump," characterized by weakness and fatigue, eventually leading to respiratory failure. They involve primarily the diaphragm but also can affect the intercostals. They are (1) *paradoxical respiration (abdominal paradox)* and (2) *respiratory alternans*.

53. What is *abdominal paradox*?

It is a sign of *diaphragmatic* fatigue. During normal respiration, the abdominal and thoracic wall are synchronized, both expanding in inspiration and contracting in exhalation (even though chest expansion is usually greater in the upright position, whereas abdominal expansion is usually greater in the *supine* position). In some conditions, however, the chest and abdomen become *asynchronous*, with the chest expanding in inspiration while the abdomen is instead being pulled in and vice versa. This "rocking motion" (labeled *abdominal paradox, paradoxical respiratory breathing,* or *respiratory paradox*) usually indicates bilateral diaphragmatic weakness or paralysis, causing the diaphragm to behave as a passive membrane, sucked up into the chest during inspiration and pushed down into the abdomen during exhalation.

54. What is the best way to detect abdominal paradox?

Bimanual palpation. Lay one hand over the patient's chest and one over the abdomen—then look for rocking motion. Note, however, that "paradox" also can be detected by simple inspection.

55. Are patients with abdominal paradox orthopneic?

Yes. Since in a supine position the abdominal content applies greater pressure on the diaphragm, patients with abdominal paradox try to compensate by assuming an upright posture.

56. How clinically valuable is this maneuver in predicting respiratory failure?

Quite valuable. Abdominal paradox has high sensitivity (95%) and good specificity (71%). In fact, in impending respiratory failure, it usually precedes deterioration of arterial blood gases.

57. What is *asynchronous breathing*?

It is a special form of abdominal paradox, seen in patients with chronic obstructive lung disease. In this case, the inward movement of the abdominal wall in *early* exhalation is almost immediately followed by an outward movement. This particular form of expiratory "rocking" reflects worse pulmonary function and prognosis, predicting respiratory failure, requirement for mechanical ventilation, and death.

58. What is *respiratory alternans*?

Another sign of respiratory muscle weakness and impending failure. It may occur in place of, or in combination with, *abdominal paradox*. Patients with *respiratory alternans* exhibit alternate use of either the diaphragm or intercostals, with the chest and abdomen first "rocking" one way, and then the other way. Occasionally, patients may cycle from respiratory alternans to abdominal paradox and vice versa.

59. How is respiration in patients with peritonitis?

Limited. In peritonitis, the abdominal wall can become quite still during respiration. This limitation in movement is *diffuse* in generalized peritonitis and *localized* in focal involvement. In diverticulitis, for example, the motionless area is the left lower quadrant; in appendicitis it is the right lower quadrant.

(4) Asymmetry in Thoracic Expansion

60. **Can inspection identify an asymmetry in thoracic expansion?**
Yes. Although not as effective as palpation, inspection *can* identify asymmetries of expansion between the two hemithoraces. These may occur in many lung conditions (including atelectasis, pneumonia, and pleural effusion), although it is only in the most *severe* cases (such as a large pneumothorax, a complete lung collapse, or a massive effusion) that the degree of change in volume of one hemithorax becomes large enough to be detectable by inspection. Protracted lung collapse may even lead to a *deviation in spinal curvature,* causing a concavity toward the side of disease.

61. **What is the best way to identify a thoracic asymmetry by inspection alone?**
Deep inspiration, since these lags are typically undetectable during quiet respiration. Hence, ask the patient to take a full deep breath and then look for a local lagging in chest expansion.

(5) Abnormalities of the Chest Cage

62. **What type of information about the chest cage should be gathered through inspection?**
Information concerning its three main components: the spine, ribs, and sternum. Some can even be gathered in fully clothed patients at the time of the interview, since abnormalities can be quite severe.

63. **What are the main chest cage abnormalities?**
It depends on whether they involve the spine, sternum, or ribs. Often, more than one component is affected.
- If the **spine** is affected, the abnormalities may be on the sagittal or frontal plane.
- If the **sternum** is involved, the two most common abnormalities are *pigeon chest* and *barrel chest*. Both may alter lung mechanics severely enough to reduce lung function.
- If **ribs** are involved, the most common abnormalities concern costal *slope* and *shape*.

Abnormalities of the Spinal Column

64. **Which spinal abnormalities can be detected by inspection?**
Abnormalities on either the *sagittal* or *frontal* plane, usually *a combination of both*.

65. **What abnormalities may be seen on the *sagittal* plane?**
These are an increase in spinal convexity (lordosis) or concavity (kyphosis)—often coexisting.

66. **What abnormalities may be seen on the *frontal* plane?**
These are *lateral* spinal curvatures, also called *scoliosis* (from the Greek word for *crookedness*). Depending on etiology, a scoliosis may have one curvature, or *two* curvatures (a primary and a *secondary*, with the latter providing a compensatory function). Scoliosis also may be *fixed* (because of muscle and/or bone deformity) or *mobile* (because of unequal muscle contraction) (*see* Fig. 13-4).

67. **What is kyphoscoliosis?**
A typical example of a mixed abnormality: scoliosis *plus* kyphosis. This is a very common problem, especially in our aging and increasingly osteoporotic population. In fact, the incidence

of spinal deformities in the United States is now 1/1000 for mild cases and 1/10,000 for more severe forms.

68. Is physical exam the best way to assess kyphoscolliosis?

No. Chest examination allows *detection* of the abnormality, but is of little value in *quantifying* its degree. To do so, you must rely on chest radiographs, and on the determination of the Cobb angle of scoliosis (Fig. 13-5). This can be calculated by drawing two lines parallel to (1) the upper border of the highest and (2) the lower border of the lowest vertebral bodies of the primary curvature, as seen on a spine anteroposterior (AP) film. The angle is then measured at the intersection points of two additional lines, drawn perpendicular to the original lines. As a rule of thumb, a Cobb's angle of 10 is considered the minimum angulation for a definition of scoliosis. Conversely, a Cobb's angle >100 degrees represents a severe deformity, one associated with higher risk for pulmonary hypertension and respiratory failure.

69. What are the most common causes of kyphoscoliosis?

Idiopathic
Neuromuscular
- Muscular dystrophy
- Poliomyelitis
- Cerebral palsy
- Friedreich ataxia
Vertebral
- Osteoporosis
- Osteomalacia
- Vitamin D-resistant rickets
- Tuberous spondylitis
- Neurofibromatosis
Disorders of connective tissue
- Marfan syndrome
- Ehlers-Danlos syndrome
- Morquio syndrome
- Thoracic cage abnormality

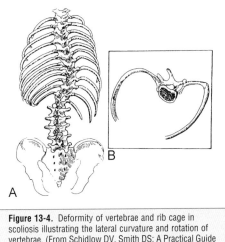

Figure 13-4. Deformity of vertebrae and rib cage in scoliosis illustrating the lateral curvature and rotation of vertebrae. (From Schidlow DV, Smith DS: A Practical Guide to Pediatric Respiratory Diseases. Philadelphia, Hanley & Belfus, 1994.)

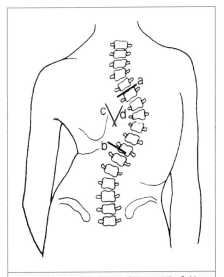

Figure 13-5. How to draw and measure the Cobb angle. (From Staheli LT: Pediatric Orthopedic Secrets. Philadelphia, Hanley & Belfus, 1998.)

- Thoracoplasty
- Empyema

70. **What is a gibbus?**
It is the Latin word for hump (or hunch), the lay term for a sharply angulated spinal deformity with the apex pointing posteriorly. In medical terminology, a hunchback (or humpback) is a severely kyphotic patient.

71. **What are the consequences of these spinal column abnormalities?**
Other than esthetic, the consequences are primarily respiratory—and often quite dramatic, too. In fact, if severe enough, any of these abnormalities can so compromise respiratory mechanics as to cause localized hypoventilation. In turn, the resulting V/Q mismatch leads to localized hypoxemia, pulmonary vasoconstriction, pulmonary hypertension, and eventually right-sided heart failure. Given its prevalence in an aging population, severe kyphoscoliosis is a common cause of *cor pulmonale*. In fact, chest cage abnormalities are among the few conditions that may result in severe right-sided failure despite lungs that are entirely normal (the others being obesity-hypoventilation and sleep apnea).

Abnormalities of the Sternum

72. **What are the two most common abnormalities of the sternum?**
They are *funnel* and *pigeon* chest, both congenital anomalies of the anterior chest wall.

73. **What is a funnel chest?**
It is a deep sternal *depression*, characterized by backward displacement of the lower half (or two thirds) of the sternum, often more visible after a deep inspiration. The alternative term, *pectus excavatum* (which is Latin for "hollow chest"), reflects the defining characteristic of this lesion (Fig. 13-6). In fact, even the upper part of the abdomen is often depressed, making it resemble a "potbelly." Note that a funnel chest may compress not only the lungs (and thus distort pulmonary mechanics), but also the *ventricles*—especially the right one because the sternal deformity is often asymmetric, displacing the heart toward the left as well as compressing the right chambers.

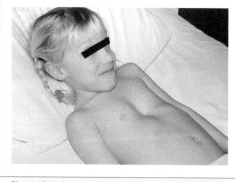

Figure 13-6. Pectus excavatum. (From James EC, Corry RJ, Perry JF: Principles of Basic Surgical Practice. Philadelphia, Hanley & Belfus, 1987.)

74. **How common is pectus excavatum?**
Quite common, present in 1 of every 300–400 births. Although occasionally associated with specific diseases (such as rickets, acromegaly, or Marfan syndrome), a funnel chest is much more likely to be sporadic or familial and thus inherited. Other musculoskeletal problems are often present, especially scoliosis, seen in approximately 20% of these patients.

75. **When does a funnel chest become recognized?**
Usually after birth, even though it often progresses with age, eventually peaking after puberty and the growth spurt. Spontaneous improvement is rare because cartilages and ligaments are fixed.

76. **What are the symptoms of a funnel chest?**
In addition to its cosmetic and psychologic implications (such as shyness and excessive reluctance toward activities where the chest is being exposed—like swimming), most symptoms tend to occur only after significant physical effort, such as the one required by athletic competition. Hence, patients often remain asymptomatic until early adulthood. Mild defects are usually associated with only decreased endurance, or easy fatigability. More severe defects can instead be associated with tachyarrhythmias caused by compression (and displacement) of the right heart and pulmonary artery. There also may be a pulmonic flow murmur and a right ventricular strain pattern on electrocardiogram (ECG). Finally, the limited movements of the chest wall can cause a compensatory increase in respiratory rate and a shift toward a more diaphragmatic respiration. This, in turn, may increase the work of breathing and thus lead to greater fatigability. Abnormal drainage of secretions also may cause respiratory infections, and even asthma.

77. **What is a pigeon chest?**
It is the opposite of the funnel chest: a sternal *protrusion* from cartilage overgrowth, with forward sternal projection and secondary flattening of either side of the chest (Fig. 13-7). This makes the sternum resemble the *keel of a ship* (*carina* in Latin), and thus the term *pectus carinatum*. As its counterpart, a funnel chest may be isolated or associated with specific diseases, like rickets, Marfan's, or Noonan's. Yet, contrary to the funnel chest, a pectus carinatum is much more of a medical oddity (with prevalence of 0.06% as opposed to 1 in 300–400 births).

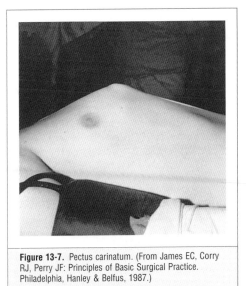

Figure 13-7. Pectus carinatum. (From James EC, Corry RJ, Perry JF: Principles of Basic Surgical Practice. Philadelphia, Hanley & Belfus, 1987.)

78. **What are the clinical consequences of a pigeon chest?**
Usually pain, due to the forward buckling of the sternum and ribs.
A pectus carinatum also produces a *rigid chest*, which is almost fixated near full inspiration. This, in turn, leads to pockets of hypoventilation, with increased frequency of respiratory infections and even asthma. It also creates the need for a greater use of both the diaphragm and accessory muscles of respiration, especially during strenuous exercise. Hence, the easy fatigability of these patients. Finally, in contrast to *pectus excavatum,* the heart of a patient with pigeon chest is normally situated, and thus there are neither murmurs nor arrhythmias.

79. **What can be done to correct these conditions?**
Surgery. Both conditions are amenable to surgical correction.

Abnormalities of the Ribs

80. **What rib abnormalities can be detected on inspection?**
    Abnormalities in *slope* and *shape*.

81. **What is the normal slope?**
    An oblique one, at a 45-degree angle—thus giving the thorax a 0.70–0.75 ratio between AP and transverse diameter.

82. **How is the rib slope modified by disease?**
    In patients with emphysema, chronic bronchitis, or status asthmaticus, the excessive pull on ribs and sternum by the accessory muscles of respiration (i.e., scalene and sternocleidomastoids) may *horizontalize the slope*. This can become severe enough to equalize the chest's AP and transverse diameters (or, at least, bring their ratio close to 0.90)—which, in turn, leads to a *barrel chest*.

83. **What is a barrel chest?**
    A chest that is almost *round*, with horizontalized ribs and an equalized thoracic ratio.

84. **How good is the interobserver reliability for the detection of this abnormality?**
    Around 70%.

85. **How are the physiologic consequences of a barrel chest?**
    Detrimental. A horizontal rib slope may compromise lung function, making ventilation less efficient.

86. **What is the clinical significance of a barrel chest?**
    Conventional wisdom links it to COPD, even though the evidence supporting this association is rather weak. Moreover, many emphysematous patients are so underweight that their flattened bellies may only give the *illusion* of an increased transverse diameter. Finally, horizontalization of the ribs (and thus a barrel chest) may simply occur as a result of aging.

87. **What are the most common abnormalities in rib shape?**
    They are deformities caused by thickening of the costochondral junction, forming two rosary-like lines of beads across the anterior chest. Common in *rickets*, these are referred to as *rachitic rosary*.

88. **What is the Harrison's groove?**
    It is another rib abnormality of rickets, first described in 1820 by the English physician Edward Harrison. The *groove* (or sulcus) is a horizontally oriented depression at the site of diaphragmatic costal insertion, caused by the phrenic pull on ribs weakened by rickets or another bone disease. The resulting indentation extends bilaterally from the xiphoid process to the axillae, making the chest resemble the body of a violin. In addition to rickets (where Dr. Harrison first described it), the "groove" also can be seen in various pediatric conditions characterized by chronic inspiratory obstruction, like, for example, laryngeal stenosis. In this case, the mechanism is not bone softening, but excessive diaphragmatic pull on bones that, albeit normal, are pliable because of growing.

89. **What is Hoover's sign?**
    It is a paradoxical *inspiratory* movement of the *lateral rib cage* in patients with COPD. It has been attributed to direct traction by the flattened diaphragm on the lateral rib margins. Since the diaphragmatic contraction of these patients pulls the lower ribs toward the midline, the

subcostal angle (i.e., the angle between the xiphoid process and the right or left costal margins) becomes more acute.

90. **What is the normal behavior of the lower rib cage during inspiration?**
Normally, the costal margins move very little during quiet respiration, but, if they do, they tend to move *outward and upward*. In some healthy subjects, they may even move a little *inward*, especially at the end of peak inspiration. This movement, however, is grossly exaggerated in patients with obstructive lung disease, with 77% of them exhibiting a large and paradoxical inward pull (Hoover's sign).

91. **Is this paradoxical inward movement also affecting the sternum?**
Yes. In patients with COPD, the paradoxical motion of the rib cage can be observed not only on lateral view (as Hoover's sign, involving the ribs), but also on the frontal plane—as a paradoxical in-drawing of the lower sternum during inspiration.

92. **What is the pathophysiology of Hoover's sign?**
In his first description, Hoover attributed the paradoxical motion of the lateral rib cage to the inward pull produced by diaphragmatic contraction. Gilmartin and Gibson found that transdiaphragmatic pressure does indeed support this hypothesis. They also found a weak correlation ($r = 0.36$) between FEV_1 and inward displacement of the lateral rib margin. Although the mean FEV_1 of obstructive patients *with* or *without* Hoover's was identical, the sign was significantly more frequent in patients with *severe airflow obstruction*. This is intuitive, since the hyperinflation of obstructive disease alters the geometry of the chest wall, especially at the level of diaphragmatic insertion. This, in turn, prevents the diaphragm from having an expanding effect on the lower ribs upon contraction. In fact, it has a *retracting* effect.

93. **Are there any other disease states characterized by Hoover's sign?**
In addition to rickets, Hoover's sign also can be seen in large pneumothoraces or large pleural effusions. Both conditions are similarly characterized by a flattening of the diaphragm. In these processes, however, the paradoxical inspiratory movement of the costal margin toward the midline occurs only *unilaterally*. Conversely, in emphysema it occurs *bilaterally*.

94. **What is Hoover's *groove*?**
It is a different term for *Hoover's sign*. It refers to the bilateral depression caused on the thoracic cage by the inward pulling of the flattened diaphragm. In rachitic children (where it was first described), this *groove* is independent of respiration, since their softened bone gets molded even by a normal diaphragmatic pull (see also Harrison's groove). Conversely, in COPD it occurs only in *inspiration*.

95. **What is the clinical and prognostic significance of Hoover's sign in COPD?**
It is associated with increased *dyspnea*—during both normal activities and exercise. It also is associated with an increased use of health care resources.

96. **What is the diagnostic accuracy and observer agreement for Hoover's sign?**
A study from Spain recently addressed these issues, and found an interobserver reliability ([kappa] statistic) of 0.74 between residents and attendings, which was as good (if not even better) as the agreement for other signs of COPD, such as wheezes, rhonchi, and distant lung sounds. Hoover's sign had an overall sensitivity for COPD of 58% and a specificity of 86%; it also had a positive likelihood ratio of 4.16, which was higher than that of the other signs (which tended to have higher specificity than sensitivity). Thus, Hoover's sign is easy to recognize and helpful in the detection of airflow obstruction. In this same Spanish series, patients with Hoover's sign also were heavier (as measured by body mass index) than the ones without it.

Hence, obesity (and its related increase in intra-abdominal pressure) may play an additional role in causing the abnormal diaphragmatic geometry that is at the root of this sign.

97. **Who was Hoover?**
Charles Franklin Hoover (1865–1927) was an American pulmonologist, who graduated from Harvard, studied in Vienna and Strasburg, and then returned to his native Cleveland, where he taught at Case Western Reserve University, studied the diaphragm, and eventually described his eponymous finding in 1920. Of interest, there are *two* Hoover's signs, the other being a neurologic maneuver aimed at separating organic hemiplegia from its hysteric variety—a common problem in Hoover's time. To carry it out, the examiner places a hand under the heel of the patient's nonparalyzed leg, and then asks the subject to *raise* the *paralyzed* leg. The pressure exercised on the examiner's hand *by the nonparalyzed heel* will be much higher in true hemiplegia than in malingering or hysteria.

98. **Are there any other bony abnormalities that should be observed?**
In addition to the static and dynamic abnormalities of the chest cage, one also should observe whether the patient is coughing or sighing, and whether there is any *pain* with that. Finally, the examiner should look for abnormalities of the chest *surface,* and even the neck and extremities.

(6) Abnormalities of the Chest Surface

99. **Why is it important to observe the characteristics of the chest surface?**
Because they can provide important diagnostic clues, such as:
- **Abnormalities in color:** Skin color helps identify patients with ineffective oxygenation and/or ventilation. *Cyanosis* is a hallmark of insufficient *ventilation* (with resulting hypercapnia and a reduced hemoglobin >5 g/100 mL). Conversely, *pallor*, diaphoresis, and agitation are the hallmarks of ineffective *oxygenation*. Neurologic repercussions are different, since hypercapnia is a central nervous system (CNS) depressor, whereas hypoxemia is a stressor.
- **Abnormalities in pigmentation:** Patients whose chests are *hyperpigmented* (especially if the skin is tightly drawn and covered with telangiectasias or vitiligo) also should have their hands and fingers evaluated for tightening. These (and a tight mouth opening) are typical features of scleroderma and important clues to the presence of underlying lung diseases, such as vasculitis, pulmonary hypertension, and cor pulmonale.
- **Expiratory bulging:** *Focal* expiratory bulging of the intercostal spaces is typical of patients with pneumothorax, whereas *diffuse* expiratory bulging occurs in patients with obstructive lung disease. Focal inspiratory *sinking* (*tirage*) is seen in patients with focal airway obstruction; diffuse tirage is seen in patients with upper airway obstruction. Finally, a localized and paradoxical motion of the thorax is observed in patients with *flail chest.*
- **Collateral circulations:** These may occur on the chest wall of patients with superior or inferior vena cava obstruction, in whom an impeded venous return creates a collateral circulation that flows, respectively, caudad or cephalad.
- **Dermatomic herpes zoster lesions**
- **Chest wall fistulas:** These may be seen in patients with *empyema necessitatis*, a form of pyothorax in which pus burrows to the outside, producing a subcutaneous abscess that finally ruptures. The drainage may actually be beneficial, allowing relief of a closed-space infection and, often, spontaneous recovery.

(7) Abnormalities of Extremities and Neck Veins

100. **Which respiratory findings can be detected on the extremities?**
Clubbing and *asterixis*. The latter is a flapping tremor often seen in hypercapnic patients (*see* Chapter 20, Coma, questions 50–52).

Clubbing

101. What is digital clubbing?

It is a bulbous swelling of the connective tissue in the terminal phalanxes, with subsequent loss of the normal angle between the nail and nail bed (Lovibond angle). It is especially prominent on the dorsum of digits.

102. What is the history of this finding?

The phenomenon has fascinated physicians since its original description by Hippocrates in a patient with empyema. Interest was rekindled in the 19th century by the German Eugen Bamberger and the Frenchman Pierre Marie and by their description of *hypertrophic osteoarthropathy* (HOA), a frequently concomitant (but separate) disorder. By the end of World War I, both clubbing and HOA had become well-known signs of chronic infection. Today, they are more commonly remembered for their association with cancer, usually bronchogenic carcinoma. In fact, this association is so strong for HOA that it has earned it the name hypertrophic *pulmonary* osteoarthropathy, even though HOA is not necessarily limited to pulmonary diseases. Still, despite increased awareness and some recent interesting twists, the pathogenesis of these two conditions remains an unsolved mystery.

103. Is clubbing painful?

No. Clubbing is never painful, although at times patients may complain of an aching discomfort in their fingertips. Conversely, HOA is typically painful.

104. Is clubbing limited to fingers?

No. It usually involves both fingers *and* toes; however, it may involve only fingers or only toes. Moreover, it can be bilateral and symmetric, or unilateral and involving a single digit.

105. Which are the causes of "differential" clubbing?

Clubbing limited to only the hands or only the feet is usually the result of a cyanotic type of congenital heart disease that selectively sends desaturated blood to either the upper or lower half of the body. The disorders most commonly responsible for *differential* clubbing (and cyanosis) include (1) *patent ductus arteriosus with pulmonary hypertension* (in which the reversed shunt limits clubbing/cyanosis to the feet and spares the hands) and (2) *right ventricular origin of the great vessels* (in which the reversed shunt limits clubbing/cyanosis to the hands and spares the feet). In this last disorder, both the aorta and pulmonary artery arise from the right ventricle, often in association with a ventricular septal defect, a patent ductus arteriosus, and pulmonary hypertension. As a result, oxygenated blood from the left ventricle enters the pulmonary trunk through the septum, shunts through the patent ductus arteriosus into the descending aorta, and eventually flows to the lower extremities. Conversely, oxygen-desaturated blood from the right ventricle enters the ascending aorta and brachiocephalic vessels, thereby reaching the upper extremities. Hence, the hands will be cyanotic and clubbed, but the feet are normal (*reversed* differential cyanosis). Finally, identical and symmetric cyanosis/clubbing of both fingers and toes indicates instead the presence of a right-to-left *intracardiac* shunt.

106. What is the cause of unilateral clubbing?

Usually, an aneurysm of the aorta or innominate/subclavian arteries. Pancoast's tumor and lymphangitis also may cause unilateral clubbing. Less common is a surgical arteriovenous fistula for dialysis.

107. What are the diagnostic features of clubbing?

They depend on whether clubbing is present alone or in association with periostosis (*see* HOA in questions 117–122). *Clubbing without periostosis*, the time-honored Hippocratic nail, has three diagnostic features (Fig. 13-8):

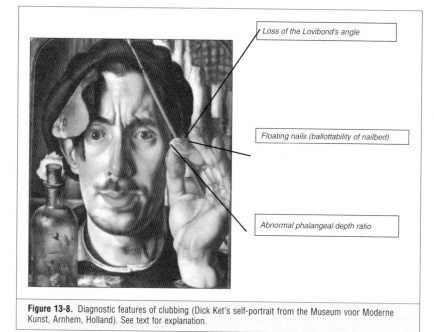

Figure 13-8. Diagnostic features of clubbing (Dick Ket's self-portrait from the Museum voor Moderne Kunst, Arnhem, Holland). See text for explanation.

1. **Loss of Lovibond's angle:** This is the angle between the base of the nail and its surrounding skin (hyponychial or unguophalangeal angle). The angle is normally <180 degrees. In clubbing, however, is either obliterated (straight line) or >180 degrees. The loss of the Lovibond's angle (Fig. 13-9) can be easily visualized by resting a pencil over the nail. Normally, there should be a clear window between the pencil and the nail. In clubbing, however, there will be none. Thus, the pencil will fully rest over the nail.

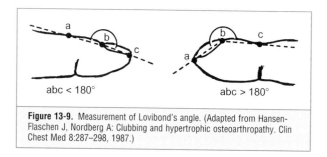

Figure 13-9. Measurement of Lovibond's angle. (Adapted from Hansen-Flaschen J, Nordberg A: Clubbing and hypertrophic osteoarthropathy. Clin Chest Med 8:287–298, 1987.)

2. **Floating nails (ballotability of the nail bed):** This refers to an increased sponginess of the soft tissue at the base of the nail. As a result, the nail plate acquires a "springy" feeling: when the skin just proximal to the nail is compressed, the nail sinks deep toward the bone; upon release, it springs backward and outward (floating fingernail base)—almost like pushing an ice cube down a pot of water. This feeling can be effectively simulated by:

- Pressing your right index finger over the skin just proximal to the nail of your left middle finger. In a normal person, the nail plate feels solidly attached to the underlying bone.
- Repeating the maneuver, but this time applying some tension to the nail by pulling downward its free edge with your left thumb, thereby increasing the natural convexity of the nail plate. After doing so, the nail plate will feel detached from the underlying bone, capable of sinking down during pressure and springing back upon release, almost as if it were floating on a spongy pad.

3. **Abnormal phalangeal depth ratio:** This consists of a greater depth of the fingertip when measured at the cuticle (distal phalangeal depth [DPD]) as compared to the interphalangeal joint (interphalangeal depth [IPD]) (*see* Fig. 13-10). The normal DPD/IPD ratio is, on

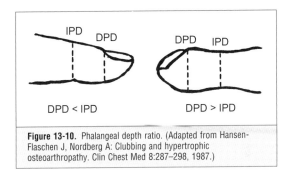

Figure 13-10. Phalangeal depth ratio. (Adapted from Hansen-Flaschen J, Nordberg A: Clubbing and hypertrophic osteoarthropathy. Clin Chest Med 8:287–298, 1987.)

average, 0.895, which means that the fingertip tends to taper going from the distal interphalangeal joint toward the end. Conversely, in clubbing it bulges, with a DPD/IPD ratio >1.0 (i.e., in excess of the norm by approximately 2.5 standard deviations). The DPD/IPD ratio is an excellent marker for clubbing, with good sensitivity and specificity. For example, a ratio >1.0 is found in 85% of children with cystic fibrosis and fewer than 5% of children with chronic asthma.

108. **Is ballotability of the nail an exclusive indication of clubbing?**
No. It also may be encountered in older patients with no clubbing. Still, ballotability remains an important and valuable sign for the diagnosis of this condition.

109. **How quickly can these changes occur?**
Rather quickly. In a setting of lung abscess, for example, loss of the unguophalangeal angle and ballotability of the nail bed have reportedly occurred within 10 days after aspiration. Once the underlying condition has been removed, changes also can quickly disappear.

110. **Is increased curvature of the nail a sign of clubbing?**
Not necessarily (*see* below, question 116). True clubbing requires accumulation of soft tissue at the base of the nail. Hence, it is defined *not* by an increase in nail convexity but by the three aforementioned characteristics.

111. **What is a drumstick finger?**
It is one of several terms used to describe the more advanced stages of clubbing (Fig. 13-11). The accumulation of connective tissue extends well beyond the base of the nail and involves the entire digit. Depending on where this accumulation predominates, a few colorful terms have been created. For example, in parrot's beak clubbing, the swelling is primarily localized to

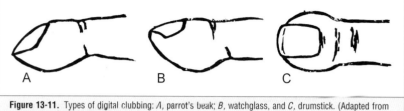

Figure 13-11. Types of digital clubbing: *A*, parrot's beak; *B*, watchglass, and *C*, drumstick. (Adapted from Hansen-Flaschen J, Nordberg A: Clubbing and hypertrophic osteoarthropathy. Clin Chest Med 8:287–298, 1987.)

the proximal portion of the distal digit; in the drumstick type, it is circumferential; and in the watchglass form, swelling is mostly at the nail base.

112. **What is Schamroth's sign?**
It is the disappearance of the diamond-shaped window normally present when the terminal phalanges of paired digits are juxtaposed (Fig. 13-12). It is just another and more recently described maneuver to confirm the loss of the Lovibond angle. It was first reported in 1976 by the South African cardiologist Leo Schamroth, who noticed it on himself during recurrent clubbing due to bouts of endocarditis.

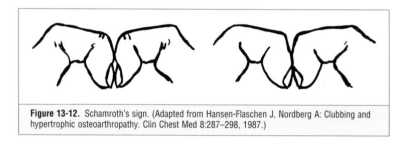

Figure 13-12. Schamroth's sign. (Adapted from Hansen-Flaschen J, Nordberg A: Clubbing and hypertrophic osteoarthropathy. Clin Chest Med 8:287–298, 1987.)

113. **What is the clinical significance of clubbing?**
Clubbing is a feature not only of lung disease, but also of several chronic inflammatory conditions not necessarily limited to the lungs. In fact, it has been described in infective endocarditis, lung abscess, bronchiectasis, and even amyloidosis. It also has been reported in chronic inflammatory bowel disease, such as Crohn's and ulcerative colitis. Although described in hypercapnia (usually from chronic bronchitis), clubbing is *not* a feature of emphysema. It is, however, encountered in hypoxemia from shunts (either cardiogenic or pulmonary) and in patients with sex hormones imbalance (because of either pregnancy or cirrhosis). Finally, clubbing has been described in various cancers, especially lung (*see* Table 13-1).

114. **What is the pathogenesis of clubbing?**
One we have recently managed to better understand. Clubbing can be *secondary* or *primary*, with the latter form including both the idiopathic and hereditary varieties (of these, *familial clubbing* is not unusual in African-Americans). Overall, 80% of *secondary* cases are due to an *underlying respiratory disorder*, either neoplastic or inflammatory. The rest is either cardiac or gastrointestinal in origin, with less than 10% being idiopathic or hereditary. The underlying mechanism is a fibrovascular proliferation of the nail bed, possibly triggered by the clumping

TABLE 13-1. DISORDERS COMMONLY ASSOCIATED WITH DIGITAL CLUBBING

Intrathoracic	Cardiovascular
Bronchogenic carcinoma*	Congenital cyanotic heart disease
Metastatic lung cancer*	Other causes of right-to-left shunting
Hodgkin's disease	Subacute bacterial endocarditis
Mesothelioma*	Infected aortic bypass graft*
Bronchiectasis*	**Hepatic and Gastrointestinal**
Lung abscess	Hepatic cirrhosis*
Empyema	Inflammatory bowel disease
Cystic fibrosis	Carcinoma of esophagus or colon
Pulmonary interstitial fibrosis	Achalasia
Sarcoidosis	Peptic ulceration of the esophagus
Pneumoconiosis	Primary biliary cirrhosis
Lipid pneumonia	Cirrhosis of the liver
Arteriovenous malformations	**Malignancies**
Miscellaneous	Thyroid cancer
Pregnancy	Thymus cancer
Acromegaly	Hodgkin's disease
Pachydermoperiostosis	Chronic myeloid leukemia
Thyroid acropachy	

(Adapted from Hansen-Flaschen J, Nordberg J: Clubbing and hypertrophic osteoarthropathy. Clin Chest Med 8:287–298, 1987.)
*Commonly associated with hypertrophic osteoarthropathy.

of large platelets in digital vessels. These are usually filtered out by the pulmonary vasculature, but in situations of pulmonary damage (from neoplastic or inflammatory disorders) or vascular shunt (from cirrhosis, pregnancy, and intracardiac defects), they manage to reach the distal digits, where they clump, release mediators, and trigger a fibrovascular response. In cases of endocarditis or infected dialysis shunts, platelet clumps would originate directly on the damaged vascular surface, detach, and eventually lodge in the digital vessels. Clubbing also may be familial, especially in African Americans.

115. **What about congenital clubbing?**
Congenital clubbing is relatively common and thus important to recognize. It may be characterized more by loss of the subungual angle than by presence of ballottement. Since many patients are unaware (and may not think of it unless asked), it should be well documented in the medical record.

116. **What is *pseudo*clubbing?**
A separate sign, characterized by an overcurvature of the nails in both the longitudinal and transverse axes ("watchglass nail") that *nonetheless preserves a normal Lovibond angle*. It is

often accompanied by hypertrophy of the distal phalanx, making the finger resemble a drumstick ("drumstick dactylitis" or "parrot beak nail"). Ironically, pseudoclubbing may be a more frequent hallmark than clubbing of a longstanding and debilitating condition, such as carcinoma of the lung, pulmonary tuberculosis, and rheumatoid arthritis. Note that nail convexity usually takes longer to develop than true clubbing, since it requires the formation of an entirely new nail plate ridge. This transverse ridge appears 1 month after the causative event, and reaches full formation at 6 months. At completion, an entirely new nail has been created, with an abnormal and more convex profile.

Hypertrophic Osteoarthropathy (HOA)

117. **What is digital clubbing with periostosis?**
It's Marie-Bamberger syndrome (from the names of its two discoverers)—a different and systemic disorder of bones, joints, and soft tissues, which can be primary but more often is *secondary* to a paraneoplastic process. Hence, the term hypertrophic *pulmonary* osteoarthropathy (HOA). In fact, the neoplasm of HOA is usually intrathoracic and typically a bronchogenic carcinoma, but it also can be a lymphoma, a mesothelioma, or a metastatic cancer. Which explains why the "P" of "pulmonary" was recently deleted from the HOA acronym. Either way, the hallmark of this condition is a chronic, symmetric, and *proliferative* periostitis of the long bones, often (*but not necessarily*) associated with clubbing. Hence, its other term of "digital clubbing with periostosis (or periostitis)."

118. **Which bones are most prominently affected by the periostosis of HOA?**
The diaphysis of the extremities. These include, in descending order, the radius and ulna, tibia and fibula, humerus and femur, metacarpals and metatarsals, and the proximal and middle phalanges. In addition to new bone proliferation, other diagnostic features of HOA include (1) symmetric arthritis-like changes in one or more joints (ankles, wrists, knees, and elbows); (2) coarsening of the subcutaneous tissue in the distal portions of the arms and legs (and, occasionally, the face); and (3) neurovascular changes in the hands and feet (with chronic erythema, paresthesias, and increased sweating).

119. **What is the boundary between HOA and clubbing?**
Fuzzy. HOA may occur in some disorders that commonly present with clubbing (thus the association), but not necessarily. For example, it can be seen in cystic fibrosis, bronchiectasis, chronic empyema, and lung abscesses (*all* typically associated with clubbing), while instead being rare in pulmonary interstitial fibrosis (also frequently associated with clubbing). Hence, HOA is in a league of its own.

120. **Is HOA symptomatic?**
Yes. In contrast to pure clubbing (which is painless), HOA is associated with aching and sometimes frank bony pain and tenderness. Moreover, the pretibial skin is *shiny* and often thickened and warm to touch. Autonomic manifestations also may be present, such as increased sweating, warmth, or paresthesias. Of interest, all these changes resolve with ablation (or cure) of the associated condition.

121. **How is the diagnosis of HOA established?**
Not by physical exam, but by bone radiography or, even better, *scintigraphy*. Both show typical evidence of periostosis. Physical exam may *suggest* the diagnosis, particularly in patients with clubbing and pretibial discomfort (whose tenderness over the long bones can be elicited by applying pressure on the wrists). Still, only the clubbing component of the syndrome is diagnosed on exam.

122. **What is *primary* HOA?**
It is a rare familial autosomal dominant disorder, often referred to as *pachydermoperiostosis*. About 3–5% of patients with HOA have *primary* HOA. Hence, the vast majority have it on a secondary basis.

123. **What is *pachydermoperiostosis*?**
From the Greek *pachys* (thick), *derma* (skin), *peri* (around), *osteon* (bone), *osis* (condition), this is a congenital and hereditary form of HOA characterized by digital clubbing and periosteal new bone formation (especially over the distal ends of the long bones). There also is coarsening of features, with thickening, furrowing, and oiliness of the facial forehead and skin, *cutis verticis gyrate,* as well as seborrheic hyperplasia (i.e., open sebaceous pores filled with plugs of sebum). In contrast to simple HOA, pachydermoperiostosis is characterized by less bony pain and greater skin changes. The syndrome is autosomal dominant, more severe in males, and with clinical evidence during adolescence.

124. **What is *cutis verticis gyrata* (CVG)?**
A descriptive term for a scalp condition characterized by thickening of the skin into convoluted folds and furrows that make it resemble a *cerebrum*. First described in 1843, it was labeled *cutis verticis gyrata* by Unna in 1907. It is probably due to increased peripheral use of testosterone, and thus almost exclusively limited to males, where it starts with puberty and may disappear with castration. It can present as either an isolated finding (rare) or in association with mental retardation, cerebral palsy, epilepsy, schizophrenia, cranial abnormalities (microcephaly), deafness, various ophthalmologic abnormalities (cataract, strabismus, blindness, retinitis pigmentosa), or a combination thereof. It is very common in institutionalized mental patients (where it's found in 0.71–3.4% of Scottish and Swedish males, and 13.4% of the Italian male psychiatric population). Secondary cases of CVG have been described in various conditions, including pachydermoperiostosis, acromegaly, diabetes, myxedema, amyloidosis, syphilis, and some skin diseases (melanocytic nevi, hamartomas, and neurofibromas/dermatofibromas).

125. **What is *thyroid acropachy*?**
It is thickening of peripheral tissues (from the Greek *acro*, distal and *pachys*, thick), which occurs in 1% of patients with Graves', often in association with other infiltrative manifestations, such as myxedema of the hands and feet and exophthalmos. Thyroid acropachy resembles HOA insofar as it is associated with clubbing and periosteal new bone formation, yet it preferentially involves the hands and feet rather than the long bones of the lower extremities. It also spares the joints and is usually painless. Graves' disease is often preexistent. In fact, patients can be hypothyroid, euthyroid, or hyperthyroid.

Inspection of the Neck

126. **What respiratory information can be gathered through neck inspection?**
Valuable information. In fact, inspection of the neck is such an integral part of the chest exam that it should be included in the evaluation of *all* patients with pulmonary diseases.

127. **Which areas should be paid attention to?**
Primarily two:
- Accessory muscles of respiration
- Neck veins

128. **What should be noted about the accessory muscles of respiration?**
First of all, whether scaleni, sternocleidomastoids, and trapezii are being used; if so, whether they appear *hypertrophic*. Normally, only the diaphragm contracts in inspiration (*expiration* is

mostly due to passive recoil), but in situations of increased work of breathing (as in chronic lung disease or respiratory distress), accessory muscles may be recruited. In fact, more than 90% of patients hospitalized for exacerbation of COPD exhibit some use of accessory respiratory muscles, even though this usually resolves with clinical improvement. Chronic use of these muscles eventually leads to hypertrophy.

129. **What are the most important of these accessory muscles?**
It depends. For *inspiration*, the most important are the scaleni and sternocleidomastoids; for *expiration*, the abdominal obliques are instead predominant. Overall, the scaleni are used before the sternocleidomastoids; both are employed in patients exhibiting retractions (Fig. 13-13).

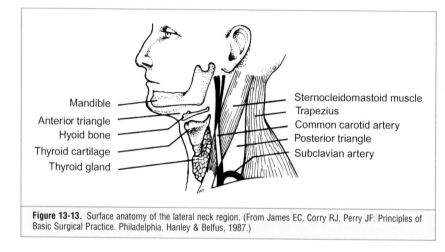

Figure 13-13. Surface anatomy of the lateral neck region. (From James EC, Corry RJ, Perry JF: Principles of Basic Surgical Practice. Philadelphia, Hanley & Belfus, 1987.)

130. **What is the physiology of these muscles?**
The sternocleidomastoids lead to an inspiratory upward motion of the clavicles (and first ribs). This may provide additional chest expansion in patients with COPD, especially those burdened with flattened diaphragms and unfavorable lung mechanics. Indeed, upward motion of the clavicle in excess of 5 mm is a valuable sign of severe obstructive disease, correlating with FEV_1 of 0.6 L. The three scalene muscles, on the other hand, connect the cervical vertebrae to the first and second ribs. Their function is to assist the intercostals in raising the rib cage.

131. **What about inspiratory retractions of the suprasternal and supraclavicular fossa?**
They may be seen in patients with COPD who have excessive swings in intrathoracic pressures. The mechanism is the same as for retraction of the intercostal spaces (*tirage*).

132. **What about accessory *expiratory* muscles?**
They primarily help exhalation (by providing an additional "push") but also may help *inspiration* (by easing the inspiratory recoil that follows expiration).

133. **Which neck vein abnormalities may provide clues to the diagnosis of lung disease?**
 ■ **Distention of neck veins:** This is seen in superior vena cava syndrome, often in association with facial, neck, shoulder, and even hand swelling. Neck vein distention also occurs in

right-sided or biventricular failure, either at baseline or after abdominal compression (abdominojugular reflux).
- **Kussmaul's sign:** This is an inspiratory bulging of neck veins and an important sign of obstruction to right ventricular filling. As such, it can be observed in many conditions, like superior vena cava obstruction, tricuspid stenosis, constrictive pericarditis, right ventricular infarction, massive pulmonary embolism, or pulmonary hypertension. Conversely, an *expiratory* bulge in neck veins is a sign of increased intrathoracic pressure and thus a good clue toward a diagnosis of COPD.

B. CHEST PALPATION

134. **What is the clinical value of palpation?**
   - To confirm, reject, or supplement information previously gathered through inspection, especially in regard to the position of the trachea and the expansion of the hemithoraces.
   - To provide *new* information, specifically concerning the status of the pleura and lung parenchyma. This is gathered through assessment of *the vocal tactile fremitus,* detection of *pleural friction rubs,* search for *bronchial fremitus* (inspiratory vibration generated by the "rattling" of intra-airway secretions), and identification of various other chest wall abnormalities (like masses and tenderness).

135. **What are the main components of palpation?**
   - Assessment of trachea
   - Assessment of vocal tactile fremitus
   - Assessment of hemithoracic expansion, with attention to possible asymmetries/asynchronies

Assessment of the Trachea

136. **How do you assess the trachea?**
   By palpating for *shifts* and *mobility*.

137. **What is the value of a tracheal shift?**
   It reflects a *mediastinal* shift. And when combined with other methods of evaluation (percussion and auscultation) it also allows for its proper *interpretation*.

138. **How do you detect a tracheal deviation?**
   First, ask the patient to sit up, lean forward, and keep the head straight. Then place the tip of your small finger in the fossa between the medial end of the sternocleidomastoid and the lateral aspect of the trachea (Fig. 13-14). Compare the depth of this fossa to the contralateral one. They should be symmetric. If not, the patient has a tracheal shift—typically toward the side with the smaller fossa.

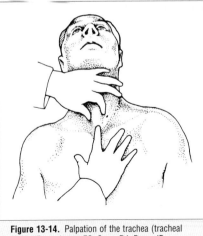

Figure 13-14. Palpation of the trachea (tracheal shift). (From James EC, Corry RJ, Perry JF: Principles of Basic Surgical Practice. Philadelphia, Hanley & Belfus, 1987.)

139. **What are the possible causes of a tracheal shift?**
(1) An *increase* in volume of the contralateral lung and/or pleural space or (2) a *decrease* in volume of the ipsilateral lung. The latter is usually due to atelectasis, whereas a volume increase is often the result of pneumothorax, large pleural effusion, or massive consolidation. Palpation of the trachea without the other steps of chest examination is usually unable to identify the reasons for a shift.

140. **How can one distinguish tracheal deviation of lung collapse from that of effusion?**
   - **Lung collapse** causes a tracheal shift that is ipsilateral to the atelectasis and its findings of dullness, decreased tactile fremitus, and auscultatory silence.
   - **Massive pleural effusion** causes instead a tracheal shift that is *contralateral* to the findings of dullness, decreased fremitus, and auscultatory silence.

141. **How do you assess for mobility of the trachea?**
It depends on the mobility:
   - **Induced mobility** can be detected by pushing the trachea sideward to see whether it is indeed mobile. A rigid and fixed trachea indicates upper mediastinal fibrosis, from mediastinitis or cancer.
   - **Spontaneous mobility** can be detected as a rostrocaudal tracheal "tug," synchronous with each heartbeat. This is often referred to as the Oliver-Cardarelli sign and usually indicates an aneurysmatic aortic arch. It is often referred to as two separate signs: Oliver's and Cardarelli's.

142. **What is *Oliver's* sign?**
A downward displacement of the *cricoid cartilage* that coincides with each heartbeat. To better detect the "tug," ask the patient to sit up with the head and chin extended, and then grasp the cricoid cartilage. Apply a gentle upward pressure with both the thumb and index finger.
A downward tug of the trachea, synchronous with each systole, suggests the presence of an *aortic arch aneurysm* that overrides the left main bronchus and pulls it down at each ejection. However, the sign also can present with mediastinal tumors or even simple COPD. First described in 1878 by the British military surgeon William S. Oliver (who served mostly in India and ended his career as surgeon general): "Place the patient in the erect position, direct him to close his mouth, and elevate his chin to the fullest extent. Then grasp the cricoid cartilage between your finger and thumb, and use gentle upward pressure on it. If dilatation or aneurism exist, the aortic pulsation will be distinctly felt transmitted through the trachea to the hand."

143. **What is *Cardarelli's* sign?**
Another sign of aortic aneurysm, and a sort of Oliver's sign on steroids. To elicit it, press on the *thyroid* cartilage, gently *displacing it toward the patient's left*. This shift in the trachea increases contact between the left main bronchus and the aorta, thus making it possible for the examiner to feel a *transverse pulsation of the trachea* in cases of aortic arch aneurysm. First described by the Italian cardiologist Antonio Cardarelli (1831–1926).

144. **What is Campbell's sign?**
A downward displacement of the thyroid cartilage during inspiration. Although also a form of *tracheal tug,* Campbell's sign is *not* due to aortic aneurysms, but to chronic airflow obstruction. To elicit it, place the tip of your index finger over the *thyroid cartilage*, and look for an inspiratory descent of the trachea >2.5 inches during inspiration. This is an accurate predictor of severity of airflow obstruction, correlating well with duration of symptoms and reduction in forced expiratory volume in 1 second (FEV_1). Still, Campbell's sign is *not* specific for COPD, since it is positive in other situations of acute respiratory distress. In fact, it is due to an excessive inspiratory pull on the trachea during strong diaphragmatic contraction.

145. What are laryngeal *height* and *laryngeal* descent?

Laryngeal height is the distance between the top of the thyroid cartilage and the suprasternal notch. Maximum laryngeal height is measured at end of *expiration*; minimum laryngeal height at end of *inspiration*. The difference between the two is the laryngeal *descent* (*see* Fig. 13-15).

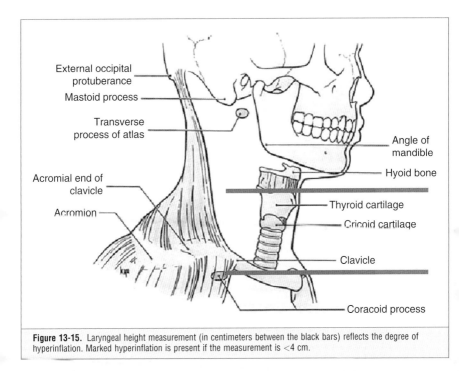

Figure 13-15. Laryngeal height measurement (in centimeters between the black bars) reflects the degree of hyperinflation. Marked hyperinflation is present if the measurement is <4 cm.

146. What is the value of laryngeal height?

It can determine both presence and severity of airflow obstruction. In fact, a laryngeal height <4 cm is a strong predictor of postoperative pulmonary risk in patients evaluated for nonthoracic surgery. In a prospective study of 272 patients by McAlister et al., three risk factors independently predicted postoperative complications: (1) age of 65 or older; (2) smoking history of 40-pack years or more; and (3) maximum laryngeal height of 4 cm or less. The latter had a *p* value <0.0001. Hence, such a simple physical sign can be highly predictive of pulmonary complications. Laryngeal height also is a strong predictor of the *presence* of obstructive lung disease (OLD). In another study by McAlister, only four clinical factors were significantly associated with a diagnosis of OLD on multivariate analysis: (1) smoking 40-pack years or more (LR, 8.3); (2) self-reported history of chronic OLD (LR, 7.3); (3) maximum laryngeal height of 4 cm or less (LR, 2.8); and (4) age of 45 or older (LR, 1.3). Patients having all four findings had an LR of 220 (ruling in OLD); those with none had an LR of 0.13 (ruling out OLD).

147. What is the value of tracheal auscultation?

It allows for recognition of *stridor* (i.e., of a "wheeze" that is present *only* in inspiration). This should not be confused with a true wheeze, which is either expiratory, or both inspiratory *and* expiratory. Still, even expiratory wheezes should be considered as originating from the upper airways when they are louder over the trachea than the chest. In fact, unless the patient is morbidly obese, these sounds usually reflect expiratory *adduction of the vocal cords* (vocal cord dysfunction) and thus should prompt laryngoscopy in all patients presenting with "refractory asthma." Finally, tracheal auscultation also allows for the measurement of the *forced expiratory time,* a valuable tool for determining the presence and severity of airflow obstruction (*see* Chapter 14, question 48).

Assessment of the Vocal Tactile Fremitus

148. **What is the vocal tactile fremitus (VTF)?**

    It is the Latin term for a palpable thrill produced by the patient's voice. This can be detected by placing the hand sequentially over various areas of the chest and by then feeling the thrill that is transmitted whenever the patient is asked to say something (Fig. 13-16). Most commonly, these sounds are "Eeee," or "1, 2, 3," or even "99"—all terms that have more historical than clinical values (they go back to the original German *neun und neunzig* [i.e., "99"]), and really matter very little, since any word or sound would probably do. And yet, it also is true that some sounds, especially the lower-pitched ones, can better pass the alveolar air filter, thus leading to a stronger tactile fremitus. This might explain why men—who have lower-pitched voices than women—have more prominent VTF.

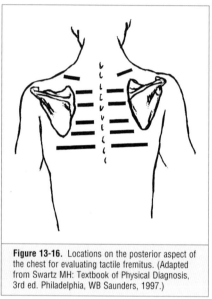

Figure 13-16. Locations on the posterior aspect of the chest for evaluating tactile fremitus. (Adapted from Swartz MH: Textbook of Physical Diagnosis, 3rd ed. Philadelphia, WB Saunders, 1997.)

149. **What is the clinical value of the VTF?**

    It provides information on sound transmission. In VTF, the larynx generates the sound; this is then transmitted downward along the tracheobronchial tree, across the pleura, through the pleural cavity/chest wall, and finally up into the hand of the examiner. Any abnormality along this way may compromise transmission, thus creating a softer and less palpable thrill. For example, an obstructed distal bronchus (because of either tumor or mucous plug), a large collection of fluid or air in the pleural space, or even a thicker skin (because of adipose tissue) will all soften the fremitus. Still, the hallmark of an abnormal VTF is the difference between the two sides of the chest—the asymmetry. Thus, each side should be compared carefully, level by level. A localized increase (or decrease) in fremitus is key.

150. **Can any disease *increase* the VTF?**

    Yes—for example, pneumonia. Note that the VTF varies, depending on whether the pneumonia is primarily alveolar or bronchoalveolar. If limited to the alveoli (i.e., patent bronchi surrounded by pus-filled parenchyma), the VTF will be increased, since fluids (or solids for that matter) transmit sound better than air. If the pneumonia extends instead to the bronchi (i.e., *broncho-pneumonia,* as typical of *Haemophilus influenzae*), the transmission of the VTF will be dampened by intrabronchial secretions, and thus softened. Hence, pneumonia increases the VTF *only if alveolar;* it decreases it if *broncho*alveolar.

151. How good is agreement for VTF among physicians?
Poor. Two studies suggest that interobserver agreement is just a little better than chance. Agreement among physicians for chest findings detected by inspection also has been shown to be poor.

Assessment of Expansion of Hemithoraces

152. What is the role of palpatory assessment of hemithoracic expansion?
It may confirm an abnormal respiratory dynamic that was suspected on inspection—for example, by observing flaring of the nostrils, or pursed-lip respiration, or asynchrony in chest/abdominal movements, or use of accessory muscles. Hence, for the detection of asymmetry/asynchrony of chest expansion, palpation of the hemithoraces is a much better tool than simple inspection. Remember that a unilateral lag on palpation is usually seen in either consolidation or effusion, whereas a *bilateral* reduction of excursion is more indicative of airflow obstruction or neuromuscular disease.

153. How do you assess hemithoracic expansion?
Stand behind the patient and grab both hemithoraces with open and extended hands. Lay your palms on the chest wall. Then ask the patient to exhale completely, while at the same time *closing in* with both hands and juxtaposed thumbs. On subsequent deep inspiration, your thumbs will move outward with the expanding chest, thus serving as pointers of the hemithoraces' symmetry, synchrony, and expansion.

Other Goals of Palpation

154. What are the other goals of palpation?
- It should identify *areas of tenderness* over the chest, ribs, or sternum. This can be encountered in neoplastic involvement, but also in atypical chest pain due to osteochondritis (Tietze syndrome).
- It should identify areas of *crepitation* (indicative of subcutaneous emphysema).
- It should identify areas of *fluctuation* or even *fistulization* (empyema necessitatis, *see* question 99)
- It should search for *pleural friction rubs* or *bronchial fremitus* (inspiratory vibration generated by the "rattling" of intra-airway secretions).
- Finally, it should systematically explore the supraclavicular and axillary fossae for the presence of *enlarged lymph nodes* (*see* Chapter 18).

C. CHEST PERCUSSION

155. How valuable is percussion?
Although less studied than auscultation, percussion remains a key component of the chest exam. Laënnec suggested that it should complement auscultation in the differential diagnosis of pleural effusion, pneumonia, pneumothorax, and emphysema—diseases in which percussion still provides crucial information (*see* also summary table at the end of Chapter 14).

156. What is the history of percussion?
Listening to sounds of the body (either spontaneous or elicited) was a truly revolutionary advance in physicians' ability to make a diagnosis. Although *succussion* had been described by Hippocrates (and so had been percussion of the *abdomen*), things really took off only in 1754–1761, thanks to Auenbrugger's work on *chest* percussion. They got even better 60 years later, when Laënnec, frustrated by percussion, added stethoscopy to the physician's toolbox (*see* Chapter 14, question 1), yet it was Giovanni Maria Lancisi (1654–1720), Roman physician

to three popes and medical historian in his own right, who first intuited (and reported) the diagnostic value of thoracic percussion.

157. **Who was Auenbrugger?**
Josef Leopold Auenbrugger (1722–1809) was an Austrian physician and the son of a wealthy innkeeper from Gratz. As a boy, little Josef used to follow his dad down to the family cellar and watch him percuss barrels of wine to see whether they were full or empty. All this paternal "tapping" must have triggered something in Auenbrugger's adolescent brain because years later, while working as an unpaid volunteer at the Spanish Military Hospital of Vienna, he concocted the cockamamy idea that human chests might similarly yield important clues about their content, thus allowing pathologic diagnoses without a need for autopsy. This novel thought was probably rooted in Auenbrugger's musical interests (he was a part-time musician, who could readily discriminate between slight changes in pitch and who later even wrote a libretto for Antonio Salieri—Mozart's menace in Peter Schaffer's *Amadeus*). Whatever the reason, Auenbrugger spent 7 years at the Spanish Military Hospital of Vienna, observing changes in sound caused by various lung or heart diseases, validating his findings with both autopsies and experiments, and even testing his sound-muffling theories by percussing variously filled barrels and cadavers. After all this cataloging, tapping, and studying, he finally published his observations in 1761, the same year Morgagni published his three-volume masterpiece of clinico-pathological correlation. Auenbrugger's opus was instead a mere 95 pages, written in Latin, and bearing the concise title, *A New Discovery that Enables the Physician from the Percussion of the Human Thorax to Detect the Diseases Hidden Within the Chest*. In this unassuming booklet, 39-year-old Auenbrugger described the various chest tones, ranging from normal (resembling that of a drum) to those produced by various thoracic diseases: (1) the *sonus altior* (high or tympanic sound); (2) the *sonus obscurior* (indistinct sound); and (3) the *sonus carnis percussae* (dull sound). He then concluded it all by announcing that simple percussion could provide physicians with pathologic information in the live patient that up to that point had been the prerogative of autopsies. It was a breakthrough. Because of this, and the work carried out in the Spanish hospital, Empress Maria Theresa eventually ordered the Viennese Faculty of Medicine to admit him at no charge as a full member. Yet, as often happens to major scientific revolutions, his little book produced a whimper and not a bang. Some even ridiculed it. Percussion remained largely underutilized and a sort of medical oddity until 50 years later, when baron Jean-Nicolas Corvisart des Marest, academician extraordinaire and personal physician to Napoleon, stumbled upon it while reading a book by Stoll, former director of the Spanish Military Hospital of Vienna. Corvisart got so intrigued by Auenbrugger's discovery, that he studied it for years and soon started teaching it to his own students. Eventually, he became so enamored with this technique as to use it regularly on rounds, predicting with remarkable and theatrical accuracy the inevitable autopsy findings. It must have been all these predictions, or Corvisart's fame, or his 1808 translation of the *Inventum Novum* (the year before Auenbrugger's death), but eventually percussion became the royal road to bedside diagnosis—"royal" until one of Corvisart's unsatisfied students (a diminutive and introverted Breton, named René Théophile Hyacinthe Laënnec) developed auscultation. The rest, as they say, is history.

158. **What is the physics behind percussion?**
It is the physics of the delivery of a fixed amount of energy to the chest wall and its back reflection as sound. The characteristics of this soundwave (*amplitude* and *frequency*) are inversely related, whereas their product remains constant. What determines these characteristics, however, remains controversial. One school of thought considers them dependent on the underlying percussed tissues. Thus, the reflected sound would have either high frequency/low amplitude or low frequency/high amplitude, based on the type of tissue percussed. In other words:

- *If the tissue is rich in air and poor in solid/fluid* (high air/fluid ratio), the percussion note will have high amplitude and low frequency. This *resonant* note is loud and typical of the normal lung.
- *If air is more abundant than normal,* the percussion note has greater amplitude and lower frequency than a resonant percussion note. It is also longer. This *hyperresonant (or tympanic)* note is typical of pneumothorax, emphysema, and big blebs—and also of the gastric bulla or a puffed cheek.
- *If the tissue ratio between air and fluid/solid is low* (i.e., there is more fluid/solid than air), the percussion note is shorter than a resonant or hyperresonant note. It also is high in frequency and low in amplitude and thus perceived as soft. In fact, *flat (or dull)* percussion notes are at times so soft that using a very light percussion technique may even fail to elicit anything audible. This technique can be used to better identify the transition between solid and aerated areas, as a change from silence (i.e., barely audible dullness) to noise (resonance). Note that, semantically, "dull" is the percussion note of consolidation and lung collapse, whereas "flat" is the note of a pleural effusion.

Hence, if the strength of striking and chest wall thickness remain constant, the *relative pitch* of the percussion note will depend on the ratio between aerated tissue/solid or liquid medium (Table 13-2 and Table 13-3).

TABLE 13-2. RELATIVE "PITCH" OF THE PERCUSSION NOTE

Normal ratio → low pitch *Resonant* percussion note (normal lung)	Increased ratio → lower pitch *Hyperresonant* percussion note (emphysema)	Diminished ratio → higher pitch *Dull* percussion note (liver)	Very diminished ratio → higher pitch *Flat* percussion note (effusion)

TABLE 13-3. SUMMARY OF FEATURES OF THE PERCUSSION NOTE

Relative Pitch	Relative Intensity	Percussion Note
Low	Loud	Resonant
Lower	Very loud	Hyperresonant
Medium	Medium	Dull
High	Soft	Flat

Yet another theory argues that the *entire* chest cage (not only the underlying tissues) resonates in response to percussion and creates the soundwave. In this sense, topographic percussion would be basically impossible, since even distant organs would participate in the sound production.

Percussion Techniques

159. What is "direct" percussion?

It is the original technique developed by Auenbrugger at the Spanish Military Hospital of Vienna. It consists of striking a clothed chest with all fingertips held firmly together. At times, prudish Auenbrugger even used a leather glove to strike the bare skin. And that is how he came to observe that a healthy thorax is *resonant,* whereas an abnormal chest has either a higher- or lower-pitched sound. Corvisart also used the *direct* method of Auenbrugger and made it a standard component of bedside examination, as a way to compare (i.e., "comparative percussion") sound characteristics between the two hemithoraces.

160. **What is the current role of *direct* percussion?**
It is still used at times for a quick screening. One form of direct percussion, for example, relies on the clavicles as pleximeters for the assessment of lung apices.

161. **What is mediated or "indirect" percussion?**
A technique developed in 1828 by the French Piorry, another of Corvisart's students and himself the inventor of "topographic" percussion—a way to map out the borders of various organs through sound. *Mediated percussion* consisted of percussing the chest—not directly— but through a solid body applied to the wall. This *mediator,* called a *pleximeter,* was to be struck with a small hammer. Piorry had initially tried lead, leather, horn, and wood but eventually settled on ivory, manufacturing a little disc that "had to be" 5 cm in diameter and 2.5 mm in thickness. Despite these guidelines, cheaper pleximeters (usually in wood) immediately flooded the market. To avoid their common loss, many of these gadgets became screwed to the end of one of Laënnec's stethoscopes. If all was lost (literally), a coin provided an easy substitute. Finally, the British William Stokes and James Hope, who had listened to Piorry's lessons in Paris (and who must have lost their pleximeters quite often), simplified the method by using instead their own middle fingers (no offense implied). Although disliked by Piorry, this variation eventually became the standard, thanks primarily to Skoda, who had become the chief advocate of mediated percussion in Vienna, and also the author responsible for the four major types of *percussion note* still taught today.

162. **What is the current technique for indirect percussion?**
It consists of laying the *pleximeter finger* (usually the middle digit of the left hand in right-handed examiners) onto the intercostal space between two ribs (and *not* on the rib, to avoid transforming it into a pleximeter itself, thus spreading the sound). To avoid dampening vibrations, only the distal interphalangeal joint of the extended pleximeter finger is allowed to touch the skin. The rest (and all other fingers) are instead lifted *off* the chest wall. The blow is then delivered via the middle finger of the opposite hand, flexed like a hammer at a 90-degree angle, and brought down over the distal interphalangeal joint of the pleximeter finger. The blow should be strong, but not too strong (to avoid setting into vibration more distant organs). In fact, a gentler tap allows better detection of the percussion note (and also a "tactile" perception of the note). This tap should be delivered by using the wrist (and not the elbow) as a fulcrum. Once delivered, the percussing finger should be lifted from the pleximeter, to avoid any sound-dampening, even though data indicate that this might not really be necessary.

163. **What is the current value of indirect percussion?**
Good but limited. The following should be kept in mind:
- A "normal" percussion note can often occur in patients with lung disease. Hence, it should not be used as an exclusion criterion.
- In its "comparative" modality, percussion complements auscultation in the differential diagnosis of *consolidation, atelectasis, pneumothorax,* and *pleural effusion.*
- In patients with fever and cough, unilateral chest dullness is a strong predictor of pneumonia (but if absent, it cannot be ruled out, given the finding's excellent specificity but poor sensitivity).
- In large pleural effusions, percussion has instead outstanding sensitivity, with unilateral dullness occurring in almost all patients (even though specificity is not as good; *see* auscultatory percussion, questions 166 and 167).

- Comparative percussion is of little or no value in detecting *circumscribed lesions,* like nodules.
- Finally, while unilateral hyperresonance suggests pneumothorax, a *bilateral* one is a strong indicator of airflow obstruction, either acute (status asthmaticus) or chronic (COPD). Even in this case, specificity is three times better than sensitivity.

164. **Are there differences between the percussion note of lung collapse from effusion and consolidation from pneumonia?**
Theoretically, yes; practically, no. In fact, this difference may be more *tactile* than auscultatory. In other words, the vibration "felt" by the pleximeter finger may be *different* depending on the characteristics of the tissue percussed. This may be intuitive for an air-filled versus a fluid-filled tissue, but it might even play a role in cases of solid tissue due to consolidation (i.e., dull), versus solid tissue due to lung compression from pleural effusion (i.e., flat). In this regard, Osler used to write, "the dullness of a pleural effusion has a peculiarly resistant, wooden quality, which is different from that of pneumonia and that can be readily recognized by skilled fingers." With all due respect for Sir William and his insistence on the role of the tactile sense in percussion, our ability to differentiate dull from flat by palpation is frustratingly limited at best.

165. **What is the current role for topographic percussion?**
Indirect percussion of the "topographic" type is mostly used to map out diaphragmatic excursion, since it has tremendous interobserver variability, making it unsuitable for defining organ borders. To map out diaphragmatic excursion, the patient's chest is percussed posteriorly, downward, and along the mid-scapular line until dullness is finally encountered. The patient is then asked to hold a deep breath while percussion is resumed. In the normal individual, there will be an additional 3–6 cm of resonance, indicative of the normal diaphragmatic movement. In situations of lung disease (or diaphragmatic paralysis), this excursion is either reduced or eliminated. In patients with COPD (whose lungs are overexpanded), diaphragmatic excursion can be limited to <2 cm. This finding has excellent specificity for COPD (>90%) but such a poor sensitivity (around 10%) to make it clinically useless.

166. **What is auscultatory percussion?**
It is a modified variety of "topographic" percussion, developed in 1940 by Camman and Clark and recently rediscovered by John Guarino as an alternative to "comparative" percussion. In either mode, detection of elicited sounds is *not* entrusted upon the unaided ear, but on the stethoscope.

167. **Is there a role for auscultatory percussion in the detection of pleural effusion?**
Yes. In fact, in its *original* form auscultatory percussion *was* advocated for the detection of pleural effusion. To do so, the patient has to be seated and the stethoscope placed in the back, 3 cm below the 12th rib. The chest is then percussed downward and posteriorly, from the apex to the base. A change in percussion note from dull to loud that is localized over the 12th rib indicates the presence of pleural fluid. In contrast to other more traditional modalities of percussion, this auscultatory variety has the same excellent sensitivity for pleural effusion (>90%), but better specificity (also >90%), being usually negative in pneumonia or atelectasis. Conversely, in its *newer and revised* modality, auscultatory percussion is practiced a little differently (Fig. 13-17). The physician taps lightly with the distal tip of one finger over the manubrium of the sternum (and thus *anteriorly*), while at the same time listening with the stethoscope over symmetric locations of the *posterior* chest wall. The theory is that sound so generated travels unimpeded through the lungs, reaching the opposite chest wall in a

symmetric fashion. Thus, any asymmetry in sound intensity is considered a sign of lung disease. By using this technique, Guarino was able to detect pulmonary lesions <2 cm in diameter (which are almost impossible to identify with conventional percussion). Studies to confirm this technique, however, have produced conflicting results.

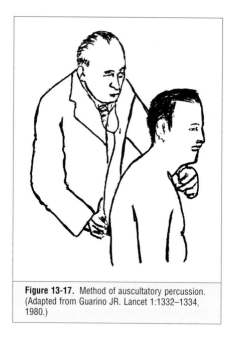

Figure 13-17. Method of auscultatory percussion. (Adapted from Guarino JR. Lancet 1:1332–1334, 1980.)

SELECTED BIBLIOGRAPHY

1. Anderson CL, Shankar PS, Scott JH: Physiological significance of sternomastoid muscle contraction in chronic obstructive pulmonary disease. Respir Care 25:937–939, 1980.

2. Andreas S, Hagenah G, Möller C, et al: Cheyne-Stokes respiration and prognosis in congestive heart failure. Am J Cardiol 78:1260–1264, 1996.

3. Barach AL: Physiologic advantages of grunting, groaning, and pursed-lip breathing: Adaptive symptoms related to the development of continuous positive pressure breathing. Bull NY Acad Med 49:666–673, 1973.

4. Bourke S, Nunes D, Strafford F, et al: Percussion of the chest revisited: A comparison of the diagnostic value of ausculatory and conventional chest percussion. Isr J Med Sci 158:82–84, 1989.

5. Brown HW, Plum F: The neurologic basis of CheyneStokes respiration. Am J Med 30:849–860, 1961.

6. Carroll DG: Curvature of the nails, clubbing of the fingers and hypertrophic pulmonary osteoarthropathy. Trans Am Clin Climat Assoc 83:198–208, 1971.

7. Cohen CA, Zagelbaum G, Gross D, et al: Clinical manifestations of inspiratory muscle fatigue. Am J Med 73:308–316, 1982.

8. Coury C: Hippocratic fingers and hypertrophic osteoarthropathy: A study of 350 cases. Br J Dis Chest 54:202–209, 1960.

9. Garcia-Pachon E: Paradoxical movement of the lateral rib margin (Hoover sign) for detecting obstructive airway disease. Chest 122:651–655, 2002.

10. Godfrey S, Edwards RH, Campbell EJ, et al: Clinical and physiological associations of some physical signs observed in patients with chronic airways obstruction. Thorax 25:285–287, 1970.

11. Guarino JR, Guarino JC: Auscultatory percussion. J Gen Intern Med 9:71–74, 1994.

12. Hansen-Flaschen J, Nordberg J: Clubbing and hypertrophic osteoarthropathy. Clin Chest Med 8:287–298, 1987.

13. Kilburn KH, Asmundsson T, et al: Anteroposterior chest diameter in emphysema. Arch Intern Med 123:379–382, 1969.

14. Mahler DA, Snyder PE, Virgulto JA, et al: Positional dyspnea and oxygen desaturation related to carcinoma of the lung: Up with the good lung. Chest 83:826–827, 1983.

15. McAlister FA, Khan NA, Straus S, et al: Accuracy of the preoperative assessment in predicting pulmonary risk after nonthoracic surgery. Am J Respir Crit Care Med 167:741–744, 2003.

16. McGee S: Percussion and physical diagnosis: Separating myth from science. Disease-a-Month 41:643–692, 1995.

17. Mueller RE, Petty TL, Filley GF, et al: Ventilation and arterial blood gas changes induced by pursed lips breathing. J Appl Physiol 28:784–789, 1970.

18. O'Neill S, McCarthy DS: Postural relief of dyspnea in severe chronic airflow limitation: Relationship to respiratory muscle strength. Thorax 38:595–600, 1983.

19. Remolina C, Khan AU, Santiago TV, et al: Positional hypoxemia in unilateral lung disease. N Engl J Med 304:523–525, 1981.

20. Robin ED, McCauley RF: An analysis of platypnea orthodeoxia syndrome, including a "new" therapeutic approach. Chest 112:1449–1451, 1997.

21. Sakula A: Pierre Adolphe Piorry (1794–1879): Pioneer of percussion. Thorax 34:575–581, 1979.

22. Shamroth L: Personal experience. South Afr Med J 50:297–300, 1976.

23. Straus SE, McAlister FA, Sackett DL, Deeks JJ: The accuracy of patient history, wheezing, and laryngeal measurements in diagnosing obstructive airway disease. JAMA 283:1853–1857, 2000.

24. Thoman RL, Stoker GL, Ross JC: The efficacy of pursed-lips breathing in patients with chronic obstructive pulmonary disease. Am Rev Respir Dis 93:100–106, 1966.

25. Yernault JC, Bohadana AB: Chest percussion. Eur Respir J 8:1756–1760, 1995.

CHAPTER 14

LUNG AUSCULTATION

Salvatore Mangione, MD

> *"Those who advise that all stethoscopes should be 'scrapped' may be influenced by the fact that they do not know how to use their own."*
>
> —Sir James Kingston Fowler of the Brompton Hospital

> *"I forthwith commenced immediately at the hospital Necker a series of observations which has been continued to the present time. The result is that I have been enabled to discover a set of new signs of diseases of the chest, for the most part certain, simple, and prominent, and calculated, perhaps, to render the diagnosis of the diseases of lungs, heart and pleura as decided and circumstantial as the indications furnished to the surgeon by the introduction of the finger. . . . Auscultation of breathing sounds with a cylinder (stethoscope) produces easily interpreted auditory signals capable of indicating presence and extent of most disorders of thoracic organs."*
>
> —R.T.H. Laënnec, 1819

GENERALITIES

Lung auscultation has long suffered from a complex and onomatopoeic terminology that goes back to the original stethoscope and its inventor. Recent application of computer technology has rekindled this art by facilitating acoustic analysis. Still, its major difficulty lies not in the identification of sounds (which is much easier than for cardiac sounds and murmurs), but in their interpretation. And despite recent attempts at standardization, terminology remains a vexing issue.

1. **Who invented lung auscultation?**
    Auscultation of the *direct* or immediate variety (that is, without the use of the stethoscope) has actually been around for a long time. References to breath sounds first appeared in the Ebers papyrus (c. 1500 BC), the Hindu Vedas (c. 1400–1200 BC), and the Hippocratic writings (4th century BC). In fact, Hippocrates himself taught and practiced auscultation, advising physicians to apply their ears to the patient's thorax in order to detect various diagnostic sounds. Since then, chest auscultation was mentioned by Caelius Aeralianus, Leonardo Da Vinci, Ambroise Paré, William Harvey, Giovanni Battista Morgagni, Gerhard Van Swieten, William Hunter, and many others. The hypochondriacal Robert Hooke, an assistant to Robert Boyle and one of the first scientists to use the word *cell* (1664), even had a good insight in describing heart sounds. He wrote, "Who knows? It may be possible to discover the motions of internal parts . . . by the sound they make." Yet, during the 18th and early 19th centuries, direct auscultation fell rapidly out of favor, being replaced by a newer diagnostic modality: chest percussion. It took a lot of serendipity (and plenty of shyness) to rekindle it as *indirect* auscultation, that is, one "mediated" by a newly invented cylindrical instrument, the stethoscope. The hero of this rediscovery was an introverted, diminutive, very asthmatic, very prudish, and very tuberculotic Breton physician, named René Théophile Hyacinthe Laënnec. In the fall of 1816 (a year after the battle of Waterloo), he was summoned to the bedside of a young woman with a chest illness. Because percussion was technically difficult (given the large size of the woman's breasts) and since direct auscultation (i.e., placing the physician's naked ear over the patient's naked chest) was, in Laënnec's own words, "inadmissible" (given the young lady's age and gender), Laënnec came up with a totally

different approach. He remembered that a few days before, while walking in the Tuileries garden in Paris, he had seen children scraping a stick of wood and listening to the other end. Imagining that something similar could be tried with patients' chests, he fetched a cardboard, rolled it into a cylinder, applied it to the lady's thorax, and to his amazement, was able to hear very distinct lung sounds. And all of this without even touching her! Being handy (he used to make flutes), Laënnec quickly manufactured a wooden contraption, shaped like a flute, which he started taking regularly on rounds. He dubbed it the cylinder (and this, in turn, gave his students a chance to dub him "the cylindromaniac"). Yet, in academic circles the tool came to be known as the stethoscope, from the Greek term for "inspector of the chest." Whatever its name, the gadget allowed Laënnec to gather over 3 years an astounding wealth of clinical–pathological correlations, which he then published on August 15, 1819—in a two-volume book titled *De l'Auscultation Mediate*. There he reported masterly descriptions of several chest diseases, many previously unheard (no pun intended), like bronchitis, bronchiectasis, pleurisy, lobar pneumonia, hydrothorax, emphysema, pneumothorax, pulmonary edema, pulmonary gangrene and infarction, mitral stenosis, esophagitis, peritonitis, cirrhosis (hence the eponym Laënnec's cirrhosis), and, of course, tuberculosis. And since autopsy was the ultimate benchmark for all these conditions, several ended up acquiring a *pathological* name. The book also presented an entirely new terminology, rooted in daily life examples and enriched by Laënnec's fascination with Greek and Latin language. Among such neologisms were stethoscope, but also auscultation, rales, rhonchus, fremitus, crackled-pot sound, metallic tinkling, egophony, bronchophony, cavernous breathing, puerile breathing, veiled puff, and bruit. The first edition of *De l'Auscultation* sold for 13 francs (16 if purchased with a wooden stethoscope) and sold quite badly. But when the considerably rewritten second edition hit the press, stethoscopy had already become the standard of chest examination. By the time of Laënnec's premature death from tuberculosis (in 1826, at age 45), many physicians were carrying stethoscopes, all personally made by Laënnec. In fact, the posthumous third and fourth editions of 1831 and 1837 sold very well, establishing the tool not only as a symbol of the art of medicine, but also as the centerpiece of bedside assessment. To reach a diagnosis, physicians could now rely on "objective" findings (instead of *subjective* symptoms reported by patients). They could finally tell their patients what they had wanted to say for a long time, "Shut up and let me listen to your lungs!" A new era had begun: one in which the patient was going to become first a sound, then a laboratory number, and, finally, a flickering computer image.

2. **How do modern stethoscopes differ from Laënnec's original cylinder?**
   Not a lot. The binaural stethoscope (invented in 1954 by Camman of New York) clearly helped. Yet, even today's expensive stethoscopes remain primarily a simple conduit for transmitting sound between the patient's chest and the examiner's ears. Even as conduits, they have flaws. For one, most of them selectively amplify specific frequencies, such as those below 112 Hz (a welcome feature for cardiologists, who deal with the low-pitched S_3 and S_4, but a not-so-welcome feature for *pulmonologists*, who deal instead with higher-frequency sounds). That is also why pulmonary auscultation has benefited so much from sound analysis through computer technology.

3. **In addition to issues of nomenclature, why is pulmonary auscultation difficult?**
   Because sounds are of too low frequency to hear well, plus they often overlap. This renders chest auscultation akin to listening to a group of people whispering at the same time. This is especially difficult in cardiac auscultation since heart sounds and murmurs have lower frequency, plus the cardiac cycle is shorter (0.8 second versus 2–3 for the respiratory cycle). To tackle these challenges, physicians develop *pattern recognition*, a crucial skill in clinical medicine, but one requiring practice.

4. **How high is the interobserver variability of chest auscultation?**
   Quite high. In a study by Shilling et al., two physicians disagreed 24% of the time in identifying the abnormal lung sounds of 187 cotton workers. A similar figure was reported by (1) Fletcher

et al. in specialists' recognition of emphysema; (2) Smyllie et al. in the assessment by nine physicians of the crackles and rhonchi of 20 patients; and (3) Schneider and Anderson for the recognition of decreased breath sounds. Although this variability seems too high to be acceptable, it is actually not much higher than that found in data collection in general, including interpretation of radiographs.

5. **What are *lung sounds*?**
They are sounds generated by the lungs. *Transmitted voice sounds* are instead sounds generated by the larynx and subsequently transmitted through the lungs (Fig. 14 1).

6. **What are the major types of lung sounds (respiratory sounds)?**
- Basic lung sounds (also called *breath sounds*)
- Adventitious (i.e., *extra*) lung sounds
Each of these subgroups contains various other sounds (Table 14-1).

7. **How are lung sounds produced?**
By two major mechanisms: (1) air movement along the tracheobronchial tree (which is responsible for basic lung sounds, or breath sounds) and (2) vibration of solid tissue (which is responsible for adventitious [or extra] lung sounds).

A. BREATH SOUNDS (BASIC LUNG SOUNDS)

8. **What are breath sounds?**
They are sounds heard over the chest of healthy (and diseased) subjects. They represent the background noise over which adventitious (or extra) sounds are occasionally superimposed.

9. **What are the major types of breath sounds?**
- Vesicular breath sounds
- Bronchovesicular breath sounds
- Tracheal breath sounds
- Bronchial breath sounds
- Amphoric (cavernous) breath sounds
This traditional division is based on the sound's site of production. Conversely, a more recent classification (based on physical characteristics) reports only two major lung sounds: (1) the normal ones (or vesicular breath sounds) and (2) the *abnormal* ones (or tubular breath sounds). The latter consist of three subvarieties: tracheal, bronchial, and amphoric. As for the bronchovesicular breath sound, it is in a league of its own and one that should probably be abandoned. (Fig. 14-2)

10. **What is the air movement responsible for the production of breath sounds?**
It depends on the size of the airway. Overall, three types of movement may take place along the tracheobronchial tree (Fig. 14-3). Some are silent and others noisy:
- **Laminar airflow** is characteristic of small peripheral airways. It is so slow that airflow in the alveoli almost comes to an end. Hence, this is a *silent* movement.
- **Vorticose airflow** is a bit faster and typical of medium-sized branching airways. "Branching" separates airflow in different layers with different velocities, whose interaction generates eddies and vortices—all *noisy*. This air movement is often called mixed (or transitional) because it resembles both laminar and turbulent airflow.
- **Turbulent airflow** is very rapid, complex, and typical of large central airways (trachea and major bronchi). Air molecules randomly collide against each other and onto the airway walls. This air movement is characteristically *noisy*.

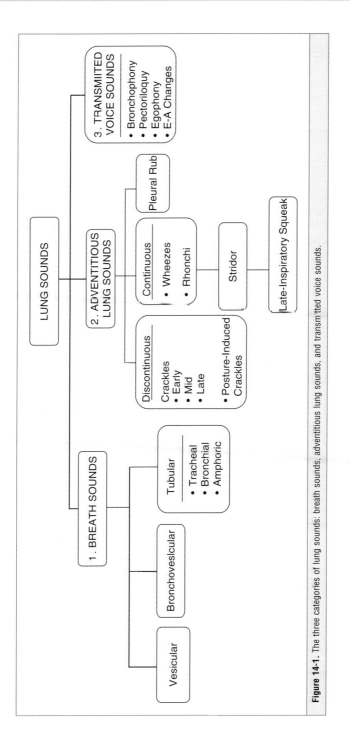

Figure 14-1. The three categories of lung sounds: breath sounds, adventitious lung sounds, and transmitted voice sounds.

TABLE 14-1.   CATEGORIES OF RESPIRATORY SOUNDS*

Respiratory Sound	Mechanisms	Origin	Acoustics	Relevance
Basic Sounds				
Normal lung sound (*vesicular*)	Turbulent flow vortices, unknown mechanisms	Central airways (expiration), lobar to segmental airway (inspiration)	Low-pass filtered noise (range <100 to 1000 Hz)	Regional ventilation, airway caliber
Normal tracheal sound (*tubular*)	Turbulent flow, flow impinging on airway walls	Pharynx, larynx, trachea, large airways	Noise with resonances (range <100 to >3000 Hz)	Upper airway configuration
Adventitious Sounds				
Wheeze	Airway wall flutter, vortex shedding	Central and lower airways	Sinusoid (range ~100 to >1000 Hz; duration, typically >80 ms)	Airway obstruction, flow limitation
Rhonchus	Rupture of fluid films, airway wall vibrations	Large airways	Series of rapidly dampened sinusoids (typically <300 Hz and duration >100 ms)	Secretions, abnormal airway collapsibility
Crackle	Airway wall stress-relaxation	Central and lower airways	Rapidly dampened wave deflection (typical duration <20 ms)	Airway closure, secretions

*This table lists only the major categories of respiratory sounds and does not include other sounds, such as squawks, friction rubs, grunting, snoring, or cough. Current concepts about sound mechanisms and origin are listed, but these concepts may be incomplete and unconfirmed.
(Adapted from Pasterkamp H, et al: Respiratory sounds. Am J Respir Crit Care Med 156: 974–987, 1997.)

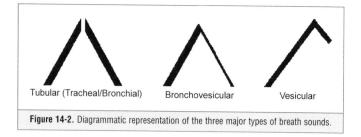

Tubular (Tracheal/Bronchial)   Bronchovesicular   Vesicular

Figure 14-2. Diagrammatic representation of the three major types of breath sounds.

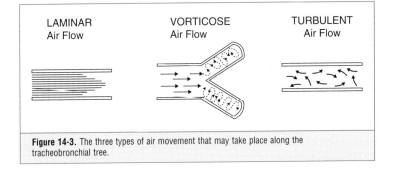

Figure 14-3. The three types of air movement that may take place along the tracheobronchial tree.

11. **How are breath sounds produced?**
Mostly by turbulent and vorticose flow in the trachea and central bronchi (*see* below, "tubular" breath sounds). Airflow in smaller and more peripheral airways is instead laminar and thus silent.

12. **Can breath sounds be heard over both the chest and mouth?**
Yes. Although produced in the central airways, they are transmitted both *downward* (to the chest) and *upward* (to the neck and mouth).

13. **Are breath sounds at the chest different from those at the mouth?**
Yes, because sounds' characteristics depend on the tissues they traverse, especially their *filtering properties*. Alveolar air, for example, is a high-frequency filter that eliminates components > 200 Hz. Since sounds transmitted to the mouth cross very little alveolar air, they will maintain all their original frequencies, including the highest. Sounds transmitted to the chest, however, traverse so much alveolar air to eventually lose most of their high frequencies. Since low frequencies are poorly perceived by the ear, sounds at the chest are typically softer than those at the mouth.

14. **What are the acoustic characteristics of breath sounds at the mouth?**
The dominant one is the high pitch (and loudness). Hence, sounds at the mouth have much wider frequencies, ranging between 200 and 2000 Hz—very much like white noise (Fig. 14-4).

15. **What is the value of comparing breath sounds at the mouth with those at the chest?**
The value of identifying airflow obstruction. Breath sounds heard at the mouth by the unaided ear have an intensity that is directly related to the spirometric degree of airway obstruction (i.e., the louder the sounds, the greater the obstruction). Conversely, breath sounds over the chest have an intensity that is inversely related to airflow obstruction, with distant sounds reflecting worse flow.

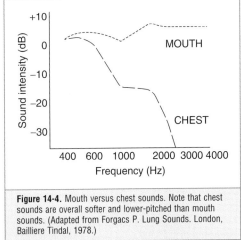

Figure 14-4. Mouth versus chest sounds. Note that chest sounds are overall softer and lower-pitched than mouth sounds. (Adapted from Forgacs P. Lung Sounds. London, Bailliere Tindal, 1978.)

16. **How do breath sounds at the mouth get produced?**

By turbulent airflow in proximal bronchi and the trachea. In normal subjects, this flow is slow enough to barely make audible any noise at the mouth. Conversely, in patients with chronic obstructive pulmonary disease (COPD), the turbulence parallels airway narrowing, eventually causing very loud mouth breathing. This increased loudness is purely limited to breath sounds and thus can occur even in the absence of crackles or wheezes. In fact, loudness can become so high that the inspiratory breath sounds of patients with COPD are often heard across the room, even in patients breathing at rest. This concept is not new, since Laënnec himself had noticed an association between noisy mouth breathing and dyspnea, reporting a patient whose breath sounds could be heard at a distance of 20 feet. In fact, he devoted a full page of *De l'Auscultation Mediate* to this phenomenon, explaining in detail that what he meant by "loud breath sounds at the mouth" was just "loud breathing," and not the noise of rattles, wheezes, or rhonchi.

17. **Are there differences in intensity of breath sounds between the various types of airflow obstruction?**

Yes (Table 14-2). In fact, the intensity of inspiratory breath sounds at the mouth can help differentiate emphysema from chronic bronchitis or asthma, since in only the last two conditions it directly correlates with (1) increased airway resistance; (2) reduced FEV_1 (forced expiratory volume in 1 sec); and (3) reduced peak expiratory flow rate (PEFR). Conversely, in emphysema, inspiratory breath sounds at the mouth are paradoxically quiet and almost silent because emphysema causes no direct narrowing of the bronchi, but only a dynamic expiratory airflow obstruction due to loss of elastic recoil.

TABLE 14-2. CHANGES IN LUNG SOUNDS WITH PULMONARY DISEASE		
Lung Disease	Breath Sounds	Adventitious Lung Sound
Pneumonia	Bronchial or absent	Inspiratory crackles
Atelectasis	Harsh/bronchial	Late inspiratory crackles
Pneumothorax	Absent	None
Emphysema	Diminished	Early inspiratory crackles
Chronic bronchitis	Normal	Wheezes and crackles
Pulmonary fibrosis	Harsh	Inspiratory crackles
Congestive heart failure	Diminished	Inspiratory crackles
Pleural effusion	Diminished	None
Asthma	Diminished	Wheezes

(From Wilkins R: Lung Sounds. St. Louis, Mosby, 1996.)

Pearl:

Noisy mouth inspiration argues in favor of asthma or chronic bronchitis, where it can predict the degree of airflow obstruction even more reliably than wheezing.

18. **Are there any other unique breath sounds' characteristics in patients with chronic bronchitis?**

The most peculiar is indeed the paradoxical behavior of inspiratory sound intensity: increased at the mouth and softened at the chest. More often, however, chronic bronchitics tend to have noisy chests, not because their breath sounds are indeed louder (in fact, they are actually softer), but because there are so many superimposed adventitious sounds to make the overall intensity *appear* louder. These extra sounds include early inspiratory crackles and rhonchi (both of which may clear with coughing), but also end-expiratory wheezes.

19. **How accurate is auscultation in identifying patients with chronic bronchitis?**
    Quite accurate, especially if computer aided. In a study of 493 subjects, computerized lung sound analysis—added to a screening program based on a symptom questionnaire plus spirometry—increased the sensitivity for detecting respiratory diseases from 71% to 87%. Half of all subjects with normal spirometry (but symptoms of chronic bronchitis) had abnormal lung sounds, primarily wheezing. Of the 24 subjects who only had abnormal lung sounds (but normal spirometry and no symptoms), three developed heart or lung disease at a 12- to 18-month follow-up.

20. **Should patients with suspected chronic bronchitis be asked to cough during exam?**
    Yes, since crackles (and rhonchi) of airflow obstruction clear with coughing. This is because they originate from air-fluid interfaces of large to medium airways. Conversely, there are some crackles that may *appear* after coughing (posttussive crackles), especially over the apical lesions of tuberculosis. Hence, the relationship with cough is a good clue to the sound's origin and should be routinely elicited. According to an old saying, you can tell a chest specialist from a generalist because the generalist never asks the patient to cough during auscultation, whereas the specialist always does.

(1) Tubular Versus Vesicular Breath Sounds

21. **What are tubular breath sounds?**
    They are sounds literally generated by air flowing through a hollow tube. In this regard, all breath sounds are indeed tubular, changing into vesicular only when filtered by alveolar air. To learn more about these sounds, listen to your own neck: tracheal sounds are classically tubular.

22. **What are the main characteristics of tubular breath sounds?**
    - *Loudness* (graphically represented by thick inspiratory and expiratory lines)
    - A brief *silent pause* between inspiration and expiration
    - A *long expiratory phase*, usually as long as inspiration (I:E ratio of approximately 1:1) (Fig. 14-5)

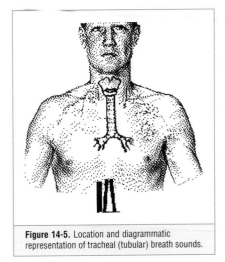

Figure 14-5. Location and diagrammatic representation of tracheal (tubular) breath sounds.

23. **Which of these characteristics is the most important?**
    The high frequency. Since they cross very little alveolar air, tracheal sounds (the quintessential tubular breath sounds) will contain higher frequencies than the vesicular ones, thus appearing louder and "hollow." In fact, they have a range between less than 100 and more than 1500 Hz, with maximal intensity at 300–800. Exhalation also has a slightly higher intensity than inspiration.

24. **What is the clinical significance of tracheal breath sounds?**
It is *indirect* and linked to their resemblance of other (and more clinically relevant) tubular sounds: the bronchial.

25. **What happens to tracheal sounds once they enter the chest?**
Once the trachea enters the chest (and branches into bronchi and bronchioli), it gets surrounded by a *mantle of alveolar air* that acts as a muffler, dampening the intensity (and frequency) of the original tubular sounds and thus transforming them into *vesicular* sounds. Hence, alveolar air acts as the equalizer of your home stereo equipment, and also as a low-pass filter: it eliminates high-frequency (and thus also louder) components, while preserving low-frequency (and softer) tones.

26. **What are the three characteristics of vesicular breath sounds?**
   - Low frequency. Hence, *soft and muffled*, graphically represented by thin respiratory lines.
   - *Absence of the silent pause* between inspiration and expiration
   - *Short duration of exhalation* because most high frequencies are concentrated in the last two thirds of exhalation and thus totally eliminated by the presence of alveolar air.

27. **Why are these sounds called vesicular?**
Because Laënnec believed they were generated by "vesicles" (the alveoli), whereas in reality they are still generated by *tubes* (i.e., bronchi and bronchioli), albeit filtered (and modified) by alveoli.

28. **What is the clinical significance of vesicular breath sounds?**
They are the normal breathing-associated sounds of healthy people. In other words, vesicular breath sounds are the same as *normal breath sounds*.

29. **Is the ability of the lung to act as a high-frequency filter a constant phenomenon?**
No, it can be eliminated by replacing the alveolar air with a medium that transmits sound better—liquid, for example. This can come as *pus* (pneumonia), *serum* (pulmonary edema), or *blood* (alveolar hemorrhage). Alternatively, air can be simply "squeezed out" of the alveoli, as in patients with alveolar collapse. Both mechanisms produce an *airless lung* (i.e., consolidation), with liquid or solid replacing alveolar air. This allows better transmission of sound, including those high-frequency components that are normally filtered out. Hence, sound will be perceived as louder.

30. **What are the acoustic differences between bronchial and vesicular breath sounds?**
Bronchial breath sounds have a peculiar quality, similar to that of tracheal breath sounds: hollow, tubular, almost Darth Vader–like. They are also louder than vesicular breath sounds—mostly because they are richer in high frequencies. Hence, their respiratory cycle is graphically represented by thicker lines. Finally, they have a silent pause between inspiration and expiration, with a longer expiratory phase. Because of longer exhalation, bronchial breath sounds also have an inspiratory-to-expiratory (I:E) ratio that is usually 1:1 (instead of 3:1 or 4:1 for vesicular sounds).

31. **What is the most striking physical characteristic of bronchial breath sounds?**
Their high frequency. This is because consolidation is associated with an overall increase in lung density, which prevents it from functioning as a low-pass filter (i.e., as an equalizer that eliminates frequencies >200 Hz). Since airless lungs allow the unaltered transmission of high-frequency sounds, bronchial breath sounds will come across as loud. Also, both inspiration and expiration have similar component frequencies (between 100 to 1200 Hz) with maximal intensity of 300–900 Hz. These frequencies are much higher than those of vesicular breath sounds and are, in fact, similar to those of other tubular breath sounds, such as the tracheal sounds.

32. **What is the clinical significance of tubular breath sounds?**
    It depends on location: they are entirely normal over the neck (i.e., originating in the trachea), but pathologic over the chest (originating in the bronchi). In this case, bronchial breath sounds (BBS) reflect absence of alveolar air and its replacement by media that better transmit high frequencies: liquid or solid (i.e., consolidation). Hence, they indicate patent airways in a setting of airless alveoli.

33. **Where are vesicular breath sounds produced?**
    In large central airways, with the inspiratory component probably originating more peripherally than the expiratory one. Sounds so produced are then transmitted through the air-filled alveoli surrounding the bronchi. Since the mantle of alveolar air acts as a "low-pass" filter, vesicular sounds only retain low frequencies (100–500 Hz), with a steep cut-off greater than 200 and maximal intensity less than 100.

34. **Are there acoustic differences in vesicular breath sounds between inspiration/expiration?**
    Expiration has lower pitch and intensity. In fact, its last two thirds are entirely silent. Hence, expiration is also shorter than inspiration, with an I:E ratio of 3:1 (in tubular sounds, it is 1:1).

35. **Do vesicular breath sounds change with age?**
    Yes. Those of children (up to age 9) are higher pitched (and louder) than adults'. In turn, vesicular breath sounds of adults are higher pitched (and louder) than those of elderly. Laënnec was the first to notice this phenomenon and called it "puerile respiration."

36. **Why does this happen?**
    Probably because of the different resonance of small thoraces, leading to less power in low frequencies for children's breath sounds (and also because of the progressive emphysema of the elderly, with an increase in "muffling" air). The smaller radius of children's airways also may be responsible for the higher turbulence and loudness of their vesicular breath sounds.

37. **Are vesicular breath sounds normally heard throughout the chest?**
    No. Although present over most lung fields of normal patients, vesicular sounds are classically absent in two narrow areas, corresponding anteriorly and posteriorly to the trachea and central bronchi (parascapular areas). Here, the vesicular sounds are replaced by bronchovesicular sounds (*see* also below, questions 60–62). Outside these narrow areas, presence of distinct vesicular sounds remains a *sine qua non* for a healthy lung (Fig. 14-6).

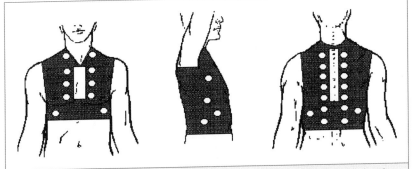

Figure 14-6. Vesicular sounds are classically absent in two narrow areas, corresponding anteriorly and posteriorly to the trachea and central bronchi (parascapular areas). (Adapted from Lehrer S: Understanding Lung Sounds, Philadelphia, WB Saunders, 1984.)

38. **What are the breath sounds characteristics of patients with pneumothorax?**
The most striking is their softening. In fact, if the pneumothorax is large enough to collapse the entire lung, the corresponding hemithorax will be silent. The distant (or absent) breath sounds of pneumothorax are not only the result of reduced sound *production* (due to diminished airflow in the collapsed lung), but also of reduced sound *transmission* (due to the cushion of air in the pleural space). The same happens with pleural effusion (of course, in pneumothorax there is an increase in intensity of the percussion note, whereas in pleural effusion there is a softening). Still, air (or fluid) in the pleural cavity forms an acoustic barrier to sound transmission that usually muffles the breath sounds. The only exception is a layer of fluid so thin as to compress only alveoli but not bronchi.

39. **Is the intensity of vesicular breath sounds important?**
Yes, since decreased intensity usually indicates reduced airflow—assuming, of course, that (1) chest wall thickness is normal (i.e., no obesity); (2) pleural space is also normal (i.e., no collection of either air or fluid); and (3) respiratory muscles are functioning normally (i.e., no weakness). Hence, distant breath sounds are typical not only of patients whose right main bronchus has been selectively intubated by a misplaced endotracheal tube, but also of patients with obstructive lung disease. In turn, vesicular breath sounds of normal intensity virtually exclude a severe reduction in FEV_1. Finally, higher intensity can also be heard during post-exercise hyperventilation.

40. **Is the intensity of breath sounds in airflow obstruction equally diminished at the mouth?**
Not at all. In fact, it's usually *increased* at the mouth.

41. **What is the best bedside predictor for the *presence* of chronic obstructive lung disease?**
A reduction in breath sound intensity (BSI). A total of 32 findings has been said to indicate COPD, with many arguing strongly for its presence (Table 14-3), yet BSI is the single best index of *emphysema*. Early inspiratory crackles also argue for obstruction (LR, 14.6), but mostly *chronic bronchitis*. If progressive over time, BSI reduction can help monitor methacholine challenge, even when wheezing is absent. Finally, any two of the following virtually rule in airflow limitation: >70-pack-years of smoking, decreased breath sounds, or history of COPD. Years of cigarette smoking, subjective wheezing, and either objective wheezing or peak expiratory flow rate also predict the likelihood of airflow limitation in males. Although other signs have been linked to obstruction (objective wheezing, barrel chest, positive match test, rhonchi, hyperresonance, and subxiphoid apical impulse), on multivariate analysis only three remain significantly associated with its diagnosis: self-reported history of COPD (LR, 4.4), wheezing (LR, 2.9), and FET >9 seconds (LR, 4.6). Patients with all three have an LR of 33 (ruling *in* COPD); those with none have an LR of 0.18 (ruling *out* COPD).

42. **How can one objectively measure breath sounds' intensity at the bedside?**
By a scoring system originally devised by Pardee:
- Ask the patient to sit up and inspire from residual volume, fast and deep, while at the same time breathing through the mouth. This generates a breath sound as loud as possible.
- Auscultate bilaterally over the upper anterior zones, the mid-axillae, and the posterior bases.
- Quantify the intensity of the inspiratory component of the vesicular breath sounds as: 0, absent; 1, barely audible; 2, faint but definitely audible; 3, normal; 4, louder than normal.
- The sum of sound intensities recorded in each area generates the BSI score. This ranges from 0 to 24 (for, respectively, scores of 0 or 4 in each of the six areas).
- To best use this method, you must disregard superimposed adventitious sounds (rhonchi, wheezes, or crackles), which, since they are louder than the underlying breath sound, would overestimate the BSI.

TABLE 14-3. ACCURACY OF BEDSIDE FINDINGS FOR THE EVALUATION OF OBSTRUCTIVE LUNG DISEASE: LIKELIHOOD RATIOS, POINT ESTIMATES, AND 95% CONFIDENCE INTERVALS

Findings	Positive LR(95% CI)	Negative LR(95% CI)
Subxiphoid cardiac impulse	7.4 (2.0, 27.1)	0.9 (0.7, 1.1)
Absent cardiac dullness	11.8 (1.2, 121.4)	0.9 (0.7, 1.1)
Hyperresonance	5.1 (1.7, 15.6)	0.7 (0.5, 1.0)
Diaphragm excursion <2 cm	5.3 (0.8, 35.0)	0.9 (0.7, 1.1)
Breath sound intensity <9	10.2 (4.6, 22.7)	–
Breath sound intensity 10–12	3.6 (1.4, 9.5)	–
Breath sound intensity 13–15	0.7 (0.3, 1.5)	–
Breath sound intensity >15	0.1 (0, 0.3)	–
Forced expiratory time <3 sec	0.2 (0.1, 0.3)	–
Forced expiratory time 3–9 sec	1.3 (0.5, 2.9)	–
Forced expiratory time >9 sec	4.8 (1.3, 17.6)	–
Early crackles, detecting obstructive disease	14.6 (3.0, 70)	0.4 (0.1, 1.4)
Early crackles, detecting severe obstruction	20.8 (3.0, 142.2)	0.1 (0, 0.4)
Unforced wheezes, detecting obstructive disease	6.0 (2.4, 15.1)	0.7 (0.6, 1.0)
Methacholine wheezes, detecting asthma	6.0 (1.5, 24.3)	0.6 (0.4, 0.9)
Diminished breath sounds, detecting asthma	4.2 (1.9, 9.5)	0.3 (0.1, 0.6)

(Adapted from McGee S: Evidence-Based Physical Diagnosis. Philadelphia, WB Saunders, 2001.)

43. **How good is interobsever reliability for BSI determination?**
Very good. It had a correlation coefficient of 0.96 in two observers examining independently 20 patients. Hence, the BSI is an accurate indicator of airflow obstruction. In fact, even unscored lung sound intensity correlates closely with FEV_1 (although the BSI correlates even better, both with FEV_1 and FEV_1/FVC [forced vital capacity]). A BSI <9 argues strongly in favor of obstruction, whereas a BSI >15 argues against it.

44. **In addition to airflow obstruction, is there any other process associated with distant breath sounds?**
Pneumonia. A reduced BSI with fever and cough is very suggestive of it.

45. **Can a change in lung sounds' intensity help monitor patients' response to airway challenge?**
Yes. In patients with a positive methacholine test, a reduced BSI is typical of asthma. In fact, a gradual reduction in BSI may even precede wheezing, thus making it a great tool for monitoring bronchial provocation. Yet, with worsening airflow, the breath sounds' pitch may paradoxically increase.

46. **What is the mechanism of decreased BSI in COPD?**
It is probably more a reduced sound *transmission* (due to parenchymal destruction, causing greater air-trapping and "muffling") than a reduced sound *production* (due to diminished airflow). This is intuitive, considering that airflow limitation in COPD is more expiratory than inspiratory.

47. **How does BSI compare to other bedside findings of airflow obstruction?**
Quite well. In a study of COPD patients, the BSI was the best indicator of "obstructive emphysema," as compared with 14 other physical findings and as judged against spirometry. The reason is its strong correlation with regional distribution of ventilation as measured by radioactive gas.

48. **What is the best bedside predictor for *severity* of airflow obstruction?**
The forced expiratory time (FET). To measure it, instruct patients to perform a forced-expiratory maneuver (i.e., to take a deep breath and blast it out as quickly and forcefully as possible) while you keep the bell of your stethoscope over the patient's suprasternal notch. Then, clock the duration of audible expiration (FETo) to the nearest half-second. An FETo >6 seconds will correspond to an FEV_1/FVC <40%. Conversely, a FETo <5 seconds will indicate an FEV_1/FVC >60%. This simple bedside test is a good and reliable "poor man's" spirometry. In a study by McAlister of 161 consecutive patients in six different countries, only three elements of the clinical exam were significantly associated with a diagnosis of COPD on multivariate analysis: self-reported history of COPD (adjusted LR, 4.4), wheezing (adjusted LR, 2.9), and FET >9 seconds.

49. **Is there any finding that argues *against* the presence of COPD?**
No single finding rules out airflow obstruction. Yet, a history of having never smoked argues strongly against it (especially if there is no wheezing on either examination or history).

(2) Bronchial Breath Sounds

50. **Are bronchial breath sounds (BBS) ever "physiologic"?**
No. Unlike other tubular breath sounds (i.e., the tracheal), BBS are always pathologic because they reflect airless parenchyma in a setting of patent bronchi, thus indicating *consolidation*. Yet, even this rule has exceptions. In fact, bronchial breath sounds can occur in normal individuals, usually over the posterior right upper chest (where the right lung is contiguous with the trachea through the first thoracic vertebra, thus allowing direct transmission of tracheal sounds). Outside of that area, bronchial breath sounds should be considered pathologic until proven otherwise.

51. **How are bronchial breath sounds produced?**
Like all other breath sounds: by air flowing rapidly through large and central airways. Their hollow quality and intensity, however, are due to better sound transmission, usually at the lung periphery.

52. **What is the cause of this improved transmission?**
1. **Consolidation** (i.e., replacement of alveolar air with a mantle of solidified lung that can better transmit higher frequencies). Consolidation reflects either alveolar *collapse* or alveolar *fluid-filling*:
   - *Alveolar collapse* (with patent airways) occurs in pleural effusions, whenever the amount of fluid is large enough to compress the alveoli but too small to compress the airways.
   - *Alveolar fluid-filling* occurs instead in situations of pneumonia (*pus* in the alveoli), alveolar hemorrhage (*blood* in the alveoli), or pulmonary edema (*serum* in the alveoli). In fact, in

patients with cough and fever, the presence of bronchial breath sounds argues strongly in favor of pneumonia. Yet, its absence cannot rule it out, since the finding is specific but poorly sensitive.
2. Bronchial breath sounds also may be heard in situations of **pulmonary fibrosis**. This mechanism, however, requires severe fibrosis and tends to be less common than simple consolidation.

53. **How deep should the consolidation be in order to generate bronchial breath sounds?**
Quite *deep*. In fact, consolidation and/or fibrosis must extend all the way from the chest surface to 4–5 cm from the hilum (where large airways are located). Only in this way is the range of transmitted frequencies increased enough to make the breath sounds resemble a tracheal sound. This also is the basis for other signs of consolidation, such as egophony, bronchophony, and pectoriloquy.

54. **Can one separate bronchial sounds of fluid-filled alveoli from those of collapsed alveoli?**
Yes, by remembering that fluid in the alveoli is often associated with fluid in the *interstitium* and that this, in turn, is associated with *adventitious lung sounds*—such as crackles. Hence, BBS without crackles are usually the result of collapsed alveoli (with patent airways), whereas BBS with crackles are more often the result of fluid-filled alveoli (also with patent airways).

55. **What is a common reason for bronchial breath sounds unaccompanied by crackles?**
A pleural effusion. Fluid occupying half of the hemithorax presents with (1) vesicular breath sounds in the upper third of the chest (reflecting normal aeration); (2) tubular (or bronchial) breath sounds in the middle third (reflecting collapsed alveoli but patent airways); and (3) respiratory silence at the bottom (reflecting collapsed alveoli *and* airways, as a result of the gravity-dependent accumulation of fluid).

56. **Other than consolidation, do bronchial breath sounds indicate anything else?**
They may help rule out an endobronchial obstruction, thus avoiding unnecessary bronchoscopies. This is because a postobstructive pneumonia is unlikely to occur in patients with densities on chest x-ray but bronchial breath sounds on examination—which is intuitive considering that tubular sounds reflect *patent* bronchi. Patency can be easily confirmed by imaging, through the presence of *air bronchograms* (i.e., air-filled airways cast against a surrounding consolidated parenchyma). Bronchial breath sounds also may be clues, albeit indirectly, to the presence of tamponade and mitral stenosis.

57. **Bronchial breath sounds can indicate tamponade and mitral stenosis?**
Yes. *Ewart's sign* (posterior dullness to percussion and bronchial breath sounds between the left scapular tip and the vertebral column) is a sign of compressive atelectasis caused by a distended pericardial sac. A similar finding occurs in the Ortner's syndrome of mitral stenosis, which is due to the raising (and squeezing) of the left main bronchus by an enlarged left atrium. This, in turn, causes (1) compression of the recurrent laryngeal nerve between the aortic arch and the pulmonary artery (with resulting hoarseness and bitonal voice); (2) left-lower lobe atelectasis (with posterior dullness and bronchial breath sounds); and (3) dysphagia (from esophageal impingement).

58. **Who was Ewart?**
A British physician (1848–1929). Born in London of a French mother (and reared in England and Paris), Ewart graduated from Cambridge and then worked in a field hospital during the

Franco-Prussian War of 1870. After the war, he lived in Berlin for a few years before returning to England, where he practiced at the Brompton and St. George's hospitals until retiring in 1907. He reported his homonymous finding in 1896. A year later, the Dutch anatomist N. Ortner reported *his* syndrome.

(3) Amphoric Breath Sounds

59. **What are amphoric breath sounds?**
They are a variant of tubular breath sounds and thus high pitched, loud, and resonant. They are typically generated by air flowing into a lung cavity, or very large cysts and blebs. "Amphoric" refers to their metallic timbre, resembling the sound produced by blowing air into a jug (*amphora* in Latin). They also are referred to as "cavernous" since they can mimic the sound of wind blowing through a "cave." They are specific for cavitary disease (often a large tuberculous *caverna*), but not sensitive.

(4) Bronchovesicular Breath Sounds

60. **What are bronchovesicular breath sounds?**
They are "transitional" sounds that may be heard over the parasternal and parascapular areas of normal people (from the third to the sixth intercostal space). They possess characteristics typical of both vesicular *and* tubular breath sounds. Many authors even dispute their existence.

61. **What are the three acoustic characteristics of bronchovesicular breath sounds?**
   - Like tubular sounds, they have long and well-preserved *expiration* (with an I:E ratio of 1:1).
   - Like vesicular sounds, they *lack a silent pause* between inspiration and expiration.
   - They are *softer/lower-pitched* than tubular sounds, but harsher/higher-pitched than vesicular.
   - These half-way characteristics are all due to the peculiar transmission of these sounds. After being produced by turbulent flow in large and central airways (distal trachea and main bronchi), bronchovesicular sounds cross only a thin mantle of alveolar air before reaching the stethoscope. Hence, in contrast to tracheal breath sounds (which are heard immediately over the neck and thus have no alveolar air to cross), bronchovesicular sounds still have to undergo some physical changes (mostly filtering of high frequencies) before reaching the chest surface. Yet this filtering is not of the same degree as that undergone by *vesicular* sounds. Hence, their hybrid features.

62. **What is the clinical significance of bronchovesicular breath sounds?**
It depends on location. If heard over the parasternal and parascapular areas (both anteriorly and posteriorly), they are normal. Anywhere else, they indicate pathology— usually *early consolidation* (with enhanced transmission of high frequencies) or a *thin pleural effusion*, partially compressing the alveoli but not the bronchi. (Fig. 14-7)

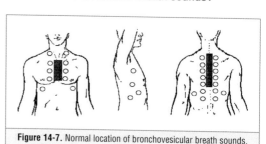

Figure 14-7. Normal location of bronchovesicular breath sounds.

B. ADVENTITIOUS LUNG SOUNDS

63. **What are adventitious lung sounds?**
They are extra (i.e., adventitious) sounds that are normally absent in a respiratory cycle but become superimposed on the underlying breath sound (vesicular or bronchial) whenever disease occurs. Theirs is a confusing alphabet soup of rubs, squeaks, crackles, wheezes, stridor, and rhonchi. (Table 14-4)

64. **How were these sounds first described?**
By Laënnec, who through painstaking clinical–pathological correlation reported many of them in his 1819 treatise *De l'Auscultation Mediate*. He called them "bruits étrangers" (i.e., foreign sounds). He also referred to them as "râles" since many of his patients had tuberculosis, and thus rattling noises (*râles* in French) were indeed the sounds he most frequently heard. Yet, realizing that râles were easier to recognize than describe, he tried to teach them by using examples from "daily" life—all actually quite bizarre. For instance, he compared fine crackles to the "crackling of salt on a heated dish," writing that these "humid râles" (or crepitations) were often present in patients with pneumonia, pulmonary edema, or hemoptysis. He then compared coarse crackles to the "gurgling of water from an upside down bottle," adding that these "mucous râles" were often heard in patients with abundant secretions of the central airways. Finally, he likened wheezes to the "chirping of little birds" and rhonchi to the "cooing of a wood pigeon"—all bizarre and confusing examples.

65. **When was the classification of adventitious lung sounds revised?**
In 1977. The problem, of course, was Laënnec's terminology and his original "daily life" examples. This was compounded by his inability to even use the term râle at the bedside, since it reminded his patients of the French expression "le râle de la mort" (the death rattle)—that is, the gurgling sound of dying people too ill to clear secretions. To avoid any bedside miscommunication, Laënnec often referred to these sounds as *rhonchi*, which was the Latin (and less scary) equivalent of rattles. Still, râles and rhonchi meant the same thing to him. This, however, escaped his first English translator, Dr. John Forbes, who decided that rhonchi should only describe *long* sounds, whereas râles should describe *short* sounds. Not all translators, however, complied with this rule, thus triggering the beginning of the end for Laënnec's classification. By the 1970s, the confusion was so bad that Fraser and Pare reported that "every physician seems to have his own classification." This eventually led to a reclassification by a team of international experts, with recommendations published in 1977, more than 150 years after Laënnec's original terminology (Table 14-5).

66. **What were the recommendations of the 1977 classification?**
The most striking was the abandonment of Laënnec's beloved term of "râle" in favor of a nomenclature based on acoustic *and* physical characteristics. Since priority was given to *duration*, adventitious lung sounds were divided into discontinuous (if lasting <250 msec) and continuous (if lasting >250 msec). The term *crackle* became the main descriptor of discontinuous sounds, replacing both the French râle and the British crepitation. Suffixes such as wet and dry were completely abandoned—as well as moist, sticky, atelectatic, close-to-the-ear, metallic, superficial, or consonating. Currently, the only acceptable modifiers for crackles are *fine* and *coarse* (in addition to indicators of the crackle's respiratory timing—such as early, mid, or late).

67. **So how should crackles be described?**
- Depending on their *number*, as either scanty or profuse
- Depending on their *predominant frequency*, as high-pitched (fine) or low-pitched (coarse)
- Depending on their *amplitude* of oscillations, as either faint or loud
- Finally, depending on their *timing* during inspiration, as either early, mid, or late inspiratory

TABLE 14-4. OUTLINE OF CLASSIFICATION OF LUNG SOUNDS

Acoustic Characteristics	Waveform	Recommended ATS* Nomenclature	Terms in some Textbooks	A British Usage	Laennec's Original Term	Laennec's Model
Discontinuous, interrupted explosive sounds Loud, low in pitch		Coarse crackle	Coarse rale	Crackle	Rale muqueux ou gargouillement	Escape of water from a bottle held with mouth directly downward
Discontinuous, interrupted explosive sounds Less loud than above and of shorter duration; higher in pitch than coarse rales or crackles		Fine crackle	Fine rale crepitation	Crackle	Rale humide ou crepitation	Crepitation of salts in a heated dish. Noise emitted by healthy lung when compressed in the hand
Continuous sounds Longer than 250 ms, high pitched; dominant frequency of 400 Hz or more, a hissing sound		Wheeze	Sibilant rhonchus	High-pitched wheeze	Rale sibilant sec ou sifflement	Prolonged whisper of various intonations; chirping of birds; sound emitted by suddenly separating 2 portions of smooth oiled stone. The motion of a small valve
Continuous sounds Longer than 250 ms low pitched; dominant frequency about 200 Hz or less; a snoring sound		Rhonchus	Sonorous rhonchus	Low-pitched wheeze	Rale sec senore ou ronflement	Snoring; bass note of a musical instrument; cooing of a wood pigeon

*American Thoracic Society

Although the terms used to name the categories of lung sounds vary widely, the categorization scheme itself has changed little since Laennec. The most recent names recommended for adoption by the American Thoracic Society and terms used by others are shown here, accompanied by acoustic descriptions and examples of typical sound wave-forms for each category.

TABLE 14-5. CLASSIFICATION OF ADVENTITIOUS LUNG SOUNDS

Acoustic Characteristics	American Thoracic Society Nomenclature	Commonly Used Synonyms (Old Terminology)	Laënnec Example
1. Discontinuous (<250 msec)	Coarse crackle	Coarse râle	Water gurgling from a bottle
	Fine crackle	Fine râle crepitation	Crackling of salt on a heated dish
2. Continuous (>250 msec)	Wheeze (high-pitched)	Sibilant rhonchus	The chirping of little birds
	Rhonchus (low-pitched)	Sonorous rhonchus	The cooing of a wood pigeon

68. **How much has this terminology been implemented?**

Not much. In common practice, outdated terms such as râles (or crepitations) are still encountered, as shown by several surveys of physicians and respiratory therapists. Even medical journals often rely on some of these old terms. A review of several case reports, for example, has shown the use of as many as 16 different terms to describe similar sounds.

69. **How are adventitious lung sounds produced?**

Mostly by *vibration of respiratory structures*, such as bronchi and pleura. This may occur in four ways:

- **Rupture of fluid films or bubbles:** This is responsible for *coarse* crackles (discontinuous adventitious lung sounds) and occurs whenever air flows through large central airways coated with thin secretions. The air–fluid interface causes the rupture of fluid films and bubbles, resulting in crackling noises. These are typical of acute and chronic bronchitis and were called by Laënnec "râles gargouillement," an expression which included the *death rattle*. (Fig. 14-8)

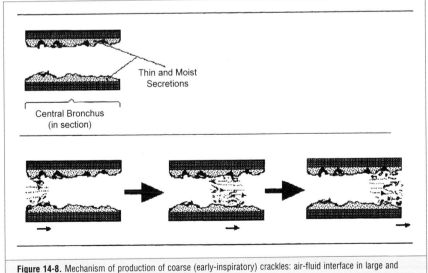

Figure 14-8. Mechanism of production of coarse (early-inspiratory) crackles: air-fluid interface in large and central airways with rupture of fluid films or bubbles.

- **Sudden equalization of intra-airway pressure:** This is responsible for *fine* crackles, which are also discontinuous adventitious lung sounds, but more typical of pneumonia, pulmonary hemorrhage, pulmonary edema, and pulmonary fibrosis. Sudden equalization of intra-airway pressure occurs whenever small airways that are partially collapsed suddenly "pop" open in inspiration. The partial collapse of distal airways is due to high interstitial pressure, the result of either scarring (pulmonary fibrosis) or fluid (pus, blood, serum). (Fig. 14-9)

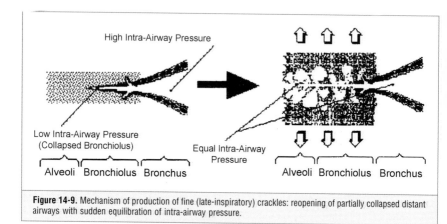

Figure 14-9. Mechanism of production of fine (late-inspiratory) crackles: reopening of partially collapsed distant airways with sudden equilibration of intra-airway pressure.

- **Fluttering of the airway wall:** This is responsible for *wheezes*, which are instead continuous adventitious lung sounds. Fluttering occurs whenever air flows rapidly through airways that have been narrowed by either bronchospasm or thick secretions/edema. The underlying mechanism is the Bernoulli principle, which also governs the water vacuum pump of many labs. In the case of the pump, it is the water rapidly flowing through a narrow tube that produces a sucking effect (which, in turn, draws-in air through a hole in the tube). In the case of wheezes, however, there is no hole in the airway wall. As a result, air flowing rapidly through a narrow bronchus will simply draw-in the airway wall, thus creating a fluttering and a wheeze (Fig. 14-10).
- **Rubbing of inflamed pleural surfaces:** This is responsible for the pleural friction rub. The two pleural layers are roughened by inflammation and covered with fibrin, and they grate against each other during respiration. This produces a leather-like sound that is typically inspiratory and expiratory.

(1) Discontinuous Adventitious Lung Sounds

70. **What are *discontinuous adventitious lung sounds* (DALs)?**
They are short (<250 msec) and explosive extra sounds that occur primarily in disease states. They are mostly inspiratory, even though they also may occur in expiration. They are called *discontinuous* because they last <250 msec, which is the cutoff for the identification by the human ear of any musical attribute. Hence, DALs are primarily noises. They are commonly referred to as crackles.

71. **How useful are crackles?**
Very useful. In fact, of all adventitious sounds, they are probably the most clinically valuable because of the strong correlation between inspiratory timing and *site* of sound production.

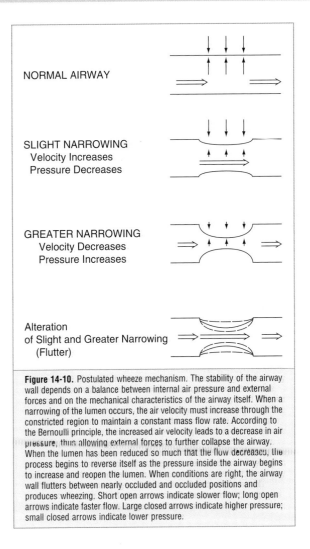

NORMAL AIRWAY

SLIGHT NARROWING
Velocity Increases
Pressure Decreases

GREATER NARROWING
Velocity Decreases
Pressure Increases

Alteration
of Slight and Greater Narrowing
(Flutter)

Figure 14-10. Postulated wheeze mechanism. The stability of the airway wall depends on a balance between internal air pressure and external forces and on the mechanical characteristics of the airway itself. When a narrowing of the lumen occurs, the air velocity must increase through the constricted region to maintain a constant mass flow rate. According to the Bernoulli principle, the increased air velocity leads to a decrease in air pressure, thus allowing external forces to further collapse the airway. When the lumen has been reduced so much that the flow decreases, the process begins to reverse itself as the pressure inside the airway begins to increase and reopen the lumen. When conditions are right, the airway wall flutters between nearly occluded and occluded positions and produces wheezing. Short open arrows indicate slower flow; long open arrows indicate faster flow. Large closed arrows indicate higher pressure; small closed arrows indicate lower pressure.

72. **What do crackles sound like?**
Forgacs vividly compared them to "miniature explosions," which is definitely better than Laënnec's "gurgling water" and "crackling salt." Williams compared them in 1828 to the sound of "rubbing a lock of one's hair between finger and thumb, close-to-the-ear." In 1876, Latham spoke of "dry and moist râles." Still, the term *crackle* is a recent addition, first introduced by Robertson and Cooper in 1957 as either coarse or fine, the latter being compared to the crushing of leaves. A more recent analogy, however—and one I particularly like—is the crepitation of Velcro, or the crinkling of cellophane, examples that would have surely defied Laënnec's wildest dreams, or nightmares.

73. **What is the underlying breath sound of crackles?**
It depends on the type of crackles. For early and mid-inspiratory ones, it is *vesicular*, whereas for late-inspiratory crackles it is either vesicular or bronchial. This distinction may help differentiate

the underlying disease. For example, a process that causes fluid-filling of the interstitium and alveoli (like pneumonia, pulmonary edema, or pulmonary hemorrhage) is much more likely to present with *late*-inspiratory crackles (due to interstitial fluid) and *bronchial* breath sounds (due to alveolar fluid). Conversely, scarring of the interstitium (i.e., pulmonary fibrosis) is much more likely to present with late-inspiratory crackles and *vesicular* breath sounds. This algorithm (Fig. 14-11) is simple but not simplistic and may be useful at the bedside.

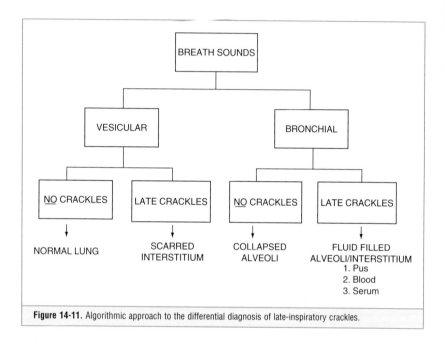

Figure 14-11. Algorithmic approach to the differential diagnosis of late-inspiratory crackles.

74. **How do crackles get produced?**
   It depends on their timing in the respiratory cycle (Fig. 14-12):
   ■ **Early and mid-inspiratory crackles** are coarse sounds produced by bubbling of air through thin secretions in large and medium-sized airways (as in, respectively, bronchitis and bronchiectasis). These crackles are superimposed on the underlying breath sound and often clear with coughing. Since they originate in large central airways, they are mostly heard over the central chest, both posteriorly and anteriorly. In addition to air-fluid interface, bronchiectatic crackles also may result from the dilation caused by destruction of the

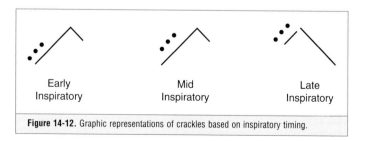

Figure 14-12. Graphic representations of crackles based on inspiratory timing.

musculoelastic framework. Loss of support causes the airway to collapse in expiration and then suddenly reopen in inspiration, in a to-and-fro cycle that produces mid-inspiratory crackles that do not clear with coughing (since they are not due to secretions).
- **Late-inspiratory crackles** are instead fine sounds that occur during the reopening of distal airways that have become partially occluded as a result of high interstitial pressure. Since the two ends of these semi-collapsed bronchioli have different intra-airway pressures (a high central and a low distal), their sudden inspiratory reopening causes rapid intraluminal equalization and, thus, a "pop." The high interstitial pressure behind them is usually due to either scarring of the interstitium or fluid-filling (such as pus, blood, or serum). Hence, late-inspiratory crackles suggest interstitial fibrosis or interstitial edema (from pneumonia, hemorrhage, or congestive failure).

75. **What are the characteristics of *early* and *mid*-inspiratory crackles?**
They are coarse, loud, low pitched, scanty, gravity independent, well transmitted to the mouth (because they originate in more proximal airways), and strongly associated with *obstructive* physiology. They vary in number, resolve with coughing, and cannot be extinguished with posture.

76. **What are the characteristics of late-inspiratory crackles?**
They are fine, soft, high pitched, profuse, gravity dependent, poorly transmitted to the mouth (because they originate in more peripheral airways), and strongly associated with *restrictive* physiology. They can be extinguished by a change in posture but not by coughing.

77. **Are there any regional preferences for late-inspiratory crackles?**
The *dependent areas*, like the posterior lung bases. These are regions of high interstitial pressure, where gravity can more easily cause the bronchiolar collapse that is key to these sounds.

78. **Can crackles occur in normal people?**
Yes. Although a sign of disease, crackles also may occur in healthy subjects. They are typically end inspiratory, high pitched, and fleeting—usually resolving after a few deep inspirations. Hence, they resemble the crackles of pulmonary fibrosis, including their predilection for lung bases, where gravity makes airway collapse more likely to occur. In fact, they indicate the reopening of atelectatic lung units, which occurs normally in most healthy subjects after a deep inspiration follows periods of quiet breathing—and especially in subjects that have been recumbent for prolonged time. Late-inspiratory crackles can be detected by careful auscultation in 63% of young nursing students, and in 92% if using an electronic stethoscope with high-pass filtration.

79. **What should one do at the bedside when confronted with crackles?**
First, separate early from mid-inspiratory and late-inspiratory crackles, since their etiology is different:
- **Early crackles** originate in large central airways and reflect *bronchitis* (acute or chronic).
- **Mid-inspiratory** crackles originate in medium-sized airways and reflect *bronchiectasis*.
- **Late crackles** arise from peripheral airways and, depending on the patients' presentation, reflect either *fluid in the interstitium* or *scarring*. In asbestos workers, for example, they indicate asbestosis; in patients with fever and cough, they suggest pneumonia; and in cardiac patients, they favor increased left atrial pressure.

80. **Summarize the characteristics of early, mid-inspiratory, and late-inspiratory crackles.**
See Table 14-6.

TABLE 14-6. CHARACTERISTICS OF INSPIRATORY CRACKLES

Early and Mid-Inspiratory	Late Inspiratory
Coarse	Fine
Low-pitched	High-pitched
Scanty	Profuse
Gravity independent	Gravity dependent
Do not change with posture	Change with posture
Clear with coughing	Do not clear with coughing
Well transmitted to the mouth	Poorly transmitted to the mouth
Associated with obstruction	Associated with restriction

81. **How good is interobserver agreement for crackles?**
Good for presence (or absence) of abnormal lung sounds and poor for grading and timing of crackles, especially the differentiation between coarse and fine. In this regard, Piirila et al. found agreement in only 60% of the cases. Differentiation between fibrosing alveolitis (i.e., late-inspiratory crackles) and bronchiectasis (i.e., mid-inspiratory crackles) was even worse. Interobserver agreement can, however, be improved by computer-assisted training.

82. **Are the crackles of pulmonary fibrosis limited to late inspiration?**
No. Although typically late in inspiration, these crackles may be mid-inspiratory or even early inspiratory. In fact, they may occur *throughout* inspiration. Their hallmark, however, is that they last until the end of inspiration. Similarly, bronchiectatic crackles predominate in mid-inspiration but may start earlier.

83. **Are late-inspiratory crackles present in all interstitial lung disease?**
No. Although reported in 65–91% of chronic interstitial pulmonary diseases (including asbestosis or idiopathic pulmonary fibrosis), they occur in only 5–20% of sarcoidosis cases. Fine crackles also are rare in other granulomatous disorders (like miliary tuberculosis, eosinophilic granuloma, or allergic alveolitis), and similarly rare in intra-alveolar processes (only 20% of pulmonary alveolar proteinosis cases). Still, whenever present, sarcoid crackles are basilar too, fine, and late-inspiratory (*see* Fig. 14-13).

84. **Why are crackles so rare in sarcoidosis but so common in other fibrotic lung diseases?**
Because of the different distribution in lung scarring, as clearly seen on high-resolution computed tomography (CT). Idiopathic pulmonary fibrosis tends to be associated with lower lobe location and subpleural scarring, which are strong radiologic predictors of the presence of crackles. Sarcoidosis is instead associated with upper lobe location and peribronchial fibrosis.

85. **How common are crackles in asbestosis?**
Very common. In large population studies, they are present in 15% of asbestos workers versus 3% of normal people. Crackles also are an early sign of disease, increasing in frequency and number with increased duration of exposure. By the time asbestosis is clinically evident, late-inspiratory, fine, and high-pitched crackles are heard in more than half of all patients. They are a good marker of disease severity, reflecting more on the *duration* of asbestos exposure than the vital capacity itself. Hence, crackles can be a valuable tool for the monitoring of exposed workers.

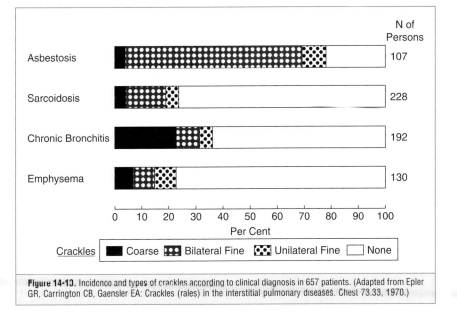

Figure 14-13. Incidence and types of crackles according to clinical diagnosis in 657 patients. (Adapted from Epler GR, Carrington CB, Gaensler EA: Crackles (rales) in the interstitial pulmonary diseases. Chest 73.33, 1970.)

86. **Where are asbestosis crackles localized?**
Usually at the *bases*, first centrally (along the mid-axillary lines) and then posterolaterally.

87. **Is there a correlation between the number of crackles and disease severity?**
Yes. In asbestosis, for example, the number of crackles correlates directly with severity of the underlying disease. This rule applies also to other interstitial processes. Automatic crackle detection and counting have indeed been developed for both diagnosis and follow-up.

88. **Are crackles common in patients with idiopathic pulmonary fibrosis (IPF)?**
Yes. In fact, so common (up to 100%) that their absence argues strongly against the diagnosis.

89. **Is there a correlation between late-inspiratory crackles and severity of IPF?**
Yes. In addition to fewer crackles, milder forms of the disease have crackles that are only late inspiratory and gravity dependent (i.e., limited to the bases in upright patients). As the disease progresses, crackles become paninspiratory (even though still predominant in end-inspiration). They may also persist despite postural changes, eventually extending to higher lung regions. Finally, they may become associated with late-inspiratory squeaks (*see* below, questions 113 and 114).

90. **Can crackles occur in exhalation?**
Crackles are primarily inspiratory, and yet 10% *do* occur in *exhalation*—usually at mid- or late-expiration in patients with either obstructive or restrictive disease.
   - In **obstructive** processes (such as bronchitis or bronchiectasis), they tend to be coarse, early expiratory, gravity independent, and profuse. They decrease in number with coughing.
   - In **restrictive** processes (such as pulmonary fibrosis or connective tissue disease), they are fine, mid- or late expiratory, gravity dependent, and scanty. They do not resolve with coughing.

91. What is the mechanism of production of late-expiratory crackles?
There are two schools of thought: (1) they are produced by the closure (not the reopening) of stiff and fibrotic small airways, and (2) they are produced by the reopening of small airways, very much like late-inspiratory crackles. Using Forgacs' model, this would occur as follows:
- High interstitial pressure (from interstitial fibrosis, for example) would collapse a small airway.
- The inspiratory traction would snap the airway open, thus creating a "pop" in late inspiration.
- The airway would then recoil in early exhalation, closing its lumen once again. This, in turn, would set up a new reopening, which this time occurs in late exhalation, when the intraluminal air exceeds pressure in the adjacent airways. The reopening produces a late-expiratory crackle.

92. What is the clinical significance of expiratory crackles?
They are an important predictor of disease severity. In patients with interstitial lung disease, for example, the number of expiratory crackles has been shown to correlate directly with a reduction in diffusing capacity. In fact, because usually fewer than inspiratory crackles (and thus easier to count), expiratory crackles may be even more valuable for the assessment of disease severity.

(2) Special Problem—Pneumonia

93. What are the traditional findings of pneumonia?
- Increased tactile fremitus
- Dullness to percussion
- Bronchial breath sounds with late-inspiratory crackles
- Egophony

Yet findings are often scanty or even absent. This argues against the original claims of physical diagnosis founders, that the bedside exam could identify *any* patient with pneumonia. The reason for this discrepancy is that modern physical exam is judged against extremely sensitive gold standards, such as roentgenograms and CT scans. Conversely, the 19th-century gold standard was autopsy, which selected the most severe forms of pneumonia, and thus the ones more likely to be associated with abnormal physical findings.

94. What is the time course of these findings?
Variable, with crackles and diminished breath sounds usually appearing first, bronchial breath sounds and egophony developing 1–3 days after onset of symptoms (i.e., cough and fever), and dullness to percussion (plus increased tactile fremitus) occurring even later. This time lag usually allows for x-ray to preempt diagnosis, thus making exam irrelevant, since early detection by imaging translates into early institution of antimicrobial therapy, which in turn leads to aborted or never-developed physical findings. Hence, physical exam may be entirely normal in patients with pneumonia.

95. What about the presence of *diminished breath sounds*?
It also can occur in pneumonia, but usually in the setting of a concomitant pleural effusion.

96. What are the most valuable bedside *predictors* in pneumonia patients?
Hypothermia and hypotension, both strong predictors of poor outcome. Improvement of blood pressure and fever—together with lowering of cardiac and respiratory rates—is instead a favorable predictor. Finally, oxygen desaturation has little prognostic value in hospitalized patients.

97. **Is there any diagnostic clue that may suggest pneumonia in ambulatory patients?**
In patients with cough, fever, sputum production, and dyspnea, the findings of egophony, bronchial breath sounds, dullness to percussion, diminished breath sounds, tachypnea, and crackles all argue (in decreasing order of importance) in favor of a diagnosis of pneumonia.

98. **What are the characteristics of *crackles* in pneumonia?**
Although Laënnec considered them very similar to those of hemoptysis and pulmonary edema, their characteristics depend very much on the *stage* of pneumonia, as demonstrated by computerized sound analysis. In the acute setting, crackles are predominantly coarse and mid-inspiratory, resembling those of bronchiectasis. During recovery, however, they tend to become shorter, more end inspiratory, and thus similar to the crackles of pulmonary fibrosis.

99. **What about crackles of congestive heart failure (CHF)?**
They are very similar to those of pulmonary *fibrosis*: profuse, fine, high pitched, and late inspiratory. Both predominate in gravity (and posture) dependent regions. In fact, they are quite difficult to separate on auscultation, even though a differentiation can usually be made on clinical grounds (or by using computerized sound analysis). Still, the examiner should be aware of their similarity, especially when considering diuresis. As a rule of thumb, bibasilar fine crackles should suggest heart failure only in patients with no other indication of pulmonary disease.

(3) Special Problem—Posturally Induced Crackles (PICs)

100. **What are posturally induced crackles (PICs)?**
Very useful findings. Crackles are quite common in CHF. Yet, if present only after recumbent position, they may have even better diagnostic/predictive value.

101. **What's the best way to elicit PICs?**
By following these steps (Fig. 14-14):

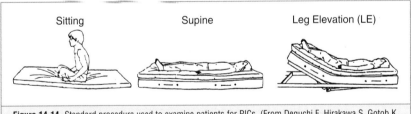

Sitting   Supine   Leg Elevation (LE)

Figure 14-14. Standard procedure used to examine patients for PICs. (From Deguchi F, Hirakawa S, Gotob K, et al: Prognostic significance of posturally induced crackles: Long-term follow-up of patients after recovery from acute myocardial infarction. Chest 103:1457–1462, 1993, with permission.)

1. Have the patient sit in bed upright for 3 minutes.
2. Listen over the eighth, ninth, and tenth interspaces along the posterior axillary line. Listen for crackles during at least five consecutive breaths. Pay special attention to late inspiration. Make sure that each breath starts from residual volume and ends in total lung capacity.
3. Have the patient assume a supine position, maintaining it for 3 minutes.
4. Listen again by using the same method outlined in step 2.
5. Have the patient elevate both legs passively at an angle of 30 degrees for 3 minutes.
6. Listen again by using the same method outlined in step 2.

102. **How should this maneuver be interpreted?**
   - If late-inspiratory crackles are absent in all positions (sitting, supine, and leg-elevated), the test is negative, and the patient receives a score of 0.
   - If late-inspiratory crackles are absent in the sitting position but become audible in the supine or leg-elevated position, the test is positive for PICs, and the patient receives a score of 1.
   - If late-inspiratory crackles are already present in the sitting position and continue throughout supine and leg-elevated changes, they are persistent, and the patient receives a score of 2.
   See Table 14-7.

TABLE 14-7. POSTURALLY INDUCED CRACKLES				
	Sitting	Supine	Leg Elevation	Score
PIC-negative	−	−	−	0
PIC-positive (1)	−	−	+	1
PIC-positive (2)	−	+	+	1
Persistent crackles	+	+	+	2

(−) = late-inspiratory and fine crackles not audible; (+) = late-inspiratory and fine crackles audible. (From Deguchi et al: Prognostic significance of posturally-induced crackles. Long-term follow-up of patients after acute myocardial infarction Chest 103:1457–1462, 1993.)

103. **What is the clinical significance of PICs?**
   Ominous, both diagnostically and prognostically. PIC-positive patients have a higher pulmonary capillary wedge pressure, lower pulmonary venous compliance, and higher mortality. Deguchi et al. monitored for 6 years 262 patients after an acute myocardial infarction. PIC-positive patients had worse long-term prognosis: 28/143 (19.6%) died of cardiac causes as compared with 3/78 (3.8%) of PIC-negative patients. Cardiac deaths were even higher in patients with persistent crackles: 15/41 (36.6%). Hence, PICs provide a noninvasive, simple, and valuable bedside test. After the number of diseased coronary vessels and the patient's pulmonary capillary wedge pressure (PCWP), PICs rank third as the most important predictor of recovery after acute myocardial infarction.

104. **Do PICs represent an independent variable?**
   Yes. In fact, when the number of disease vessels is constant, PICs consistently predict a lower survival rate. They do the same when PCWP is high ($\geq$13 mmHg). Hence, the lower survival of PIC-positive patients does not simply reflect an increased number of diseased vessels or a greater PCWP, but represents instead an independent variable.

(4) Continuous Adventitious Lung Sounds (CALS)

105. **What are continuous adventitious lung sounds?**
   They are musical extra sounds superimposed on the underlying breath sound. Usually expiratory, they also may occur in inspiration, or even throughout the respiratory cycle, but *never in inspiration only*. If high-pitched, they are called *wheezes* (dominant frequency >400 Hz), and if low-pitched, they are called *rhonchi* (dominant frequency <200 Hz). Note that they

are called continuous not because they cover the entire length of the respiratory cycle, but simply because they are *long*. In fact, longer than the discontinuous adventitious lung sounds (i.e., crackles). Hence, they are perceived by the human ear as "musical."

106. **How long should these sounds be in order to qualify as "continuous"?**
According to American Thoracic Society Guidelines, they should last >250 ms. In reality, CALs are rarely that long, lasting instead 80–100 ms.

107. **What are the physical characteristics of CALs?**
In addition to their long duration, they have a high-frequency range: from <100 to >1000 Hz. They have even higher frequency when recorded directly from within the airway.

108. **What are monophonic and polyphonic CALs?**
CALs that can be compared to either a solo singer (monophonic wheezes) or a polyphonic choir.
- **Monophonic wheezes** consist of single or multiple notes starting and ending at different times. A good example is the rhonchus produced by a tumor almost completely occluding a bronchus.
- **Polyphonic wheezes** contain instead several notes, all starting and ending at the same time, like a chord. These can occur in healthy people at the end of a forceful exhalation, but are usually more typical of asthma, where narrowing of multiple airways produces a real polyphonic choir: the so-called "concertus asthmaticus." Because fluttering of large airway walls is diffuse in asthma, CALs occur throughout the lung fields (*see* expiratory polyphonic CALs in question 113).

109. **If a polyphonic CAL may have more than one frequency, how does one determine its pitch?**
By its fundamental. A wheeze may contain several harmonically related frequencies, but its pitch is always determined by its lowest (or fundamental) frequency.

110. **How are wheezes produced?**
Not like the tone of an organ pipe (i.e., by vibration of air within the pipe, so that the pipe's length and diameter correlate with the tone's pitch [with larger and longer pipes producing the lower pitch]). If wheezes were generated this way:
- Airways would have to be 4–8 feet long, which is the necessary length for producing some of the lowest-pitched wheezes of asthma. Instead, the bronchial tree is <1 foot long.
- The frequency of a wheeze generated by a particular airway would stay constant throughout respiration (while instead it differs by as much as 1 octave between inspiration and expiration).
- The pitch of a wheeze would change when breathing a mixture of helium and oxygen (just as the pitch of an organ pipe would rise when blown with helium). Instead, the pitch is constant.

Hence, wheezes are not generated like tones of organ pipe, but rather like notes of a toy trumpet's reed—or, even better, like sounds of a harmonica's reeds. In this model (first suggested by Forgacs in the 1960s), airflow sets each individual reed into oscillation between opening and closure, thus generating a note of constant frequency. Air flowing at high velocity through a narrow bronchus has a similar sucking effect on the airway wall, by pulling it inward and thus initiating a flutter (i.e., a wheeze) of closing and opening, resembling very much the vibration of a toy trumpet's reed. This fluttering typically delivers a note of constant frequency that depends on the mass and elasticity of the bronchial walls, the tightness of the narrowing, and the rate of gas flow through it.

111. **What is the physical principle behind this mechanism?**

It is the Bernoulli principle, which centers on a local drop in intra-airway pressure whenever air flows at high velocity through narrowed pipes. The faster the flow at point of constriction, the lower the local pressure. Eventually, the drop in pressure becomes severe enough to collapse the airway. Since the collapse also reduces flow, the airway reopens and the fluttering cycle starts anew, repeating itself indefinitely (*see* Fig. 14-5). Thus, wheezes are *not* produced by vibration of air (as in organ pipes or woodwind instruments), but by vibration (fluttering) of airway walls. This is facilitated by fast jets of air, forced by high expiratory pressures through tightly compressed airways.

112. **Is the pitch of a wheeze related to its site of production?**

No. This widely held belief is based on the erroneous analogy with an organ pipe. Yet, wheezes are not the sounds of organ pipes. Hence, their pitch does not depend on the diameter and length of the airway, but on the degree of airway narrowing at the site where the sound is being generated. In other words, wheezes are generated whenever the bronchial diameter is narrowed to the point of dynamic compression. That's why, in contrast to late-inspiratory crackles (and the high-frequency tones of an organ pipe), high-pitched wheezes do not originate in small peripheral airways. And low-pitched wheezes do not originate in large central bronchi.

113. **How are CALs classified?**

In addition to being classified according to dominant frequency (in either wheezes or rhonchi), CALs are also divided into:

- **Expiratory polyphonic CALs** are multiple musical tones that occur only in exhalation. Each component has constant frequency and similar duration, but all have a high-pitched hissing quality that earns them the name of *wheezes*. Although typical of mild asthma, they also may be heard in healthy subjects at the end of a forced exhalation. Because each tone has its own frequency, their summation generates a polyphonic sound, like the one of a chorus. Since they reflect widespread alteration of airway mechanics, they are present throughout the lung fields. (Fig. 14-15)

- **Random monophonic CALs** are single or multiple musical tones of various frequency and duration that occur randomly throughout respiration. They are produced by fluttering of central airways, narrowed by bronchospasm or inflammation. They have a high-pitched hissing quality and are often referred to as *multiple monophonic*

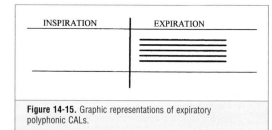

Figure 14-15. Graphic representations of expiratory polyphonic CALs.

wheezes. They are typical of severe asthma (status asthmaticus), where they occur throughout the chest. Like expiratory polyphonic CALs, they can occur in exhalation, though they more typically tend to cover the entire respiratory cycle. Yet, in contrast to stridor and squeaks, they are never limited to inspiration.(Fig. 14-16)

- **Fixed monophonic CALs** are single musical tones of constant frequency and long duration that are generated by the vibration of a large and partially obstructed bronchus because of tumor, inflammation, secretions, or a foreign body. They are low pitched and snoring and often are referred to as *rhonchi*. Change in posture may soften or eliminate them. Still, a localized and persistent rhonchus should arouse suspicion, since it can be the earliest and only abnormal finding of an endobronchial lesion. Auscultatory site usually reflects the location of the process.

- **Sequential inspiratory CALs** are also called *late-inspiratory squeaks*, or squawks (in John Earis' 1982 description). They are produced by the reopening of partially collapsed airways and thus are common in interstitial lung diseases (especially at

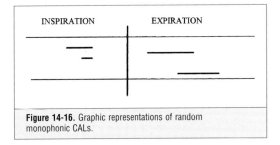

Figure 14-16. Graphic representations of random monophonic CALs.

the bases), where they coexist with late-inspiratory crackles. Except in the case of squeaks, the airway has a very irregular lumen, usually due to regenerating mucosa (as in bronchiolitis obliterans). It's this irregularity (and the resulting narrowing) that is responsible for the high-pitched and squeaky characteristics of the sound. Hence, air passing through a newly reopened but still partially narrowed airway (because of the irregular lumen) will cause both a crackle (as the airway opens abruptly) and a wheeze (as the air rushes through the narrowing). Squeaks can be simple (monophonic) or multiple (polyphonic), musical, and of various duration and frequency. Most often, they are single, short, high pitched, and resembling a late-inspiratory wheeze. Laënnec called it "le cri d'un petit oiseau" (the chirp of a little bird).

114. **What are the causes of a late-inspiratory squeak?**
The three most common are pulmonary fibrosis, allergic alveolitis, and bronchiolitis obliterans. Still, any interstitial lung disease can produce them.

115. **How are CALs graphically represented?**
By bars, in a way very similar to the representation of musical notes:
- The pitch of the CALs is graphically indicated by the height of the bar (i.e., the vertical location of the bar above the respiratory cycle; the higher the pitch, the higher the bar and vice versa),
- The loudness is represented by the thickness of the bar (thicker bars, louder sounds),
- The duration is represented by the length of the bar (the longer the bar, the longer the sound).
- Finally, the timing of the CALs is represented by their location within the respiratory cycle. CALs may be early or late expiratory, and even panrespiratory (i.e., throughout the cycle).

116. **What are the most common causes of airway narrowing responsible for wheezes?**
Bronchospasm, peribronchial edema (from left ventricular failure), accumulation of secretions, and airway closure by a partially obstructing tumor.

117. **Does the presence of wheezing rule *in* bronchial narrowing?**
Not necessarily. Since wheezes reflect the degree of dynamic narrowing of the airway (and its flow rate, according to the Bernoulli principle), an expiratory flow that is forceful enough will produce a wheeze even in an entirely normal airway. This is why a forced expiratory maneuver has no value in unmasking "subclinical" asthma. In fact, wheezing on maximal forced exhalation has such a low sensitivity and specificity for asthma (57% and 37%, respectively) as to be completely unreliable for diagnosing subclinical airflow obstruction. Conversely, a weak expiratory flow might remain totally silent, even though the airway is quite narrowed (i.e., "beware of the asthmatic who stops wheezing while turning blue"). Thus, presence of wheezing does *not* rule-in bronchial narrowing. And its absence does *not* exclude it.

118. **What are the underlying breath sounds of asthmatic patients?**
They vary, depending on the degree of airway narrowing. In fact, one of the first signs of bronchospasm is an increase in frequency of the underlying vesicular breath sound—which takes place even before wheezes develop (especially in children). The opposite occurs during bronchodilator therapy. Thus, breath sounds of asthmatics tend to have higher frequency than regular vesicular breath sounds, but also lower intensity.

119. **Asthmatics have breath sounds of lower intensity?**
Yes. Even though wheezing during bronchial challenge is very suggestive of asthma, a softening of the breath sound may be the earliest (and only) manifestation of positive bronchoprovocation. In fact, this is as common as the appearance of a wheeze. An increase in *frequency* of breath sounds also is a useful clue to the unfolding of an asthmatic attack. Thus, the breath sounds of bronchospasm are indeed *higher pitched* (because of the effect of stiffer and narrowed airways on sound transmission) but also *softer* (because of diminished regional air flow).

120. **Are there any wheeze characteristics that correlate with the degree of airflow obstruction?**
One is the *pitch*. Shim and Williams have indeed shown that the worse the asthmatic attack, the higher the pitch of its wheezes. This is also why bronchodilator therapy lowers the frequency of wheezes. If pitch is a good indicator of asthma severity, length, however, is even better.

121. **So how can wheezing help assess the severity of airflow obstruction?**
This question was answered by Baughman and Loudon, who studied patients admitted to the emergency department for status asthmaticus. They recorded sounds at four standard chest sites and correlated findings with FEV_1 and FVC, both prior to and after treatment. In their analysis, neither the wheezing intensity nor the simultaneous presence of wheezes of different pitch (polyphonic wheezing) correlated with severity of obstruction. Instead, only two variables were consistently related to the degree of airway narrowing: (1) the proportion of the respiratory cycle occupied by the wheeze and (2) the frequency content of the highest-pitched wheeze. Hence, only *pitch* and *length* are useful predictors of airway narrowing: higher-pitched and longer wheezes reflect worse obstruction.

122. **How does one express the length of a wheeze?**
By the proportion of the respiratory cycle occupied by the wheeze (T_w/T_{tot}). In adults with moderate to severe obstruction, T_w/T_{tot} is inversely related to FEV_1. Hence, wheezing that occurs only in exhalation is *not* as severe as wheezing occurring both in exhalation *and* in inspiration; similarly, longer expiratory wheezes reflect worse obstruction than shorter ones.

123. **What are then the acoustic characteristics of a resolving asthma attack?**
A decrease in frequency of the highest-pitched wheeze component, and a decrease in T_w/T_{tot}.

124. **Summarize the time course of status asthmaticus based on auscultation.**
Findings depend primarily on the degree of obstruction. The most prominent is a high-pitched wheeze, first heard in exhalation, and then (as disease worsens) both in inspiration *and* exhalation. These wheezes are initially monophonic, but become polyphonic with progression:
- In **mild asthma,** the site of dynamic obstruction is in the central airways. The bronchial fluttering generates random monophonic wheezes that are loud and well transmitted, both upward (to the mouth) and downward (to the chest wall).
- In **worse asthma,** the site of dynamic obstruction is instead peripheral. Because airflow in small airways is too slow to cause major fluttering, the sounds generated will be

random monophonic wheezes, barely audible at the chest wall and too weak to reach the mouth.

- Finally, in **status asthmaticus,** the airflow obstruction is due to a combination of bronchial edema, bronchospasm, and mucous plugging. These changes start in the central airways and cause at first only expiratory, random, monophonic CALs (i.e., wheezes). Subsequently, however, the site of airway fluttering moves gradually toward the periphery of the tracheobronchial tree, where airflow rate is too low to generate adequate vibration. Hence, the chest of patients with advanced status asthmaticus may become paradoxically silent.

125. **How sensitive and specific are wheezes for the diagnosis of airflow obstruction?**
Neither sensitive nor specific. Although wheezing on forced exhalation can occur even in healthy subjects (as long as they exhale with enough force), *unforced* wheezing argues strongly for chronic airflow obstruction. Still, it can be absent in 30% of patients with $FEV_1 < 1$ L. It also may resolve in acute asthmatics whose FEV_1 remains at 63% of predicted value. In fact, in status asthmaticus, wheezing is the least discriminating factor in predicting hospital admission or relapse. Yet, its absence in acute asthma may be ominous. For instance, it may indicate flow rates too low to generate sound (a reminder of the lack of correlation between asthma severity and wheezing intensity, and of the time-honored dictum, "beware of the quiet asthmatic"). Thus, wheezes, although useful, are not that great diagnostically. They are much less valuable than crackles.

126. **What about pulsus paradoxus?**
Pulsus paradoxus has a significant and direct relation with hypercapnia in children with status asthmaticus and may thus serve as an indirect monitor when CO_2 cannot be measured.

127. **And how about diaphoresis and orthopnea in asthma?**
Diaphoresis and orthopnea on admission to an emergency center predict worse peak expiratory flow rates and greater need for admission.

128. **What is the differential diagnosis of wheezes?**
It is a rather broad one. Overall, wheezes are more frequent in asthma than COPD. Still, the old saying, "Not all that wheezes is asthma" is an important reminder that we should always exclude other etiologies before concluding that a wheezy patient is indeed asthmatic (Table 14-8). In a large epidemiologic study, for example, wheezes were present in 25% of the population, whereas the prevalence of asthma was only 7%. Among the extrathoracic causes of wheezing, vocal cord dysfunction is a particularly common one. And, of course, stridor is important, too.

129. **What is cardiac asthma?**
It's wheezing in association with left ventricular failure. The traditional explanation is airway narrowing due to peribronchial and interstitial edema. In reality, cardiac asthma is indeed asthma. In fact, patients who wheeze when in pulmonary edema have positive methacholine challenge. The proposed mechanism is therefore a heightened airways reactivity, which leads to dynamic airflow obstruction whenever triggered by interstitial and peribronchial edema. That's why only a minority of patients in left ventricular failure develop wheezing. The rest have crackles.

130. **What about wheezes over the neck?**
Wheezes louder over the neck may reflect *upper airway obstruction*. Note that even though stridor is primarily inspiratory, the wheezing of vocal cord dysfunction may be either inspiratory or expiratory. This might be misleading, unless coupled with careful auscultation of the neck. Exertional inspiratory stridor that spontaneously resolves with rest can occur in

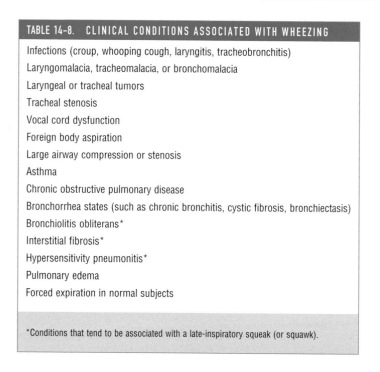

TABLE 14-8. CLINICAL CONDITIONS ASSOCIATED WITH WHEEZING

Infections (croup, whooping cough, laryngitis, tracheobronchitis)

Laryngomalacia, tracheomalacia, or bronchomalacia

Laryngeal or tracheal tumors

Tracheal stenosis

Vocal cord dysfunction

Foreign body aspiration

Large airway compression or stenosis

Asthma

Chronic obstructive pulmonary disease

Bronchorrhea states (such as chronic bronchitis, cystic fibrosis, bronchiectasis)

Bronchiolitis obliterans*

Interstitial fibrosis*

Hypersensitivity pneumonitis*

Pulmonary edema

Forced expiration in normal subjects

*Conditions that tend to be associated with a late-inspiratory squeak (or squawk).

5% of athletes (as compared to 2.5% in the general population), and is a manifestation of vocal cord dysfunction too, even though it is frequently misdiagnosed as exercise-induced bronchospasm.

(5) Stridor

131. **What is stridor?**
It is a loud, long, high-pitched, and inspiratory sound that always indicates upper airway obstruction. Although resembling a wheeze, stridor differs because it is (1) louder over the neck and (2) inspiratory (whereas wheezing is either expiratory, or, in the more severe cases, both inspiratory and expiratory). With the sole exception of the late-inspiratory squeak, "wheezes" heard only in inspiration are stridor.

132. **Are there any acoustic differences between wheezes and stridor?**
Definitely not pitch. The best discriminators are instead timing and location. Baughman and Loudon have analyzed the physical characteristics of these two sounds and found that stridor is exclusively inspiratory (and more prominent over the neck), whereas wheezes are more predominant over the chest (and never inspiratory only). Otherwise, there are no major acoustic differences.

133. **What is the time course of stridor due to posttracheostomy tracheal stenosis?**
A slow time course. First, the patient complains of dyspnea, cough, or problems with throat clearing. Only much later, stridor appears, usually indicating a critical tracheal narrowing <5 mm.

(6) Pleural Rub

134. **What is a pleural rub?**
It is a special type of adventitious lung sound: loud, creaky, grating, and often compared to the sound of leather. It is generated by two inflamed pleural surfaces rubbing against each other.

135. **What does a rub sound like?**
It has been compared to a violin bow striking a string in a to-and-fro motion. According to this model, the chest wall, because of its large mass and springiness, behaves like the body of a string instrument, continuing to vibrate for a short time after each impulse transmitted by the pleural friction. Hence, the various components of the rub lengthen and even merge into a continuous and often musical sound, similar to a rhonchus or a wheeze.

136. **Are rubs inspiratory or expiratory?**
Usually *both*, because rubs are caused by the sliding on each other of both pleural layers. Since sliding is faster during inspiration, the inspiratory component of a rub is usually louder. At times, it may even be the only one audible. The expiratory component, on the other hand, is usually a bit longer, accounting for 65% of the entire rub duration. Overall, two thirds of rubs are present in inspiration and expiration. Some are inspiratory only. Very few are limited to exhalation.

137. **How can one differentiate rubs from crackles?**
With great difficulty. Rubs, in fact, are often misdiagnosed as crackles because they share similar characteristics. To help differentiate them, remember that in contrast to crackles, rubs: (1) occur both in inspiration and expiration; (2) do not change with coughing; (3) are usually longer, louder, lower pitched, and often *palpable*; and (4) are usually localized to a very small area.

138. **How can one differentiate rubs from wheezes?**
This is a bit easier. Although rubs can be confused with polyphonic wheezes (either medium- or low pitched), they can be easily separated by remembering that they never occur in expiration only, whereas most wheezes do. Hence, an adventitious sound that is audible (or louder) only in inspiration is more likely to be a rub, whereas an adventitious sound that is audible only in exhalation is more likely to be a wheeze (or a rhonchus).

139. **How can one separate pleural from pericardial rubs?**
By asking patients to hold their breath. If the rub persists, it is more likely to be pericardial.

140. **What is the natural history of a pleural rub?**
Rubs are fleeting. They usually disappear as soon as the amount of pleural fluid gets large enough to separate the two layers, thus preventing them from rubbing against each other. Hence, if not carefully (and frequently) sought, transient rubs may be easily missed.

141. **What is the histology underlying a pleural rub?**
In normal subjects, the visceral and parietal pleura are lined by a single layer of flat mesothelial cells. These layers are smooth and lubricated by a thin film of fluid that allows them to slide easily and silently on each other during respiration. Yet, this smoothness is immediately lost as soon as fibrin and cells (neoplastic or inflammatory) cover the two pleural layers. As a result, the roughened pleural surfaces will rub against each other during respiration, thus creating a

friction that is responsible for the pleural rub. The separation of the two pleural layers (because of fluid accumulation in the pleural cavity) will make the rub disappear. Pleural rubs, therefore, are pathognomonic of pleural inflammation. Noninflammatory effusions, such as those associated with congestive heart failure, nephrotic syndrome, or cirrhosis, are never associated with a rub.

142. **What are the most common causes of a pleural rub?**
Cancer, pneumonia, and pulmonary embolism. Serositis (as in collagen vascular diseases) may also produce one, despite an entirely normal chest radiograph. In this regard, rubs are common in lupus pleuritis but rare in rheumatoid effusion. They also are common in thromboembolic disease and parapneumonic pleuritis, but rare in tuberculous pleurisy. Similarly, rubs have variable frequency in neoplastic involvement. Cancers may produce a rub, either directly (through invasion of pleural layers) or indirectly (though inflammation of the pleura overlying a lung cancer). Finally, rubs often occur in lobar pneumonia (pneumococcal, staphylococcal, or gram-negative).

143. **What are the physical characteristics of a rub?**
The hallmark is a series of short, loud, creaky, and high-frequency sounds. These can be visualized as tall "spikes" superimposed on the underlying breath sound (Fig. 14-17). Hence, the soundwave of a rub is very similar to that of a crackle (although the rub tends to span throughout inspiration and expiration, whereas crackles predominate in inspiration). The frequencies of these spikes are medium to high pitched, but not as

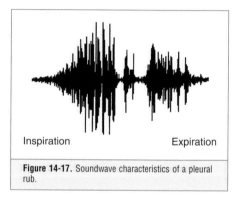

Inspiration   Expiration

Figure 14-17. Soundwave characteristics of a pleural rub.

high as those of crackles. Still, rubs are well perceived by the human ear and appear loud. Their inspiratory components usually have higher intensity and sometimes may be the only audible sounds. Finally, the rub is characterized by what Forgacs defines as the "mirror image effect," which refers to the apparent reverse sequence of the expiratory component of the rub as compared with the inspiratory component.

C. TRANSMITTED VOICE SOUNDS

144. **What are transmitted voice sounds? Why are they important?**
They are sounds that are not produced by the patient's lungs, but by the *larynx*. This is unlike other acoustic respiratory events, whether breath sounds or adventitious lung sounds. Voice-induced sounds may become abnormally transmitted in certain diseases, thus providing a valuable clue.

145. **What are the most important transmitted voice sounds?**
They are three, and all originally described (and named) by Laënnec. There also is a fourth and more recent type (the E-to-A change), but still a variation of Laënnec's original description:

- **Bronchophony** (Greek for "sound of the bronchi") indicates a clear voice sound—at least as clear as a voice sound heard over the bronchi or larynx (in bronchophony, however, this sound is heard over chest areas that are remote from either the bronchi or larynx). The words spoken by the patient remain nonetheless unintelligible; only the sound becomes clear and loud.

- **Pectoriloquy** (Latin for "the voice of the chest") indicates clear and intelligible words over the chest of patients either whispering (whispered pectoriloquy) or speaking (spoken pectoriloquy).
- **Egophony** (Greek for "the voice of the goat") is the goat-like and bleating sound produced by the patient's voice when heard over an area of consolidation.
- **E-to-A changes** are a more recent variant of egophony.

146. Is there any magic word that one should ask patients to say in order to elicit these sounds?

Not really. In the United States, we ask them to say "ninety-nine" (which is the same number used to elicit tactile fremitus). In Italy (smaller country), "thirty-three" is the number of choice. As Sapira points out, "ninety-nine" is nothing more than the translation of the German "neun und neunzig" (akin to the onomatopeic "oink-oink"), which actually changed the physical characteristics of the original sound, making it possibly less fit for the task. An alternative is to ask the patient to say, "one, two, three." Still, for eliciting abnormally transmitted voice sounds, any sound will do (except, of course, for eliciting E-to-A changes; *see* below, questions 151–155).

147. What is the significance of these maneuvers?

They all mean the same thing: an abnormal transmission of spoken (or whispered) words across the lungs. More specifically, they indicate airless and consolidated lung parenchyma.

148. Are the bronchi of patients with abnormally transmitted voice sounds open or closed?

Open. If closed, there would be no sounds transmission across the chest.

149. When should one check for the presence of these sounds?

When suspecting abnormal sound transmission along the tracheal bronchial tree and across the lungs. In general, when suspecting consolidation.

150. How do voice sounds get produced and transmitted?

They are produced by vocal cords set in vibration by exhaled air. Normal voice sounds are then transmitted upward toward the mouth, and downward toward the chest. There, the air-filled lungs act as a low-pass filter, eliminating high-frequency components (>300 Hz) and allowing instead passage of only lower-pitched tones (100–300 Hz), which are eventually most of the sounds that reach the chest wall. This low-pass filtering also eliminates the higher-frequency components of the vowels, the so-called *formants*. Because recognizing vowels is essential to the comprehension of words (vowels have been called the spice of a language), the elimination of formants by the normal (and aerated) lung transforms voice sounds into a muffled, low-pitched, and unintelligible mumble. Since solids and fluids can transmit higher frequencies better than air, a consolidated (and airless) lung improves transmission of vowels, thus making voice sounds louder, clearer, and *intelligible*.

151. Who first described egophony?

Laënnec, who also introduced its complicated Greek term. "Egophony," he wrote, "possesses one constant characteristic from which it has seemed to me suitable to name the phenomenon; it is quavering and jerky like the bleating of a goat." The E-to-A changes were instead described later.

152. Who came up with the idea of asking patients to say "E"?

Good point. In fact, why not "U," or "A," or "O"? Whenever questions of this sort come up in history of medicine, there are usually three major requirements: a British missionary, a far-flung land, and lots of serendipity. In the case of E-to-A changes, the British missionary was a chap named Shibley, who in the 1920s was practicing missionary medicine in China. Part of his job consisted of auscultating chests while patients were saying "one, two, three"—which, since the patients were Chinese, was appropriately said in Mandarin, as "i, er, san." Since the Mandarin for "one" ("i") was pronounced "E" in the province where Shibley was working at the time, that "E" turned into an "A" whenever there was either pneumonia or pleural effusion. In fact, all five vowel sounds (A, E, I, O, U) became "A" in cases of effusion or consolidation. Shibley reported this "E-to-A change" in the *Chinese Medical Journal* in 1922. That same year, the Viennese Froschels and Stockert reported a similar observation (of course, their Austrian patients did not speak Mandarin, but still experienced a similar transformation of one vowel sound into another whenever "consolidated"). Of interest, "one" in Cantonese would have been "iat," thus making Shibley's "E-to-A change" a much less appealing "E-AT to A-AT change," which would have never worked out.

153. What is the mechanism behind E-to-A changes?

It is, of course, consolidation—more precisely, consolidation that extends from the auscultated chest wall to the tracheobronchial tree. A less extensive process (as, for example, the consolidation of a pulmonary nodule) would not create a bridge long enough to cause egophony.

154. What are the most common causes of extensive consolidation?

The most common are either filling of the alveoli by a medium that transmits sound better than air (such as pus, blood, or serum) or collapse of the alveoli. In cases of pleural effusions, the layer of fluid must be thick enough to compress the alveoli (and thus make them airless) but also thin enough to leave the airways patent. Although generally valid (and intuitive), this rule has exceptions. There are, in fact, patients who have obstructed or collapsed bronchi and yet still manage to transmit the high frequencies of egophony and tubular respiration. In this case, the transmission does not occur along the airways but directly through the lung parenchyma.

155. How does consolidation transform an "E" into an "A"?

By changing the filtering properties of the lung, thus allowing it to transmit higher-frequency sounds. The fact that an "E" may turn into an "A" when heard over a consolidated focus remains, nonetheless, an acoustic paradox. In fact, when heard at the mouth, "E" is higher pitched than "A." Thus, it seems counterintuitive that a consolidated lung (which is capable of transmitting higher frequencies better than a normal lung) should change a high-pitched sound like "E" into a low-pitched one like "A." The explanation is that the sound "E" is a mixture of both high and low frequencies. The high frequencies are in the 2000–3500 Hz range, whereas the low are in the 100–400 Hz range. "A" also has low and high frequencies, but its low frequencies have a range that is a bit higher than that of the low-frequency components of "E" (in "A" they reach 600 Hz). When "E" or "A" is heard over the chest, none of its high-frequency components comes across, regardless of whether the underlying lung is consolidated. Thus, even though a consolidated lung can transmit higher frequencies better than a normal lung (close to 1000 Hz instead of 400), it still cannot transmit the highest frequencies (such as the 2000–3500 frequencies) that are so typical of "E." In other words, a consolidated lung better transmits the low frequencies that are important features of "A" (the ones up to 600 Hz), but still cannot transmit the higher frequencies that are unique to "E." As a result, "E" becomes "A," as so do all other vowels when similarly analyzed.

156. **What is the mechanism of production for whispered pectoriloquy?**
It is still consolidation. Remember that whispered sounds consist almost entirely of high-frequency components. Thus, they are not transmitted by the aerated lung, but become audible only when the loss of alveolar air (due to consolidation) allows their transmission.

157. **What breath sounds accompany these transmitted voice sounds?**
Tubular (bronchial) breath sounds, because both transmitted voice sounds and tubular sounds reflect improved conduction of high-frequency components, typical of consolidation. Consolidation from alveolar fluid-filling is characterized by tubular sounds and late-inspiratory crackles, whereas consolidation from alveolar collapse is characterized by pure tubular sounds. In patients with cough and fever, the presence of egophony increases the likelihood of pneumonia.

158. **What is the radiologic equivalent of abnormally transmitted voice sounds?**
Air bronchograms. These are patent and air-filled bronchi silhouetted out against the white background of airless and consolidated alveoli. This radiographic finding is nonspecific and may be seen with atelectasis, lung hemorrhage, pneumonia, or pulmonary edema.

159. **What is the most useful of all these transmitted voice sounds?**
Probably egophony, closely followed by whispered pectoriloquy. In some patients, whispered pectoriloquy may be the first finding to appear in cases of consolidation.

160. **Summarize disease processes associated with lung auscultation findings.**
See Table 14-9.

TABLE 14-9. CHEST EXAMINATION FINDINGS OF COMMON DISEASE PROCESSES

Disease	Trachea	Fremitus	Percussion Note	Breath Sounds	Adventitious Breath Sounds	Transmitted Voice Sounds
Normal lung	Midline	Normal	Resonant	Vesicular	Late-inspiratory crackles at bases (resolve with deep breaths)	Absent
Consolidation (pneumonia, hemorrhage)	Midline	Increased	Dull	Bronchial	Late-inspiratory crackles	All present
Pulmonary fibrosis	Midline	Normal/increased	Resonant	Bronchovesicular	Late-inspiratory crackles	Absent
Bronchiectasis	Midline	Normal	Resonant	Vesicular	Mid-inspiratory crackles	Absent
Bronchitis	Midline	Normal	Normal to hyperresonant	Vesicular	Early inspiratory crackles Possible rhonchi and wheezes	Absent
Emphysema	Midline	Decreased	Hyperresonant	Diminished vesicular	Usually absent	Absent
Large pleural effusion	Shifted to the opposite	Decreased to absent over the effusion	Dull to flat	Bronchial immediately above the effusion Absent over the effusion	? Rub above the effusion	May be present above the effusion Absent over the effusion
Pneumothorax	Shifted to the opposite	Absent	Tympanic	Absent	Absent	Absent
Atelectasis (patent bronchi)	Shifted to the same side	Increased	Dull	Bronchial	Absent	All present
Atelectasis (plugged bronchi)	Shifted to the same side	Absent	Dull	Absent	Absent	Absent
Status asthmaticus	Midline	Decreased	Hyperresonant	Vesicular	Inspiratory/expiratory wheezes	Absent

SELECTED BIBLIOGRAPHY

1. Baughman RP, Loudon RG: Quantitation of wheezing in acute asthma. Chest 86:718–722, 1984.
2. Baughman RP, Loudon RG: Sound spectral analysis of voice-transmitted sound. Am Rev Respir Dis 134:167–169, 1986.
3. Baughman RP, Loudon RG: Stridor: Differentiation from asthma or upper airway noise. Am Rev Respir Dis 139:1407–1409, 1989.
4. Baughman RP, Shipley RT, Loudon RG, Lower EE: Crackles in interstitial lung disease: Comparison of sarcoidosis and fibrosing alveolitis. Chest 100:96–101, 1991.
5. Bohadana AB, Peslin R, Uffholtz H: Breath sounds in the assessment of airflow obstruction. Thorax 33:345, 1978.
6. Bohadana AB, Kopferschmitt-Kubler MC, Pauli G, et al: Breath sound intensity in patients with airway provocation challenge test positive by spirometry but negative for wheezing. Respiration 61:274–279, 1994.
7. Brenner BE, Abraham E, Simon RR, et al: Position and diaphoresis in acute asthma. Am J Med 74:1005–1009, 1983.
8. Cugell DW: Lung sounds: Classification and controversies. Semin Respir Med 6:210–219, 1985.
9. Deguchi F, Hirakawa S, Gotoh K, et al: Prognostic significance of posturally induced crackles. Long-term follow-up of patients after recovery from acute myocardial infarction. Chest 103:1457–1462, 1993.
10. Earis JE, March K, Pearson MG, Ogilvie CM: The inspiratory "squawk" in extrinsic allergic alveolitis and other pulmonary fibroses. Thorax 37:923–926, 1982.
11. Epler GR, Carrington CB, Gaensler EA, et al: Crackles (râles) in the interstitial pulmonary disease. Chest 73:333–339, 1978.
12. Forgacs P, Nathoo AR, Richardson HD: Breath sounds. Thorax 26:288–295, 1971.
13. Forgacs P: Crackles and wheezes. Lancet 2:203–205, 1967.
14. Forgacs P: Lung Sounds. London, Bailliere Tindall, 1978, pp:34.
15. Forgacs P: The functional basis of pulmonary sounds. Chest 3:399–405, 1978.
16. Gavriely N, Nassan M, Cugell W, Rubin AH: Respiratory health screening using pulmonary function tests and lung sound analysis. Eur Respir J 7:35–42, 1994.
17. Godfrey S, Edwards RH, Campbell EJ, et al: Repeatability of physical signs in airways obstruction. Thorax 24:4–9, 1969.
18. Hidalgo HA, Wegmann MJ, Waring WW, et al: Frequency spectra of breath sounds in childhood. Chest 100:992–1002, 1991.
19. Holleman DR Jr, Simel DL: Does clinical examination predict airflow limitation? JAMA 273:313–319, 1995.
20. King DK, Thompson BT, Johnson DC: Wheezing on maximal forced exhalation in the diagnosis of atypical asthma: Lack of sensitivity and specificity. Ann Intern Med 110:451–455, 1989.
21. Lal S, Ferguson AD, Campbell EJ, et al: Forced-expiratory time: A simple test for airway obstruction. BMJ 1:814, 1964.
22. LeBlanc P, Macklem PT, Ross WR, et al: Breath sounds and distribution of ventilation. Am Rev Respir Dis 102:10–16, 1970.
23. Marini JJ, Pierson DJ, Hudson LD, Lakshminarayan S: The significance of wheezing in chronic airflow obstruction. Am Rev Respir Dis 120:1069–1072, 1979.
24. Martell JA, Lopez JG, Harker JE, et al: Pulsus paradoxus in acute asthma in children. J Asthma 29:349–352, 1992.
25. McFadden ER, Kiser R, DeGroot WJ: Acute bronchial asthma: Relations between clinical and physiologic manifestations. N Engl J Med 388:221–224, 1973.
26. McGee S: Evidence-Based Physical Diagnosis. Saunders, Philadelphia, 2001.
27. Meslier N, Charbonneau G, Racineuz JL: Wheezes. Eur Respir J 8:1942–1948, 1995.
28. Murphy RL, Gaensler EA, Holford SK, et al: Crackles in the detection of asbestosis. Am Rev Respir Dis 129:375–379, 1984.
29. Nath AR, Capel LH: Lung crackles in bronchiectasis. Thorax 35:694–699, 1980.
30. Nath AR, Capel LH: Inspiratory crackles: Early and late. Thorax 29:223–227, 1974.
31. Pardee NE, Martin CJ, Morgan EH: A test of the practical value of estimating breath sound intensity. Breath sounds related to measured ventilatory function. Chest 70:341–344, 1976.

32. Pasterkamp H, Kraman SS, Wodicka GR, et al: Respiratory sounds. Am J Respir Crit Care Med 156:974–987, 1997.

33. Rundell KW, Spiering BA: Inspiratory stridor in elite athletes. Chest 123:468–474, 2003.

34. Scheider IC, Anderson AE: Correlation of clinical signs with ventilatory function in obstructive lung disease. Ann Intern Med 62:477–485, 1965.

35. Schilling RS, Hughes JP, Dingwall I, et al: Disagreement between observers in an epidemiologic study of respiratory disease. BMJ 1:65, 1995.

36. Shim CS, Williams MH: Relationship of wheezing to the severity of obstruction in asthma. Arch Intern Med 143:890–892, 1983.

37. Shiral F, Kudoh S, Shi A, et al: Crackles in asbestos workers. Br J Dis Chest 75:383–396, 1981.

38. Straus SE, McAlister FA, Sackett DL, et al: CARE-COAD2 Group. Clinical Assessment of the Reliability of the Examination-Chronic Obstructive Airways Disease: Accuracy of history, wheezing, and forced expiratory time in the diagnosis of chronic obstructive pulmonary disease. J Gen Intern Med 17:684–688, 2002.

39. Thatcher RE, Kraman SS: The prevalence of auscultatory crackles in subjects without lung disease. Chest 81:672–674, 1982.

CHAPTER 15

THE ABDOMEN

Salvatore Mangione, MD

GENERALITIES

Conventional teaching has long recognized the abdomen as "the grave of the internist," since in contrast to the chest, this cavity has been quite unyielding to physical exam. Although maneuvers devised by generations of physicians to unlock the secrets of its many organs have been for the most part wanting, there are still a few golden nuggets worth learning about. This chapter reviews sequentially the bedside examination of the abdomen, as applied to (1) the abdominal wall, (2) liver, (3) gallbladder, (4) spleen, (5) stomach, (6) pancreas, (7) kidneys, (8) urinary bladder, (9) evaluation of ascites, and (10) evaluation of peritonitis.

A. THE ABDOMINAL WALL

"Here too their sisters dwell.
And they are three, the Gorgons, winged,
With hair of snakes, hateful to mortals.
Whom no man shall behold and draw again
The breath of life"

Aeschylus, Prometheus Bound

Although many maneuvers belong more to the art (and folklore) than to the science of medicine, inspection, palpation, and auscultation of the abdominal wall (actually, *auscultation*, percussion, and palpation—since the order in this case is different from that of other organs) still allow the detection of useful findings. Abdominal percussion as applied to selective organs (mainly the liver, spleen, kidneys, and bladder) is discussed separately.

(1) Inspection

1. **Outline the topographic divisions of the abdomen.**
    See Figure 15-1.

I. Evaluation of the Abdominal Contour

2. **What are the most important contours of the abdomen?**
    On frontal inspection, the most clinically important is a *scaphoid* contour (i.e., an abdomen *shaped like a boat* [from the Greek *skaphe*, boat]). This is typical of supine cachectic patients, with rib margins representing the stern, iliac spines and symphysis pubis representing the bow, and the sunken abdominal wall representing the hulk.

3. **What are the most important contours on lateral inspection?**
    -   A *Cupid's bow* profile is typical of acute *pancreatitis*, with the midpoint between the two bow branches coinciding with the umbilical retraction from localized peritonitis (Fig. 15-2).
    -   A discrete *bulge* in the *epigastric* area is seen in large pericardial effusions (*Auenbrugger's sign*, from the name of the inventor of percussion). This *lopsided* protuberance should not be

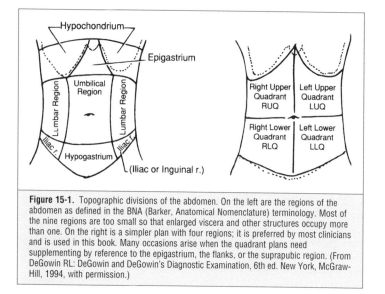

Figure 15-1. Topographic divisions of the abdomen. On the left are the regions of the abdomen as defined in the BNA (Barker, Anatomical Nomenclature) terminology. Most of the nine regions are too small so that enlarged viscera and other structures occupy more than one. On the right is a simpler plan with four regions; it is preferred by most clinicians and is used in this book. Many occasions arise when the quadrant plans need supplementing by reference to the epigastrium, the flanks, or the suprapubic region. (From DeGowin RL: DeGowin and DeGowin's Diagnostic Examination, 6th ed. New York, McGraw-Hill, 1994, with permission.)

confused with a fat belly, which on lateral view appears instead as a convex arching of the abdominal contour, peaking at the umbilicus.

- A localized bulge over the *hypogastric* area is typical of a distended urinary bladder (*see* Fig. 15-2).
- A bulge over the two upper quadrants is seen in hepatosplenomegaly (Fig. 15-3).
- A "ladder" pattern of abdominal distention is typical of *small* bowel obstruction (*large* bowel obstruction produces instead an inverted-U pattern) (*see* Fig. 15-4). Visible peristaltic waves also can occur in intestinal obstruction, and when associated with abdominal distention and hyperactive bowel sounds, they argue favorably for the presence of the condition. Unfortunately, visible peristalsis is only present in 6% of patients, and decreased or absent bowel sounds are present in one quarter of cases. In fact, more than one third of intestinal obstructions do not even have abdominal distention.

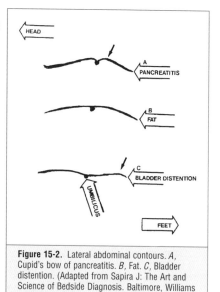

Figure 15-2. Lateral abdominal contours. *A,* Cupid's bow of pancreatitis. *B,* Fat. *C,* Bladder distention. (Adapted from Sapira J: The Art and Science of Bedside Diagnosis. Baltimore, Williams & Wilkins, 1990.)

II. Evaluation of the Umbilicus

4. **What are the major abnormalities of the umbilicus?**

   Appearance of the umbilicus can provide valuable information (Fig. 15-5). There are three possible abnormalities: (1) protuberances, (2) purplish discolorations, and (3) a shift along the vertical line.

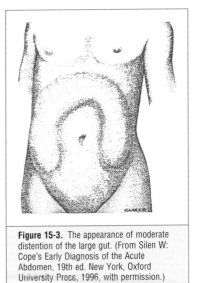

Figure 15-3. The appearance of moderate distention of the large gut. (From Silen W: Cope's Early Diagnosis of the Acute Abdomen, 19th ed. New York, Oxford University Press, 1996, with permission.)

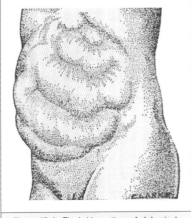

Figure 15-4. The ladder pattern of abdominal distention dictating obstruction of the lower ileum. (From Silen W: Cope's Early Diagnosis of the Acute Abdomen, 19th ed. New York, Oxford University Press, 1996, with permission.)

5. **What are the most common protuberances?**
   Primarily two: (1) an *eversion* of the umbilical scar and (2) the Sister Mary Joseph nodule.

6. **What is an eversion of the umbilical scar?**
   It is the most common of all umbilical protuberances, usually due to increased intra-abdominal pressure from either fluid or masses, the most frequent cause being ascites. Eversion, however, also can occur with simple obesity and a very lax abdominal wall.

7. **What is Sister Mary Joseph's nodule?**
   It is the most ominous of all umbilical protuberances, since it represents a metastatic node by an intra-abdominal malignancy (*see* Chapter 18, questions 45 and 46). It presents as a nontender, irregular, and often exfoliative protuberance, either completely replacing the umbilicus or being palpable through it. It should not be confused with an *omphalith,* which is another umbilical nodule, but due instead to poor personal hygiene, resulting in collection of sebum and keratin.

8. **What is the significance of a purplish discoloration of the umbilicus?**
   It is a sign of subcutaneous intraperitoneal bleed, usually from *acute hemorrhagic pancreatitis.* A periumbilical ecchymosis is commonly referred to as *Cullen's sign,* and it is often encountered in association with *Grey Turner's,* a bilateral reddish/purplish discoloration of the flanks. Both are poorly sensitive and poorly specific markers of hemorrhagic pancreatitis (*see* below, questions 13 and 116).

9. **What are the most common vertical shifts of the umbilicus?**
   - The most common is a **downward** displacement, usually seen in ascites or hepatosplenomegaly, especially if long standing.
   - Less common is an **upward** displacement, often seen in pregnancy, but also in cases of pelvic tumors.

10. **What other important points should be included in the inspection of the abdominal wall?**
    In addition to an overall evaluation of abdominal contour and the umbilicus, general inspection of the abdomen should include an assessment of (1) *abdominal respiratory motion* (i.e., abdominal

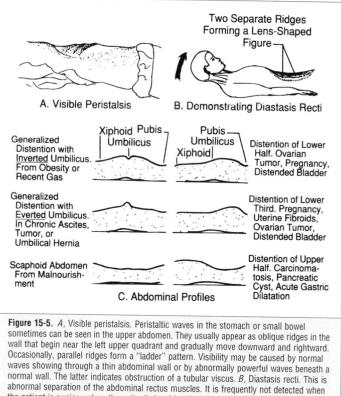

Figure 15-5. *A,* Visible peristalsis. Peristaltic waves in the stomach or small bowel sometimes can be seen in the upper abdomen. They usually appear as oblique ridges in the wall that begin near the left upper quadrant and gradually move downward and rightward. Occasionally, parallel ridges form a "ladder" pattern. Visibility may be caused by normal waves showing through a thin abdominal wall or by abnormally powerful waves beneath a normal wall. The latter indicates obstruction of a tubular viscus. *B,* Diastasis recti. This is abnormal separation of the abdominal rectus muscles. It is frequently not detected when the patient is supine unless the patient's head is raised from the pillow so the abdominal muscles are tensed. *C,* Abdominal profiles. Careful inspection from the side may give the first clue to abnormality, directing attention to a specific region and prompting search for more signs. (From DeGowin RL: DeGowin and DeGowin's Diagnostic Examination, 6th ed. New York, McGraw-Hill, 1994, with permission.)

paradox, respiratory alternans, and the still abdomen of peritonitis); (2) *abnormal skin markings* (such as ecchymoses, striae, and surgical scars); and (3) *abnormal venous patterns*.

III. Abdominal Respiratory Motion

11. **How should the abdominal wall behave during normal respiration?**
    It should be synchronized with the chest wall, so that both expand in inspiration and contract in exhalation. In respiratory muscle weakness (and impending respiratory failure), the two become instead asynchronous, with *respiratory alternans* and *abdominal paradox* (*see* Chapter 13, questions 52–59).

IV. Abnormal Skin Markings

12. **What kind of skin markings can be seen on the abdominal wall?**
    The most common are *ecchymoses* and *striae.* An *abnormal venous pattern* is a different type of abdominal marking and will be discussed separately.

13. **What are ecchymoses?**
    They are soft tissue bruises, caused by bleeding into the subcutaneous fascial planes. These are commonly seen with retroperitoneal or intraperitoneal hemorrhage. Frequent in the *periumbilical*

and *flank* areas, they often carry the names of physicians who first reported them—like the Canadian gynecologist T.S. Cullen (who in 1922 described *periumbilical ecchymosis* in a case of ruptured ectopic pregnancy) and the British surgeon Gilbert Grey Turner (who in 1920 reported *flank ecchymosis* in a case of hemorrhagic pancreatitis).

> **Pearl:**
> These bruises are quite rare, occurring in <1% of ruptured ectopic pregnancies and only 3% of acute pancreatitis (usually 2–6 days after the event). Their specificity is also low, since they can occur in other intra-abdominal and intrapelvic catastrophes, such as ischemic bowel, strangulation of the ileum or an umbilical hernia, hemorrhagic ascites, bilateral salpingitis, hepatic hemorrhage from tumor, splenic rupture, perforated duodenal ulcer, ruptured abdominal aortic aneurysm, and even following percutaneous liver biopsy.

14. **What are striae?**
    They are *stretch marks,* usually located on either flanks or lateral aspects of the abdomen. They are 1–6 cm long, often multiple, and typically presenting in other regions of chronic stretching—such as the shoulders, thighs, and breasts. Although usually due to rapid weight gain (and loss), they also may represent a sequela of pregnancy. They can be seen, though, in *Cushing's syndrome* too, including its iatrogenic variety. Yet, since Cushing presents with erythrocytosis, the striae of this condition tend to be *purplish,* a hue usually absent in weight loss or pregnancy.

15. **What about surgical scars?**
    Every surgical scar should be investigated and inquired about, since they can often be the telltale sign of old (and possibly current) pathology. Scars also should be reported in the patient's record, by using a sketch to indicate their location in the four abdominal quadrants (Fig. 15-6).

V. Abnormal Venous Patterns

16. **What are the collateral venous circulations of the abdominal wall?**
    They are abnormal venous networks that appear on the wall in cases of obstruction to (1) the superior vena cava, (2) the inferior vena cava, and (3) the portal venous system (Fig. 15-7).

17. **How can you distinguish them?**
    By identifying their location and direction of blood flow (Fig. 15-8):

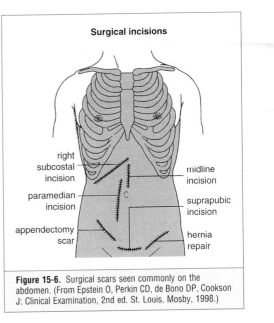

Surgical incisions

right subcostal incision

midline incision

paramedian incision

suprapubic incision

appendectomy scar

hernia repair

Figure 15-6. Surgical scars seen commonly on the abdomen. (From Epstein O, Perkin CD, de Bono DP, Cookson J: Clinical Examination, 2nd ed. St. Louis, Mosby, 1998.)

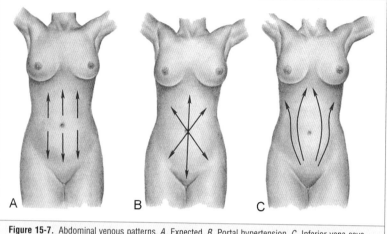

Figure 15-7. Abdominal venous patterns. *A*, Expected. *B*, Portal hypertension. *C*, Inferior vena cava obstruction. (From Seidel HM, Ball JW, Dains JE, Benedict GW: Mosby's Guide to Physical Examination, 3rd ed. St. Louis, Mosby, 1995.)

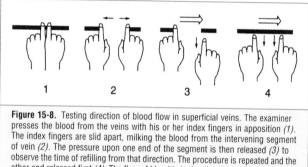

Figure 15-8. Testing direction of blood flow in superficial veins. The examiner presses the blood from the veins with his or her index fingers in apposition *(1)*. The index fingers are slid apart, milking the blood from the intervening segment of vein *(2)*. The pressure upon one end of the segment is then released *(3)* to observe the time of refilling from that direction. The procedure is repeated and the other end released first *(4)*. The flow of blood is in the direction of the faster flow. (From DeGowin RL: DeGowin and DeGowin's Diagnostic Examination, 6th ed. New York, McGraw-Hill, 1994, with permission.)

- A **superior vena cava obstruction** creates a venous engorgement of the *upper* abdominal wall that has a downward flow.
- An **inferior vena cava obstruction** creates a venous engorgement of the *lateral* abdominal wall (flanks) that has an upward flow.
- A **portal system obstruction** creates instead a *periumbilical* network of veins, with the most rostral draining upward and the most caudal draining downward.

18. **How can you assess the direction of blood?**
By "milking" the vein. To do so, place your two index fingers over the engorged vein, and collapse it. Then slide the fingers apart, producing a 1-inch stretch of empty vein. Now, release first the pressure on the caudal end of the vein, and then on the rostral end. By doing so, it will be easy to visualize whether the direction of *refilling* is upward or downward.

19. **What is caput medusae?**
It is the name given to the abnormal venous networks of portal hypertension. It is most commonly seen in cirrhotics whose umbilical vein has reopened (*see* Cruveilhier-Baumgarten

murmur, disease, and syndrome, discussed in question 34). This presents with a tuft of veins radiating from the umbilicus as spikes of a wheel or a *nest of snakes*; hence, the name. Some of these engorged veins drain rostrally into the internal mammary, whereas others drain caudally into the inferior mammary.

20. Who was Medusa?
She was one of the three Gorgon sisters, and a rather wicked figure in Greek mythology. Her hair was made of snakes (hence, the expression "caput medusae" [i.e., *Medusa's head* in Latin]), and her face was so horrifying that whoever gazed upon it turned into stone. Perseus was eventually able to slay her by looking at her image across a specially polished shield he had received from Athena, goddess of wisdom (a metaphor for the value of rationality as defense against the wickedness of life). Afterward, Perseus pinned Medusa's head on his shield, using it as a primitive biologic weapon to turn enemies into stone. Many Greek foot soldiers followed his lead, painting the Gorgon's head on their hoplite shield. Yet, today Medusa is much more famous for being the trademark of the Versace Fashion & Design Company.

(2) Auscultation

21. What is the value of abdominal auscultation?
Limited. In fact, more limited than its thoracic counterpart and mostly aimed at (1) bowel sounds, (2) murmurs and bruits, (3) venous hum, (4) friction rubs, and (5) succussion splashes.

Bowel Sounds

22. Should bowel sounds be pursued before or after palpating/percussing the abdomen?
Definitely *before*, since palpation (and percussion) may silence the belly.

23. Where are these bowel sounds produced?
Mostly in the *stomach*, with the rest originating in the *large* and, for a lesser part, *small intestine*.

24. Is the abdominal location indicative of the production site?
No. Bowel sounds can be transmitted very well across the abdomen, and so detecting them in a particular quadrant doesn't necessarily reflect the site of production. Hence, the need for a thorough examination of *all* quadrants (and also the little clinical value of these findings).

25. What causes these sounds?
It is not entirely clear. The most likely explanation is the propulsion of food through the various segments of the gastrointestinal tract, as suggested by the tendency of bowel sounds to become more prominent after meals. Still, a rise in the *tone* of bowel loops also is important, which explains why these sounds tend to increase in intestinal obstruction. (Yet, years ago the author—asked to produce a recording of increased bowel sounds for a board examination question—was unable to elicit enough noise for a decent tape, even though he had ingested a concoction that made him detonate several times. This unfortunate experience confirms how unpredictable these sounds can be.)

26. What is the significance of increased bowel sounds?
It is in the ears of the beholder, since even normal individuals may exhibit great variation from time to time. For example, it is not unusual to have no sounds for 5 minutes and then experience a burst of as many as 30 sounds per minute. Still, the increased bowel sounds of small intestinal obstruction (described as frequent and high-pitched rushes interspersed with periods of silence) are poorly sensitive for this condition, even though quite *specific*. This may be due to their fleeting nature (in animal models they increase in number only during the first 30 minutes after obstruction, eventually abating over time). This is probably why bowel

sounds are *increased* in only one half of small intestinal obstructions, and diminished or absent in one quarter.

> **Pearl:**
>
> Bowel sounds lack sensitivity and specificity for intestinal obstruction. Hence, they are not useful.

I. Murmurs and Bruits

27. What is the difference between an abdominal murmur and a bruit?
Both are arterial in origin, and yet a *murmur* is usually systolic, whereas a *bruit* typically extends beyond the second heart sound and thus is *continuous.*

28. How frequent are these findings?
They have been reported in 4–20% of healthy individuals and 1–2% of unselected patients on a medical ward. Prevalence *declines* as a result of age.

29. What is the significance of an abdominal murmur/bruit?
It depends on its location. This may be either epigastric or right/left upper quadrant.

30. What is the significance of an *epigastric* murmur?
A systolic, medium- to low-pitched murmur over the epigastrium is not uncommon in healthy individuals. It occurs especially often in pregnancy, and, in fact, as many as one fifth of normal and thin women may have it, too (this frequency is a little lower in men). In contrast to a pathologic finding (like the murmur of renal artery stenosis, which tends to be louder *outside* the epigastrium [*see* below, questions 122 and 123]), a benign murmur is characteristically limited to the area between the xiphoid process and umbilicus. It usually originates from a normal celiac tripod.

31. What is the significance of a *right or left upper quadrant* murmur/bruit?
- When over the *right upper quadrant,* it often indicates a hepatic tumor, typically a hepatoma but also a metastasis. It is due to tumoral neovascularization or extrinsic vascular compression by the cancer, but also can reflect hepatitis, cirrhosis, an arteriovenous malformation, or, occasionally, simple tricuspid regurgitation.
- When over the *left upper quadrant,* it indicates instead cancer of the pancreas or a vascular anomaly of the spleen. Less frequent causes of a left (or right) upper quadrant murmur/bruit are aneurysmatic lesions of the abdominal aorta or of renal, celiac, and mesenteric vessels.
- Finally, *renal vascular disease of the right (or left) kidney* also may produce a systolic murmur in the upper quadrants. Yet, these lesions are more commonly associated with a *continuous* murmur (i.e., a bruit). This can be heard, albeit less strongly, over the epigastrium, too.

> **Pearl:**
>
> A continuous murmur (bruit) in patients with severe and refractory hypertension should suggest renovascular disease until proven otherwise.

II. Venous Hums

32. What is the significance of a venous hum?
If heard over the epigastric and umbilical areas, it reflects the *caput medusae* of cirrhotic patients with portal hypertension. More than a murmur, this is indeed a "hum," that is a *continuous sound* of *venous* origin. It also is referred to as the Cruveilhier-Baumgarten murmur (or sign).

33. **What is the mechanism of production of this sound?**
The *recanalization* of the umbilical vein caused by portal hypertension. This results in reverse flow (from a cirrhotic liver into the abdominal wall veins), with final decompression into various portosystemic shunts. The Cruveilhier-Baumgarten murmur softens with epigastric pressure, while intensifying with the forced expiratory phase of Valsalva (which increases back-flow to the umbilical vein through reduced right-sided venous return). It is often accompanied by a *thrill*.

34. **What are Cruveilhier-Baumgarten disease and Cruveilhier-Baumgarten syndrome?**
They are both characterized by "feeding" of the *caput medusae* through the (para)umbilical vein. Yet the *disease* and the *syndrome* may actually be two separate entities:
- The **disease** is a *congenital* patency of the umbilical vein, even though portal hypertension may be absent. Patients with this condition do *not* have ascites, but may have a small and atrophic liver—like the first patient described by Cruveilhier (*see* below, question 35).
- The **syndrome** is instead typical of portal hypertension from cirrhosis and consists of either an *acquired* reopening of the umbilical vein or high flow in paraumbilical/anastomotic veins.

35. **Who were these guys?**
Léon Jean Baptiste Cruveilhier (1791–1874) was a French pathologist and the son of an army surgeon. Raised by Mom (because Dad was away fighting the Napoleonic wars), little Cruveilhier developed a strong interest in priesthood and very little stomach for medicine. This got him into trouble when Dad eventually came home, determined more than ever to turn his reluctant son into a well-respected physician. Forced to enter medical school, Cruveilhier fled after his first autopsy, finding temporary refuge in the nearby St. Sulpice seminary. Chased by Dad (and forced to re-enter medical school), he was finally entrusted to an old family friend, Baron Guillaume Dupuytren. This turned out to be a good idea, since Dupuytren became a mentor to Cruveilhier and a lifelong inspiration for the study of pathology. After graduating from Paris in 1816 (the same year Laënnec invented the stethoscope), Cruveilhier practiced in Limoges before becoming professor of surgery at Montpellier in 1823. Two years later, he moved to Paris, where in 1836 he took the chair of the newly created department of pathological anatomy. A modest man with neither clinical acumen nor eloquence, he was primarily a researcher who owed his fame to the books he wrote rather than the teaching he imparted. Author of a popular pathology textbook, he eventually reported the case of a French soldier who in 1813 had been captured by Hungarian troops, beaten with rifle butts to the belly, and left for dead. After spending 6 months in the hospital, he developed abdominal swelling and a loud umbilical murmur. Following his death in 1833, the autopsy had revealed a small and noncirrhotic liver, with a portosystemic shunt operated by large umbilical veins. Cruveilhier interpreted this as either a congenital variant or an acquired lesion provoked by war trauma.
Paul Clemens von Baumgarten (1848–1928) was a German pathologist. Also the son of a physician, he graduated from Leipzig a year before Cruveilhier's death, and from 1874 to 1889, he taught at Königsberg, until moving to Tübingen, where he remained for the rest of his life. He also is famous for describing the tubercle bacillus in 1882, the same year as Koch but independently.

III. Friction Rubs

36. **What is the significance of friction rubs?**
It depends on their location. Rubs over the left (or right) upper quadrants usually indicate infarcts (or tumors) of the spleen and liver, respectively.

IV. Succussion Splash

37. **What is a succussion splash?**
It is the noise of shaking a body cavity with a large amount of air and water. Hippocrates was the first to describe it, probably in reference to a *hydropneumothorax*. Stressing its diagnostic value,

he wrote: *"You shall know that the chest contains water but not pus, if in applying the ear during a certain time on the side, you perceive a noise like that of boiling vinegar."* If elicited in the abdomen, it reflects instead an intestinal obstruction or a gastric dilation (*see* below, question 114). Although often detected by the unaided ear, it usually requires a stethoscope.

(3) Percussion

38. What is the value of abdominal percussion?
It helps in identifying both the *amount* and *localization* of abdominal gas. It also can help detect intra-abdominal fluid (ascites, distended bladder) or outline solid organs (liver, spleen, masses). Hence, it will be described in greater detail in the corresponding sections.

39. How should one percuss?
Usually, lightly and in all four quadrants. Percussion should guide palpation, by eliciting *tympanitic* notes over gas-filled areas, and *dull* notes over *solid* areas. It should always be performed *after* auscultation, since doing otherwise might alter bowel sounds.

(4) Palpation

40. How should the abdomen be palpated?
In a clockwise sequence: start from the right upper quadrant, move to the left upper quadrant, then down to the left and right lower quadrants, and finally ending with the periumbilical region, where you should give special attention to palpating aorta and navel (look for Sister Mary Joseph's nodule!). Use first a lighter and then a deeper technique. Leave areas of tenderness last. In this regard, cross-palpation (such as testing for pain in the right lower quadrant while palpating the *left* lower quadrant, see Rovsing's sign) can be an even better way to detect intra-abdominal pathology. In addition to areas of tenderness, look for masses, hernias, aneurysms, and organomegaly. Minimize abdominal wall tension by having the patient bend knees and thighs.

41. What is the difference between a light and a deep palpation?
- In **light palpation**, the palm of the hand rests gently on the wall, while the fingers are pressed *into* the abdomen at a depth of 1 cm.
- **Deep palpation** is the same as light palpation, except that the examiner presses his or her fingers more deeply than 1 cm. This technique is usually carried out by *reinforced palpation* (i.e., by pushing on the fingers of the palpating hand with the fingers of the other hand [bimanual palpation]; Fig. 15-9).

42. How can one distinguish between an intra-abdominal and an intramural mass?
By palpating the mass while the patient is raising the head from the pillow. This tenses the abdominal wall muscles, thus pushing away an intra-abdominal mass but *not* an intra-mural mass (i.e., one localized in the abdominal wall). This technique also can be used to separate the abdominal wall from peritoneal tenderness (*see* below, questions 153–160).

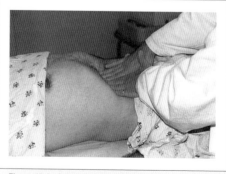

Figure 15-9. Technique for deep palpation.

Examples of Abnormalities Detectable On Palpation

43. How can one detect an abdominal aortic aneurysm?

By placing the hands over the epigastric area, parallel to the *recti* muscles and with the fingers pointing toward the patient's head. This position is a must since the aortic bifurcation is *above* the umbilical region. Then feel for an *expansile* pulsation that pushes your hands *apart*. This horizontal expansion is the *sine qua non* for a positive aortic finding, since prominent (but *not* expansile) pulsations may often occur in normal and thin patients.

44. When is this maneuver considered positive?

It depends on the abdomen, since fat bellies are more difficult to examine than thin ones. Overall, the test is positive when the diameter of the expansile mass is >3 cm (with diameter of pulsation reflecting the diameter of the aneurysm). In cases of *small* aneurysms (3–5 cm in diameter), the finding is very specific, with the few false positives usually reflecting a tortuous aorta (yet, it is also poorly sensitive, detecting only one of five cases). In patients with *large* aneurysms (>5 cm), sensitivity increases to four out of five patients. In fact, lack of expansile pulsation in a thin patient should strongly argue against the presence of a large aneurysm.

B. LIVER

> *"Zeus' winged hound, an eagle red with blood,*
> *Shall come a guest unbidden to your banquet.*
> *All day long he will tear to rags your body,*
> *great rents within the flesh,*
> *feasting in a fury on the blackened liver.*
> *Look for no end to this agony,*
> *Until a God will freely suffer for you,*
> *will take on Him your pain, and in your stead*
> *Descend to where the sun is turned to darkness,*
> *the black depths of death."*
>
> Aeschylus, Prometheus Bound

45. What are the two goals of bedside evaluation of the liver?

- To palpate the liver edge and identify its characteristics
- To determine the hepatic size

Yet the role of physical diagnosis has become increasingly questionable. Assessment of hepatomegaly, for example, has proven highly unreliable, and some authors have even suggested scrapping it altogether.

(1) Palpation of the Liver

46. Which edge can be palpated? How?

Only the *lower edge* is accessible, since the upper border is tucked deep into the rib cage and thus beyond the reach of the examiner's fingers. To access the lower margin, ask the patient to lie supine, ideally with flexed hips and knees to better relax the abdominal wall (Fig. 15-10). To feel the edge, you can use one of three strategies, differing more in personal preference than value:

- **Cephalad approach:** Place one hand on the patient's abdomen, keeping the edge parallel to the rectus muscle and the fingers pointing toward the head. Place the other hand behind the patient's back, to help support it. Then, while the patient is taking a deep breath, press the anterior hand downward and cephalad, so that the respiratory excursion of the diaphragm displaces the liver edge downward, bringing it into contact with the fingertips.
- **Transverse approach:** Place your hand *parallel* to the costal margin (with fingers pointing toward the patient's flank). This is probably not as good a maneuver as the other two,

since it relies primarily on the hand's margin, which is not as sensitive as the fingertips.
- **Hook technique:** Point your fingers toward the patient's *feet*, while trying to gently hook the liver with both hands.

If you cannot feel the edge, you should probably end your liver exam at this point. If instead you do feel the edge, then determine its characteristics, and finally listen for rubs or bruits.

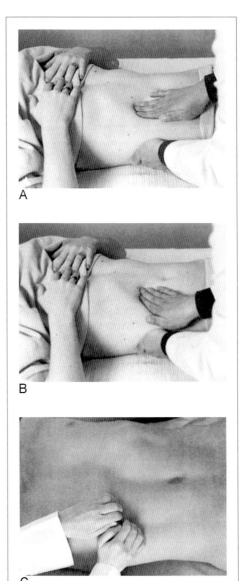

47. **What can be learned from palpation of the liver?**
What *cannot* be learned is the presence (or absence) of hepatomegaly, since palpation allows only an assessment of lower liver edge *characteristics*, such as (1) consistency and contour, (2) abnormalities of surface (e.g., presence of nodules), (3) tenderness, (4) presence of systolic pulsations, and (5) presence of frictions and thrills.

48. **How reliable is palpation of the liver edge as a measure of hepatic *consistency*?**
Not reliable at all. Interobserver variability is in fact huge. In two studies of alcoholic and jaundiced patients, multiple experts had a mere 11% chance-corrected agreement for abnormal consistency of a palpable liver edge, and a 26–29% agreement for the presence of nodules. Only agreement on tenderness reached a more acceptable 49%.

Figure 15-10. Palpating the liver. *A*, Fingers are extended, with tips on the right midclavicular line below the level of liver tenderness and pointing toward the head. *B*, Alternative method with fingers parallel to the costal margin. *C*, Palpating the liver with fingers hooked over the costal margin. (From Seidel HM, Ball JW, Dains JE, Benedict GW: Mosby's Guide to Physical Examination, 3rd ed. St. Louis, Mosby, 1995.)

49. **What is the significance of liver *tenderness*?**
It usually indicates distention of the hepatic capsule, as may be encountered in patients with passive liver congestion. It is, however, a nonspecific finding that also may be due to inflammation, or even tension, of the abdominal wall muscles.

50. **What is the significance of a *firm and hard* liver edge?**
    A *very hard* edge suggests tumor, whereas a *sharp* one suggests cirrhosis. A *firm* liver, neither sharp edged nor stone hard, is usually passively congested. *Nodules* may indicate cirrhosis but are more often related to cancer. The size of the *nodules* also may help distinguish the two conditions (with larger nodules being more likely neoplastic).

51. **What is the significance of a *pulsatile* liver edge?**
    It may represent transmission of aortic pulsations through an enlarged liver, but usually indicates one of two conditions: (1) constrictive pericarditis or (2) tricuspid regurgitation (where it is encountered in 30–90% of cases, usually indicating moderate to severe disease).

52. **How can one distinguish these two entities?**
    By an inspiratory increase in magnitude of pulsations. This occurs in tricuspid regurgitation (TR) (especially in held mid- or end-inspiration), but *not* in constrictive pericarditis. In TR, the hepatic pulsations are felt as a double movement of the liver edge, usually synchronous with a giant jugular "V" wave at the neck and a strong diastolic dip immediately after the carotid pulse. *Pulsatility in a setting of hepatomegaly* is instead such a good indicator of *constrictive pericarditis* (present in 65% of patients) that its absence argues strongly against the diagnosis.

53. **What is the hepatojugular reflux?**
    More of a cardiac than an abdominal maneuver. In fact, it is commonly used to unmask *subclinical congestive heart failure* (for its description and clinical significance, *see* Chapter 10, questions 106–114).

(2) Percussion of the Liver

54. **Is assessment of liver *size* another goal of palpation?**
    No, since it cannot be accomplished by palpation alone, but by a combination of *percussion* and palpation (with the possible addition of the *scratch test*).

55. **Does a palpable liver edge reflect hepatomegaly?**
    Not at all. Although many physicians do indeed screen for hepatomegaly by checking whether the liver is palpable at peak inspiration (and, if so, by measuring the number or centimeters—or finger breadths—below the costal margin), palpability of the edge is a highly inaccurate marker of organomegaly. A normal liver, for example, may become palpable simply because it is pushed down by an emphysematous lung. In fact, Palmer found a palpable edge in 57% of military personnel with normal liver tests and no history of liver disease (in 28% the edge was palpable $\geq$2 cm below the costal margin). Similarly, Riemenschneider found hepatomegaly at autopsy in less than one half of all patients with palpable liver on exam. In fact, there is no correlation between edge palpability and liver scan/autopsy data because palpability may have more to do with *consistency* of the edge, with the firmer liver of cirrhotics being more easily palpable.

> **Pearl:**
> Palpability of the lower hepatic margin is a common and nonspecific finding that cannot be used to estimate liver size since half of all palpable livers are not enlarged and half of truly enlarged livers are not palpable. Although palpable livers are more likely to be enlarged (whereas nonpalpable livers are more likely to be normal), palpability of the edge does not necessarily indicate hepatomegaly. Hence, the primary value of palpation is *localization* (and *description*) of the lower hepatic border. Palpability of the edge can be used for estimating liver span only after being linked to percussion of the superior hepatic border.

56. **Should the lower liver edge then be assessed by percussion alone?**
This has indeed been suggested. It is, however, counterintuitive, considering that percussion is notoriously inaccurate even in locating the *upper* liver border, especially when done with light intensity. Indeed, most errors in measuring liver span occur when the lower margin is not palpable and the examiner has to rely on percussion alone to locate both the upper *and* lower edge.

57. **So what is the best way to determine liver size on physical exam?**
There is no best way. Definitely *not* palpation alone, since half of all palpable livers are not enlarged and half of truly enlarged livers are not palpable. Hence, to guestimate size, measure the longitudinal (or vertical) liver span (i.e., the distance in centimeters between the lower and upper borders along the midclavicular line [MCL]). These can be located as follows:
- The **lower liver border** by palpation, percussion, or scratch test. The last two maneuvers are usually conducted along the MCL—an important point since otherwise inaccuracies may lead to an interobserver variability of as much as 10 cm.
- The **upper liver border** is located by percussion alone.

58. **How can one best determine hepatic size by percussion?**
Through *direct* or *indirect* percussion (Fig. 15-11). Both are carried out during quiet respiration. The direct technique consists of a light abdominal percussion by the index finger alone. *Indirect* percussion is instead the more traditional combination of plexor and pleximeter, as, respectively, the striking and stricken finger. The pleximeter (usually the middle finger of one hand) is applied to the abdominal wall only by its distal interphalangeal joint (to avoid dampening of vibrations); the middle finger of the other hand is then used as a plexor against the pleximeter, usually tapping along the right MCL. Even when performing indirect percussion, it is important that you tap *lightly*, making the note barely audible to only yourself. By doing so, you can more easily identify the hepatic area as a change in percussion note, from resonant (pulmonary parenchyma), to dull (liver), and to resonant again (air-filled bowel loops). Yet, even this may lead to inaccuracies.

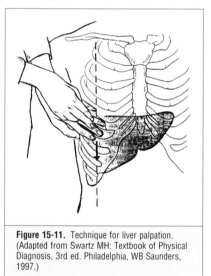

Figure 15-11. Technique for liver palpation. (Adapted from Swartz MH: Textbook of Physical Diagnosis, 3rd ed. Philadelphia, WB Saunders, 1997.)

Vertical liver span is the distance between two resonant points along the MCL, detected during either quiet breathing, or at the same phase of respiration. Direct percussion performed by gastroenterologists has been found to be more accurate than *indirect* percussion, yet a normal range of liver span for this technique has not been determined. Thus, indirect percussion should still be the maneuver of choice.

59. **What is a normal liver span?**
A variable figure, since it depends on body size and shape. Overall, a normal liver span is <12–13 cm on MCL, as assessed by indirect percussion or a combination of percussion/palpation.

60. **What is the scratch test?**
It is a combined auscultatory/percussive maneuver aimed at localizing the inferior hepatic border (Fig. 15-12). Place the stethoscope either beneath the xiphoid or over the liver, just above the costal margin of the MCL. Then administer "scratches" in a cephalad fashion, by moving the

finger along the MCL—from the right lower quadrant toward the costal margin. The point at which the scratching sound intensifies indicates a change in underlying tissue, and thus the presence of the lower liver edge. A variation of the test is *auscultatory percussion*, in which the examining finger does *not* scratch the abdominal wall but gently percusses it (or flickers it).

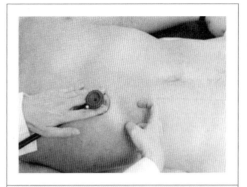

Figure 15-12. Scratch technique for auscultating the liver. With the stethoscope over the liver, lightly scratch the abdominal surface, moving toward the liver. The sound will be intensified over the liver. (From Seidel HM, Ball JW, Dains JE, Benedict GW: Mosby's Guide to Physical Examination, 3rd ed. St. Louis, Mosby, 1995.)

61. **How reliable is the scratch test in localizing the lower liver edge?**
One study found it to be more accurate than percussion or palpation. Others have found it to be instead more wanting, especially when compared to palpation, or *ultrasound*.
Moreover, there is very little consensus about the technique, in terms of positioning the stethoscope (near the umbilicus, on the liver, or at the costal margin?), scratching methodology (finger alone, finger plus pleximeter, a bristle brush or a corrugated rod?), and direction of the stroke (circular, left to right, longitudinal?). Thus, additional validation is needed before the scratch technique may become more than a simple adjunct to either palpation or percussion.

62. **How accurate are these bedside techniques in diagnosing hepatomegaly?**
Poorly accurate. Palpation of the lower liver edge has interobserver variability of 6 cm and intraobserver variability of 1–2 cm. Determination of liver span by percussion alone has interobserver variability of 2.5–8 cm, and intraobserver variability of 1–2 cm. Variability in measurement by percussion is usually due to changes in *intensity* of percussion, which may yield differences in span as great as 3 cm, primarily because of the difficulty in localizing the upper edge through interposed lung tissue. Direct percussion was shown by Skrainka et al. to be as accurate as ultrasound in estimating liver span, but this relied on skilled consultants. Other studies conducted among general practitioners, however, have yielded disappointing results. Overall, *indirect* percussion *underestimates* liver size (the lighter the percussion, the greater the underestimation). This may be overcome by using a firm technique and by comparing the measured span to the span predicted by nomograms, which take into account patients' weight and height. A span >95% confidence intervals predicted by these tables most likely represents hepatomegaly. Nomograms also are available for a light percussive maneuver.

> **Pearl:**
> Because each clinician's technique may be so different (and interobserver variability as high as 30–50%), measurement of liver size by physical diagnosis represents only an index, not a true measurement. Some authors have recommended abandoning it altogether.

63. **In summary, what are the pros and cons of bedside assessment of liver size?**
- When compared with firm percussion, *light* percussion underestimates liver size, yet it is still closer to ultrasonic evaluation.

- Measurements by direct and indirect percussion vary significantly.
- Palpability of the lower liver edge is a totally inaccurate marker of hepatomegaly.
- The scratch test needs further validation.
- Liver span measured by physical exam does not correlate with the actual size of the liver. Hence, bedside examination of the liver provides highly inaccurate information about organ's size. Based on this disappointing evidence, one can make the following recommendations:
  1. Because of the low *intraobserver* variability (which permits accurate follow-ups), a physician may use serial examinations of the liver to detect changes *over time*.
  2. Given the high *interobserver* variability, a physician *cannot* use physical examination alone to objectively and accurately assess liver size. The gold standard should then become ultrasound, which not only allows a quantitative and reproducible estimate of liver span, but also permits a calculation of total liver volume by means of reconstruction techniques.
  3. The primary role of physical examination of the liver should therefore remain the determination by palpation of the lower edge's characteristics and consistency.

(3) Auscultation of the Liver

64. What is the role of auscultation of the liver?
In addition to the *scratch test* (previously discussed), its role is mostly limited to detecting (1) friction rubs, (2) arterial murmurs (i.e., sounds limited to systole), and (3) venous hums.

I. Hepatic Friction Rubs

65. What is the significance of hepatic friction rubs?
They can occur in hepatomas, but also in 10% of metastatic tumors. Instead, they are much less common in localized or disseminated inflammatory processes, like liver abscesses or hepatitis. Overall, they are rare and nonspecific findings.

II. Hepatic Arterial Murmurs

66. What is the significance of an arterial murmur over the liver?
It suggests a hepatic tumor (primary or metastatic), but also hepatitis. Since prevalence in the general population is low (<3%), but high (10–56%) in liver cancer, you should look for hepatic murmur(s) only in patients whose history and exam increase the pretest probability of disease.

67. What is the significance of a hepatic murmur associated with a rub?
It should be considered cancer until proven otherwise.

III. Hepatic Venous Hums

68. What is the significance of a hepatic venous hum?
It indicates the presence of portal venous hypertension (previously discussed).

69. How can one differentiate a venous hum from an arterial murmur?
By the presence (or absence) of a diastolic component. Whereas arterial murmurs are primarily systolic, venous hums are both systolic and diastolic (and thus they resemble *bruits* more than murmurs). Hums originate in a communication between the umbilical veins and the abdominal wall veins. They do *not* originate in arteriovenous fistulas or hepatic hemangiomas—lesions that are instead responsible for the production of true arterial continuous murmurs (i.e., bruits).

(4) Special Problems

70. **What is jaundice?**
It is an abnormal yellowish-to-orange discoloration of skin and mucous membranes produced by accumulation of bile pigment. It is usually first detected in the eyes, even though the traditional reference to "scleral icterus" is incorrect, since most of the bilirubin is actually accumulated in the *conjunctiva* (the sclera has no vascular supply). By the time blood concentration of bilirubin increases, both skin and mucous membranes become pigmented.

71. **Is there any diagnostic difference in the hue of pigmentation?**
Although some differences have been traditionally reported between various types of jaundice (pale-yellow = *hemolytic jaundice*; orange-yellow = *hepatocellular jaundice*; yellow-green = *prolonged obstructive jaundice*), these differences are not clinically relevant. It is instead important to separate jaundice from *pseudojaundice*. The latter is usually due to:
   - **Subconjunctival fat:** This can be yellowish and often misinterpreted as jaundice, except that the yellow of fat is confined to the conjunctival folds and never to the pericorneal region.
   - **Hypercarotenemia:** This may result from excessive ingestion of carrots or pigmented fruits and vegetables (oranges and tomatoes). In this case, the yellowish discoloration spares the conjunctiva while affecting predominantly the palms, soles, and nasolabial folds.
   Once jaundice and pseudojaundice have been differentiated, bedside evaluation should search for extrahepatic findings of hepatocellular but *not* obstructive disease.

72. **How can you separate obstructive from hepatocellular jaundice?**
Obstructive jaundice usually presents acutely or subacutely—often with a dilated and palpable gallbladder (Courvoisier's sign). Hepatocellular jaundice presents instead more slowly, often with the following signs of chronic liver disease: (1) spider telangiectasias, (2) palmar erythema, (3) dilated abdominal veins, (4) palpable spleen, (5) asterixis, and (6) fetor hepaticus.

73. **What are spider nevi (telangiectasias)?**
They are dilated blood vessels that primarily affect areas of intense blushing, like the face and neck, but also the shoulders, arms, hands, and torso (they are instead quite rare on the palms, scalp, and below the umbilicus, probably reflecting regional differences in neurohormonal control of the microcirculation). They should not be confused with *cherry angiomas,* which are instead round, venous, and commonly encountered as a result of aging. *Spider angiomata* are *spider-like,* insofar as they consist of a central arteriole (the spider) with radiating thin-walled branches (the legs). They have a surrounding area of erythema (with a temperature 2–3°C higher than the surrounding skin), and vary in size from a tiny pinhead to a diameter of 0.5 cm. When the "body" is compressed with a cover glass slide, it appears to pulsate and eventually blanches. The body and branches then refill rapidly upon release of pressure.

74. **Can spider nevi occur in normal individuals?**
Yes, they may occur in 10–15% of healthy adults and young children, but usually in fewer number (average three) and smaller size. When not congenital, spider nevi suggest four conditions:
   - **Liver disease, especially alcoholic:** Alcohol plays an important role, since lesions are indeed more frequent in alcoholic cirrhosis (and cirrhosis due to hepatitis C *and* alcohol) than in cirrhosis due solely to hepatitis C. In male cirrhotics, the angiomas tend to correlate with an abnormally increased serum ratio of estradiol to free testosterone. They also correlate with higher levels of substance P, which may play a vasodilator role through its release of nitric oxide. They typically wax and wane according to disease severity, and can predict both the stage of hepatitis C and the presence of hepatopulmonary syndrome.
   - **Pregnancy:** Spiders appear during the second to fifth months of gestation and quickly disappear after delivery. Same with oral contraceptives.
   - **Thyrotoxicosis**
   - **Malnutrition**

75. **What is the hepatopulmary syndrome (HPS)?**
    A condition seen in 8% of cirrhotics and characterized by hypoxemia and spider nevi. The mechanism is bibasilar intrapulmonary arteriovenous shunt, due to multiple "spider angiomata." These, in turn, cause clubbing, orthodeoxia, and platypnea (*see* Chapter 13, questions 46 and 47). Diagnosis is confirmed by a positive bubble echocardiogram, and liver transplant is often curative. HPS should not be confused with portopulmonary hypertension (PHTN), which is instead a condition of cirrhotics with portal *and* pulmonary hypertension (the latter being akin to primary pulmonary hypertension). Oxygenation is normal at rest, but not on exercise; there is orthopnea (but not platypnea), plus right-sided failure. Pulmonary hypertension does not respond to transplant.

76. **What is palmar erythema?**
    Another vascular anomaly of liver disease. It is characterized by symmetric reddening of the palms, mostly over the *thenar and hypothenar* eminences. In fact, it often *coexists* with spider nevi, waxes and wanes together with them, and is frequently associated with the same underlying conditions. When examining the palm of cirrhotic patients, also look for Dupuytren's contracture.

77. **What is Dupuytren's contracture?**
    It is a benign and slowly progressive fibroproliferative disease, characterized by thickening of the palmar fascia on the ulnar side, eventually leading to flexural contraction of the digits, especially the fourth and fifth (the index finger and thumb are instead typically spared) (Fig. 15-13). In

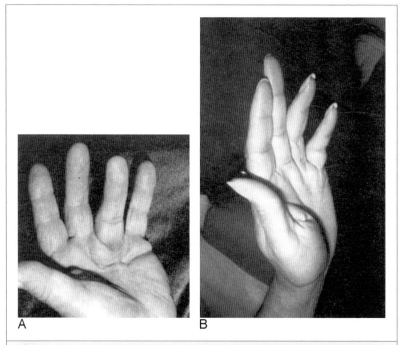

A   B

Figure 15-13. In Dupuytren's contracture, fibrous bands of diseased palmar fascia can contract to pull the finger into flexion. *A*, The fibrous band can be seen at the level of the proximal palmar crease of the ring finger. *B*, Early Dupuytren's contracture producing flexion of the fifth finger. (From Concannon MJ: Common Hand Problems in Primary Care. Philadelphia, Hanley & Belfus 1999.)

addition to the *flexion deformity* of the metacarpophalangeal (MCP) and the proximal interphalangeal (PIP) joints, there also may be *firm palmar nodules* (possibly tender to palpation) and *palpable "cords"* (proximal to the nodules and usually painless). Most patients are bilaterally affected (65%), whereas unilateral cases tend to be mostly right sided. The hand of Dupuytren is so typical to have been dubbed "the hand of Papal benediction" (which is different from the "obstetrician's hand" of Trousseau's sign—*see* Chapter 2, questions 104–107). Dupuytren's also is familial (27–68% of cases), with males more frequently and more severely affected. It is very common in northern Europe and the United Kingdom, and especially in countries with large immigration from these areas. In Scotland, for example, it affects 39% of males and 21% of females older than 60. In the United States, it affects instead 5–15% of males older than 50. The basic pathophysiology is uncontrolled fibroblast proliferation of the palmar fascia. Etiology is unknown, but several associations *are* known: (1) 18–66% of patients with alcoholic liver disease (either cirrhotic or noncirrhotic); (2) 13–42% of patients with chronic pulmonary tuberculosis; (3) 8–56% of epileptics on treatment; (4) 35% of smoker males older than 60, usually. In some studies, manual laborers (and brewery workers) have a slightly higher predominance, but this is still controversial. Prior hand trauma is, however, a risk factor, present in 13% of cases. In addition, 31–48% of Dupuytren patients are just alcoholics (with or without liver disease); 10–35% have either peptic ulcer disease or cholecystitis; 6–25% have diabetes mellitus (strongly correlated with retinopathy); 93% have glucose intolerance; and 2.5% have Peyronie's disease. Famous sufferers have included former British Prime Minister Margaret Thatcher and the late U.S. President Ronald Reagan, suggesting that conservative views might represent an additional risk factor.

78. **Who was Dupuytren?**
A very weird character. Guillaume Dupuytren (1777–1835) was born just 1 year after the American Revolution, but some of the ideas of his times must have definitely rubbed off on him, since he remained all his life an eccentric and flamboyant character. For one, he was famous for operating in a cloth cap and carpet slippers. But he also was famous for being abrasive, cynical, and vindictive. Born of humble origins, he was an attractive and intelligent child, to the point of being kidnapped at age 4 by a rich lady from Toulouse (who later returned him to his family— probably after realizing what kind of "pain" the kid could be). As a teenager, he moved to Paris, where at age 24 he became prosector at the local School of Health. This gave him the opportunity to work directly with two of the giants of his time, Laënnec and Bayle, but this soon backfired, since Laënnec, realizing that Dupuytren was trying to gain credit for Bayle's work, stopped any interaction. This did not prevent Dupuytren from joining the Paris Hôtel Dieu, where he eventually made a name for himself as a skilled surgeon and a gifted speaker. He remained, however, as obnoxious as ever, to the point of being called "first of surgeons and last of men." Still, he *was* a great surgeon: he not only described his eponymous contracture, but even devised an operation to cure it. He also was the first to create a classification system for burns, and one of the first great promoters of plastic surgery. A workaholic rumored to see an average of 10,000 patients per year, Dupuytren also was very cheap. These two traits contributed to make him very rich, but not too popular. His motto was "fear nothing but mediocrity," which, of course, did not win him many friends either, but contributed nonetheless to make him famous well beyond the borders of France and rendered him more arrogant than ever. When King Charles X got dethroned and needed money, Dupuytren even offered him 1 million francs, stating that he was keeping aside 2 more million: one for his daughter and the other for his own old age. The king graciously declined. In 1833, Dupuytren suffered a stroke while delivering a lecture. He did manage to finish it, but emerged from the experience as an invalid. Eventually, he developed aspiration pneumonia and empyema. Offered surgery, he refused, claiming that he "would rather die at the hands of God than of surgeons." He died 12 days later, at 58. His description of the clinical manifestations and surgical management of the eponymous contracture was published in 1832, mostly by his students, since the Baron had a profound distaste for writing. Yet, it had already been reported by Felix Plater of Basel in 1614, and by

Henry Cline Senior in 1777, the year of Dupuytren's birth. Still, it was Dupuytren who established the palmar fascia as its site of origin. The familial nature of the disease was instead recorded by the French surgeon Jean-Gaspard-Blaise Goyrand, soon after Dupuytren's report.

79. **What is asterixis?**
A common (and early) finding of hepatic encephalopathy and a classic sign of hepatocellular disease. Since it requires some degree of voluntary muscular contraction, it disappears in comatose patients. It is demonstrated by asking patients to stretch the arms while at the same time holding their fingers spread apart, as if they were "stopping traffic." In the case of asterixis, the fingers and hands will start "flapping" in a myoclonic fashion, with brisk movements occurring at intervals of less than 1 second to more than 1 second (*see* Chapter 20, questions 50–52).

80. **What is fetor hepaticus?**
It is a sign of a severe portosystemic shunt from advanced hepatocellular disease. It is due to the accumulation of dimethyl sulfide in the breath, with an odor that has been compared to rotten eggs and garlic. Since it is caused by parenchymal disease (and not necessarily hepatic encephalopathy), it may be present in noncomatose patients.

81. **What other physical findings can be encountered in patients with portal hypertension?**
In addition to dilated abdominal wall veins (previously discussed), patients with portal hypertension from severe hepatocellular disease also present with *an enlarged spleen*.

> **Pearl:**
> In jaundice, the presence of splenomegaly is a good predictor of hepatocellular disease.

C. GALLBLADDER

In contrast to the liver, the gallbladder has escaped much indictment and still occupies an important role in abdominal exam. The organ is usually not palpable but becomes detectable in case of pathology. Two maneuvers/findings have been traditionally linked to the assessment of a diseased gallbladder: (1) Murphy's sign and (2) Courvoisier's law.

(1) Murphy's Sign

82. **What is Murphy's sign?**
It is a painful arrest in inspiration, triggered by palpation of the edge of an inflamed gallbladder. To elicit it, ask the patient to lie supine and take a deep breath, while you press your fingers under the right lower costal margin and along the midclavicular line (point of location of the gallbladder). Aim toward the patient's head. If the gallbladder is inflamed, the encounter between your fingertips and the fundus will cause pain and a reflex arrest in inspiration.

83. **What are Murphy's signs?**
Additional maneuvers that, in addition to "the" original sign, also carry Dr. Murphy's name. In fact, he humbly considered these techniques "the most valuable contributions I have made to medicine and surgery in the way of aids to diagnosis." One of them (percussion of the costovertebral angle for presence of kidney pathology, especially a perinephric abscess) has long lost its linkage with Murphy's name, even though it is still routinely used (*see* below, questions 118–120). The other ones are:

- *Deep-grip palpation of the gallbladder* (the real Murphy's sign, or at least its forebear)
- *Hammer stroke percussion of the gallbladder*

Murphy used the latter on more obese patients and considered it indisputably "the best test of all." In his original description:

> [T]he examiner sitting at the right side of the recumbent patient presses the tip of the 2nd finger of the left hand, flexed at a right angle, firmly up under the costal arch at the tip of the 9th cartilage... The patient is instructed to take a deep breath, and at the height of the inspiration, when the gall bladder is forced below the costal guard, the flexed finger is struck forcibly with the ulnar side of the open right hand of the examiner, and if there be an inflammation or a retention in the biliary tract, the patient will announce that the blow caused him severe pain, since one is striking an overdistended, inflamed viscus that contains sensitive nerve filaments.

Dr. Murphy used deep-grip palpation routinely in the examination for suspected biliary disease, even though he did not consider it to be "as good a test as the perpendicular finger percussion test, i.e., the hammer stroke percussion." Dr. Murphy described deep-grip palpation in 1903:

> Hypersensitiveness of the gallbladder is present in all varieties of infection and calculous obstruction, but not in the neoplastic, torsion, flexion, cicatricial, or valvular obstructions. The hypersensitiveness is elicited by deep palpation just below the right ninth costal cartilage, or in a line from that point to the middle of Poupart's ligament, as this is the common track of gallbladder enlargement. Deep percussion along the same line, with the patient in forced inspiration, gives pronounced pain. The most characteristic and constant sign of gallbladder hypersensitiveness is the inability of the patient to take a full, deep inspiration, when the physician's fingers are hooked up beneath the right costal arch below the hepatic margin. The diaphragm forces the liver down until the sensitive gallbladder reaches the examining fingers, when the inspiration suddenly ceases as though it had been shut off. I have never found this sign absent in a calculous or infectious cause of gall bladder or duct disease.

Notice that the current Murphy's sign is not elicited by the original "hook" technique of Dr. Murphy (i.e., the deep-grip palpation), but by a variation, in which the examiner's fingers are distended and pointed toward the head of the supine patient.

84. **Who was Dr. Murphy?**
John B. Murphy of Chicago (1857–1916) was an acclaimed leader in American surgery, who trained in Vienna with Billroth and established himself as the greatest surgical teacher of his day. A tall man with a parted red beard and a flamboyant character, Dr. Murphy linked his name to several diagnostic maneuvers for the evaluation of the acute abdomen, but also was the first to introduce in the United States the artificial immobilization and collapse of the lung for the treatment of pulmonary tuberculosis, a technique pioneered in Pavia by the Italian Carlo Forlanini.

85. **How accurate is Murphy's sign in predicting cholecystitis?**
Decently accurate, with sensitivity and specificity of 50–80% (specificity usually a little higher than sensitivity). Its significance increases in patients whose presentation is consistent with cholecystitis (i.e., nausea, vomiting, and right upper quadrant pain), whereas it decreases in patients with back tenderness, where other conditions (pancreatitis/renal disease) become more likely.

86. **What is the current role of Murphy's sign in the evaluation of acute cholecystitis?**
A helpful but limited role. In a 1914 article, Murphy had boasted that "you can make the differential diagnosis at the bedside. You do not have to go home for your instruments; you do not have to have a blood count made. You just have to use your brain and your fingers." This is mildly exaggerated. A century later, his sign remains helpful if present, but nonetheless

limited. Ultrasound can help more, by identifying cholelithiasis and eliciting a *sonographic Murphy's*.

87. **What is the sonographic Murphy's sign?**
It is a sort of Murphy's on steroids. Since discovering stones by ultrasound (U/S) does not, in and of itself, link an episode of acute abdominal pain to cholecystitis, a sonographic Murphy's has been proposed to confirm the diagnosis. Under U/S guidance, the examiner locates the gallbladder and then ascertains whether it corresponds to the point of maximal tenderness by pressing directly with the ultrasound transducer over the gallbladder. A positive sonographic Murphy's has an accuracy of 87% for acute cholecystitis, suggesting that the lower sensitivity of the plain Murphy's sign might reflect difficulty in localizing the gallbladder's fundus.

88. **Do patients with cholecystitis exhibit other findings?**
They also may have an area of hypersensitivity over the right costophrenic angle (Boas' sign; *see* acute abdomen) and, at times, an audible rub over the edge of the gallbladder. Still, they rarely have a palpable and tender right upper quadrant mass (*see* Courvoisier's law).

(2) Courvoisier's Law

89. **What does Courvoisier's law state?**
It states that in cases of *painless* jaundice, an enlarged, palpable, and nontender gallbladder is *not* due to *cholelithiasis,* but to *cancer* of either the biliary tract or the pancreatic head.

90. **Why should the gallbladder of patients with cholelithiasis remain small?**
Two possibilities, the first proposed by Courvoisier himself and probably not as accurate:
- Recurrent biliary colic caused by stone migration tends to lead to chronic cholecystitis and thus to a *stiffening of the gallbladder wall*. This, in turn, prevents the gallbladder from enlarging whenever the passing of new stones causes additional obstruction. Conversely, the slow growth of a biliary duct cancer (or of a cancer of the head of the pancreas), coupled with the pliability of the gallbladder, leads to painless jaundice and a palpable, enlarged gallbladder. This hypothesis, however, conflicts with experimental data indicating a similar stiffness in gallbladders that are either dilated or nondilated.
- Biliary colic from stones is less likely to produce a *complete* ductal obstruction. It also is more likely to be *symptomatic* and thus acted upon quickly, whereas malignant obstructions tend to be more severe, cause higher intraductal pressures, and last longer.

91. **How accurate is Courvoisier's law?**
Not much. In fact, it is a law that may not be as written in stone as originally claimed. To his credit, even Courvoisier had no intention to *legislate* when he first reported his original observation. The "law" was written later, and by other authors. What Courvoisier had written was a simple observation: that jaundiced patients with common duct obstruction were more likely to have a palpable and nontender gallbladder *if afflicted by stones rather than cancer*. In his original 187 cases of jaundice from common duct obstruction (87 due to stones and 100 to other causes), only 20% of cholelithiasis patients had an enlarged gallbladder, as opposed to 92% of those with other problems (of which malignancy was the most common). More recent series, however, suggest a lower sensitivity for malignant obstruction (25–50%), but still a good specificity (80–90%). In one study, only one half of patients with jaundice due to pancreatic carcinoma had a clinically palpable gallbladder (an incidence that increased considerably if operative or autopsy enlargement was taken into consideration—in this case, 80% of pancreatic cancers had an enlarged gallbladder at surgery, as opposed to 42% of common duct stones).

92. **In the final analysis, what is the significance of Courvoisier's sign?**
A palpable and nontender gallbladder in a jaundiced patient strongly suggests that the jaundice is *not* due to hepatocellular disease, but to an *extrahepatic* obstruction of the biliary tract. Albeit

not too sensitive, this finding is highly specific. Whether the obstruction is caused by tumor or stone is instead more difficult to say, even though the likelihood of tumor is a bit higher.

93. **Is right upper quadrant tenderness indicative of cholelithiasis?**
No. In cases of biliary colic, right upper quadrant tenderness does not separate patients with cholelithiasis from those without. U/S is the gold standard, with 95–99% accuracy for stones.

94. **Who was Courvoisier?**
Not a cognac. In fact, despite his French-sounding name, Ludwig G. Courvoisier was from *Basel*, Switzerland, where he had been born in 1843. Not only was he not French, but he actually *fought* the French during the Franco-Prussian war of 1870. Afterward, he became professor of surgery at the local university, where he published extensively on the biliary tract. Courvoisier's law originated in a monograph titled "The Pathology and Surgery of The Biliary Tract," a review of more than 100 patients with jaundice.

D. THE SPLEEN

"The neighbouring organ [the spleen] is situated on the left-hand side, and is constructed with a view of keeping the liver bright and pure, like a napkin always ready prepared and at hand to clean the mirror."

Plato, *Timaeus* 72 C.

95. **How effective is abdominal examination in assessing the spleen?**
Not too effective. The spleen is another subdiaphragmatic structure that, like the liver, does not lend itself easily to outside evaluation, especially in regard to size assessment. Both palpation and percussion have good specificity in detecting splenomegaly, but variable sensitivity. These techniques also are among the most difficult to master in the entire physical diagnosis repertoire. Examiners' skills, therefore, play an important role.

(1) Palpation of the Spleen

96. **Is there any contraindication to palpating the spleen?**
A relative one is infectious mononucleosis, which may carry a small risk of splenic rupture in cases of palpations conducted too enthusiastically.

97. **What can be learned from palpation?**
The major piece of information, of course, is to see whether the spleen is palpable—at least its tip. If so, you should conclude that splenomegaly is indeed present and then proceed with assessing the *characteristics* of its tip, such as *consistency*. In this regard, a *firmer* spleen indicates a more protracted and possibly fibrotic splenomegaly, as, for example, in cirrhosis.

98. **What is the best way to palpate the spleen?**
It varies, depending on the examiner. As for the patient's position, some physicians prefer the supine approach (from either the right or the left side), whereas others have the patient in right lateral decubitus position. These have all been compared and found to be equivalent; hence, personal preference remains the major factor (Fig. 15-14). Overall, there are as many as *four* techniques: (1) bimanual, (2) ballottement, (3) palpation from above, and (4) one-hand hook technique. As in the case of the liver exam, any of these would benefit from having the patient flex the knees and hips.

- **Bimanual palpation:** Stand at the right side of the supine patient, and apply gentle pressure with your *right* hand to the left upper abdominal quadrant, keeping the fingers parallel to the rectus muscle and pointing toward the patient's head. Place your *left* hand on the lower left rib cage. Then instruct the patient to breathe in slowly, so that at peak inspiration the splenic edge will touch your fingers. If you cannot feel the edge, end the examination there. If you *do* feel it, determine its *consistency* and *contour*, and then listen for rubs and bruits.

- **Ballottement:** Use your left hand to reach over and around the supine patient's left hemithorax, lifting it up. Use your *right* hand to feel for transmission of impulses by a large spleen.

- **Palpation from above:** The patient lies either supine or in the right lateral decubitus position, while you stand on the left side of the bed, pointing all fingers toward the patient's feet, trying to hook the spleen gently with both hands while asking the patient to take a deep breath.

- **One-hand hook technique:** Although not validated, this method should detect an enlarged spleen weeks before it becomes palpable by more conventional maneuvers. In the words of Dr. Hedge, who first described it:

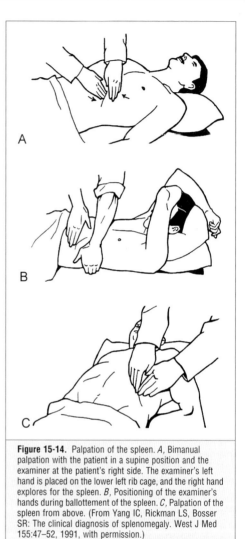

Figure 15-14. Palpation of the spleen. *A,* Bimanual palpation with the patient in a supine position and the examiner at the patient's right side. The examiner's left hand is placed on the lower left rib cage, and the right hand explores for the spleen. *B,* Positioning of the examiner's hands during ballottement of the spleen. *C,* Palpation of the spleen from above. (From Yang IC, Rickman LS, Bosser SR: The clinical diagnosis of splenomegaly. West J Med 155:47–52, 1991, with permission.)

> The examiner stands on the left side of the bed, facing the patient's head at the level of his chest. The patient should be in right lateral decubitus. The examiner's left hand is placed on the patient's left costal border. The fingers should be flexed around the left subcostal margin, with the middle finger around the top of the 11th rib. The patient is then asked to breathe slowly and deeply, and early splenic enlargement may be noted when the soft splenic edge hits the tip of one of the flexed fingers of the examiner's left hand.

99. **If the splenic tip is palpable, can you conclude that the spleen is enlarged?**
Yes, detecting a splenic tip has high specificity for splenomegaly. This is in contrast to liver examination, where palpation of the edge does not necessarily indicate organomegaly.

100. Does lack of a palpable spleen rule out splenomegaly?

No, since many large spleens are not detectable. Hence, palpation has high specificity for splenomegaly, but variable sensitivity (20–70%), which depends not only on the operator's skills but also the organ's size (with larger spleens being more easily detectable). To better quantify size, Hacket has proposed a semiquantitative assessment that refers to three lines, passing respectively through the left costal margin, umbilicus, and symphysis. Spleen size is progressively numbered from 0–5, as not palpable (0), palpable only after deep inspiration (1), reaching between the left costal margin and a line halfway to the umbilical line (2), reaching the umbilical line (3), halfway between the umbilical line and the symphysis (4), or beyond the umbilical line (5). This method not only helps sharing information but also standardizes chart documentation.

101. How accurate are these bedside maneuvers in diagnosing splenomegaly?

Once again, they are more specific than sensitive. Yet, detecting splenomegaly should always raise two questions: (1) is it real, and (2) is it pathologic or just an incidental finding? Indeed, some "palpable spleens" are just a conglomerate of colonic feces, miraculously melting with enemas. Still, the specificity of bedside detection remains a respectable 90%, so that a palpable spleen should always be taken seriously. Yet, even truly enlarged spleens may not be pathologic. For example, they can be found in 3% of college students, 12% of postpartum women, 10.4% of hospitalized patients undergoing liver scans, and 2.3–3.8% of ambulatory patients.

> **Pearl:**
>
> Palpation has good specificity for splenomegaly (89–99%), but wide sensitivity, which is directly proportional to the size of the organ, increasing from 50% (for spleens of 600–750 gm) to almost 100% (for spleens >2350 gm). False positives may occur in chronic obstructive lung disease, where the spleen is pushed downward into the abdomen. False negatives may occur in obesity, ascites, or narrow costal angles. Finally, interobserver variability is rather low. In a study of 32 patients, four observers agreed 88% of the time on the presence or absence of splenomegaly.

102. Which other findings may help identifying the *cause* of splenomegaly?

- Concomitant *hepatomegaly* suggests primary liver disease (causing splenomegaly through portal hypertension).
- *Lymphadenopathy excludes* primary liver disease and makes hematologic or lymphoproliferative disorders more likely.
- *Massive splenomegaly* (or left upper quadrant tenderness) also argues in favor of a myeloproliferative etiology.
- Finally, *Kehr's sign* suggests impending splenic rupture.

103. What is Kehr's sign?

It is referred pain (or hyperesthesia) to the left shoulder—a sign of left diaphragmatic irritation, usually from splenic rupture, with intraperitoneal spillage of blood. Since they represent "referred" symptoms, pain and hyperesthesia are *not* elicited by pressure or movement of the shoulder. Instead, they are induced by asking the patient to lie supine for 10–15 minutes in reverse Trendelenburg, so that the intraperitoneal blood can more easily reach the diaphragm.

(2) Percussion of the Spleen

104. How do you percuss the spleen?

- **Nixon's technique** (Fig. 15-15A) percusses the entire spleen outline while the patient is in the right lateral decubitus position. This allows the spleen to lie above the stomach and colon, thus permitting determination of both upper and lower margins. Nixon described it in 1954 as follows:

> Percussion is initiated at the lower level of pulmonary resonance in approximately the posterior axillary line and carried down obliquely on a general perpendicular line toward the lowest mid-anterior costal margin. Normally, the upper border of dullness is measured 6–8 cm above the costal margin. In the adult, dullness over 8 cm indicates splenic enlargement.

- **Castell's technique** (Fig. 15-15B) percusses the lowest left intercostal space (eighth or ninth) along the anterior axillary line. The patient is instructed to breathe in deeply and then exhale, while percussion is carried out during both inspiration and exhalation. This should normally yield a resonant note, even on deep inspiration. However, enlarged spleens (even those missed on palpation, or just barely palpable) would yield a dull percussion note at peak inspiration. Castell described this technique in 1967 as follows:

> With the patient in supine position, percussion in the lowest intercostal space (8th or 9th) in the left anterior axillary line usually produces a resonant note if the spleen is normal in size. Furthermore, the resonance persists with full inspiration. As the spleen enlarges, the lower pole is displaced inferiorly and medially. This may produce a change in percussion note in the lowest left interspace in the anterior axillary line, from resonance to dullness with full inspiration. The percussion sign is considered positive when such a change is noted between full expiration and full inspiration.

- **Percussion of Traube's semilunar space** (Fig. 15-15C): Described by Barkun et al. in 1989, Traube's space is a triangular area bordered by the left sixth rib superiorly, the left midaxillary line laterally, and the left costal margin inferiorly. In the original description, dullness in this area suggested a pleural effusion. More recently, it has been thought to indicate splenomegaly.

Pearl:

Barkun compared percussion of Traube's space with ultrasonography and found it 62% sensitive and 72% specific for the detection of splenomegaly. But Traube's dullness becomes much less sensitive after meals or in patients who are overweight.

---

105. **Who was Traube?**

Ludwig Traube (1818–1876) was a member of the 19th-century school of great German clinicians, who also were excellent pathologists and often outstanding bacteriologists, too. Trained at the Berlin clinic, Traube was especially interested in the pathology of fever and the connections between diseases of the heart and kidneys. He introduced the thermometer into the clinic and described the peculiar dullness over the gastric bubble area (otherwise tympanitic) that still carries his name. He originally described this as a sign of left pleural thickening (caused, in his days, by tuberculous empyema) but did not name it after himself, nor did he associate dullness of the left upper quadrant with splenomegaly.

106. **What are the limitations of percussion in detecting splenomegaly?**

It is not that reliable. In a study of 65 patients undergoing liver scan, Sullivan and Williams compared percussion to palpation (using Nixon's and Castell's). Castell's was more sensitive than palpation (82% versus 71% false negative rate) but less specific (16% versus 10% false positive rate). Nixon's was instead less sensitive than palpation (59% versus 71%), but more specific (6% versus 16%). Castell's technique appeared, therefore, to be more sensitive than Nixon's (82% versus 59%, respectively). Still, Castell's and Nixon's had an overall combined false positive rate of 16.6%. In another study comparing physical exam with nuclear scintigraphy, Halpern et al. found a sensitivity of only 28% (and a specificity of 1.4%)

for the bedside detection of splenomegaly. This study, however, was flawed by lack of a standardized method for physical exam. Hence, the best comparison of palpation, percussion, and technology-based assessment remains the study by Sullivan and Williams.

Although still widely cited, Castell's technique was validated in only 10 male patients who had a positive percussion sign and an otherwise nonpalpable spleen. In this study, the gold standard was nuclear scan, and controls were males whose disease made hepatosplenomegaly not "expected." It also is uncertain whether the percussion technique (light versus heavy) interferes with the sensitivity of this maneuver. Castell himself wrote a paper demonstrating that this variable is indeed important in determining liver size by percussion.

107. **What are the recommendations for the bedside assessment of spleen size?**
Both percussion and palpation have better specificity than sensitivity, with palpation being overall the most accurate. Hence, percussion should serve as an *adjunct* to palpation. The two techniques are indeed complementary, since each may fail to detect splenomegaly and thus be rescued by the other. Moreover, percussion by the Castell's technique may even be more sensitive than palpation alone and thus unmask patients with barely palpable spleens. Yet, having to choose between the two, palpation should be the clear choice.

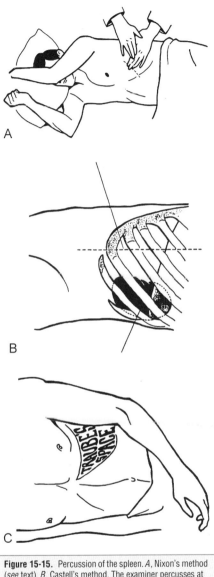

Figure 15-15. Percussion of the spleen. *A*, Nixon's method (*see* text). *B*, Castell's method. The examiner percusses at the intersection of the left anterior axillary line and ninth intercostal space (marked). The lower diagonal line points to the normal spleen. *C*, Traube's space is shown, as defined by Barkun et al. (From Yang JC, Rickman LS, Bosser SK: The clinical diagnosis of splenomegaly. West J Med 155:47–52, 1991, with permission.)

108. **What are the technologic alternatives for assessing the spleen?**
Given the limitations of physical diagnosis, imaging provides a very attractive alternative. Plain films of the abdomen are, however, poorly sensitive and unreliable for assessing

splenomegaly, only helpful in cases of gross enlargement. *Ultrasonography* is instead the gold standard: quick, reliable, cheap, noninvasive, safe, and highly sensitive and specific. In a study of more than 3000 patients, Leopold and Asher found ultrasonic assessment to be a reliable index of splenomegaly in more than 90% of patients. *Nuclear scintigraphy* also is highly accurate in predicting and assessing splenic size, although limited by long acquisition time, need for immobility, vascular integrity and function of the spleen, and cost. *Computed tomography (CT) scan* is a highly accurate (albeit expensive) method to assess splenomegaly, producing a mean error of 3.59% (using 1-cm cuts) or 3.65% (using 2-cm cuts). Its major limitations are cost and exposure of the patient to radiation. *Magnetic resonance imaging* seems to offer no clear advantage over CT scanning.

109. **Summarize bedside and technology-based methods of assessing splenomegaly.**
See Table 15-1.

TABLE 15-1. BEDSIDE AND TECHNOLOGY-BASED METHODS TO ASSESS SPLENOMEGALY

Examination	Reference	Sensitivity (%)	Specificity (%)
Palpation	Holzbach et al. (1962)	—	62
	Halpern et al. (1974)	28	99
	Sullivan and Williams (1976)	71	90
Percussion			
Nixon's method	Sullivan and Williams (1976)	59	94
Castell's method	Sullivan and Williams (1976)	82	83
Traube's method	Barkun et al. (1989)	62	72
Plain film	Whitley et al. (1966)	—	—
Ultrasonography	Leopold and Asher (1975)	—	>90
Nuclear scans	Rollo and DeLand (1970)	93	—
Computed	Heymsfield et al. (1979)	>95	—
tomography	Breiman et al. (1982)	96.4	—

(3) Auscultation of the Spleen

110. **What is the role of auscultation of the spleen?**
It should be limited to the detection of *rubs* (usually indicative of splenic infarcts) or *murmurs*. The latter can be encountered in patients with massive splenomegaly, or, more commonly, in cases of carcinoma of the pancreas compressing the splenic artery (sensitivity, 39%).

E. THE STOMACH

"The stomach is what distinguishes animals from vegetables;
for we do not know any vegetable that has a stomach, nor any animal without one."
J. Hunter, 1728–1793, Principles of Surgery

111. **What is the role of physical diagnosis in assessing the stomach?**
Very small, and usually limited to detecting gastric stasis or retention. The stomach traditionally has been off limits to physical diagnosis. It still is. The major value of the bedside

exam may be in auscultation, which can indirectly confirm the position of endotracheal or nasogastric tubes.

112. What maneuvers can be used to test for gastric retention?
Clapotage and succussion splash.

113. What is clapotage?
It is a "splashing sound" produced by fluid moving around in the stomach (from the French *clapotage*—or *clapotement*—the whoosh of water after a passing boat). It can be elicited by tapping a relaxed epigastrium with fingertips held together, even though the tapping should first begin in the lower abdomen (slightly to the left of the midline) and then move gradually up to the xiphoid process. The *splash* should be detected as soon as the first few blows are struck because otherwise muscle guarding by the patient will interfere with the test.

114. What is a succussion splash?
It is another splashing sound, but this time elicited by first placing the stethoscope over the epigastrium and then rapidly jerking the patient from side to side (I am not making this up). Absent in an empty stomach, the splash indicates a delay in gastric emptying if present 5 hours after a full meal, and 2 hours after a simple glass of water. In addition to being a little rude, it is neither sensitive nor specific since the abdomen (as opposed to the chest) contains many viscera that might cause a "succussion." Overall, a flat and upright film (which in gastric stasis will show air–fluid levels) is more valuable and dignified. Still, the splash has a (limited) role as a frugal way to screen for gastroparesis—especially in patients who get on our nerves.

115. Is there any role for auscultating the stomach?
Only to determine whether a nasogastric tube has been successfully placed in the stomach (if the tube is placed correctly, air injected through the tube produces a gurgling sound over the stomach). This maneuver, however, has limitations. Similarly limited is auscultation over the stomach (and lungs) after placement of an endotracheal tube.

F. THE PANCREAS

"Many a diabetic has stayed alive by stealing the bread denied him by his doctor."
M. H. Fischer (1879–1962), *Principles of Surgery*, Chapter V

116. What is the role of physical diagnosis in assessing the pancreas?
A very limited one since the organ traditionally has been off limits to physical diagnosis and still is. The major value of exam is in the occasional detection of massive pancreatic enlargements, such as pseudocysts and possibly cancer. As for acute pancreatitis, the role of bedside diagnosis is also limited, since *retroperitoneal subcutaneous hemorrhages* (traditional findings of acute hemorrhagic pancreatitis, visible on the abdominal wall as either Cullen's or Grey Turner's signs), are neither sensitive nor specific. Other findings of pancreatitis include:

- *Arching of the abdominal wall*, or Cupid's bow profile (*see* also question 3 and Fig. 15-2)
- *Tenderness to percussion of the thoracolumbar spine* (or to palpation of the left upper quadrant). The latter is seen in patients lying in the right lateral decubitus position and with knees flexed to the chest (Mallet-Guy's sign, from the French surgeon who first described it).
- *Sequelae of pancreatitis*. The most common is a pseudocyst, which may manifest as a visible deformation of the abdominal wall—palpable in 50% of the patients.

G. THE KIDNEYS

> *"Bones can break, muscle can atrophy, glands can loaf, even the brain can go to sleep,*
> *without immediately endangering our survival; but should the kidneys fail. . .*
> *neither bone, muscle, gland, nor brain could carry on."*
>
> Homer Smith, *From Fish to Philosopher,* Chapter 1

117. **What is the best way to assess renal size?**
Not physical exam. This is because the kidneys are hidden within the retroperitoneal fat, far from reach of prodding fingers (especially in the typical and overweight patient). Hence, exam should concede to ultrasound the assessment of renal size and keep for itself the detection of costophrenic tenderness in acute renal inflammation and the identification of arterial bruits in renal vascular disease.
   In the absence of ultrasound, various maneuvers of kidney palpation may be tried. Although these may detect polycystic kidney disease (*bilateral* renal enlargement) or hydronephrosis and carcinoma of the kidney (*unilateral* renal enlargement), they are difficult to perform and have low yield in patients who are not very thin.

118. **What is the value of testing for costophrenic tenderness?**
It is a good value. Percussion of costophrenic (or costovertebral) angles remains an excellent way to identify pyelonephritis or other conditions that distend the renal capsule and pelvis (like perinephric abscess and renal infarction, but stones, too—in fact, renal colic also may present with flank and costovertebral tenderness). Pioneered by J. B. Murphy, this technique served him well in differentiating renal from biliary, appendiceal, and pancreatic pathology.

119. **How do you percuss the costophrenic angle?**
By striking with the ulnar aspect of your hand the patient's flanks (between the lumbar column and costal margin). Alternatively, in Dr. Murphy's original method you could use both hands:

   [P]lace the left hand flat upon the back of the patient over the kidney region, care being taken to have the hand pressed firmly upon the back. The clenched right hand is then brought down *with considerable force* upon the dorsum of the fixed hand, and if an acute congestion, or urethral obstruction exists in that kidney, *the patient will cry out with the pain of the blow.* [Note that Prof. Murphy had probably studied at the Dr. Mengele's School of Medicine. Hence, be gentle....]

120. **What is the thumb pressure test?**
A variation on the theme, wherein costophrenic angle pressure is carried out by using the thumb. This maneuver may separate *renal* from *abdominal wall* tenderness; yet, like all other maneuvers, it has much greater specificity (80–100%) than sensitivity (15-80%).

121. **What are the physical findings of a renal colic?**
The most common is flank and costovertebral tenderness—a finding that also has greater specificity than sensitivity.

(1) Auscultation of the Kidneys

122. **What is the role of renal auscultation?**
An important one for detecting *renovascular* disease. Approximately one half of such patients will indeed have a systolic murmur, whose significance depends on *location* and characteristics:

- **Anterior systolic murmurs** are heard along an anterior horizontal band that crosses the umbilicus. Although quite sensitive, these have disappointing specificity for renovascular disease, with false positive rates as high as 30%—especially in hypertensive patients.
- **Posterior systolic murmurs** are instead localized to the area between the lumbar column and the costal margins. They are valuable only if present, since they have high specificity for renovascular disease (close to 100%), but very low sensitivity (10%).

123. What is the significance of anterior *bruits*?
Bruits (i.e., murmurs that typically extend beyond the second heart sound and thus are *continuous*) have a sensitivity of approximately 50% for renovascular disease, but this may reach 80–90% in hypertensive patients with fibromuscular hyperplasia of the renal artery. The bruit also is much more specific than the *systolic anterior murmur*, with false positive rates less than 7%.

Pearl:

Posterior murmurs are specific but not sensitive. Anterior murmurs are sensitive but not specific. Anterior bruits (i.e., continuous murmurs) are both specific and sensitive.

H. THE URINARY BLADDER

"You notice that the tabetic has the power of holding water for an indefinite period. He is also impotent—in fact two excellent properties to possess for a quiet day on the river."
Dr. Dunlop, Teaching at Charing Cross Hospital, London

124. What is the main purpose of physical diagnosis in assessing the urinary bladder?
Physical diagnosis can still detect a full bladder. Tools include *"subjective" palpation* and percussion, aided or unaided by auscultation (i.e., *auscultatory percussion*).

125. Is the urinary bladder palpable?
Only when distended—and only in thin patients or bladders fibrotic from radiation therapy.

126. What is "subjective" palpation of the bladder?
A good way to detect a full bladder. To carry it out, push *perpendicularly* (and gently) one finger into the patient's lower abdomen, starting at the umbilicus and then down toward the pubis in stepwise fashion. The test is positive when it causes an urge to urinate, indicating that the fundus of the bladder has been touched, and thus identifying the level of its distention.

127. How accurate is this technique?
It was evaluated in 50 consecutive patients undergoing cystoscopy. All 20 patients who experienced an urge to urinate after suprapubic palpation had at least 100 mL of urine in their bladder, and this even though only two of the bladders were objectively palpable and percussable. None of the 25 patients with negative findings had >200 mL of urine. Hence, when suprapubic pressure evokes a call to micturition, the bladder probably contains >100 mL of urine; whereas if it does *not* evoke an urge, the bladder probably contains <200 mL of urine.

128. What is the physical diagnosis gold standard for detecting a *full* bladder?
It remains percussion—either alone or coupled with auscultation:
Plain percussion: To carry this out, percuss rostrocaudally along the midline, from the umbilicus to the symphysis, until you reach a level of suprapubic dullness (corresponding to the fundus of the bladder). This is neither sensitive (it requires 400–600 mL of urine) nor

specific (many patients with suprapubic dullness do *not* have an enlarged bladder). And yet, in cases of sizable distention, the extent of suprapubic dullness *does* indeed correlate with bladder volume.

Auscultatory percussion: This is a combined percussive *and* auscultatory maneuver that can be used to localize the upper border of the bladder. To carry it out:

- Place the diaphragm of your stethoscope along the midline, just above the symphysis pubis.
- Administer "scratches" in a rostrocaudal fashion, by moving your finger along the vertical midline—from the umbilicus downward, 1 cm at a time.
- The point at which the scratching sound intensifies indicates a change in underlying tissue and thus locates the upper edge of the bladder.

129. **How accurate is auscultatory percussion?**
It depends. The likelihood of identifying a "full" bladder (defined as ≥250 mL of urine on catheterization) directly correlates with the distance above the symphysis pubis at which the percussion note changes. A distance of 6.5 cm or less has 0% likelihood, whereas a distance of 6.5–7.5 cm has 43% likelihood and >7.5 cm has 91% likelihood.

130. **How accurate is *plain* percussion in diagnosing a full bladder?**
Less sensitive than auscultatory percussion, since it requires at least 400–600 mL in order to yield suprapubic dullness. It also is nonspecific.

I. ASCITES (DROPSY)

"I walk as I were girdled with my spleen
And look as if my belly carried twins
Wretch that I am! I fear me I shall burst."

Plautus, Curculio, Act II, Scene I

131. **How useful is physical diagnosis of ascites?**
Quite useful. Maneuvers that can help physicians identify patients with ascites are still quite valuable, especially if combined.

132. **What is ascites?**
It is the presence of free fluid in the abdominal cavity. This is an important clinical finding, and like pleural effusion is usually the result of one of three problems: (1) *increased hydrostatic pressure* (from either right-sided or biventricular failure); (2) *decreased oncotic pressure,* from either protein loss (as in nephrosis and enteropathy)—or reduced synthesis (as in malnutrition and cirrhosis); or (3) *peritoneal inflammation* (either neoplastic or infectious).

133. **What are the best tools for diagnosing ascites?**
A focused history for sure, since this may provide important diagnostic information *even before resorting to physical exam.* Inquire about (1) *any current (or past) history of liver disease,* since this greatly increases the pretest probability of ascites and (2) *recent weight gain,* especially a change in abdominal girth or a new ankle edema. If absent, these two symptoms strongly argue against ascites, particularly in cases of an already low pretest probability of disease. For example, in patients with less than a 20% chance of having ascites (because of no liver disease by history), absence of recent ankle swelling lowers the likelihood to less than 2.5%.

> **Pearl:**
> Ascites is very unlikely in the absence of a recent increase in abdominal girth and extremely unlikely in the absence of recent ankle edema (particularly in male patients).

134. **What are the causes of ankle edema in ascites?**
They are both *hydraulic causes* (compression of leg veins by the ascitic fluid) and *oncotic* (concomitant hypoalbuminemia, frequently encountered in either hepatic or renal disease).

135. **What is the role of physical diagnosis in assessing ascites?**
It provides a quick, convenient, and inexpensive tool. Yet, exam is only valuable for large volumes of fluid (500–1000 mL). For smaller amounts, the gold standard remains ultrasound, which can detect as little as 100 mL of fluid at a cheaper cost than CT.

136. **What bedside maneuvers may be used to detect ascites?**
The classic four are: (1) inspection for bulging flanks, (2) percussion for flank dullness, (3) the shifting-dullness maneuver, and (4) the fluid-wave test. In addition, three other maneuvers have been found to be useful: the ballottement sign and two maneuvers that are instead an application of *auscultatory percussion* (the puddle sign and Guarino's variation).

137. **What are *bulging flanks*?**
They are not a reference to Mae West's silhouette, but rather to the peculiar abdominal shape of a supine patient with ascites. Because of the weight of intra-abdominal fluid (and the effect of gravity on fluid), the flanks of ascitic patients who lay supine are pushed outward, almost like the belly of a frog. This same shape, however, also may be seen in patients who are simply obese. To separate them, one has to resort to the flank-dullness maneuver.

138. **How does one percuss for *flank dullness*?**
By tapping the abdomen in a radiating pattern, from the umbilicus toward the flanks and symphysis. Since gas-filled intestinal loops (resonant) float on top of ascites (dull), the maneuver reveals a periumbilical rounded area of tympany, flanked by two areas of dullness. Tympany and dullness are separated by a *horizontal* border.

> **Pearl:**
> Bulging flanks and flank dullness are both very sensitive ($\geq$72% and $\geq$80%, respectively) but poorly specific for ascites, thus unable to separate it from other conditions.

139. **How is the *shifting-dullness* maneuver performed?**
Ask the patient to lie supine. Then percuss the abdomen along one flank—from the umbilicus downward. Mark the level at which the percussion note turns from resonant to dull, and then ask the patient to roll over on the right side. Once the patient is in the right lateral decubitus position (and supported by a 45-degree–angle pillow), restart the percussion sequence. A gravity-dependent shift in dullness of at least 1 cm (with the shifting border still remaining horizontal) indicates that the dullness is due to fluid, whereas absence of a shift indicates that the dullness is due to a solid organ. Once again, tympany and dullness remain separated by a *horizontal* border (Fig. 15-16).

140. **How accurate is this test?**
It, too, has good sensitivity ($\geq$83% in two separate studies, indicating the presence of at least 500–1000 mL of fluid), but low specificity (although one study yielded 90% specificity, a more accurate figure is probably 50%, with the most common confounder being the colonic fluid accumulation of patients with diarrhea). Nonetheless, due to its high sensitivity, a negative shifting dullness *argues strongly against the presence of gross ascites*.

141. **How is the *fluid-wave* maneuver performed?**
It requires two examiners, or one examiner assisted by the patient. With the patient supine, place one hand on one flank and tap gently on the opposite flank. In the meantime, ask the

other examiner (if available) to place the ulnar surface of *both* hands over the patient's umbilicus and along the abdominal vertical midline (from the xiphoid process to the symphysis pubis). This is done to prevent a false positive fluid wave, which may occur whenever flickering of the abdominal wall creates ripples of mesenteric fat (not of ascites) toward the contralateral side. If an assistant is unavailable, ask the patient to place the ulnar surface of one hand vertically over the umbilicus. The test is positive when you feel a fluid wave emanating into the contralateral side. This has to be of moderate to strong intensity. *Slight* fluid waves have high interobserver variability and should not be relied on for diagnosing ascites (*see* Fig. 15-17).

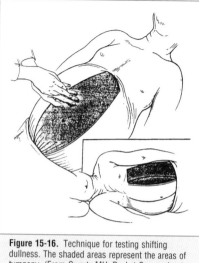

Figure 15-16. Technique for testing shifting dullness. The shaded areas represent the areas of tympany. (From Swartz MH: Pocket Companion to Textbook of Physical Diagnosis. Philadelphia, WB Saunders, 1995.)

142. **How reliable is this test?**
    Quite reliable, with specificity of 80–90%. In fact, this is probably *the only truly specific* bedside test for ascites. Hence, a positive fluid wave can help *ruling in* the disease. If negative, though, it should *not* exclude it, since its sensitivity is just 50% (it detects only large volumes).

143. **What is the *ballottement* (or dipping) maneuver?**
    Another bedside test for ascites, and not a particularly sensitive one. To carry it out, roll the patient's body toward the side of the organ to be palpated (usually the liver or spleen). Then apply with your fingers a quick pushing motion to the chosen organ. The test is positive when it elicits a feeling of displaced fluid before your fingers can actually touch the organ in question.

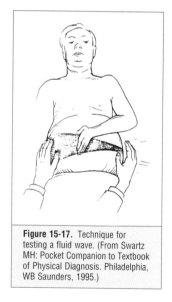

Figure 15-17. Technique for testing a fluid wave. (From Swartz MH: Pocket Companion to Textbook of Physical Diagnosis. Philadelphia, WB Saunders, 1995.)

144. **What is the *puddle sign*? How is it elicited?**
    It is a sign of *auscultatory percussion,* performed by asking patients first to lie on their belly for 5 minutes and then eventually to raise themselves by supporting their body weight on the knees and stretched forearms (Fig. 15-18). As a result, the middle portion of the abdomen becomes pendulous and dependent. At this point, you should place the diaphragm of your stethoscope over the lowest abdominal area, while at the same time flicking a finger over a localized flank area. Then gradually move your stethoscope over the opposite flank. The test is positive when there is a sudden increase in intensity and clarity of the sound, signaling that the stethoscope has passed the edge of the peritoneal fluid.

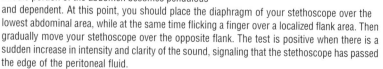

Pearl:

> This test was initially reported as having high sensitivity (capable of detecting as little as 140 mL of fluid). In reality, the sensitivity is much lower (40–50%), especially for small amounts of ascites. Moreover, the test is cumbersome and difficult to perform. Therefore, it cannot be recommended in the routine evaluation of patients with ascites.

145. **What is the *Guarino's variation*?**
It is a maneuver that has been reported too recently for adequate validation. It consists of having the patient sit or stand for 3 minutes after voiding. This allows free abdominal fluid to gravitate into the pelvis. The examiner then places the stethoscope in the abdominal midline, immediately above the pubic crest, while at the same time percussing the abdomen (by finger-flicking) from the costal margin downward and perpendicularly toward the pelvis, along three or more vertical lines. Normally, the level where the percussion note turns from dull to loud is the pelvic border, just where the stethoscope resides. In patients with free fluid, however, this level is clearly raised above the pelvic baseline.

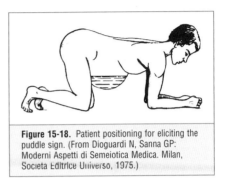

Figure 15-18. Patient positioning for eliciting the puddle sign. (From Dioguardi N, Sanna GP: Moderni Aspetti di Semeiotica Medica. Milan, Societa Editrice Universo, 1975.)

146. **What is the overall accuracy of these signs for ascites?**
No single sign is both sensitive *and* specific. Many, however, are quite sensitive *or* quite specific. Moreover, their detection has little interobserver variability, suggesting that physicians tend to agree on their presence or absence. Overall, the two most useful signs to *rule in* ascites in patients with abdominal distention are (1) a positive fluid wave and (2) a history of ankle edema. The least useful signs to *rule in* a diagnosis of ascites are (1) the puddle sign and (2) auscultatory percussion. Conversely, the two most useful signs to *rule out* ascites are: (1) absence of ankle swelling (or increased abdominal girth) and (2) absence of flank dullness.

147. **How can one improve the diagnostic accuracy of these maneuvers?**
By combining them. For example, fluid-wave has low sensitivity (50%) but high specificity (80–90%), whereas shifting-dullness has high sensitivity (≥83%) but low specificity (55%).

Pearl:

> Hence, combining these maneuvers provides a decent bedside tool for the diagnosis of ascites, with overall accuracy of 80%. Still, the amount of volume necessary for them to become positive (500–1000 mL) is much larger than that detected by ultrasound alone (100 mL).

148. **What is the role of the Bayes' theorem in diagnosing ascites at the bedside?**
A very important one, since interpreting each maneuver in light of the pretest probability of disease is the best way to improve accuracy. Because the predictive value of any test (including

physical diagnosis) depends on the prevalence of the disorder in the population undergoing the test, a positive test in patients with low prevalence of the disease is more likely to represent a false positive than a true positive (like a positive pregnancy test in a man). This can be extended to the positive predictive values of shifting-dullness and fluid-wave for ascites. Hence, a prominent fluid wave has a high positive predictive value for ascites (96%) in patients with prolonged prothrombin time (PT), but a much lower one (48%) in patients with normal PT. Conversely, absence of shifting dullness makes ascites very unlikely in patients with normal PT (2%). Thus, a focused physical examination based on just two maneuvers (shifting-dullness and fluid-wave) and interpreted In light of patients' pretest probability of disease (as based on PT) can allow physicians to use ultrasound more judiciously and cost effectively (*see* Table 15-2).

TABLE 15-2. DIAGNOSIS OF ASCITES		
Maneuver	Sensitivity (%)	Specificity (%)
History		
Increased abdominal girth	90	60
Recent weight gain	60	70
Ankle swelling	100	60
Physical examination		
Bulging flanks	70	60
Flank dullness	80	60
Shifting dullness	90	60
Fluid wave	60	90
Puddle sign	50	70

Pearl:

In summary, patients with history of liver disease, prolonged PT, and positive fluid wave are very likely to have ascites and do not need an ultrasound for confirmation. Conversely, patients with normal PT and no shifting dullness are unlikely to have ascites even if they have a history of liver disease. Thus, they do not need an ultrasound.

J. THE ACUTE ABDOMEN (PERITONEAL SIGNS)

*"The abdomen is like a stage
enclosed within a fleshy cage,
The symptoms are the actors who
Although they are a motley crew
Act often with consummate art
The major of the minor part;
Nor do they usually say
Who is the author of the play.
That is for you to try and guess
A problem which, I must confess*

is made less easy for the fact
You seldom see the opening act,
And by the time that you arrive
The victim may be just alive"
      Sir Zachary Cope, *The Acute Abdomen in Rhyme*, 5th ed. London, HK Lewis, 1972

149. Summarize the role of physical examination in patients with peritonitis.
It is crucial for the identification of surgical "abdomens." To this end, a set of bedside maneuvers has been developed over the years to help diagnosis, and remains valuable even in our times of magnetic resonance imaging (MRI) and CT scan. Still, individual capabilities play an important role in the success (or failure) of these techniques.

150. What are the most commonly used maneuvers for the bedside evaluation of peritonitis?
- Guarding/rigidity
- Abdominal wall tenderness
- Rebound tenderness

151. What is *guarding*?
It is a diffuse (or localized) tension of the abdominal wall. This muscular stiffness can be *involuntary* (and thus commonly referred to as *rigidity*) or *voluntary*. In the latter case, it is usually elicited by pressure from the examiner's fingertips. Voluntary guarding does not necessarily indicate peritoneal inflammation, since it also can result from the patient's anxiety or the examiner's cold hands. As a peritoneal sign, it is more sensitive than *rigidity* but less specific.

152. What is the significance of *"localized"* rigidity?
It refers to a focal area of peritonitis. In this case, the stiffness of the abdominal wall is limited to the region overlying the inflamed viscus. A good example of localized rigidity is the absence of respiratory motion in selective parts of the abdominal wall.

153. What is "induced guarding"? How can it be triggered?
Induced guarding is an *induced tension of the abdominal wall*. To trigger it, ask the patient to raise the head above the pillow until (s)he can touch the chest with the chin. This tenses the abdominal musculature, forming a sort of cuirass that protects any inflamed intra-abdominal organ against the examiner's hand. Induced guarding can be used for eliciting Carnett's sign.

154. What is Carnett's sign?
It is a maneuver that uses *induced guarding* to differentiate the abdominal tenderness of an inflamed intra-abdominal *viscus* from that of an inflamed abdominal *wall*. To carry it out, first localize by palpation the area of tenderness. Then ask the patient to contract his or her abdominal muscles by raising the head from the couch. While the patient does so, maintain pressure on your examining fingers, and then ask whether there was any change in tenderness. An abdominal wall pain would *increase* (positive Carnett's sign), whereas pain from an intra-abdominal viscus would *decrease* (negative Carnett's sign). The sign was first described by Carnett in 1926.

155. What is *abdominal wall tenderness* (AWT)?
It is a variation of Carnett's sign, also called *modified induced guarding*. As for the previous maneuver, first identify the site of maximal abdominal tenderness with the patient lying flat and relaxed. Then, with your examining hand still in place, ask the patient to cross arms and sit forward. While the patient is *midway between a sitting and recumbent position* (and with the

anterior abdominal wall muscles being tensed), renew pressure on the previously tender spot. The test is positive when pain is increased at midway (positive abdominal wall tenderness) but negative if the pain is actually improved (negative abdominal wall tenderness).

156. What is the significance of a positive abdominal wall tenderness?

Very much the same as Carnett's sign. Pain on palpation may arise from the abdominal wall, the parietal peritoneum, or an underlying viscus. Tensing the abdominal muscles allows the physician to separate the first from the other two. If tenderness on palpation is increased by abdominal muscular tension (positive abdominal wall tenderness), the pain originates from the abdominal wall itself because tensing the wall will protect the parietal peritoneum and the intra-abdominal viscera against the prodding of the examiner's hand.

157. What are the causes of abdominal wall tenderness?

They are mysterious. A common one is diabetic neuropathy of the lower thoracic segments, associated with abdominal wall hyperesthesia and weakness. Other causes include muscular strain, viral myositis, fibrositis, nerve entrapment, and trauma. Still, the most important value of a positive AWT is that it argues against intra-abdominal or peritoneal pathology.

158. Does the AWT maneuver have limitations?

1. It should not be used in children or elderly patients (because of the risk of misinterpretation).
2. It is useless and inhumane in patients with diffuse abdominal pain who already have rigidity.
3. It is possibly dangerous in patients with intra-abdominal abscess, since this may burst.

159. When should one use the AWT maneuver?

Whenever laparotomy is considered in patients with acute abdominal pain, and always in the clinical context and in the setting of periodic reexaminations.

160. How accurate is the modified induced guarding technique (AWT)?

The AWT sign has been extensively studied and found to be clinically useful in the evaluation of either *acute* or *chronic* abdominal pain. Thomson and Francis used it in 120 patients admitted as surgical emergencies for acute localized abdominal pain. Only 1 of the 24 patients with positive AWT had an intra-abdominal inflammatory process (acute appendicitis). Conversely, all 96 with a negative test had intra-abdominal pathology. Gray et al. studied 158 patients admitted for acute abdominal pain. They found AWT to be less accurate, being present in only 28% of patients *without* intra-abdominal pathology (true positive) and 5% of patients with intra-abdominal pathology (false positive). They also found a predominance of young females among patients with positive AWT and no intra-abdominal pathology. Finally, Thomson et al. revisited this sign for the evaluation of chronic abdominal pain. Patients with positive AWT tended to undergo a great deal of studies (including surgical procedures) but only a minority turned out to have serious pathology. Hence, *the AWT sign is quite useful in differentiating peritonitis or intra-abdominal pathology from inflammation of the abdominal wall.*

161. What is *rebound tenderness*?

It is severe pain of the abdominal wall that is indirectly elicited by the *sudden release of hand pressure*. This maneuver (also called Blumberg's sign) is carried out by palpating an area of tenderness as gently but as deeply as allowed, and by then suddenly releasing pressure. This will make the elastic abdominal wall spring back into its baseline position, thus eliciting an exquisite (and localized) pain whenever there is localized peritonitis (with the pain being caused by the sudden tension of the inflamed peritoneum). A less painful alternative may be a *light indirect percussion* over the area of pain. Still, rebound tenderness has modest sensitivity and specificity, is painful, and is totally unnecessary in patients who already have guarding or rigidity.

162. **Who was Blumberg?**

Jacob Moritz Blumberg (1873–1955) was a German surgeon and gynecologist, who trained both in Germany and England, where he investigated methods of surgical sterilization and even invented a type of rubber glove that became widely used. He fought with the German Army during World War I, managing to control a typhus epidemic in a prisoners of war camp by delousing 10,000 Russian prisoners in only a few days. After the war, he returned to his surgical practice in Berlin, where he founded a radiology institute and organized many prenatal clinics. With the rise of the Nazis, he eventually left Germany and moved to England, where he resumed his medical work with considerable success.

163. **What is the *referred* rebound tenderness test?**

It is a more humane variant of Blumberg's sign and also a more correct application of the original technique. In this case, the examiner first compresses and then releases the abdominal wall of the quadrant *contralateral* to the one where the patient has pain. The maneuver is positive only when it elicits pain *in the site where the patient originally felt it*. Pain at the site of palpation represents instead a negative test. Yet, this should not rule out localized peritonitis and thus must be followed by a rebound tenderness maneuver *over the painful area*.

164. **What is a cough test?**

It is the sudden increase in abdominal pain caused by a brisk rise in intra-abdominal pressure, such as the one elicited by coughing. The maneuver is indicative of peritonitis, but since it has greater sensitivity than specificity, is more valuable when absent than present.

165. **What is jar tenderness?**

It is another maneuver aimed at detecting (and localizing) peritoneal irritation, very much like the cough test. First described by Dr. Markle, it is carried out in the ambulatory setting by asking the patient to first stand on outstretched toes and then let his or her body weight fall on the heels. The maneuver sets the abdominal wall into motion, thus allowing the patient to localize any area of pain. In addition to being a bit cruel, it is of obvious limited value in patients too ill to stand.

166. **What is the role of a Valsalva maneuver in patients with acute abdomen?**

It is another way to heighten peritoneal pain by inducing a sudden distention of the abdominal wall. This, in turn, may help the patient better identify a particular area of tenderness. For example, a 20-second Valsalva may allow someone with acute appendicitis to pinpoint the area of pain. Hence, it may be used to screen (very much like the cough test and the jar tenderness) and to guide (and possibly avoid) more painful tests—like rebound tenderness.

167. **What is the stethoscope sign?**

It is a sign elicited by palpating the abdomen twice, first with your hands and then with your stethoscope. When doing it with the stethoscope, you should preinform the patient that you are only trying to listen to the abdomen. This seems to have a distracting effect, often allowing you to compress the anterior abdominal wall all the way down in cases of unreal or exaggerated pain, when just a few seconds before there was flinching, grimacing, complaining, and quick abdominal tension in preparation for even the lightest finger touch.

168. **How reliable is this sign?**

It has not been studied prospectively. There is, however, a case report of a false positive outcome in a patient with acute appendicitis. As always, things should be evaluated in the context of the clinical picture and within the realm of periodic observation.

169. **While performing these maneuvers, should you look at the patient's face or abdomen?**
At the patient's face. It is essential that you observe facial expression while testing for guarding or rebound tenderness. Any grimacing/reaction is often the only clue to an acute abdomen.

170. **What is the closed-eyes sign?**
It is the peculiar face of patients with nonspecific abdominal pain (i.e., without a clear-cut intra-abdominal pathology), who often keep their eyes closed during abdominal palpation, with an embalmed and almost beatific smile. This is quite different from patients with true intra-abdominal pathology, who keep their eyes wide open, always monitoring what you are doing.

171. **Explain the use and cause of a closed-eyes sign.**
It is a relatively accurate test for nonspecific abdominal pain. It is not clear why patients with no intra-abdominal pathology should keep their eyes closed. It may be because, unlike patients with true pathology, they might not need to monitor the physician's hand to avoid unnecessary pain. It also is possible that they may be aware (either consciously or unconsciously) that palpation will *not* produce severe pain, implying that their pain has a psychologic cause. Either way, a positive closed-eyes sign suggests no intra-abdominal pathology.

172. **How accurate is the closed-eyes sign in diagnosing nonspecific abdominal pain?**
Gray et al. studied it in 158 consecutive patients admitted for acute abdominal pain. Eyes were closed in 6/91 patients with true pathology (6.5%) and 22/67 patients with no pathology (33%); 22/28 patients with closed-eyes were females (p <0.01), usually young. In summary, the predictive power of a positive closed-eyes test is 79% and that of a negative test is 65%.

173. **What is abdominal hyperesthesia?**
It is hypersensitivity (hyperesthesia) to light touch in areas that overlie an inflamed viscus.

174. **How can one detect abdominal hypersensitivity?**
One can easily identify areas of *hyperalgesia* (increased pain) by lightly drawing across the abdominal wall with a cotton wisp, a pin, or even a fingernail. Head was the first to describe these areas of hypersensitivity. Since then, they have been referred to as *Head's zones* (*see* Fig. 15-19).

175. **Is abdominal hyperesthesia specific to localized peritonitis?**
No. It also may occur in herpes *zoster* (where it precedes the cutaneous rash by several days) and at times even in *peptic ulcer disease* (as an area of localized midepigastric tenderness).

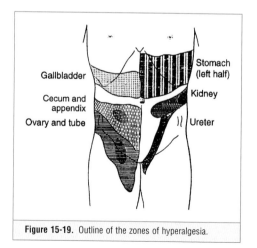

Figure 15-19. Outline of the zones of hyperalgesia.

> **Pearl:**
> In an endoscopic study of 88 patients with peptic ulcer disease, this sign was found to be an insensitive indicator, being present in many normal people and patients with either functional disorders or abdominal wall tenderness.

176. **What is Boas' sign?**
It is abdominal hyperesthesia as applied to the gallbladder. In Boas' sign, patients with acute cholecystitis experience referred pain and hyperesthesia of the right costophrenic angle (which is indeed the referred site for gallbladder pain). Even a light touch in this area will elicit exquisite tenderness. The sign, unfortunately, has very low sensitivity (only 7%).

177. **Who was Boas?**
Ismar I. Boas (1858–1938) was a German gastroenterologist and the author of an acclaimed textbook on stomach diseases. After a brief stint in general practice, he joined the Augusta Hospital Faculty in Berlin, where building on Kussmaul's recently introduced gastric tube, he used the test-meal to measure gastric secretion. He also became the first to recognize "occult blood" and its diagnostic importance. A world leader in his field, Boas was the founder of the German Gastroenterological Society. After Hitler's ascent to power, he left Berlin for Vienna in 1936, dying there the year Austria was annexed to the Reich.

K. SPECIAL PROBLEMS—APPENDICITIS

178. **Which maneuvers can be used for evaluating patients with suspected appendicitis?**
- McBurney's sign
- Rovsing's sign
- Obturator test
- Reverse psoas maneuver
- Rectal tenderness

179. **What is McBurney's sign?**
It is maximum tenderness and rigidity elicited by pressure of one finger over McBurney's *point*. This is located 1.5–2 inches medial to the right anterosuperior iliac spine, on a line that joins it to the umbilicus. Although most patients with appendicitis have right lower quadrant tenderness, tenderness in the McBurney's point has slightly better specificity (75–85%).

180. **Who was McBurney?**
Charles McBurney (1845–1913) was a graduate of Harvard and the New York College of Physicians, who became one of the leaders of 19th-century American surgery. Surgeon-in-chief at the Roosevelt Hospital of New York, he presented his classic report on the advantages of early intervention in patients with appendicitis before the 1889 meeting of the New York Surgical Society. In it he described the area of greatest abdominal pain that still carries his name. Five years later, he described instead the incision he used for patients with appendicitis, still called McBurney's incision. An avid hunter and fisherman, McBurney died of myocardial infarction at age 68, while on a hunting trip.

181. **What is Rovsing's sign?**
It is pain in the *right* iliac fossa, elicited by pressure over the *left* lower quadrant (indirect tenderness). This finding has similar specificity, but slightly lower sensitivity than McBurney's.

182. **Who was Rovsing?**

Neils T. Rovsing (1862–1927) was a professor of surgery at the University of Copenhagen, who wrote extensively on gallbladder and bladder diseases, eventually becoming a surgical leader in Denmark. He also was an entrepreneur, who acquired a financial interest in a medical journal that he subsequently owned and finally presented to the Danish Medical Society. Forced to retire in 1926 due to heart disease, he died 1 year later of carcinoma of the larynx.

183. **What is the *obturator test*?**

It is a test carried out by asking patients to flex the hip and rotate it internally while lying supine. Examiners can help this movement by pulling the patient's ankle toward themselves while pushing the knee away. The maneuver should be carried out on both thighs and should remain painless. Pain (usually referred to the suprapubic region) indicates inflammation in one of the organs surrounding the *obturator internus muscle* and is therefore specific (but poorly sensitive) for retrocaecal appendicitis. The obturator test (*see* Fig. 15-20) also may be positive in various obstetric-gynecologic conditions of intrapelvic pus; yet in these cases the test is usually positive in *both* legs, whereas in appendicitis, it is only positive in the right leg.

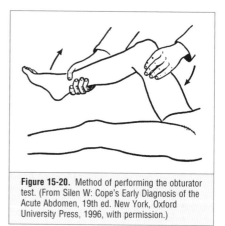

Figure 15-20. Method of performing the obturator test. (From Silen W: Cope's Early Diagnosis of the Acute Abdomen, 19th ed. New York, Oxford University Press, 1996, with permission.)

184. **What is the *reverse psoas maneuver*?**

It is another test of irritation of the iliopsoas muscle, either because of retrocaecal appendicitis or some other localized collection of pus and blood. It is performed by having the patient roll toward the left side and hyper-extend the right hip (*see* Fig. 15-21). The test is positive when it elicits pain. Like the obturator test, it has very low sensitivity for appendicitis, but high specificity. Still, given the low sensitivity, both maneuvers are of limited clinical value.

185. **What is *rectal tenderness*?**

It is tenderness on rectal exam elicited in patients with appendicitis confined to the pelvis. It is only helpful in patients with perforation, whose rectal exam reveals a right-sided tender mass representing the pelvic abscess.

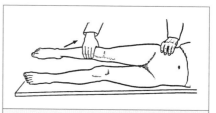

Figure 15-21. Method of performing the iliopsoas test. (From Silen W: Cope's Early Diagnosis of the Acute Abdomen, 19th ed. New York, Oxford University Press, 1996, with permission.)

SELECTED BIBLIOGRAPHY

1. Aldea PA, Meehan JP, Sternbach G, et al: The acute abdomen and Murphy's signs. J Emerg Med 4:57–63, 1986.

2. Arkles LB, Gill GD, Molan MP: A palpable spleen is not necessarily enlarged or pathological. Med J Aust 145:15–17, 1986.

3. Ashby EC: Detecting bladder fullness by subjective palpation. Lancet 2:936–937, 1977.

4. Barkun AN, Camus M, Meagher T, et al: Splenomegaly and Traube's space: How useful is percussion?. Am J Med 87:562–566, 1989.

5. Barkun AN, Camus M, Green L, et al: Bedside assessment of splenic enlargement. Am J Med 91:512–518, 1991.

6. Castell DO, O'Brien KD, Muench H, Chalmers TC: Estimation of liver size by percussion in normal individuals. Ann Intern Med 70:1183–1189, 1969.

7. Castell DO: The spleen percussion sign. Ann Intern Med 67:1265–1267, 1967.

8. Cattau EL Jr, Benjamin SB, Knuff TE, et al: The accuracy of the physical examination in the diagnosis of suspected ascites. JAMA 247:1164–1166, 1982.

9. Chen JJ, Changchien CS, Tai DI, et al: Gallbladder volume in patients with common hepatic duct dilatation: An evaluation of Courvoisier's sign by ultrasonography. Scand J Gastroenterol 29:284–288, 1994.

10. Chervu A, Clagett GP, Valentine RJ, et al: Role of physical examination in detection of abdominal aortic aneurysms. Surgery 117:454–457, 1995.

11. Chung RS: Pathogenesis of the Courvoisier's gallbladder. Dig Dis Sci 28:33–38, 1983.

12. Cummings S, Papadakis M, Melnick J, et al: Predictive value of physical examination for ascites. West J Med 142:633–636, 1985.

13. Dowdall GG: Five diagnostic methods of John B. Murphy of Chicago. Arch Diag 3:18–21, 1910.

14. Espinoza P, Ducot B, Pellettier G: Interobserver agreement in the physical diagnosis of alcoholic liver disease. Dig Dis Sci 32:244–247, 1987.

15. Gray DW, Dixon JM, Seabrook G, et al: Is abdominal wall tenderness a useful sign in the diagnosis of non-specific abdominal pain?. Ann Coll Surg Engl 70:2333–2334, 1988.

16. Gray DW, Dixon JM, Collin J, et al: The closed eyes sign. BMJ 297:837, 1988.

17. Guarino JR: Auscultatory percussion to detect ascites. N Engl J Med 315:1555–1556, 1986.

18. Guarino JR: Auscultatory percussion of the bladder to detect urinary retention. Arch Intern Med 145:1823–1825, 1985.

19. Halpern S, Coel M, Ashburn W, et al: Correlation of liver and spleen size: Determinations by nuclear medicine studies and physical examination. Arch Intern Med 134:123–124, 1974.

20. Kelley ML: Discolorations of flanks and abdominal wall. Arch Intern Med 108:132–135, 1961.

21. Lawson JD, Weissbein AS: The puddle sign—an aid in the diagnosis of minimal ascites. N Engl J Med 260:652–654, 1959.

22. Lederle FA, Simel DL: Does this patient have abdominal aortic aneurysm?. JAMA 281:77–82, 1999.

23. Lipp WF, Eckstein EH, Aaron AH, et al: The clinical significance of palpable spleen. Gastroenterology 3:287–291, 1944.

24. Ludwig Courvoisier (1843–1918). Courvoisier's sign. JAMA 204:165, 1968.

25. McGee S: Percussion and physical diagnosis: Separating myth from science. Disease-a-Month 41:643–692, 1995.

26. McGee S: Evidence-Based Physical Diagnosis. Philadelphia, WB Saunders, 2001.

27. McLean ACJ: Diagnosis of ascites by auscultatory percussion and hand-held ultrasound. Lancet 2:1526–1527, 1987.

28. Mellinkoff SM: Stethoscope sign. N Engl J Med 271:630, 1964.

29. Meyers MA, Feldberg MA, Oliphant M: Grey Turner's and Cullen's sign in acute pancreatitis. GI Radiol 14:31–37, 1989.

30. Naylor CD: Physical examination of the liver. JAMA 271:1859–1865, 1994.

31. Nixon RK: The detection of splenomegaly by percussion. N Engl J Med 250:166–167, 1954.

32. Parrino TA: The art and science of percussion. Hosp Pract 99:25–36, 1987.

33. Ralls PW, Halls J, Lapin SA, et al: Murphy's sign in cholecystitis. Radiol Clin North Am 21:477–493, 1983.

34. Simel DL, Halvorsen RA Jr, Feussner JR, et al: Clinical evaluation of ascites. J Gen Intern Med 3:423–428, 1988.

35. Tucker WN, Saab S, Rickman LS, et al: Scratch test is unreliable for detecting liver edge. J Clin Gastroenterol 25:410–414, 1997.

36. Williams JW, Simel DL: Does this patient have ascites? JAMA 267:2645–2648, 1992.

37. Zoli M, Magalotti D, Grimaldi M, et al: Physical examination of the liver: Still worth it? Am J Gastroenterol 90:1428–1432, 1995.

CHAPTER 16

MALE GENITALIA, HERNIAS, AND RECTAL EXAM

Salvatore Mangione, MD

> *"God gave Man the penis and the brain as His two greatest gifts.*
> *Unfortunately, He made it so that Man could only use one at a time."*
>
> —Robin Williams

GENERALITIES

Examination of male genitalia and the rectum is an important but often overlooked part of physical examination, usually conducted rather quickly at the end. There is no gain in being prudish about it (or, even worse, skipping it altogether, while documenting in the chart: *patient refused*). In fact, a wealth of information can be garnered.

A. MALE GENITALIA

1. **What are the main components of the male reproductive system?**
   The penis, the scrotum (with testicle, epididymis, and deferens), the seminal vesicles, and the prostate (Fig. 16-1).

2. **What is the best technique for examining male genitalia?**
   The same as for examining the rectum: with the patient either standing up or lying down on one side. Still, it is probably easier to assess the testes (and search for hernias) with the patient standing up and the examiner seated in front of him.

3. **What should I focus on during inspection of this region?**
   - Any obvious penile, scrotal, or perineal abnormalities
   - Inguinal bulges/scars suggestive of current or past hernias

(1) Penis

4. **Describe the anatomy of the penis.**
   The penis consists of a *shaft,* formed by three juxtaposed columns of spongy and vascular tissue: the *corpora cavernosa.* These can be temporarily filled with blood, thus providing a unique erectile capacity to the organ. The distal tip of the penis consists of a cone-shaped structure called the *glans* ("acorn" in Latin), which contains the vertical slit-like opening of the urethra *(urethral meatus).* The glans is separated from the shaft by a circular sulcus called the *corona* ("crown" in Latin), which in uncircumcised men is covered in a hood-like fashion by the *prepuce or foreskin,* a fold surgically removed during circumcision. All areas must be examined (*see* Fig. 16-2).

5. **What steps should I take to properly examine the penis?**
   The first, of course, is precautionary: put on a pair of gloves because some sexually transmitted diseases (including syphilis) can be acquired through simple skin abrasions. With

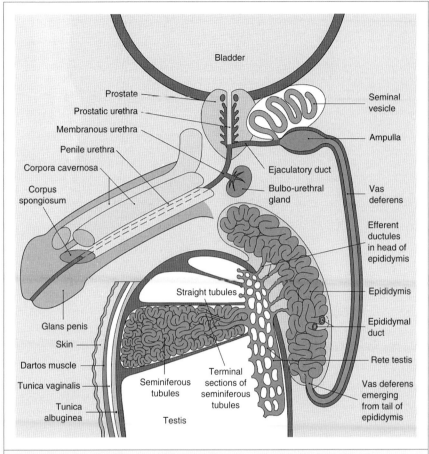

Figure 16-1. Male pelvic anatomy. (From Meszaros G: Crash Course Endocrine and Reproductive Systems. St. Louis, Mosby, 2006.)

gloves on, examine the penis by first palpating the shaft, and then by carefully looking for areas of induration or tenderness. Then, look for unusual curvatures (*see* Peyronie's disease, question 47). Retract the prepuce to gain access to the *glans,* and inspect it for abnormalities. After completing the exam, return the foreskin to its original position since failure to do so may cause severe edema in unconscious patients. Finally, gently compress the glans between your thumb and forefinger to visualize the urethral meatus, and possibly express secretions. Note that this maneuver may be unyielding *even in patients with a history of penile discharge.* In this case, milk the shaft of the penis (from its base to the glans), since this may produce a few precious drops for analysis. Finally, examine the base of the penis for hair or skin abnormalities.

6. **What is priapism?**
   A fancy term for a protracted erection, usually associated with pain. If we look back at the American presidency, we might conclude that priapism qualifies as a White House

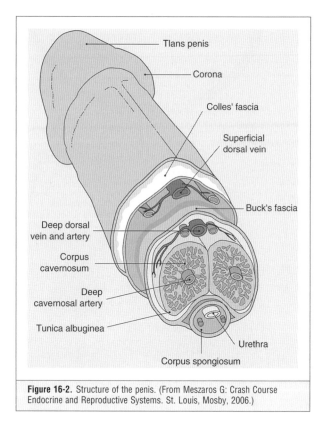

Figure 16-2. Structure of the penis. (From Meszaros G: Crash Course Endocrine and Reproductive Systems. St. Louis, Mosby, 2006.)

occupational hazard, were it not for the fact that this condition is usually *not* associated with sexual desire. The term "priapism" is actually rooted in Greek mythology, specifically in Priapus, one of the many illegitimate sons of Zeus, King of the Gods (which confirms our suspicion that power and sex may be linked, at least among American presidents and Greek deities). According to tradition, Hera (Zeus' unfortunate wife) found out about this umpteenth illicit affair of her husband and decided to attend the child's birth, to cast a mortal spell on the baby. Things, however, did not go as expected, since Priapus was born so well endowed that Hera, taken by surprise, completely missed her chance. Hence, the baby was rushed to safety, and a new medical term was born. Priapism eventually came to signify a condition characterized by chronic, protracted, and painful erections. Still, Priapus also prompted great respect for the penis, which became a symbol not only of fertility, but also of luck, since it had literally saved his owner's life. From that time on, Romans developed a penchant for wearing little phalluses around their neck, usually made in coral (because of its apotropaic virtue [i.e., the ability to ward off the evil eye]), but occasionally also in gold. They also carved phalluses on buildings—as hopeful lucky charms. For example, the great Roman wall erected (no pun intended) in England by Emperor Hadrian during the 1st century AD was riddled with various penile carvings, still visible today and accurately catalogued in local museums by serious British archeologists. Stone phalluses were supposed to bring good luck to the wall's defenders but unfortunately fell short of expectations: Hadrian's wall was pierced by raiding Scots and Picts and eventually abandoned. The reverence for the penis, however, continued unabated throughout the Mediterranean basin. Indeed, in some parts of Italy and Greece (not to mention South

Philadelphia) it is still possible to see golden pricklets hanging from people's necks, a reminder of the long-lasting value of Greek mythology and penile lore.

7. What is the pathophysiology of priapism?
It is a persistent erection of the corpora cavernosa of the penis, due to disturbances in the mechanisms controlling penile detumescence.

8. Does priapism involve all erectile tissue?
No. Only the corpora cavernosa of the penis. The one surrounding the urethra and the corpus spongiosum of the glans remains instead flaccid.

9. What is the cause of priapism?
Often idiopathic. Yet, priapism also may reflect systemic or local abnormalities:
- **Local conditions** are usually neoplastic or inflammatory diseases of the shaft, but also thrombotic and/or hemorrhagic processes of the penile vasculature (i.e., *arterial* high-flow priapism).
- **Systemic conditions** are instead either neurologic lesions (spinal cord injury and spinal anesthesia) or various hematologic disorders that predispose to thrombosis, like leukemia or sickle cell anemia (which are therefore responsible for *veno-occlusive* priapism). In one study, close to one half of sickle cell patients reported at least one episode of priapism. Finally, the condition also has been reported after recent infection by *Mycoplasma pneumoniae*, possibly because of secondary hypercoagulability.

10. And what about drugs?
Many drugs can cause priapism. In addition to the various products that release *nitric oxide* into the corpora cavernosa (e.g., sildenafil [Viagra]) or the intracavernosal injection of medications for impotence, drugs that can induce priapism include:
- Psychotropics (chlorpromazine, trazodone, and thioridazine, and even serotonin reuptake inhibitors such as citalopram)
- Calcium channel blockers
- Anticoagulants (both warfarin and heparin)
- Vasodilators (hydralazine and prazosin, especially in patients with renal failure)
- Various others (metoclopramide, omeprazole, hydroxyzine, tamoxifen, testosterone, and androstenedione in athletes)
- "Recreational" drugs such as cocaine, marijuana, ecstasy, and alcohol (which should instead be called *destructive* drugs, since they kill you, make you destitute, or both)

11. What is phimosis?
From the Greek *phimos* (muzzle or snout), this is a narrowed opening of the prepuce, so that the foreskin cannot be retracted over the glans penis (Fig. 16-3). Usually *congenital* (from membranes binding the prepuce to the glans), phimosis also may result from *acquired* adhesions, often the sequela of poor hygiene, previous infections (chronic balanoposthitis), or a too-forceful retraction of a congenital phimosis. If untreated, it can degenerate into squamous intraepithelial cancer of the penis.

12. Is a phimosis always pathologic?
No. A congenital phimosis can be quite physiologic in children, in fact well into the teenage years. In a recent study from Japan (where circumcision is *not* routinely done), a congenital phimosis was seen in 88.5% of children aged 1–3 months, and 35% of those aged 3 years. In fact, only 39.7% of these children had foreskins *fully* retractable by 3 years of age. Other studies have shown persistence of congenital phimoses in 6% of boys aged 8–11, and 3% of those aged 12–13. Only 20% of 200 boys aged 5–13 years had fully retractable foreskins.

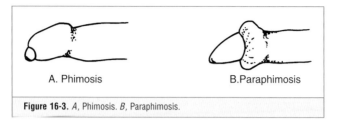

A. Phimosis   B.Paraphimosis

Figure 16-3. *A*, Phimosis. *B*, Paraphimosis.

13. **What is paraphimosis?**
A condition related to, but actually different from, a phimosis. Once a phimotic prepuce is forcibly retracted over the glans, the edematous foreskin cannot be brought forward again, thus resulting in *paraphimosis*, a tight band of retracted foreskin *behind the coronal sulcus* (*see* Fig. 16-3). This is a very painful condition, which, if unrelieved, can cause urinary tract obstruction, venous engorgement, edema, and even necrosis of the foreskin and glans.

14. **What are the causes of paraphimosis?**
The same as those of phimosis: an uncircumcised or incorrectly circumcised penis. In fact, both conditions are often indication for circumcision to prevent vascular or infectious complications. In children, the narrowed preputial opening of a congenital phimosis often results in paraphimosis, especially if parents forcibly retract the foreskin while attempting to clean the glans. In adults, there is often a history of catheterization (without allowing the foreskin to return over the glans) or poor hygiene (with *balanoposthitis* eventually leading to phimosis and then to paraphimosis). Vigorous sexual activity can predispose to paraphimosis, too. Finally, body piercing with penile rings that prevent the reduction of a retracted foreskin can be a unique, but not too uncommon, cause.

15. **What is balanoposthitis?**
It is the inflammation of the glans (*balanos* is Greek for acorn) and prepuce (*posthe* is Greek for foreskin) due to a wide variety of organisms. This is often seen in uncircumcised males because of poor local hygiene, with accumulation of (and irritation by) *smegma*—a mix of desquamated epithelial cells, sweat, debris, and transudated oils (from the Greek term for "soap"). Examination of prepuce and the glans reveals a red, moist, and macular lesion, at times with areas of yellow-to-black discoloration. Irregular borders and lichenification suggest instead *human papillomavirus* or a chronic bacterial process, eventually leading to phimosis. Ulceration and deep erosion occur only with fungal infection in immunocompromised hosts.

16. **What are the causes of balanoposthitis?**
The most common is infection, either by bacteria (staphylococci and streptococci, but also anaerobes, *Gardnerella* sp., and *S. pyogenes* sp.) or yeasts (usually candidal). This is usually facilitated by poor hygiene and poorly retractile foreskin. Contact dermatitis also may cause it, and in one third of cases no specific etiologies are established. Associations with ulcerative colitis and Crohn's disease also have been reported. Refractory or recurrent forms may benefit from circumcision. Still, do *not* confuse balanoposthitis with *balanitis*.

17. **What is balanitis?**
An inflammation of the *glans*, usually in uncircumcised men with poor personal hygiene. It is common, affecting 11% of American men in a urology clinic. Irritation from smegma causes edema and inflammation of the glans, with eventual adherence of the foreskin to the penis (i.e., phimosis). Local burning and a red rash also are common. The skin may appear to peel off,

as if scalded. Predisposing conditions include diabetes, but also morbid obesity, edema (nephrosis, cirrhosis, and heart failure), and old age. Seborrheic and contact dermatitis can do it, too. Given its frequent infectious nature, it may be sexually transmitted.

18. **What is Reiter's syndrome? What are its manifestations?**
Reiter's is a reactive arthritis, usually triggered by an infection. This may be *sexually transmitted* (*Chlamydia,* genital mycoplasmas, and, to a lesser degree, gonococci) or *enteric* (*Shigella, Salmonella, Yersinia,* and *Campylobacter* spp.). Its clinical manifestations include acute arthritis/arthralgia, lower urogenital tract inflammation, mucocutaneous lesions, and conjunctivitis/iridocyclitis. One quarter of affected men have small, ulcerated plaques around the glans and foreskin. In fact, the most common mucocutaneous lesion involves the penis and is called *circinate balanitis* (*circinata* means round in Latin, and *balanitis* is the Greek term for inflammation of the glans). This is a painless inflammation of glans, sulcus, and corona, which starts as tiny blebs, eventually merging into a larger ring of inflammatory tissue that may completely circumscribe the glans. In addition, Reiter's patients often have mucocutaneous lesions of the mouth, palms, and soles. Over the hands and feet, these tend to be scaly, sometimes pustular, and frequently resembling severe psoriasis (*keratoderma blennorrhagica*). Whether initial infection was sexually transmitted or enteric, there also may be urethritis with discharge. This is scanty, thin, and whitish—hence, quite different from the profuse, thicker, and more purulent discharge of gonorrhea. In fact, the discharge of Reiter's resembles that of other nongonococcal urethritides (like chlamydia) insofar as it is usually clear. Acute Reiter's also can present with systemic symptoms (fever, malaise, anorexia, and weight loss). Most cases resolve in 2–6 months with annual risk of recurrence of mucocutaneous manifestations around 15%, at intervals of months or years. The arthritis is usually persistent.

19. **Who was Reiter?**
Hans C. Reiter (1881–1969) was a German physician and the son of a rich Leipzig industrialist. He described his famous syndrome in 1916, while serving with the Hungarian Army in the Balkans during World War I. There, he encountered a young lieutenant affected by diarrhea, urethritis, arthritis, and conjunctivitis. Reiter first thought that the patient might have had syphilis but eventually changed his diagnosis and recognized the new syndrome. The same constellation of findings was described 2 years later by Sir Benjamin Brodie in his textbook, *Diseases of the Bones and Joints.* Reiter also is famous for having identified the spirochete causing Weil's disease while being stationed on the Western front. He later became a member of the Nazi party, was appointed minister of health for Mecklenburg, and even signed an oath of allegiance to Adolf Hitler—hence the recent calls to remove his name from medical textbooks.

20. **What about gonococcal urethritis?**
It is the hallmark of gonorrhea, characterized in men by urethritis with thick and profuse discharge, urethral itch, dysuria, and epididymal pain (although more than *one half* of all men and women with gonorrhea are asymptomatic). If untreated, gonorrhea can lead to major sequelae, such as epididymo-orchitis and possibly infertility.

21. **What kind of skin lesions can be seen on the penis?**
The most common are classified on the basis of appearance (Table 16-1):
1. **Ulcerating:** Skin craters filled with serum, pus, or crust. They represent a full-thickness loss of epidermis and can be single or multiple.
2. **Non-ulcerating:** Further divided into:
   - *Papules*: Small (<1 cm in diameter) lesions, *raised* above the skin surface
   - *Plaques*: Larger (>1 cm in diameter) lesions, flat-topped

TABLE 16-1. PENILE LESIONS

Ulcerating			Non-Ulcerating	
Single	Multiple			
	Acute	Chronic	Papules	Plaques
Primary syphilis	Secondary syphilis	Pemphigus	Hair follicles and sebaceous glands	Psoriasis
Chancroid	Aphthous ulcers	Behçet's disease	Pearly penile papules	Balanitis and posthitis
Granuloma inguinale	Herpes simplex	Reiter's syndrome	Fordyce spots	Zoon's plasma cell balanitis
Lymphogranuloma venereum			Psoriasis	Erythroplasia of Queyrat
Penile cancer			Molluscum contagiosum	Lichen sclerosus and balanitis xerotica obliterans
			Genital warts	
			Secondary syphilis	

22. **How do *ulcerating lesions* present?**
As single or multiple. The single are more serious, since they reflect sexually transmitted diseases such as primary syphilis, chancroid, granuloma inguinale, and lymphogranuloma venereum. Penile cancer also can present as a painless, irregular, genital ulcer.

23. **Describe the ulcerating lesion of primary syphilis.**
It is a single, round, nontender, and painless ulcer (often called a chancre) with bilateral lymphadenopathy.

24. **Describe the ulcerating lesion of chancroid.**
It is a painful, single ulcer, at times multiple, with lymphadenopathy.

25. **Describe the ulcerating lesion of granuloma inguinale.**
It is a single, painless ulcer without lymphadenopathy.

26. **Describe the ulcerating lesion of lymphogranuloma venereum.**
It is a small, nontender ulcer with unilateral tender lymphadenopathy.

27. **Which other dermatoses can be transmitted through sexual contact?**
Definitely scabies and pediculosis. In both cases, *itching* is the prevalent symptom, and *redness* the predominant finding. Note that whereas *scabies* burrow under the skin to lay eggs, *lice* bite into the skin to draw blood. Hence, lice present with red and scaly areas of skin or hair where insects and eggs may be visible. Scabies, on the other hand, present with little bumps, blisters, and crusting in areas of pruritus.

28. **What about *multiple* ulcerating lesions?**
These are more common than single ulcers and may have less serious causes. Based on duration, they can be *acute* (<2-week course) or *chronic* (>2-week course).

29. **What are the most important *acute* multiple ulcerating lesions?**
- Secondary syphilis
- Aphthous ulcers
- Herpes simplex

30. **Describe the multiple ulcerating lesions of secondary syphilis.**
Secondary syphilis is characterized by a papulosquamous rash involving not only the penis but also the palms and soles. Multiple, irregular, shallow, *painless*, and gray ulcers (often described as "serpiginous" since they move like a snail track along the penis) are usually present. There also may be a flu-like illness and a blotchy, red body rash.

31. **What are aphthous ulcers?**
Small, shallow, *painful* ulcers that most commonly appear in the mouth but also can affect the penis. Typically, they have a gray center surrounded by a bright red halo, occur in crops, and resolve without treatment. They can easily be confused with herpes simplex ulcers, so laboratory tests are necessary to reliably distinguish the two. They are not infectious, and their cause is unknown.

32. **Describe the multiple ulcerating lesions of herpes simplex.**
They appear as small, multiple vesicular skin lesions that are *painful*, in clusters, and *not* associated with adenopathy. Note that *chancroid* lesions also can be multiple.

33. **Are genital herpetic lesions due to HSV-1 or HSV-2?**

Usually to *herpes simplex virus* type *2*, the leading cause of infectious genital ulceration in the United States (HSV-1 is instead the most common cause of *oral* infections). Although one out of five American adults is seropositive for this virus, more than one half remain asymptomatic and yet capable of shedding and transmitting the virus. Lesions present as small, clustered vesicles on an erythematous base, rapidly progressing into pustules and painful ulcers, and eventually forming a crust. Since lesions follow the distribution of a sensory nerve, they tend to recur at (or near) the same site. Fever, malaise, and acute toxicity also may occur—especially in primary infections.

34. **What are the most important *chronic* multiple ulcerating lesions?**
- **Pemphigus:** These are fragile, thin-walled blisters that eventually break down to form ulcers. Often painful and itchy. Note that pemphigus usually affects other parts of the body (frequently starting in the mouth) but also may involve only the penis.
- **Behçet's disease**: An inflammatory and noninfectious multisystem disease that involves the skin, joints, nerves, and eyes. Genital lesions present as large, deep, and painful penile/scrotal ulcers, always accompanied by mouth ulcers.
- **Reiter's syndrome** (circinate balanitis)

35. **And what about *non*ulcerating lesions?**
They consist of *papules* and *plaques*.

36. **Describe penile *papules*. What are the most important lesions of this sort?**
Papules are usually benign, although a few are infectious and some are early and preulcerating cancers.
- **Hair follicles and sebaceous glands** are completely normal and frequently found on the penile shaft, particularly its ventral surface. Sebaceous glands can be either *seen* (as small and yellowish nodules, homogenous, and rather symmetrically distributed) or *palpated* (as small skin lumps). They are often referred to as *Fordyce spots* (*see* question 53). Hair follicles, on the other hand, typically contain hair. Neither should be confused with *genital warts* (which are asymmetric and heterogeneous, with a cauliflower-like presentation) or *molluscum contagiosum* (which presents as fleshy, rounded, and umbilicated lesions).
- **Pearly penile papules** are multiple, tiny (1–3 mm), pearly appearing, and skin-colored papules around the circumference of the glans' crown. They typically develop in men ages 20 to 40, with 10% of all subjects being affected, especially if uncircumcised. Although often mistaken for warts (which instead are asymmetric, heterogeneous, and with a

cauliflower-like presentation), pearly papules are neither infectious nor symptomatic. Hence, their only "treatment" is reassurance. They are still referred to as *preputial* or *Tyson's glands,* since initially they were believed to be *smegma*-producing glands.

- **Fordyce spots** (*see* also question 53)
- **Lichen planus** and **psoriasis**
- **Molluscum contagiosum**
- **Genital warts**
- **Secondary syphilis**

37. **How does lichen planus present on the penis?**
The most common form is classical papules and patches, mostly clustered in a circle on and around the glans. These are purple colored or white, ring shaped, and often resembling thrush. Unlike other patches of lichen planus (LP), they rarely itch. White streaks and erosive lesions are much less common presentations.

38. **What are the characteristics of penile psoriasis?**
Like lichen planus, psoriasis of the genital area may present with atypical features—usually because of moisture and maceration. The classic psoriatic *scale,* for example, is often rare (except in uncircumcised men). Instead, genital psoriasis presents as thickened red papules or plaques with well-defined edges and is rarely associated with irritation. Although psoriasis most commonly affects other parts of the body (especially the knees, elbows, and scalp), it can first appear on the penis, usually on the glans or inner surface of the foreskin. This may require differentiation from syphilis.

39. **What is molluscum contagiosum?**
A benign and common *viral* disease of skin and mucous membranes. In children, it is acquired through peer contact, whereas in adults, it may be sexually transmitted. *Penile molluscum* presents as multiple, small, soft, and spherical papules of penis or scrotum, often with a central depression or plug. If squeezed, lesions can express a curd-like discharge. Usually a marker for "unsafe" sexual practices (hence, test for HIV), molluscum lesions may disappear without treatment, although freezing or cautery is often curative.

40. **And what about genital *warts*?**
These also are quite common, and in fact increasing in prevalence, especially in young and sexually active people. *Condylomata acuminata* are arbor-like (acuminata) lesions caused by the human papillomavirus virus (the *condylomata lata* of syphilis are instead *flat—see* question 41). Usually more wart-like than ulcerating, *condylomata acuminata* usually occur in moist areas (such as the corona or sulcus), but also may affect the penis's tip and shaft, plus scrotum, anus, and mouth. They appear as tiny and skin-colored genital warts, isolated or in clusters, and with a shiny surface. These may become fleshy and cauliflower-like. Highly infectious, genital warts can be latent, subclinical, and clinical—very much like herpes. Hence, asymptomatic infection (and shedding) is frequent. The most common agents are low-risk human papillomavirus (HPV) 6 and 11; high-risk HPV types 16 and 18 are less common but are associated with premalignant and malignant degeneration (i.e., squamous cell carcinoma of the penis, anus, and cervix). They may be confused with pearly penile papules.

41. **What are condylomata lata?**
They are flat (*lata* in Latin), multiple lesions of secondary syphilis. They present as flat-topped, soft, moist or macerated, reddish-brown to grayish genital papules or, more rarely, nodules. These may eventually coalesce into larger plaques, often cauliflower-like. Differential diagnosis includes the nonulcerating and papular lesions of psoriasis, lichen planus, scabies, squamous cell carcinoma (which usually presents as an indurated and nontender *nodule,* but at times may even ulcerate), and Reiter's (which also may present with a nonulcerating penile lesion).

42. **What about penile *plaques*?**

They are usually benign (like *psoriasis* and *Zoon's plasma cell balanitis*) and often infectious (*balanitis* and *posthitis, see* questions 15–17). Still, three of these lesions (erythroplasia of Queyrat, lichen sclerosus, and balanitis xerotica obliterans) are quite serious since they may degenerate into penile cancer. Finally, diffuse red plaques with a poorly defined edge and finely scaled surface (eczema-like) may be due to allergic contact dermatitis. Although often the result of lubricants, condoms, spermicides, and feminine deodorant sprays, they are more frequently caused by poor hygiene, with persistent moisture and maceration. They are quite irritating and usually respond to topical steroids.

43. **What is Zoon's balanitis?**

A noninfectious condition characterized by a brightly red and shiny plaque on either the glans or inner foreskin. It is histologically characterized by a plasma cell infiltrate. Etiology is unknown and prognosis benign, even though it often prompts a differential diagnosis with the much more serious *erythroplasia of Queyrat*. Usually painless, it may be itchy and often recurrent, despite topical steroids. It always responds to circumcision.

44. **What is the erythroplasia of Queyrat?**

A sharply demarcated red plaque, bright, painless, and not itchy—often with a typical velvety surface. It is seen almost exclusively in uncircumcised men, and, unless excised, it eventually progresses to invasive cancer. Hence, it is an *in situ* form of squamous cell carcinoma. Queyrat lesions may be solitary or multiple, typically circumscribed, minimally raised, and with variegated erythematous plaques that may be smooth, scaly, crusty, or verrucous. It is typically located at the mucocutaneous junction of the penis or prepuce, but also can involve the mouth and vulva. Ulceration or distinct papillomatous papules within a plaque may indicate progression to invasive squamous cell carcinoma. Still, its nondescript look may lead to a lengthy period of misdiagnosis. Biopsy of any suspicious lesion is always the best approach. The lesion was originally described by Tarnovsky in 1891, and subsequently reported by Fournier and Darier as a penile disease in 1893. The French dermatologist Queyrat described in 1911 *erythroplasia* of the glans penis, and correctly identified it as precancerous. Hence, the eponym.

45. **What about squamous cell carcinoma of the penis?**

It is the most common penile cancer. Human papillomavirus, precancerous lesions, and poor hygiene from phimosis are all predisposing factors. Hence, it is almost absent in circumcised males. Rare before age 40, it presents with lymphonodal spread and proliferative glans lesions.

46. **What is lichen sclerosus et atrophicus?**

A lymphocyte-mediated chronic inflammation of the glans, foreskin, or shaft, presenting with atrophic white plaques that are usually asymptomatic, although irritation and burning also can occur. Its most severe form is *balanitis xerotica obliterans (BXO),* a condition affecting the prepuce of uncircumcised men, giving it a firm, whitish, and scarred appearance that may interfere with urination or sex. Indurated, flat, shiny, and white patches with an erythematous halo may eventually lead to foreskin depigmentation, atrophy, scarring, and eventually phimosis. Hence, the term of "obliterans." BXO also may cause dysuria, progressive stenosis of the urethral meatus, stricture, and even penile cancer. Steroid creams may help, but the condition often recurs.

47. **What is Peyronie's disease (PD)?**

A peculiar disease of unknown etiology, at times associated with Dupuytren's contracture, and often referred to as *penile fibromatosis*—or van Buren's disease, from the Philadelphia surgeon of Dutch descent, William Holme Van Buren (1819–1883). It presents with plaques (or strands) of dense fibrous tissue around the corpora cavernosa, possibly the result of trauma. These may be detectable by palpation and often cause penile deformity, with crooked and painful erections. Note that the penis of Peyronie patients is entirely normal at rest; only when erected does it appear bent and deformed. Although its major significance is psychologic, in some extreme cases the deformity is severe enough to interfere with erection, penetration, orgasm, and even fertility. Peyronie's disease also was the condition rumored to affect the presidential penis of Bill Clinton, based on descriptions filed by Paula Jones in her lawsuit for sexual harassment.

48. **Who was Peyronie?**
François Gigot de La Peyronie (1678–1747) was a well-respected Montpellier surgeon and the personal physician to the Sun King, Louis XIV. He astutely used his connection to have the king pass a law banning barbers and wigmakers from practicing medicine, thus eliminating with the stroke of a pen the main competition to the surgical community. He subsequently founded the French Academy of Surgery and became one of the forces in the establishment of Paris as *the* world center of surgery. An immensely rich man, Peyronie described his eponymous lesion at the end of his life, in 1743, in a patient who had "rosary beads of scar tissue to cause an upward curvature of the penis during erection."

49. **Define hypospadias and epispadias.**
   - **Hypospadias** is a developmental anomaly characterized by a defect on the lower (ventral) surface of the penis. Consequently, the urethral meatus is more proximal than normal, opening on the ventral aspect of the penis rather than on the glans.
   - **Epispadias** is a defect on the upper (dorsal) surface of the penis. Hence, the urethral meatus opens *dorsally*.
   Both these congenital malformations (Fig. 16-4) may lead to fertility problems. They also represent a clue to other underlying abnormalities, such as undescended testis (cryptorchidism), Klinefelter's syndrome, or other chromosomal disorders. Hypospadias may be induced by the mother's ingestion of estrogens or progesterone or congenital adrenal hyperplasia.

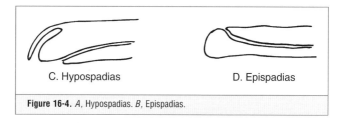

C. Hypospadias   D. Epispadias

Figure 16-4. *A,* Hypospadias. *B,* Epispadias.

(2) Scrotum

50. **Describe the anatomy of the scrotum.**
The scrotum consists of a skin pouch, divided in the midline by a raphe extending from the ventral surface of the penis to the perineum. It is internally subdivided into right and left compartments, housing, respectively, the testes, epididymis, and the various spermatic cord structures (vas deferens with its vascular and nervous supply).

51. **Which scrotal abnormalities can be identified through inspection?**
Mostly skin abnormalities, including sexually transmitted or fungal lesions. *Tinea cruris* is especially common, presenting as large erythematous areas involving the scrotum and adjacent thighs. Lesions are often scaly and with ragged margins. *Candidal infection* also may cause scrotal lesions, particularly in grossly overweight and diabetic patients. Finally, *lice* (or

sometimes even *scabies*) can be visualized in scrotal and pubic areas, often heralded by excoriations. Fordyce "lesions" and "spots" are also important and yet benign findings.

52. What are Fordyce *lesions*?

They are small, pin-sized (2–5 mm), *bright red or purple* papules that may occur on the scrotum, but occasionally on the glans and shaft, too, and even the inner thigh or lower abdomen. First described in 1896 by the American dermatologist John Addison Fordyce (on the scrotum of a 60-year-old man), they are still referred to as Fordyce's angiokeratomas. They are *not* infectious but vascular. Hence, they should *not* be biopsied. In fact, they may even bleed after the minimal trauma of intercourse. At times solitary, they usually present as clusters of 50 to 100 asymptomatic lesions. They are benign and common, being present in as many as one of six men older than 50 (conversely, they are quite rare in men younger than 40). Since they reflect a congenital predisposition, they often occur in families, and yet remain primarily a by-product of age. Although often a cause of embarrassment or concern, they just represent abnormally dilated capillaries covered by thickened skin. They should not be confused with *Fordyce spots (or granules)*.

53. What are Fordyce *spots*?

They are very common (80–95% of adults) *yellowish/white* papules, 1–3 mm in diameter, that occur on the *shaft* of the penis (or the labia of women), but also the tongue, vermillion border of the lips, and the inner surface of the cheeks. Usually clustered in 50 to 100, they are probably present at birth, even though they become bigger and more visible from puberty on. They represent enlarged ectopic sebaceous glands and are just of cosmetic concern.

54. What are the causes of scrotal swelling?

It depends on whether the swelling is bilateral or unilateral:

- **Bilateral** scrotal edema, diffuse and painless, is usually a feature of *systemic* disease, most commonly anasarca. Ascites, pleural effusion, and scrotal edema are commonly seen in severe congestive heart failure, nephrotic syndrome, or cirrhosis.
- **Unilateral** scrotal edema, on the other hand, is a sign of *local* pathology. The most common is a *varicocele,* from the Latin *varix* (dilated vein) and Greek *kele* (tumor).

55. What is a varicocele?

A condition caused by incompetent valves in the internal spermatic veins, resulting in *engorgement along the spermatic cord*. Hence, a varicocele resembles a nest of worms, which only presents upon standing and resolves with either a supine position or scrotal elevation. Easily identifiable on exam, a varicocele is quite common, occurring in 15% of the general male population and 40% of men evaluated for infertility. It is, in fact, a common cause of reversible sterility (due to the increased testicular temperature of the affected testis). This was intuited by the first century A.D. Roman physician Celsus, who described the condition as "veins that are swollen and twisted over the testicle, which thus becomes smaller than its fellow inasmuch as its nutrition has become defective." Note that because of the drainage characteristics of the testicular veins, a varicocele is much more common on the left than on the right. Accordingly, a *right* varicocele should prompt investigation to exclude either anatomic abnormalities or an alternative diagnosis. Other than a varicocele, localized and painless scrotal swelling usually reflects pathology of the testis or epididymis (*see* questions 63 and 64). Conversely, *painful and tender scrotal swelling* usually indicates a much more acute process, such as torsion of the spermatic cord, strangulated inguinal hernia, acute orchitis, or acute epididymitis.

Pearl

The sudden appearance of a varicocele in a patient with nephrotic syndrome suggests renal vein thrombosis until proven otherwise.

56. What are the normal characteristics of testes and epididymides?

- **Testes** are paired organs, 2–3 cm in thickness, and 3.5–5.5 cm in length. They have the shape of an egg, with the vertical axis being the longest. All but the posterior surfaces are wrapped by a folded serous sheath with a potential cavity: the *tunica vaginalis*.
- **Epididymides** (in Greek, "the ones on top of the testicles") are two elongated structures attached to the posterior surface of the testes (even though in 7–10% of normal adults the epididymides are located *anteriorly* to the testicles). Each structure consists of a head (caput epididymidis), body (corpus epididymidis), and tail (cauda epididymidis). The tail turns sharply upon itself to become the *ductus* (or *vas*) *deferens*. Both the tail and the beginning of the ductus deferens serve as reservoir for spermatozoa. Secretions from the ductus deferens, seminal vesicles, and prostate form the semen.

57. How should the testes and epididymides be examined?

With great care, since these organs (especially the testes) are exquisitely sensitive, not only to touch but also to temperature. In fact, in a cold room they may even retract toward the inguinal canal. Hence, to best palpate them, use your thumb plus index finger, or thumb plus index and medium fingers. This also allows you to gauge the length and thickness of each testicle, although for more accurate measurements, you will need a caliper. Note any discrepancy in consistency or size, and, if present, ask how long this has been so. If ruling out a congenitally undescended testis, examine the inguinal canal for localized swelling. Search for testicular lumps or bumps, which, if present, should be considered neoplastic until proven otherwise. Still, keep in mind that *diffuse* testicular enlargement usually reflects either a *hydrocele* (*see* question 59) or a *varicocele* (previously discussed, *see* question 55). Note that the left testis lies a bit lower in the scrotum than its counterpart (the reverse would suggest *situs inversus*). Also note that, although the testicles can be examined in either the standing or supine position, a search for hernias or varicoceles requires the patient *to stand*. Finally, move cephalad and gently assess the upper and posterior poles of the testes and adjacent heads of the epididymides. Examine the *spermatic cord,* which goes from the epididymis all the way up into the inguinal canal. This contains the vas deferens, the testicular artery/vein, the ilioinguinal nerve, plus lymphatic vessels and fat tissue. Of all these structures, only the vas can be easily recognized, based on its firm and wire-like feel and the location along the posterior aspect of the bundle. Identify any lumps or bumps in the cord, and then note their relationship to the testes and inguinal canal. Note that a varicocele will be palpable not only in the testes, but also throughout the length of the cord, since it represents a varicose dilation of the spermatic vein.

58. What is transillumination of a scrotal mass?

A good way to find out whether a localized scrotal swelling is solid or liquid. To do so, shut off the lights in the exam room, raise the penis (to better visualize the scrotum), and shine a penlight from behind the scrotal mass. Inability of the mass to transmit light suggests a solid lesion, whereas transmission of the light beam favors instead a fluid-filled lesion—like a *hydrocele* or *spermatocele*. Note, however, that a *hematocele* (a fluid-filled lesion caused by accumulation of blood) and a *varicocele* (varicose veins of the spermatic cord) are transillumination-negative because blood does *not* transmit light.

59. What is a hydrocele?

A collection of serous fluid in either the tunica vaginalis or in a separate pocket along the spermatic cord (literally, a *water tumor* in Greek). This presents as a unilateral and painless scrotal swelling. Since a hydrocele has different consistency from that of testicular tissue, it can be easily recognized by transillumination.

60. **What is a spermatocele?**
A spermatozoa-filled cyst of the epididymis (literally, a *sperm tumor*). It presents as a unilateral, painless, and movable scrotal mass, just above the testis and identifiable by transillumination. A true epididymal cyst is clinically similar but does *not* contain sperm.

61. **What is cryptorchidism?**
A condition characterized by failure of one or both testes to descend (literally, the *invisible testis* in Greek). The undescended testicle lies in the inguinal canal or abdomen and eventually atrophies from high surrounding temperatures. It may even undergo neoplastic degeneration. Yet, since the other testis remains fully functional, cryptorchidism does *not* affect fertility. It may, however, cause emotional repercussions. For example, it has been suggested that Adolf Hitler's psychopathology could have been due to cryptorchidism, a condition documented by a urologist he consulted before rising to power (the Brits even wrote a song, titled "Hitler Has Only Got One Ball," later set to the tune of *Colonel Bogey March*). Napoleon was cryptorchic, too. As a result, both men decided to screw the world.

62. **What about small testes?**
"Small" is a testis <3.5 cm in length. Its most common cause is *atrophy*. This may be either congenital (as in Klinefelter's syndrome) or acquired (as in alcoholic cirrhosis). Klinefelter's testicles tend to be small and firm, whereas those of cirrhosis are small and *soft*. Atrophy also may result from inflammatory or infectious processes (i.e., orchitis), often due to viruses (mumps), but also syphilis, filariasis, and even trauma.

63. **What are the causes of an enlarged and solid testis?**
Cancer for sure. Hence, an enlarged and firm testis should always be transilluminated to exclude a fluid-filled mass, such as a hydrocele, spermatocele, or epididymal cyst. A confirmed solid lesion increases the likelihood of testicular cancer, which is the most common tumor in men between the ages of 20 and 35. Solid testicular lesions should be actively sought out, not only by physicians but also by patients through self-examination.

64. **What are the causes of a tender epididymis?**
The most common is *acute epididymitis,* which may be associated with such a swelling that separation from the testis may be difficult to detect. In addition to edema, these patients also will have tenderness of the epididymal head and *vas deferens*. Occasionally, there is even swelling and redness of the overlying skin. Acute epididymitis is often the result of urinary tract infection (especially in men >35 years), whereas in younger men, it is usually due to sexually transmitted urethritis (by chlamydia or gonococcus) with prostatitis. Still, epididymitis occurs in less than 1% of all cases of identified sexually transmitted urethritis. Finally, an enlarged, nodular, beaded, and nontender epididymis should suggest *tuberculous epididymitis,* often the complication of renal tuberculosis.

B. HERNIA EXAMINATION

65. **What are the two possible sites of groin hernias?**
- **Inguinal hernias:** More common than femoral hernias and the most frequent of *all* abdominal hernias. They may occur medially (*direct* hernias) or laterally (*indirect* hernias). Both present as a bulge in the inguinal crease. *Indirect hernias* are the most frequent, affecting patients of both sexes and all ages, although typically more common in children. They originate above the inguinal ligament (near its midpoint [i.e., the internal inguinal ring]) and are due to a defect in the abdominal ring, through which the spermatic cord exits the scrotum and enters the pelvis. Hence, they follow the testicular embryologic pathway, descending from the abdomen into the scrotum. *Direct hernias* also originate above the inguinal ligament, but in a congenital defect near the external inguinal ring and pubis tubercle.

They usually affect men 40 years of age or older (since the abdominal wall weakens with age), rarely progress into the scrotum, and on examination bulge anteriorly, pushing the side of the finger forward.

- **Femoral hernias** are less common, especially in males. They originate *below* the inguinal ligament and are located laterally to the site of inguinal hernias. They often are confused with femoral lymph nodes. They do not progress into the scrotum and on examination are associated with an empty inguinal canal (Fig. 16-5).

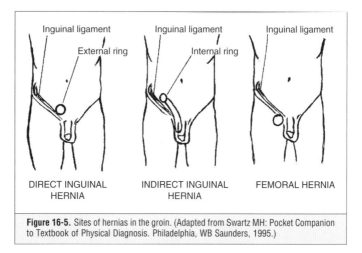

Figure 16-5. Sites of hernias in the groin. (Adapted from Swartz MH: Pocket Companion to Textbook of Physical Diagnosis. Philadelphia, WB Saunders, 1995.)

66. **What is the best way to detect a hernia?**

Start with *inspection*. Ask the patient to stand while you comfortably sit in a chair. Observe the external inguinal ring, looking for a localized bulge. If not visible, elicit the bulge by asking the patient to either cough or perform a Valsalva maneuver. After inspection, palpate the patient's right inguinal region with your right index finger and the patient's left inguinal region with your left index finger. Gently insert the finger along the spermatic cord, through the invaginated scrotum (Fig. 16-6), aiming for the external ring of the inguinal canal (from where the cord emerges). As your fingertip reaches into the external ring, put the fingers of your opposite hand over the inguinal canal, or over any noticeably swollen area. Ask the patient to cough or strain and see whether you can feel, with either hand, any bulging/impulse suggestive of hernia.

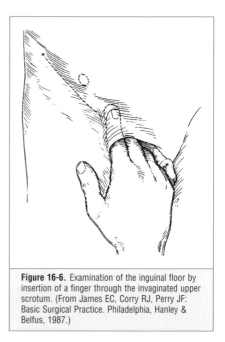

Figure 16-6. Examination of the inguinal floor by insertion of a finger through the invaginated upper scrotum. (From James EC, Corry RJ, Perry JF: Basic Surgical Practice. Philadelphia, Hanley & Belfus, 1987.)

- A *strong* palpable impulse that pushes your finger *out* argues for a *direct* inguinal hernia
- A *soft* impulse without any bulging suggests instead an *indirect* inguinal hernia, gently descending the inguinal canal
- Finally, an empty inguinal canal argues for a femoral hernia. This can be substantiated by placing the index and middle fingers into the triangle lying medially to the femoral artery. A palpable bulge in this area after straining or coughing confirms a femoral hernia.

67. How do you separate indirect from direct inguinal hernias?
With great difficulty. Which is not a great loss, since both types usually need repair, treatment is the same, and identification is eventually carried out at surgery.

68. Should one auscultate over a hernia?
Yes, since presence of bowel sounds would confirm bowel herniation.

69. Should the patient always be standing?
Not necessarily. If the patient is unable to do so, examination *can* be definitely carried out in a supine position. This is preferable when evaluating the inguinal canal for an undescended testicle.

70. Are hernias painless?
Yes. In fact, pain and tenderness (plus evidence of local inflammation, such as skin edema or redness) always suggest an incarcerated/strangulated hernia—a surgical emergency.

71. How large are inguinal hernias?
Some are small enough to barely allow access to your fingertip; others are instead so massive to make it impossible to tell apart the structures of the spermatic cord (and testis) from the contents of the hernia (although the testis usually lies at the bottom of the scrotum).

72. What is Zieman's tridigital examination for hernia?
A procedure used to identify both femoral and inguinal hernias (direct and indirect). The examiner stands at the right side of the patient (who also is standing) and places the palm of the right hand over the patient's right lower abdomen, with fingertips near the right inguinal ligament: the tip of the long finger in the *external* inguinal ring; the tip of the index finger near the *internal* inguinal ring; and the tip of the ring finger in the *femoral triangle*. The patient then either strains or performs a Valsalva maneuver. The increase in intra-abdominal pressure will cause a hernia in any of these three sites to manifest itself as either a gliding motion of the walls of the empty sac or as an impulse caused by the protrusion of the viscus into the sac. The maneuver is then repeated for the other side.

C. DIGITAL RECTAL EXAMINATION (DRE)

73. What is the role of the digital rectal exam?
It is an essential part of any comprehensive examination. Not only in regard to genital/pelvic evaluation (i.e., prostate and gynecologic organs), but also for the assessment of many gastrointestinal, infectious, and oncologic problems.

74. Is it routinely performed?
Not really. Up to two thirds of patients presenting with anorectal and urogenital tract symptoms do *not* undergo a DRE before being referred to a specialist, and more than one half of all inpatients in a teaching hospital do not receive a DRE as part of their admission examination. Rates in community hospitals may be even lower: 25% in one study and 36% among elderly

patients. This is concerning, since one third of all *rectal* cancers are palpable. Hence, lack of DRE may delay referral for resectable disease.

75. **Is the rectal exam performed with the patient standing or in the lateral decubitus position?**

Either. As for the rest of the genital exam, there are two schools of thought: one prefers a standing patient (and a seated physician), and the other opts instead for a standing physician and a recumbent patient (i.e., lying on one side, with knees tucked up toward the chest and body as close as possible to the table edge to facilitate the physician's job). There are no data supporting one approach versus the other, and so it comes down to individual preference. Yet a lateral decubitus position is clearly a must in patients too weak to stand. Still, it is probably easier to perform a rectal exam (especially for its receiving end) with the patient lying down. Conversely, it is better to evaluate testes and inguinal hernias with the patient standing up. Hence, its choice for the genital exam.

76. **What are the steps to follow in a rectal exam?**

If you elect to have the patient standing, instruct him to turn around and rest his chest on the exam table. This will ease both the examiner's and examinee's job. Then sit down, put on gloves, and gently spread the patient's buttocks. Evaluate the perianal area, and look for any skin abnormalities. Having done so, adequately lubricate your index finger and tell the patient that pretty soon you will be inserting it into his rectum. Place your finger against the anus and ask the patient to bear down as if he were having a bowel movement. This will relax the sphincter and allow you to insert the finger more easily. Aim your index finger toward the patient's umbilicus, enter through the anus, and assess its sphincter tone. Palpate the prostate gland through the wall of the rectum. Using the palmar aspect of your index finger, you will be able to examine the posterior and lateral aspects of the gland, but not its anterior surface since this is inaccessible. Then, advance your index finger as far (and as gently) as you can toward the umbilicus, aiming for the seminal vesicles. These are usually not palpable, unless there is disease. Once you have done so, rotate your finger in order to reach upward, posteriorly, and laterally for rectal-based masses or lesions. Then withdraw and inspect the stool on your gloved finger for any evidence of mucus, blood, or tarry color (which would indicate a bleeding site above the ligament of Treitz, whereas obvious blood would point instead to rectal or anal sources). Afterwards, dab some of the stool on a guaiac card, and test it for occult blood. Finally, hand the patient a box of tissues for cleaning.

77. **What perianal findings can be detected by rectal examination?**

Skin lesions caused by sexually transmitted diseases (i.e., papillomavirus or herpes), parasitic infestations (pinworms), or fungi (*Candida* sp.). Fissures or fistulas also may be visualized (usually suggesting Crohn's disease), and so are bleeding sites and tumors. Hemorrhoids are occasionally visible (especially if prolapsing), but usually require palpation.

78. **How do you assess a reduced sphincter tone? What is its significance?**

Look for degree of spontaneous resistance to your finger. Alternatively, ask the patient to contract the sphincter by trying to "hold on" to your finger. A reduced tone may reflect a central or peripheral nervous system compromise, disrupting sphincter innervation and causing rectal incontinence. For example, a neoplastic cord compression of sacral roots.

Pearl

A rectal exam can be important in appendicitis, especially the retrocecal variety, since this variant does not produce the classic abdominal findings.

79. **What characteristics of the prostate should you assess?**
You should appreciate the two lobes and the longitudinal cleft between them. Assess size, symmetry, consistency, and surface characteristics, especially nodularities and tenderness (the latter usually indicates prostatic infection). A normal gland is small, rubbery, with symmetric and smooth lobes and a well-demarcated median cleft. A *firm* gland suggests instead malignancy, but also may indicate chronic prostatitis. A gland that has become *fixed to the pelvis* signals extension of tumor (and so does palpability of seminal vesicles).

80. **What causes prostatic nodules?**
A common cause is benign prostatic hyperplasia. Nodules also may reflect various inflammatory processes, and even infarct. Of course, a nodule should always raise concern about prostatic *cancer*. Since tumors often originate in the posterior lobe, which is accessible to the finger, they may indeed present as palpable hard nodules.

81. **What causes a tender prostate?**
The most common cause is *infection* (i.e., prostatitis and prostatic abscess). Patients with these conditions also may have palpable prostatic nodules.

82. **What does the normal prostate look like?**
It has the shape of a *heart* (which makes it especially endearing to those of us who are romantically inclined) and the size of a *walnut*. Enlargement does not necessarily indicate cancer but is instead a common sign of *benign prostatic hypertrophy*—a frequent by-product of aging. Nodules, on the other hand, are invariably suspicious and thus should always be biopsied. Still, only 50% of all nodules eventually turn out to be neoplastic, with the rest usually reflecting benign prostatic hypertrophy (hence, the low positive predictive value for cancer—*see* questions 83 and 84). Also, a localized area of induration is not necessarily typical of *early* cancer, but more of a late neoplastic process.

83. **What is the diagnostic value of DRE in primary care screening for cancer?**
Limited. In a meta-analysis of 14 studies, DRE had high specificity and negative predictive value for detecting prostate cancer (94% and 99%, respectively), but low sensitivity and positive predictive value (59% and 28%). Since false negative results are rare in the outpatient setting (given the small prevalence of cancer in an unselected population), DRE may have value for initial screening. Yet, given its moderate sensitivity (and very low positive predictive value), a positive DRE should not be used to rule in prostate cancer. Hence, further confirmation must be carried out. This includes measurement of serum *prostatic specific antigen (PSA)* and transrectal ultrasonography with possible biopsy. Still, DRE alone allows detection of almost one out of five cancers with "normal" PSA levels. These are usually small and confined.

84. **What are the limitations of DRE for the screening of prostatic cancer?**
In addition to examiner's experience and interobserver variability on what constitutes an abnormal finding, the major limitation is access to only the posterior and lateral aspects of the gland. As a result, an overview of studies of screening suggests that DRE alone detects fewer than 60% of prostate cancers. Adding DRE to PSA does appear to increase the yield of screening; in a large study of volunteers, the combination of DRE and PSA detected 26% more cancers than PSA alone. However, combining DRE and PSA also increases the rate of false positive results. Note that in 2002 the U.S. Preventive Services Task Force (USPSTF) concluded that there was not enough evidence to recommend for, or against, routine screening for prostate cancer by DRE or PSA.

85. **How about the effectiveness of DRE for the detection of colorectal cancer?**
Questionable, since fewer than 10% of all colorectal cancers arise within reach of the examining finger (and some of these lesions will already be symptomatic). The same can be said for a

single office-based *fecal occult blood testing* (FOBT) that relies on a stool sample obtained on DRE: the sensitivity of this test is substantially lower than that of screening protocols involving multiple cards (in one study the first test card would have missed 42% of cancers detected by multiple test cards). In addition to being a one-shot deal, FOBT on samples collected by DRE may be invalidated by inadequate amount of stool or trauma from the exam. Specificity, on the other hand, is usually high. Overall, sensitivity of a single test has been estimated at 40%, whereas specificity can be as high as 96–98%. Hence, in 2002, the USPSTF *did* recommend periodic fecal occult blood testing as a way to reduce mortality from colorectal cancer.

86. **Should rectal exam be deferred in patients with a myocardial infarction?**
No. Although conventional teaching suggests that a rectal examination may worsen ischemia (and even trigger arrhythmias in patients suffering an acute myocardial infarction), no scientific data support this assumption. In fact, a prospective study by Akhtar et al. of 480 intensive care unit and telemetry patients showed that none of the patients developed sustained arrhythmias during the test. There also was no change in vital signs. Conversely, DRE was able to detect significant clinical findings in 11% of all patients. Note that digital rectal exam may increase the *acid prostatic phosphatase*, but it will do so only in patients with prostatic cancer, not in patients with benign prostatic hypertrophy. Hence, when screening for cancer, you should obtain the serum acid phosphatase *after* a rectal exam, not before.

SELECTED BIBLIOGRAPHY

1. Akhtar AJ, Moran D, Ganeson K, et al: Safety and efficacy of digital rectal examination in patients with acute myocardial infarction. Am J Gastroenterol 95:1463–1465, 2000.
2. Buechner SA: Common skin disorders of the penis. BJU Int 90:498–506, 2002.
3. DeGowin RL: DeGowin and DeGowin's Bedside Diagnostic Examination, 6th ed. New York, McGraw-Hill, 1994.
4. Edwards S: Balanitis and balanoposthitis: A review. Genitourin Med 72:155–159, 1996.
5. Gairdner D: The fate of the foreskin: A study of circumcision. BMJ 2:1433–1437, 1949.
6. Gerber GS: Carcinoma in situ of the penis. J Urol 151:829–833, 1994.
7. Guinan P, Bush I, Ray, V, et al: The accuracy of the rectal examination in the diagnosis of prostatic carcinoma. N Engl J Med 303:499–583, 1980.
8. Hennigan TW, Franks PJ, Hocken DB, Allen-Mersh TG: Rectal examination in general practice. BMJ 301:478–480, 1990.
9. Hoogendam A, Buntinx F, de Vet HC: The diagnostic value of digital rectal examination in primary care screening for prostate cancer: A meta-analysis. Fam Pract 16:621–626, 1999.
10. Imamura E: Phimosis of infants and young children in Japan. Acta Paediatr Jpn 39:403–405, 1997.
11. Oster J: Further fate of the foreskin: Incidence of preputial adhesions, phimosis, and smegma among Danish schoolboys. Arch Dis Child 43:200–203, 1968.
12. Sapira JD: The Art and Science of Bedside Diagnosis. Baltimore, Urban & Schwarzenberg, 1990.
13. Singhal VK, Razdan JL, Gupta, SN, et al: Carcinoma of the penis. J Ind Med Assoc 89:120–123, 1991.
14. Willms JL, Schneidermann H, Algranati PS: Physical Diagnosis. Baltimore, Williams & Wilkins, 1994.

CHAPTER 17

FEMALE GENITALIA AND THE PELVIS

Salvatore Mangione, MD

"A child of our grandmother Eve, a female; or, for thy more sweet understanding, a woman."
—Shakespeare, Love's Labour's Lost, Act I

1. **What is the role of the pelvic exam?**
   To provide an essential component of the female exam, which, when well performed, allows for "low-tech" cancer screening plus the detection of various obstetric-gynecologic conditions—including pregnancy.

2. **How can I make my patient as comfortable as possible during the pelvic exam?**
   By following a few simple steps:
   - Instruct her to void prior to the exam, since a full bladder can often be confused for a pregnant uterus or an ovarian cyst.
   - Ideally have her empty her bowels, too.
   - Raise the table back to a comfortable height so that you can maintain eye contact at all time.
   - Offer a pillow for her back.
   - Place a drape over her abdomen, thighs, and knees.
   - Before performing each step of the exam, inform her about it.
   - Instruct her to relax the perineal muscles through appropriate breathing.
   - Always wash your hands in the presence of the patient.
   - Warm the speculum before using it.
   - Watch your terminology during the exam. Never say you are going to "feel" something since this has sexual connotations. Use instead "check." Also, do not refer to "foot rests" as "stirrups." And more importantly, keep them out of sight until you are ready to use them.
   - Always explain your findings, even if normal.
   - Continuous communication is paramount. Provide your patient with a sense of control by reassuring her that she will be able to stop the exam at any time if it were to become too uncomfortable. Also, offer her a hand-held mirror so that she can become more of a participant. By following these guidelines, pelvic exams should cause minimal discomfort or embarrassment. They should *never* be painful, except for tenderness from underlying pathology.

3. **When should a chaperone attend the pelvic exam?**
   - Whenever the examiner is male
   - If the patient is a minor
   - If the patient requests it
   - At the examiner's discretion when the patient is particularly anxious

4. **What circumstances can make pelvic exams difficult for women?**
   For one, it may be their very first exam and, hence, totally unfamiliar. In this case, explain very clearly what you are going to do, and show the equipment you will use. Secondly, the patient might have never had intercourse and thus presents with a small vaginal opening that makes speculum insertion rather difficult. Postmenopausal women, especially if not sexually active, also may present with a small (and atrophic) introitus. In addition, women

from various cultures might have undergone some type of "circumcision" that altered their anatomy and rendered the examination more difficult. Finally, the patient might have a background of childhood/adult sexual abuse—even rape. This can often cause panic (or dissociation) during the exam. Hence, it is essential that you elicit information of this sort during history-taking, especially while the patient is still clothed and comfortably seated—*not* while she is on the exam table.

5. **What are some techniques that can assist you in a difficult exam?**
The most valuable, definitely, is *communication*—and observation, too. For example, if at the beginning of the exam you see the patient bring her knees together, immediately stop and allow her to sit up comfortably. Put a drape on her lap, and then ask about her concerns. *If the exam is not urgently needed, reschedule it.* For women who are anxious because they are undergoing their first evaluation, ask them to return, but also instruct them to practice by inserting tampons or a disposable speculum. Instruct postmenopausal women with atrophy to apply an estrogen vaginal cream during the week preceding the rescheduled exam. Ask sexual abuse survivors if they feel *safe* about undergoing a pelvic exam. In fact, you may even want to offer them preparatory counseling. Finally, ask patients who have experienced "female circumcision" (i.e., female genital mutilation [FGM]) to contact the *RAINBO Foundation*, which can provide them with useful information.

6. **Who is qualified to perform a pelvic exam for sexual assault victims?**
Only individuals with training in forensic techniques, because an incomplete exam might prevent law enforcement authorities from arresting (and convicting) the perpetrator. Hence, when confronted with these situations, immediately contact local officials, who will provide you with qualified examiners, evidence-collecting kits, and appropriate forms for documenting the history and pelvic exam. Always be as supportive of the victim as possible—yet, do not allow her to change (or bathe) until the forensic exam has been completed. Otherwise, valuable evidence might get lost, including fibers, hairs, fingernail scrapings, blood, or body fluids.

7. **What are the tools needed for a pelvic exam?**
   - Padded exam table with padded foot rests (quilted oven mitts do nicely)
   - Good and adjustable light source (gooseneck or fiberoptic lamp)
   - Examination gloves
   - Plastic (or metal) vaginal specula of various sizes and types, including Pedersen's, Graves', and pediatric
   - Water-soluble lubricant
   - Tissues
   - Although a simple direct exam can provide lots of information, a few bedside diagnostic procedures are routinely added. These include occult blood testing, microbiologic assessment, and performance of the Papanicolaou smear (which provides a simple cytologic exam for cervical inflammation, atypia, or dysplasia). To carry out these procedures you will need:
     - Glass slides for Pap smear and wet mount
     - Cytological fixative
     - A small test tube with a few drops of normal saline for the wet mount
     - pH paper
     - Cytobrush and wooden spatula for collecting the Pap smear
     - Cotton-tipped applicators and specimen collection tubes for gonococcal and chlamydial testing by DNA probe analysis
     - Fecal occult blood testing card and hemoccult developer

8. **What are the components of the pelvic exam?**
   - Inspection and palpation of external genitalia
   - Examination with speculum
   - Bimanual palpation
   - Rectovaginal palpation

A. INSPECTION/PALPATION OF EXTERNAL GENITALIA: VULVA AND PERINEUM

9. **What is the anatomy of the vulva?**
   The vulva comprises several anatomic structures: (1) the mons veneris (or pubis), (2) the labia majora and minora, (3) the clitoris, (4) the urethral meatus, (5) the Skene's glands, (6) the vaginal vestibule and introitus, and (7) the vestibular (Bartholin's) glands. All should be inspected. Any lesion should be palpated.

10. **What should you look for in the external genitalia?**
    It depends on the structure. Inspect (1) the *vulvar skin* (for redness, nodules, swellings, excoriations, ulcerations, and changes in pigmentation/leukoplakia); (2) the *mons veneris* (for lesions and swelling); and (3) the *hair* (for lice and nits). By gently spreading the labia majora and minora, you will then get access to the vaginal vestibule. Inspect (and palpate) the *urethral* meatus (for purulent discharge) and the Skene's glands. Inspect the *clitoris, perineum,* and *anus*. Look for masses, scars, fissures, and fistulas. Finally, check for hemorrhoids, and palpate any visible lesions.

11. **Where are the openings of *Skene's (paraurethral) glands*?**
    On either side of the urethral meatus. Inspect them, and palpate them. Then, insert your index finger into the vagina, press up onto the urethra, and milk it for possible discharge.

12. **Who was Skene?**
    Alexander J. Skene (1838–1900) was a Scot, who at the age of 18 moved to Canada and then to New York, where he obtained his medical degree in the midst of the American Civil War. He did serve in that war (even planning an army ambulance corps), eventually going back to the practice of gynecology and becoming one of the founders of the American Gynecological Society. Still, his call to fame was the 1880 description of the homonymous glands, which was nothing new, since they had already been reported in 1672 by Reiner de Graaf, in an observation that (as often happens in medicine) had been totally forgotten.

13. **What important information can be gained by inspecting the vulva?**
    Mostly the degree of estrogenization of the urogenital tract, which is reflected by the presence of mucus and by the thickness and rugation of the vulvar/vaginal mucosae.

14. **What is the *female escutcheon?***
    It is the triangular pattern of pubic hair that is unique to adult females (i.e., with apex pointing *down* toward the pubis). The male escutcheon is instead a *reverse* triangle, with apex pointing *up* toward the umbilicus. A masculine escutcheon in a woman is usually a sign of virilization, even though it also may be a normal variant.

15. **What are Tanner's stages of sexual maturation?**
    They are a way to assess sexual maturation by following the growth of *breast* and *pubic hair*. They are mostly used in pediatric and adolescent medicine, but also can be helpful in evaluating patients with primary amenorrhea (Table 17-1).

TABLE 17-1. TANNER STAGES OF SEXUAL MATURATION IN GIRLS

Stage	Description	Mean Age	Age Range (5–95%)
Pubic Hair			
I	None	—	—
II	Countable; straight; increased pigmentation and length; primarily on medial border of labia	11.25	9–13.5
III	Darker; begins to curl; increased quantity on mons pubis	12	9.5–14.25
IV	Increased quantity; coarser texture; labia and mons well covered	12.5	10.5–15
V	Adult distribution with feminine triangle and spread to medial thighs	14	12–16.5
Breast Development			
I	None	—	—
II	Breast bud present; increase areolar size	11	9–13
III	Further enlargement of breast; no secondary contour	12	10–14
IV	Areolar area forms secondary mound on breast contour	13	10.5–15.5
V	Mature; areolar area is part of breast contour; nipple projects	15	13–18
Menarche		12.8	11–14.5

(From Polin RA, Ditmar MF: Pediatric Secrets, 2nd ed. Philadelphia, Hanley & Belfus, 1997.)

16. **What is the differential diagnosis of *enlarged inguinal nodes*?**
The major one is *infection* of the genital area, lower extremities, or nodes per se. *Cancer* should also be ruled out, either primary (lymphoma) or metastatic.

17. **What is the significance of *white* vulvar lesions?**
They may be benign, premalignant, or malignant.

18. **What are the *benign white* lesions of the vulva?**
They are mostly vitiligo and inflammatory dermatitis, like psoriasis.

19. **What are the most common *premalignant white* lesions?**
Vulvar dystrophies, such as *hyperplastic dystrophy* (squamous cell hyperplasia) and *lichen sclerosus et atrophicus* (LS&A). LS&A is an atrophic condition of the vulva and perianal skin that can occur alone or in association with other cutaneous lesions. It presents as patches of reddened and thin skin, which evolve into yellowish-bluish papules/macules, eventually coalescing into areas of atrophic, grayish, and crinkling mucosa—smooth, thin, fragile. Itching and burning are common, and so is secondary infection. Other symptoms may include

dyspareunia (pain during intercourse) and skin splitting and bleeding. The condition may eventually lead to resorption of the clitoris and labia minora. It also may progress to malignancy, usually squamous cell carcinoma. Although LS&A may occur in all age groups, it is more common in postmenopausal women (especially Caucasian and Latino), where extensive lesions can even narrow the introitus. *Hyperplastic dystrophy* can present quite similarly, as a pruritic grayish-whitish plaque, but it does *not* lead to resorption of the labia and clitoris. Moreover, it is microscopically differentiated from LS&A because of its squamous cell hyperplasia/atypia. Vulvar dystrophies represent a continuum from benign to malignant, with white lesions of both kinds frequently coexisting in the vulva. Hence, the need to biopsy any white and dystrophic area.

20. **What are *malignant white* lesions?**
    Mostly two: vulvar intraepithelial neoplasia and Bowen's disease.

21. **What are other vulvar malignancies?**
    The most common is squamous cell carcinoma. Of interest, melanoma is the next most common. Hence, both patients and physician should be quite attentive to vulvar "moles" and include this area in their regular examination for nevi. Other histologic types include adenocarcinoma (of Bartholin's gland), basal cell carcinoma, and sarcoma.

22. **What is the differential diagnosis of a *painful* vulvar ulceration?**
    A painful (and multiple) vulvar ulceration is usually due to ruptured and coalescent herpes simplex lesions or chancroid.

23. **What is the differential diagnosis of a *painless* vulvar ulceration?**
    A painful (and solitary) vulvar ulceration is usually due to syphilis. A painless but longstanding ulcer should raise the suspicion for a vulvar carcinoma.

24. **What is a labial hernia?**
    The uncommon occurrence of the herniation of a bowel loop into one of the *labia majora*, analogous to an inguinal hernia in a male.

25. **Where are Bartholin's glands located?**
    Deep in the lateral walls of the vulva, close to the posterior fornix.

26. **How do you examine them?**
    By placing a gloved index finger just inside the vaginal opening (near the posterior end of the introitus) and the thumb on the outside. Then, to examine the right Bartholin's gland, grasp the posterior portion of the right major labium between the index finger and the thumb. Palpate gently for enlargement or tenderness. Do the same for the contralateral gland. Note that in the absence of disease, Bartholin's glands should be neither visible nor palpable.

27. **What is the differential diagnosis of a mass or swelling of the Bartholin's gland?**
    The most common is cysts or abscesses of the glands. These are quite common and present as indurated (and often tender) enlargement of one or both labia majora. More rarely, adenocarcinoma of the gland also can be responsible.

28. **Who was Bartholin?**
    Caspar Bartholin (1655–1738) was a Danish physician and the son of a famous anatomist (who provided the first description of intestinal lymphatics and their drainage into the thoracic duct). Caspar managed to outdo his dad, not only because of his description of the homonymous glands (and their possible cystic degeneration), but also because of his discovery of the *sublingual glands* and their ducts, which still carry his name. During the last

part of his life, he left medicine for politics, becoming Denmark's procurator general and deputy of finance.

29. **What is the hymen? What are the myths surrounding it?**
From the Greek *humen* (membrane), the hymen is a ring of tissue around the vaginal opening. Contrary to popular belief, a normal hymen does *not* completely occlude the introitus (*see* question 30) but simply surrounds it as an *annular* structure. Hymens also can be *septate* (with one or more bands across the opening) or *cribriform* (completely stretching across the opening, but with several perforations). After pregnancy, they are usually reduced to a few remnants around the vaginal opening or to a ragged and irregular outline. Yet completely intact hymens have been reported after delivery. They also have been reported after intercourse. In fact, bleeding may *not* occur at all after the first vaginal penetration, and if it does, it may not be due to laceration of the hymen, but to trauma of nearby tissues. Finally, the infamous straddle injuries of old (such as horseback riding or falling on the horizontal bar of a bicycle) do *not* traumatize the hymen.

30. **What is an imperforate hymen?**
A congenital abnormality that often goes unrecognized until puberty, when the patient becomes symptomatic from retained menses. On exam, the hymen appears as an intact and completely closed membrane, bulging with retained menstrual products. If untreated, this can lead to hematometrium and hematosalpinx. Treatment is *hymenotomy,* which also is the treatment of choice for unusually thick hymens, another congenital abnormality, often responsible for dyspareunia.

31. **What is the normal size of the glans clitoris?**
Around 3–4 mm.

32. **What is the clitoral index (CI)? How do you calculate it?**
The CI is a "poor man's" bioassay of androgenic stimulation since it reflects the stimulation of the clitoris by both testosterone and 17-ketosteroids. It is calculated by multiplying the sagittal and transverse diameters of the glans, with the normal range being 9–35 mm. A CI of 36–99 mm is usually borderline, whereas one >100 mm is considered abnormal. Enlargement of the clitoris indicates virilization and thus should prompt a search for sources of androgenization.

33. **What is the appearance of the clitoris and vulva in congenital adrenal hyperplasia?**
Virilized. This is usually apparent from birth, including clitoral hypertrophy and fused labia. In untreated females, secondary sex characteristics fail to develop.

34. **What is congenital adrenal hyperplasia?**
The generic term for hereditary deficiency of a number of enzymes of glucocorticoid synthesis—the most common being 21-hydroxylase and 11-B-hydroxylase. The resulting decrease in hydrocortisone levels leads to greater adrenocorticotropic hormone (ACTH) production, which, in turn, causes a secondary increase in adrenal androgens. Hence, the virilization. A very famous patient with this condition was probably Queen Christina of Sweden, whose sexuality has been a subject of speculation from the very day of her birth, when she was indeed mistaken for a boy (the cannons at the royal palace saluted her as such). Some have even suggested that she may have been a *female pseudohermaphrodite*. Christina was the cultured and intellectual daughter of Gustavus Adolphus, a war-mongering Protestant king and the Catholics' scourge during the Thirty Years War. After her father got himself killed in battle, young Christina invited Descartes to Stockholm to spruce up the local cultural scene. Unfortunately, he soon caught pneumonia and died, which convinced the queen that it was finally time to move to

more southern and warmer climates. In a few months, she abdicated, became a Catholic, and relocated in Rome. Some historians have even speculated that the real reason behind this surprising decision was that she did not want to take a husband, possibly as a result of her congenital adrenal hyperplasia. Either way, she spent the rest of her life in Italy, pursuing culture, beauty, and romantic liaisons—mostly with women. After her death, she was buried in St Peter's Basilica, not too far from Michelangelo's Pietà—the only woman (?) to this day to have had such an honor. Of interest, she also was portrayed in a homonymous movie by another enigmatic Swede, Greta Garbo, who also was rumored to like women better than men. In 1965, Christina's body was disinterred and examined, but because of decomposition (and the fact that the embalmers had removed the internal organs), no final conclusions could be drawn on her sexuality. She remained as elusive in death as she had been in life.

35. **What should one look for when inspecting the labia?**
For warts (*see* questions 36 and 37), ulcers, masses, discharge, atrophies, and swellings. Note that yellow-white asymptomatic papules may occasionally be noted on the inner aspect of the labia minora. They represent ectopic sebaceous glands (Fordyce's spots), like those seen in the mouth and penile shaft (*see* Male Genitalia and HEENT chapters). They are entirely normal.

36. **What are condylomata *lata*?**
They are *flat* warts typical of secondary syphilis.

37. **What are condylomata *acuminata*?**
They are *genital warts* due to the human papillomavirus (HPV). They present as flesh-colored papules with cauliflower-like papillations that can degenerate into cervical cancer. There are more than 70 serotypes of HPV. Of these, serotypes 16, 18, 45, and 56 have the highest malignant potential.

38. **How does genital herpes simplex present?**
With clusters of small (<1 mm) fluid-filled vesicles on an erythematous base. These may rupture or coalesce, eventually resulting in a *painful* vulvar ulceration (*see* question 22).

B. EXAMINATION WITH SPECULUM—THE VAGINA

39. **What is a speculum?**
A metal (or plastic) tool that is used to hold back the walls of the vagina in order to visualize the cervix and collect specimens. Specula come as small, medium, and large, and all consist of a handle and two blades (or bills). Before using them, always practice with the handle mechanism, and *always warm the blades with warm water*. Never use jelly lubricant, since this may interfere with cytologic determination and gonococcal cultures (*see* questions 59–64).

40. **What are *Pedersen's* and *Graves'*? What are their differences?**
They are the two main specula types. Pedersen's is 0.5-inch *narrower* than Graves' and with *flat* blades. Although it provides a more comfortable fit for women, it is mostly suited for patients with a small, (and at times) atrophic introitus, such as the young (nulliparous) and the elderly (menopausal). The Graves' speculum is instead *wider* than Pedersen's and with blades that are *biconcave*. It is more commonly used, especially in multiparous women, or women in whom Pedersen's is unable to retract the vaginal wall adequately enough to visualize the cervix. Both Pedersen's and Graves' may be made of metal or clear plastic.

41. **How do you insert the speculum?**
Use your *left* index and middle fingers to separate the labia and depress the perineum. Ask the patient to take a deep breath, and then use your *right* hand to gently insert the closed

speculum into the introitus, pointing the handle down at *an oblique angle of 45 degrees* (inserting it vertically may traumatize urethra or meatus). Slide the speculum over your left fingers, and while inserting it, *rotate it downward to 90 degrees*— eventually pointing the handle vertical to the floor. Gently open the blades by squeezing on the handle mechanism. This will open the vaginal walls and hold them apart, allowing you to inspect the lateral walls of the vagina and the cervix. If made of clear plastic, the speculum also will allow you to inspect the vaginal *vault*. Once in good position (i.e., with the cervix in clear view), keep the speculum open by tightening the set screw.

42. **When do you withdraw the speculum? How?**
    The speculum can be withdrawn once you are done with cervical inspection and Pap sampling. To do so:
    1. *Hold the blades open while releasing the screw* (otherwise the blades might painfully close on the cervix).
    2. Once the speculum is safely away from the cervix, allow the blades to partially close, so that you can still inspect the vaginal walls. Look for bleeding, ulcers, tumors; also note the amount, color, and character of any discharge.
    3. Finally, as you further withdraw the speculum, allow the blades to close completely.

43. **What is a *colpocele*?**
    From the Greek *kolpos* (vagina) and *kele* (bulging), a colpocele is a vaginal prolapse, often the result of hysterectomy.

44. **What is a *cystocele*? How can you detect it?**
    A cystocele is a bulge in the *anterior* wall of the vagina, caused by weakening of the wall and protrusion of the bladder. It can be detected by observing through the speculum the anterior vaginal wall with the patient either bearing down or coughing. In more severe cases, it can even be observed at the vestibule, after separating the minor labia. Finally, it can be palpated, too.

45. **What is a *rectocele*? How can you detect it?**
    A rectocele is a bulge in the *posterior* wall of the vagina, caused by weakening of the wall and protrusion of the rectum. Like the cystocele, it can be detected through inspection or intravaginal palpation while the patient is bearing down or coughing.

46. **What are the clues to the presence of a rectovaginal fistula?**
    A history of fecal contamination in the vagina. The fistula also may be *palpable,* as an indurated area in the posterior vaginal wall.

47. **What is *Chadwick's sign*?**
    The bluish-violet appearance of vagina or cervix. This is a sign of pregnancy (usually occurring after the seventh week of gestation), but it also may occur in association with a pelvic tumor. It results from mucosal congestion and is most notable in the anterior vaginal wall.

48. **Who was Chadwick?**
    James R. Chadwick (1844–1905) was an American gynecologist. Born in Boston and schooled at Harvard, Chadwick traveled extensively in Europe after graduation, visiting the medical centers of Vienna, London, Paris, and Berlin. He eventually returned to his native Boston, where he went on to become one of the founding fathers of the Boston Medical Library and the president of the American Gynecological Society.

49. **What is diethylstilbestrol (DES)? What is the vaginal appearance of women with prenatal exposure to it?**
DES was an oral synthetic nonsteroidal estrogen, which was used from 1938 to 1972 to prevent miscarriage, until found to cause vaginal changes in women who had been exposed to it in utero. The most common of these is *adenomyosis* (90% of the cases), which consists of a glandular columnar epithelium of the vagina. This is not premalignant, but can be associated with clear cell adenocarcinoma. Hence, DES patients must be followed serially, with exams and colposcopy.

50. **What is a *Gartner's duct cyst*?**
A benign tumor arising in the anterior or lateral wall of the vagina. It is a congenital lesion caused by retained epithelial remnants of the Wolffian duct.

51. **Who was Gartner?**
Hermann T. Gartner (1785–1827) was a Danish surgeon. A native of St. Thomas, West Indies (when this was still a Danish possession), Gartner eventually returned to Denmark, graduated from Copenhagen Medical School, and worked as an army surgeon for most of his professional life.

52. **What is the normal vaginal pH?**
Acid, because vaginal secretions are in the acidic range, with pH <4.5.

53. **What is the significance of tenderness in the vaginal fornices?**
It depends. Tenderness in either the left or right vaginal fornix usually indicates ipsilateral salpingitis, but tenderness of the *right* fornix also may represent a sign of retrocecal appendicitis.

C. EXAMINATION WITH SPECULUM—THE CERVIX

54. **What is the best way to visualize the cervix?**
Through the speculum. Note that cervical visualization may be difficult in patients with either retroverted uterus or displacement by prolapse. To improve vision, reposition the speculum by slowly pulling it back. You also may want to gently turn the bills in various directions. Yet, remember that the most common reason for not visualizing the cervix is an *incomplete insertion of the speculum*. If still unable to locate the cervix, perform first the bimanual exam by lubricating your gloved fingers with water (other lubricants may ruin the Pap smear). Once you have palpated the cervix, it will be easier to aim the speculum toward the correct direction.

55. **How does a normal nonparous cervix appear?**
It looks round, pink, and with a central *os* (this in the *parous* cervix is horizontal and possibly "fishmouthed"). A darker and reddish columnar epithelium at the *os* is a normal variation, as are the presence of small and yellowish nabothian cysts. Inspect the cervix for color, size, configuration, discharge, erosions, ulcerations, cysts, polyps, leukoplakia, and masses.

56. **What are *endocervical polyps*? What is their significance?**
They are small pedunculated masses that protrude from the endocervical canal and are composed of columnar epithelium. Although at times friable and bleeding, they are invariably benign.

57. **What is the cause of cervical duplication?**
Common in animals, a cervical (and uterine) duplication is usually due to failure of Müllerian duct fusion. It is often associated with a partially or fully septate vagina. On physical exam, the two cervices are often different in size, appearing side by side in the coronal plane.

58. **What is the *squamocolumnar junction*?**
It is the meeting of the *columnar* endothelium of the *endocervical* canal with the external pink mucosa of the *ectocervix* (which is covered by *squamous* cells). This transition zone is a crucial area, since 95% of all cervical cancers originate from it. Yet, the junction may or may not be visible on speculum examination. Note that for an adequate evaluation of the cervix, you *must* sample cells from all three layers: ectocervix, transition zone, and endocervix.

59. **What is a Pap smear? What is the best way to obtain it?**
The Pap smear is a preparation of *endocervical* canal cells. These are obtained by inserting a brush into the endocervical canal, and rotating it 180 degrees (a 360-degree rotation is more likely to cause bleeding). The brush is then withdrawn and either run across a slide (standard method) or agitated in a tube of medium (thin prep method). Squamous cells from the *ectocervix* are instead obtained by scraping the cervix circumferentially with a wooden spatula, and then spreading the sample on either a slide or a tube medium. Pap smear slides must be fixed with cytology fixative as quickly as possible.

60. **Which patients benefit from regular Pap smear screening?**
Mostly two groups of patients:
  - Women who are sexually active (since they are the ones mostly at risk for HPV infection). They should undergo vaginal Paps either yearly or biennially.
  - Women who have had hysterectomies for malignant disease. Conversely, women who have had hysterectomies for *benign* reasons (such as myomata) no longer need Pap screening.

61. **Who was "Pap"?**
George N. Papanicolaou (1883–1962) was an American pathologist. A native of Greece and a graduate of Athens University, Papanicolaou gained a medical degree only because of his father's wishes and only as a prerequisite to then be free to pursue a career in history and philosophy. The Balkan Wars of 1912–1913 (and the outbreak of World War I) totally changed his plans, pushing him to emigrate to the United States, where he went on to become chair of pathology at Cornell. A soft-spoken and modest man, he always maintained a very thick Greek accent.

62. **What is the significance of a purulent cervical discharge?**
It is usually the harbinger of purulent cervicitis, most often caused by gonorrhea or chlamydia. If untreated, this may result in pelvic inflammatory disease and its various sequelae.

63. **What is the significance of cervical motion tenderness?**
It suggests pelvic inflammatory disease. Informally known as the "chandelier sign," since patients "hit the chandelier" whenever their tender cervix is palpated.

64. **What additional laboratory tests should be obtained from the cervix?**
In high-risk populations, some clinicians routinely culture for gonorrhea and chlamydia because chlamydial infection may be relatively asymptomatic, and if undiagnosed, can lead to serious sequelae—such as infertility. Hence, the low threshold for screening, especially in cases of any of the aforementioned signs of purulent cervicitis.

D. BIMANUAL PALPATION—THE UTERINE CORPUS

65. **What is the normal shape and location of the uterus?**
The uterus has the shape and size of a small pear. It is *anteverted* and *anteflexed* in approximately 80% of women.

66. **What is the best way to examine the uterus?**
    Bimanually—a technique used not only to palpate the uterus, but also the adnexa (*see* questions 77–82). Prepare the patient by first lowering the head of the exam table to 15 degrees or flat, and by then having her lay the arms on either the chest or sides (which will relax the abdominal muscles). While standing next to the patient, insert then the gloved middle finger and forefinger of one hand (usually your right) into the vagina, in a downward and posterior direction, with gentle pressure toward the *posterior* fornix. Try to avoid the periurethral area. With fingers half in, rotate your hand 90 degrees clockwise, so that your palm faces upward, the thumb is extended, and the fourth and fifth fingers are pushed against the palm. Continue to insert the fingers into the vagina until you reach the cervix. At this point, palpate the vaginal walls and rugae, looking for nodules, scarring, and induration. Also assess the cervix for configuration, consistency, and tenderness. Once done, place your *other* hand (usually the left) on the abdominal wall, starting from the umbilicus and moving downward to the symphysis. Reach through the wall for both the uterus and adnexa. Use your vaginal hand to push the pelvic organs *up*, making them accessible (and palpable) to the abdominal hand. Note size, position, configuration, consistency, and sensitivity of the uterus. Remember that throughout the exam you should keep your eyes *on the patient*, looking for any signs of discomfort.

67. **What is *Goodell's sign*?**
    The softening of the cervix that usually occurs at 8 weeks of gestation. While the cervix of a *non*pregnant woman feels like the tip of the nose, the softer cervix of a pregnant woman feels like a *lip*.

68. **Who was Goodell?**
    William Goodell (1829–1894) was an American gynecologist. Born in Malta (where his missionary father was temporarily stationed), he graduated from Jefferson Medical College in 1854. After practicing in Constantinople for 3 years (where he also married), he returned to the United States and went on to become chair of gynecology at the University of Pennsylvania. A wealthy clinician and a refractory insomniac, Goodell suffered all his life from gout.

69. **What is *Hegar's sign*?**
    It is a peculiar softening of the uterus at the junction between cervix and fundus, typical of the first trimester of pregnancy. It may be elicited by placing two fingers in the posterior vaginal fornix, and then compressing the uterus gently down by using the other hand.

70. **What is the difference between uterine retroversion and retroflexion?**
    Retroversion is a posterior angulation of the *entire uterus*, including the cervix. **Retroflexion** is a posterior flexion of the uterine *corpus*, while the cervix remains in its usual position. Both are normal variants, occurring in about 20% of women (Fig. 17-1).

71. **What is uterine *prolapse*?**
    It is a downward sagging of the uterus caused by gravity and a weak pelvic floor musculature. In *first-degree prolapse*, the uterus has slipped downward but is still palpable relatively high in the vaginal vault. In *second-degree prolapse*, the uterus has descended the length of the vagina and the cervix presents at the introitus. *Third-degree prolapse* (also known as *procidentia uteri*) is instead a descent of the uterus beyond the vaginal opening.

72. **What is *fundal height*? How does it change with weeks of gestation?**
    Fundal height is the vertical dimension of the pregnant uterus. After 12 weeks of gestation, the uterine fundus is palpable above the pelvic brim. At 18 weeks it is palpable at the umbilical level.

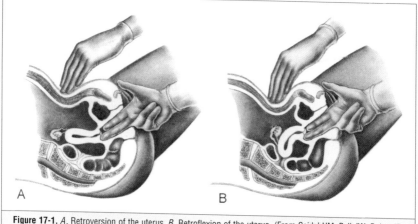

Figure 17-1. *A*, Retroversion of the uterus. *B*, Retroflexion of the uterus. (From Seidel HM, Ball JW, Dains JE, Benedict UW: Mosby's Guide to Physical Examination, 3rd ed. St. Louis, Mosby, 1995.)

73. **What are *Leopold's maneuvers*?**
They are four sequential palpations of the pregnant abdomen to determine the intrauterine position (and presentation) of the fetus after the 28th week of gestation. They are difficult to perform in obese women, thus making ultrasound a necessity.

74. **Who were Hegar and Leopold?**
They were both German gynecologists who lived during the second half of the 19th century and died at the beginning of the 20th century. Hegar also is famous for the dilators that still carry his name.

75. **What are *leiomyomata*?**
Also known as uterine myomas (or "fibroids"), leiomyomata are benign muscular tumors of the uterus. They may range in size from impalpable to very large. Size is usually notated in *weeks of gestation* (e.g., a myomatous uterus that is as enlarged as an 18-week pregnancy may be described as an "18-week size fibroid"). Leiomyomata on the lateral aspect of the uterus may be indistinguishable from adnexal masses. Large leiomyomata may be easily palpable in the lower abdomen.

76. **Are "fibroids" ever malignant?**
Rarely. Leiomyosarcomas account for less than 1% of uterine tumors.

E. BIMANUAL PALPATION—THE ADNEXA

77. **What are the adnexa?**
They are ovaries, oviducts (Fallopian tubes), and supporting tissues.

78. **When do you examine them?**
During the bimanual examination and after completing the uterine evaluation. To do so, shift the fingers you are holding in the vagina from the posterior fornix to each *lateral* one, while at the same time sweeping with your abdominal hand medially and inferiorly from the pelvic brim, toward the left lower abdominal quadrant. Gently compress the tissues between your

fingertips. Look for ovaries, adnexal masses, and tenderness. Beware that this part of the exam is markedly limited in obese patients.

79. **How large are the ovaries?**
In young women, they are usually 3.5–4 cm in the longest diameter, and thus often palpable in a thin subject—like a small almond sliding between your fingers. In postmenopausal women, on the other hand, they shrink to 2 cm in diameter, so that they become impalpable.

80. **What is the differential diagnosis of adnexal *masses*?**
It includes physiologic cysts (follicular or corpus luteum cysts), polycystic ovaries, ectopic pregnancy, and endometriomas; also, benign tumors (such as teratomas, serous or mucinous cystadenoma, or Brenner tumor); malignant ovarian tumors; tubo-ovarian abscesses; hydrosalpinx or hematosalpinx. In some cases, an adnexal mass is actually *not* adnexal, but instead a uterine myoma that is lateral or pedunculated; an appendiceal mass or abscess; a pelvic kidney; or some other abdominal tumor.

81. **What is the differential diagnosis of adnexal *tenderness*?**
The major are (1) ectopic pregnancy and (2) tubo-ovarian abscesses. Other less common causes include ovarian cysts, endometriomas, and other intra-abdominal pathology—such as appendicitis.

82. **What are the physical characteristics of *malignant ovarian tumors*?**
Bilateral, large, less mobile, and with a nodular/irregular quality on palpation. Ovarian cancers also may be associated with other suggestive findings, such as abdominal distention and ascites.

F. BIMANUAL PALPATION—THE CUL-DE-SAC

83. **What is the cul-de-sac?**
Also called the *pouch of Douglas*, this is the parietal peritoneum-lined space behind the uterus. It can be evaluated at the end of the bimanual exam, by moving the vaginal fingers to the posterior fornix. This allows you to palpate the uterosacral ligaments and the posterior uterine aspect (including the cul-de-sac) for fluid or tenderness.

G. RECTOVAGINAL PALPATION

84. **What is rectovaginal palpation?**
It is an assessment of the rectovaginal *septum*. To do so, first change your gloves (not to spread infection from the vagina to the rectum), then inspect the anus for external lesions, lubricate your gloved index and middle fingers, and ask the patient to bear down while you insert the middle finger into the rectum and the *index* finger into the vagina. Palpate the *rectovaginal septum* looking for tenderness, thickness, nodularities, or masses. Also palpate the cul-de-sac.

85. **What is the role of rectovaginal examination?**
It allows for a better assessment of the posterior aspect of the pelvis and cul-de-sac. For example, tenderness in this area suggests endometriosis, especially if associated with nodularity.

86. **When is the rectovaginal exam carried out?**
Usually when (1) the uterus is retroverted, (2) a malignancy is suspected, (3) the patient is older than 40. Otherwise, it is not necessary.

ACKNOWLEDGMENT

The author gratefully acknowledges the contributions of Carol Fleischman, MD, to this chapter in the first edition of *Physical Diagnosis Secrets*.

SELECTED BIBLIOGRAPHY

1. Bastian I A, Piscitclli JT: Is this patient pregnant? Can you reliably rule in or rule out pregnancy by clinical examination? JAMA 278:586–591

2. Bates B: A Guide to Physical Examination and History Taking. Philadelphia, JB Lippincott, 1991.

3. De Gowin E, DeGowin R: Bedside Diagnostic Examination. New York, Macmillan, 1976.

4. Frederickson HL, Wilkins-Haug L: Ob/Gyn Secrets. Philadelphia, Hanley and Belfus, 1997.

5. Mayeaux EJ, Spigener S: Epidemiology of human papillomavirus infections. Hosp Pract 15:39–41, 1997.

6. Moore K: The Developing Human. Philadelphia, WB Saunders, 1982.

7. Pearce KF, Haefner HK, Sarwar SF, et al: Cytopathological findings on vaginal Papanicolaou smears after hysterectomy for benign gynecological disease. N Engl J Med 335:1559–1562, 1996.

8. Robbins S, Cotran R: The Pathologic Basis of Disease. Philadelphia, WB Saunders, 1979.

CHAPTER 18

LYMPH NODES

Salvatore Mangione, MD

> *"Whatever the date may be, this unfortunate foot-soldier and bearer of misfortune entered the city with a large bundle of clothes bought or stolen from German troops. He went to stay at the house of relations in the district round the Porta Orientale, near the Capuchin convent. Scarcely had he arrived, that he fell ill. He was carried to the hospital, where a bubonic tumour found under the arm-pit made the attendant suspect what was, in fact, the truth. On the fourth day he died."*
>
> –Alessandro Manzoni (1785–1873), *The Plague of Milan*, from *The Betrothed*

A. GENERAL CONSIDERATIONS

Lymph nodes are important. A methodical search may yield invaluable clues in cancer or systemic disease. Some "sentinel" nodes have even entered medical folklore, forever linked by eponyms to the physicians who first described them.

1. **Which nodes are normally palpable in the healthy individual?**
   Out of a total of 600, only the *submandibular*, *axillary*, or *inguinal* nodes may at times be felt. Examiner's skill is, of course, paramount, usually improving with time.

2. **What is *lymphadenopathy*?**
   The presence of abnormal nodes, because of size, consistency, or number. Adenopathy can occur in various conditions, affecting individuals of any age, and with or without symptoms. It may be happenstance (as incidental detection by the physician or patient during routine exam) or the first sign of malignancy, the presenting manifestation of a complex systemic disorder or a self-limited finding. The differential diagnosis is always challenging.

3. **How many adenopathies turn out to be "bad"?**
   Difficult to say, since data are scarce. In a Dutch study of 2556 patients presenting with unexplained lymph nodal enlargement to a primary care office, 10% were eventually referred to subspecialists, and 3.2% ultimately underwent biopsy. Only 29/2556 (1.1%) had a final diagnosis of malignancy. This low prevalence was confirmed by two separate U.S. studies, suggesting that the much higher neoplastic prevalence of 40–60% reported by many textbooks refers only to the 3% who underwent biopsy, thus grossly overestimating the likelihood of cancer. Hence, in primary care settings, unexplained adenopathy has a neoplastic risk of only 4% in patients 40 years or older and 0.4% in those younger than 40.

4. **What is the first approach to adenopathy?**
   To sort out "serious" from benign. To do so, first separate *generalized* from *localized*, since these are distinct conditions with unique differential diagnoses.

5. **What is a generalized adenopathy?**
   One that involves two or more noncontiguous sites (conversely, a *localized* adenopathy is one that involves only one site). Always make sure that the "localized" ones are not instead

part of a *generalized* process. This may not be necessarily self-evident, since only 17% of all generalized adenopathies are correctly identified by primary care physicians. Hence, whenever you find an abnormal site, always evaluate all others.

6. **Where should you look for enlarged nodes?**
   - Submandibular and submental areas
   - Anterior and posterior cervical regions
   - Supraclavicular fossa
   - Axilla
   - Epitrochlear space
   - Inguinal/femoral sites

   Important nodes also can be found in the popliteal fossa and paraumbilical region. Deeper ones (hilar, mediastinal, abdominal, and pelvic) are important, too, but inaccessible.

7. **Which parts of the exam should be emphasized in cases of generalized adenopathy?**
   Those that may uncover signs of *systemic disease*, such as skin rash, mucous membrane lesions, hepatomegaly, splenomegaly, and arthritis.

8. **What is the differential diagnosis of a *generalized* adenopathy?**
   One of three processes: (1) *a disseminated malignancy,* especially hematologic (lymphomas, leukemias, and angioimmunoblastic lymphadenopathy); (2) *a collagen vascular disorder* (sarcoidosis, rheumatoid arthritis (RA), and systemic lupus erythematosus [SLE]); or (3) *an infectious process* (mononucleosis, cytomegalovirus [CMV], AIDS, toxoplasmosis, syphilis, tuberculosis, histoplasmosis, coccidioidomycosis, brucellosis, and bubonic plague). Drug reaction can do it, too, and so can intravenous abuse. Some medications (e.g., phenytoin) specifically cause lymphadenopathy; others (e.g., cephalosporins, penicillins, or sulfonamides) do it instead in the context of a serum sickness-like syndrome, with fever, arthralgias, and skin rash (*see* Table 18-1).

TABLE 18-1. MEDICATIONS THAT MAY CAUSE LYMPHADENOPATHY

Allopurinol (Zyloprim)	Penicillin
Atenolol (Tenormin)	Phenytoin (Dilantin)
Captopril (Capozide)	Primidone (Mysoline)
Carbamazepine (Tegretol)	Pyrimethamine (Daraprim)
Cephalosporins	Quinidine
Gold	Sulfonamides
Hydralazine (Apresoline)	Sulindac (Clinoril)

(Adapted from Ferrer R: Lymphadenopathy. Am Fam Physician 58:1313–1323, 1998.)

9. **Should a biopsy be done in patients with generalized lymphadenopathy?**
   Yes, especially considering the often serious (and systemic) character of the condition. Remember to always biopsy the *largest* node. If nodes are of similar size, choose in descending order: the supraclavicular, cervical, axillary, epitrochlear, and inguinal stations. The latter is the

least helpful, since it often shows only reactive hyperplasia. Yet, do not disregard it. In one retrospective study (with careful patient selection), 53% of inguinal biopsies turned out to be diagnostic. Also, beware that some sites may be more prone to surgical complications than others. Sampling the parotid area, for example, can damage the facial nerve or its branches, while biopsying the posterior cervical triangle may injure the spinal accessory nerve.

10. **Which is more common, localized or generalized adenopathy?**
    Localized. In a primary care setting, 75% of patients will present with localized involvement (head and neck, 55%; supraclavicular, 1%; axillary, 5%; inguinal, 14%).

11. **Can the region of involvement narrow the diagnosis?**
    Yes. As in real estate, location is very important for nodes (as applied, of course, to *regional* or *localized* adenopathies). For the *generalized* form, differential diagnosis is another ballgame). Overall, *regional* adenopathy reflects localized infection or neoplasm. For instance, cat-scratch disease for *cervical* or *axillary* nodes, sexually transmitted diseases for the *inguinal ones*, and infectious mono for the *cervical* station. Finally, *preauricular* nodes (of any size) are usually more significant than similarly sized nodes in other locations.

12. **Should one know the regions drained by the various lymphonodal stations?**
    Yes, since this may unlock the underlying cause. After detecting an enlarged node, always examine the region drained by it (*see* Table 18-2). Look for infections, skin lesions, or tumors.

13. **What are the general characteristics that can help interpret an abnormal node?**
    The mnemonic is **ALL AGES**:
    - **A** = **A**ge of patient
    - **L** = **L**ocation of the abnormal nodes
    - **L** = **L**ength of time the nodes have been present
    - **A** = **A**ssociated signs or symptoms, whether *local* or *extranodal*
    - **G** = Presence or absence of **g**eneralized lymphadenopathy
    - **E** = **E**xtranodal associations
    - **S** = Presence or absence of **s**plenomegaly and/or fever

14. **Why does the patient's age help?**
    Because it is the most important predictor of malignancy. Although lymphoproliferative disorders also may affect younger individuals, neoplastic nodes are usually more common in those older than 40 years (Table 18-3). Yet some malignant-looking nodes may actually be benign. Infectious mononucleosis, for example, may often resemble Hodgkin's disease.

15. **What about *associated signs and symptoms*?**
    They can be "local" or systemic (Table 18-4). *Local* findings suggest infection or neoplasm in a specific site (like the swollen nodes and lymphangitic streaks of a skin infection). Conversely, *systemic* symptoms (such as fever, fatigue, night sweats, and unexplained weight loss) argue in favor of a collagen vascular, lymphoproliferative, or infectious disorder (e.g., tuberculosis [TB]). Still, lack of associated signs or symptoms does *not* exclude malignancy and thus should *not* stop a work-up. Finally, remember that the adenopathy of Hodgkin's disease may become painful after alcohol ingestion.

16. **What about *splenomegaly*?**
    It occurs in only 5% of adenopathies, and when it does it argues in favor of sarcoidosis, acute leukemia, chronic lymphocytic leukemia, Hodgkin/non-Hodgkin lymphoma or a mononucleosis-like syndrome. It is instead uncommon in metastatic cancer.

TABLE 18-2. LYMPH NODE GROUPS: LOCATION, LYMPHATIC DRAINAGE AND SELECTED DIFFERENTIAL DIAGNOSIS*

Location	Lymphatic Drainage	Causes
Submental	Lower lip, anterior floor of mouth, tip of tongue, skin of cheek, teeth, nose	Mononucleosis-like syndromes, Epstein-Barr virus, CMV, toxoplasmosis
Submandibular	Tongue, submaxillary gland, lips and mouth, conjunctivae	Infections of head, neck, sinuses, ears, eyes, scalp, pharynx
Anterior cervical (jugular)	Tongue, tonsil, pinna, parotid, larynx, thryroid, upper esophagus	Pharyngitis organisms, rubella, upper respiratory infections, cancer of tongue, larynx, thyroid and cervical esophagus
Posterior cervical	Scalp and neck, middle ear, skin of arms and pectorals, thorax, cervical and axillary nodes	Mononucleosis, toxoplasmosis, tuberculosis, rubella, otitis media, scalp infections and dandruff, Kikuchi's disease, lymphoma, head and neck malignancy
Preauricular	Eyelids and conjunctivae, temporal region, pinna	Disease external auditory canal, ipsilateral conjunctivitis (Parinaud's syndrome), lymphoma
Postauricular	External auditory meatus, pinna, scalp	Local infection, but also rubella
Occipital	Scalp and head	Local infection
Right supraclavicular node	Breast, lungs, esophagus mediastinum,	Lung, breast, mediastinum
Left supraclavicular node	Breast, lungs, abdomen via thoracic duct, and pelvis	Lymphoma, thoracic, retroperitoneal, gastrointestinal or pelvic cancer, bacterial or fungal infection
Axillary	Arm, thoracic wall, breast	Arm infections, cat-scratch disease, tularemia, lymphoma, breast cancer, silicone implants, brucellosis, melanoma
Epitrochlear	Ulnar aspect of forearm and hand	Infections, lymphoma, sarcoidosis and connective tissue diseases, tularemia, secondary syphilis, leprosy, leishmaniasis, rubella
Inguinal	Penis, scrotum, vulva, vagina, perineum, gluteal region, lower abdominal wall, lower anal canal, extremities (benign reactive in shoeless walkers)	Infections of the leg or foot, STDs (e.g., herpes simplex virus, gonococcal infection, syphilis, chancroid, granuloma inguinale, lymphogranuloma venereum), lymphoma, pelvic malignancy, bubonic plague

STDs = sexually transmitted diseases.
*Modified from Ferrer R: Lymphadenopathy. Am Fam Physician 58:1313–1323, 1998.

TABLE 18-3. LYMPH NODE BIOPSY FINDINGS (%)[*]

	Benign	Carcinoma	Lymphoma
Nodes			
All (n = 925)	60	28	12
Abdominal (n = 51)	63	33	4
Thoracic (n = 149)	73	26	1
Peripheral (n = 653)	56	29	15
Unspecified (n = 72)	61	25	14
Ages[†]			
All	57	28	15
<30	79	6	15
31–50	59	30	11
51–80	40	44	16

[*]From Habermann TM, Steensma DP. Mayo Clin Proc 75:723–732, 2000.
[†]Age distribution based on 628 patients with peripheral lymph node biopsies.

17. **What about *fever*?**
It usually suggests infection or lymphoma. Still, the differential diagnosis can be quite wide, since many *infectious processes* may present with febrile adenopathy (TB, mononucleosis, toxoplasmosis, histoplasmosis, salmonellosis, AIDS, CMV, syphilis, and subacute bacterial endocarditis). Many *cancers* can do it, too (chronic lymphocytic leukemia [CLL], Waldenström's, multiple myeloma, and Kaposi's sarcoma), and so can *systemic disorders* (sarcoid, SLE, RA, Kawasaki, and Whipple disease).

18. **Are there any epidemiologic clues that might narrow the differential diagnosis?**
Yes. Occupational exposure, recent travel, or high-risk behavior may all contribute (Table 18-5).

19. **Which node characteristics can be clinically helpful?**
In addition to *location*, six features may help the diagnosis:
- **Size:** This is easily measured by a plastic caliper or ruler. It can predict its nature and guide biopsy. Although there is no "normal" size (since this depends on age and background antigenic exposure), some authors have defined the upper limits of normal as a node >1 cm that has been present outside the inguinal region for more than 1 month. Yet, *inguinal* nodes can be normal up to 1.5 cm, whereas *preauricular* and *epitrochlear* nodes are suspicious even if 0.5–1 cm. Moreover, large but benign nodes are quite common in IV drug users. In fact, some authors have even suggested raising the threshold of suspicion to 1.5 × 1.5 cm. Finally, although no specific diagnosis can be based on size, some valuable predictions can be inferred. For example, in 213 *adults* with unexplained lymphadenopathy, nodes <1 cm were never neoplastic. Conversely, cancer was the final diagnosis in 8% of 1–1.5 cm nodes and 38% of >1.5 cm. In children, nodes >2 cm (along with an abnormal chest x-ray and absence of ear, nose, and throat symptoms) argue in favor of *granulomatous* diseases (TB, cat-scratch disease, sarcoid) or *cancer* (mostly lymphomas).
- **Duration:** The longer the node has been present, the less its risk of being neoplastic or granulomatous. Still, lymphomatous nodes *can* regress, albeit temporarily.

TABLE 18-4. LYMPHADENOPATHY—ASSOCIATED SIGNS AND SYMPTOMS

Disorder	Associated Findings
Common Causes of Lymphadenopathy	
Mononucleosis-type syndromes	Fatigue, malaise, fever, atypical lymphocytosis
Epstein-Barr virus[*]	Splenomegaly in 50%
Toxoplasmosis[*]	80–90% asymptomatic
Cytomegalovirus[*]	Often mild symptoms; patients may have hepatitis
Initial stages of HIV infection[*]	"Flu-like" illness, rash
Cat-scratch disease	Fever in 30%; cervical or axillary nodes
Pharyngitis (group A *Streptococcus*, gonococcus)	Fever, pharyngeal exudates, cervical nodes
Tuberculosis lymphadenitis[*]	Painless, matted cervical nodes
Secondary syphilis[*]	Rash
Hepatitis B[*]	Fever, nausea, vomiting, icterus
Lymphogranuloma venereum	Tender, matted inguinal nodes
Chancroid	Painful ulcer, painful inguinal nodes
Lupus erythematosus[*]	Arthritis, rash, serositis; renal, neurologic, hematologic disorders
Rheumatoid arthritis[*]	Arthritis
Lymphoma[*]	Fever, night sweats, weight loss in 20–30%
Leukemia[*]	Blood dyscrasias, bruising
Serum sickness[*]	Fever, malaise, arthralgia, urticaria; exposure to antisera or medications
Sarcoidosis	Hilar nodes, skin lesions, dyspnea
Kawasaki disease[*]	Fever, conjunctivitis, rash, mucosal lesions
Less Common Causes of Lymphadenopathy	
Lyme disease[*]	Rash, arthritis
Measles[*]	Fever, conjunctivitis, rash, cough
Rubella[*]	Rash
Tularemia[*]	Fever, ulcer at inoculation site
Brucellosis[*]	Fever, sweats, malaise
Plague	Febrile, acutely ill with cluster of tender nodes
Typhoid fever[*]	Fever, chills, headache, abdominal complaints
Still's disease[*]	Fever, rash, arthritis
Dermatomyositis[*]	Proximal weakness, skin changes
Amyloidosis[*]	Fatigue, weight loss

[*]Causes of generalized lymphadenopathy.
(Adapted from Ferrer R: Lymphadenopathy. Am Fam Physician 58:1313–1323, 1998.)

TABLE 18–5. EPIDEMIOLOGIC CLUES TO THE DIAGNOSIS OF LYMPHADENOPATHY

Exposure	Diagnosis
General	
Cat	Cat-scratch disease, toxoplasmosis
Undercooked meat	Toxoplasmosis
Tick bite	Lyme disease, tularemia
Tuberculosis	Tuberculous adenitis
Recent blood transfusion or transplant	Cytomegalovirus, HIV
High-risk sexual behavior	HIV, syphilis, herpes simplex virus, cytomegalovirus, hepatitis B infection
Intravenous drug use	HIV, endocarditis, hepatitis B infection
Occupational	
Hunters, trappers	Tularemia
Fishermen, fishmongers, slaughterhouse workers	Erysipeloid
Travel-related	
Arizona, southern California, New Mexico, western Texas	Coccidioidomycosis
Southwestern United States	Bubonic plague
Southeastern or central United States	Histoplasmosis
Southeast Asia, India, Central or West Africa	Scrub typhus
Central or West Africa	African trypanosomiasis (sleeping sickness)
Central or South America	American trypanosomiasis (Chagas' disease)
East Africa, Mediterranean, China, Latin America	Kala-azar (leishmaniasis)
Mexico, Peru, Chile, India, Pakistan, Egypt, Indonesia	Typhoid fever

HIV = human immunodeficiency virus.
(Adapted from Ferrer R: Lymphadenopathy. Am Fam Physician 58:1313–1323, 1998.)

- **Consistency:** Soft nodes are usually infectious or inflammatory, whereas *rock-hard* ones tend to be neoplastic, often metastatic. Exceptions include the nodes of Hodgkin's, which are firm but rubbery. *Fluctuant* nodes reflect instead bacterial lymphadenitis with necrosis. They feel like a tense balloon or grape, are typically tender, and may even fistulize through the skin, forming open sinuses that are a common feature in TB. Nodes of this type, especially in groins or axillae, are often referred to as *buboes* (from the Greek term for swollen groin) and used to be typical of infectious processes, such as gonorrhea, syphilis, TB, and, of course, the "bubonic" plague of old.
- **Matting:** Fusion into a scalloped mass transforms individual nodes into large conglomerates. This is usually a neoplastic feature (metastatic carcinoma or lymphomas), but also can

occur in inflammatory processes (like sarcoid) and chronic infections (like TB and lymphogranuloma venereum).

- **Relationship to surrounding tissues:** Adherence to overlying skin, subjacent tissues, or both does not separate inflammation from neoplasm but does exclude benignity.
- **Pain/tenderness:** This reflects rapid growth with painful capsular stretching. It is a sign of suppurative inflammation but also may reflect hemorrhage into the necrotic center of a rapidly expanding neoplastic node. Hence, tenderness does *not* reliably differentiate benign from malignant ones. The same applies to sinus tract formation, which can occur in infections (actinomycosis and TB) as well as cancer.

Pearl. *Benign nodes* tend to be small, soft, nontender, mobile, and discrete (well demarcated). *Neoplastic nodes* are large, nontender, matted, fixed, and rock-hard. *Inflammatory nodes* are tender, firm (but not rock-hard), occasionally fluctuant, and often matted and fixed.

20. **What is the best way to deal with adenopathy?**
    - Start with history and physical exam (H&P), since they can often identify the etiology (upper respiratory infection [URI], pharyngitis, periodontal disease, conjunctivitis, insect bites, focal infection, recent immunization, cat-scratch disease, tinea, or dermatitis), thus preempting the need for further work-up.
    - H&P also can offer a *presumptive* diagnosis and guide the work-up (EBV, HIV, lymphoma, syphilis).
    - Once the initial evaluation is complete, some patients may still have either *unexplained* lymphadenopathy or a presumptive diagnosis unconfirmed by labs and clinical course. In this case, if the adenopathy is *localized* (and the clinical picture is reassuring [i.e.,a benign history, an unremarkable exam, and no constitutional symptoms]), allow 3–4 weeks of observation before resorting to biopsy. If the clinical picture is instead worrisome (risk factors for malignancy, constitutional signs/symptoms) or the lymphadenopathy is *generalized,* do further testing and get a biopsy. Still, avoid biopsy in patients with probable viral illness, since their pathology may simulate lymphoma.

21. **What is *unexplained lymphadenopathy*?**
    One that remains perplexing after initial evaluation. In this case, pursue a specific diagnosis based on the patient's age, but also the nodes' duration, characteristics, and location.

22. **What is the differential diagnosis of an unexplained lymphadenopathy?**
    Usually *infectious, neoplastic,* or *autoimmune*—which also is the differential diagnosis for fever of unknown origin or an elevated sedimentation rate. A helpful mnemonic is **CHICAGO**:
    - **C** = **C**ancers: hematologic malignancies (Hodgkin's disease, non-Hodgkin's lymphoma, acute and chronic leukemia, Waldenström's macroglobulinemia, multiple myeloma [uncommon], systemic mastocytosis) and metastatic "solid" tumors (breast, lung, renal cell, prostate, other)
    - **H** = **H**ypersensitivity syndromes: serum sickness, drug sensitivity (diphenylhydantoin, carbamazepine, primidone, gold, allopurinol, indomethacin, sulfonamides, others), silicone reaction, vaccination-related, and graft versus host disease
    - **I** = **I**nfections: viral (infectious mononucleosis [Epstein-Barr virus], cytomegalovirus, infectious hepatitis, postvaccinal lymphadenitis, adenovirus, herpes zoster, HIV/AIDS, human T-lymphocyte virus 1), bacterial (cutaneous infections [staphylococci, streptococci], cat-scratch fever, chancroid, melioidosis, TB, atypical mycobacteria, primary and secondary syphilis), chlamydial (lymphogranuloma venereum), protozoan (toxoplasmosis), mycotic (histoplasmosis, coccidioidomycosis), rickettsial (scrub typhus), helminthic (filariasis)
    - **C** = **C**onnective tissue disorders: rheumatoid arthritis, systemic lupus erythematosus, dermatomyositis, mixed connective tissue disease, Sjögren syndrome
    - **A** = **A**typical lymphoproliferative disorders: angiofollicular (giant) lymph node hyperplasia (Castleman disease), angioimmunoblastic lymphadenopathy with dysproteinemia, angiocentric immunoproliferative disorders, lymphomatoid granulomatosis, Wegener granulomatosis

- **G = G**ranulomatous lesions: TB, histoplasmosis, mycobacterial infections, cryptococci, silicosis, berylliosis, cat-scratch fever
- **O = O**ther unusual causes of lymphadenopathy: inflammatory pseudotumor of lymph nodes, histiocytic necrotizing lymphadenitis (Kikuchi lymphadenitis), sinus histiocytosis with massive lymphadenopathy (Rosai-Dorfman disease), vascular transformation of sinuses, progressive transformation of germinal centers

23. **Which clinical presentations may help identify the cause of lymphadenopathy?**
   - **Mononucleosis-type syndromes:** Adenopathy plus fatigue, malaise, fever, and increased atypical lymphocyte count. Differential diagnosis includes Epstein-Barr virus (mononucleosis), toxoplasmosis, CMV, streptococcal pharyngitis, hepatitis B, and acute HIV.
   - **HIV infection:** Any *persistent generalized lymphadenopathy* (i.e., one of at least 3 months' duration, involving two extrainguinal sites or more) should suggest an early stage of HIV infection. Generalized adenopathy in HIV suggests Kaposi, CMV, toxoplasmosis, TB, cryptococcosis, syphilis, and lymphoma.
   - **Ulceroglandular syndrome:** Regional adenopathy plus skin lesions. The classic cause is tularemia, acquired by contact with an infected rabbit or tick. More common, however, are streptococcal infection (impetigo) and cat-scratch and Lyme diseases.
   - **Oculoglandular syndrome:** Preauricular adenopathy with conjunctivitis. Common causes include viral keratoconjunctivitis and cat-scratch disease from ocular lesions.

B. CERVICAL AND SUPRACLAVICULAR NODES

24. **How do you palpate cervical nodes?**
   By using the pads of your fingertips, the hands' most sensitive parts. Examine both sides of the head and neck *simultaneously*, by sliding your fingers over the area of attention. Apply steady and gentle pressure. Explore all cervical sites by following the anterior and posterior aspects of the underside of the jaw and neck. Large nodes are often *visible*, presenting as localized skin bulging. Involvement of only one side of the neck makes these swellings even more visible.

25. **What are the important head and neck stations?**
   There is a fair amount of variability and overlap in pathways of drainage (Fig. 18-1). Overall, you should examine nodes in the following order:
   - **Submental:** Just below the chin. They drain the teeth and intra-oral cavity.
   - **Submandibular:** Along the underside of the jaw, on either side. They drain the structures in the posterior floor of the mouth.
   - **Anterior cervical** (both superficial and deep): Also called "jugular chain nodes," these lie on top of and beneath the sternocleidomastoid muscles (SCM) on either side of the neck, from the angle of the jaw to the top of the clavicle (the SCMs allow the head to rotate to the opposite side and can be easily identified by asking the patient to turn the head). They drain the internal structures of the throat as well as part of the posterior pharynx, tonsils, and thyroid gland.
   - **Posterior cervical:** Also called "posterior triangle nodes," these extend in a line posterior to the SCMs, but in front of the trapezius, from the mastoid bone to the clavicle. They drain the skin on the back of the head and are frequently enlarged during upper respiratory infections (mononucleosis).
   - **Tonsillar:** Just below the angle of the mandible. They drain the tonsillar and posterior pharyngeal regions.
   - **Preauricular and postauricular:** Respectively, anterior and posterior to the ear. Swelling of the pre-auricular node in a setting of conjunctivitis-like "pink eye" represents *Parinaud's*

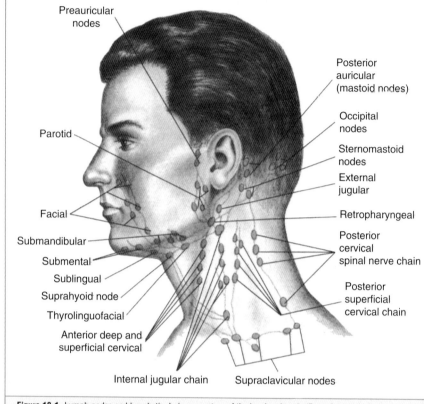

Figure 18-1. Lymph nodes and lymphatic drainage system of the head and neck. (From Seidel HM, Ball JW, Dains JE, Benedict GW: Mosby's Guide to Physical Examination, 3rd ed. St. Louis, Mosby, 1995.)

(oculoglandular) syndrome, occurring in various conditions, including Tularemia and Catscratch disease (Bartonellosis).

- **Occipital:** Common in childhood infections, but rare in adults—except in a setting of either banal scalp infection or, more ominously, generalized lymphadenopathy from systemic disease *(HIV).*
- **Supraclavicular:** In the hollow above the clavicle, just lateral to where it joins the sternum. They drain part of the thoracic cavity and abdomen (*see* questions 31–36).

  Palpation of other cervical groups also may be indicated in cases of disease affecting specific regions. For example, *preauricular and postauricular nodes* (just in front or behind the ears) may enlarge because of infections of the external ear canal.

26. **And so, what is the overall significance of *cervical* lymphadenopathy?**
    It depends on location, but may suggest either *infection* or *malignancy.*
    - **Infections:** Bacterial pharyngitis, dental abscesses, otitis media or externa, infectious mono, gonococcal pharyngitis, CMV, HIV, TB, rubella, toxoplasmosis, hepatitis, and adenovirus
    - **Malignancies:** Non-Hodgkin lymphoma, Hodgkin's disease, and squamous cell carcinoma of the head and neck

Note that one of the processes responsible for isolated posterior cervical and occipital adenopathy is Kikuchi disease (histiocytic necrotizing lymphadenitis). This is a syndrome of unknown etiology first described in 1972 in Japan. The classic patient is a young woman who presents with unilateral painless lymphadenopathy of the posterior cervical region, typically resolving in 3 months.

27. **Can cervical nodes remain permanently enlarged after an infection?**
Yes. In this case, they are rather small (<1 cm), never tender, and with a rubbery consistency. For example, small palpable nodes in the tonsillar submental and submandibular regions may often occur in otherwise healthy individuals, representing the sequelae of past pharyngitis or dental infections. Conversely, rock-hard nodes should always suggest malignancy, whose location depends on the site drained by the corresponding nodes.

28. **What are "shotty" nodes?**
They are small nodes that feel like shotgun pellets, or tiny peas. They are typically nontender, firm but not stony-hard, small but equal, mobile, round, and well demarcated. Usually found in the cervical chain of children with *viral illnesses* (with location reflecting the original site of infection), they may outlast the illness by several weeks and are usually of no clinical consequence. The expression "shotty" was commonly used in 19th-century lay language but is now quite obsolete—except, of course, for medical jargon.

29. **What is *scrofula*?**
An old term for *cervical tuberculous lymphadenitis:* swollen nodes that make the patient's neck resemble that of a piglet (*scrofa*, sow in Latin). Scrofula used to be very common in children, since it was spread by unpasteurized milk from infected cows. It was typically treated by the *king's touch,* which consisted in having the children's neck healed by the laying on of his/her majesty's hands (usually of either England or France). This "cure," of course, reflected the overall benign nature of the disease rather than the healing power of royalty. Note that chronic mycobacterial (or fungal) infections also can cause *supraclavicular* adenopathy.

30. **What are Delphian nodes?**
A cluster of small and midline prelaryngeal nodes (Fig. 18-2). These are typically located on the thyrohyoid membrane—just anterior to the cricothyroid ligament, and just above the thyroid isthmus. Given their pretracheal and superficial location, they are easily palpable if enlarged, even though at times they may be confused with the pyramidal lobe of the gland. They drain

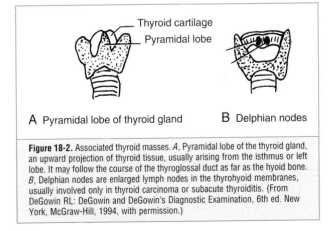

Figure 18-2. Associated thyroid masses. *A,* Pyramidal lobe of the thyroid gland, an upward projection of thyroid tissue, usually arising from the isthmus or left lobe. It may follow the course of the thyroglossal duct as far as the hyoid bone. *B,* Delphian nodes are enlarged lymph nodes in the thyrohyoid membranes, usually involved only in thyroid carcinoma or subacute thyroiditis. (From DeGowin RL: DeGowin and DeGowin's Diagnostic Examination, 6th ed. New York, McGraw-Hill, 1994, with permission.)

the *thyroid* and *larynx*, and like Delphi in ancient Greece, they have traditionally been considered an oracle—of thyroid disease or laryngeal malignancy (even though objective supportive data are lacking). They also are the first to be exposed during surgery, thus foretelling the nature of the underlying illness. Delphian nodes reflect a range of thyroid involvement, including subacute thyroiditis, Hashimoto's, and thyroid cancer. If due to laryngeal carcinoma, they give the disease a more ominous connotation.

31. **What is the clinical significance of a palpable *supraclavicular* node?**
An ominous one. A localized node in either the right or left supraclavicular fossa carries a 90% risk of malignancy for patients older than 40 and a 25% risk for younger patients.
   - **Right supraclavicular nodes** usually indicate metastatic involvement from ipsilateral *breast* or *lung* (but also mediastinum and esophagus). Because of bilateral crossed drainage, a *right* node also may reflect lung cancer of the *left* lower lobe.
   - **Left supraclavicular nodes** have instead a much wider differential diagnosis, since the left supraclavicular fossa not only drains the thorax, but also various abdominal and pelvic sites. Hence, it functions as a *sentinel* for distant metastases.

32. **What is Troisier's node? What is its significance?**
Troisier's node (or sign) is another name for a palpable single *left* supraclavicular node. Frequently located just behind the clavicular head of the sternocleidomastoid, it suggests metastasis from a deep-seated carcinoma. Sources include not only the *thorax* (esophagus or ipsilateral breast and lung), but also the *abdomen* (stomach, liver, gallbladder, pancreas, kidneys, intestine) and *pelvis* (ovaries, endometrium, testes, and prostate).

33. **Who was Troisier?**
Charles E. Troisier (1844–1919) was a graduate of the University of Paris and, subsequently, a professor at the same institution. A well-respected pathologist and clinician, he mostly contributed to the understanding of lymphatic spread by cancer, but also rheumatoid nodules, meningitis, venous thrombosis, and hemochromatosis. In fact, bronzed diabetes (or hemochromatosis) is still referred to as Troisier's syndrome.

34. **What is Virchow's node?**
A left-sided Troisier's node due to *gastric* carcinoma.

35. **Who was Virchow?**
Rudolf Ludwig Karl Virchow (1821–1902) was a graduate of the Friedrich-Wilhelm Institute for Army Doctors in Berlin, which he joined after realizing that his voice was not strong enough to support a career as a preacher. Preaching, however, remained one of his lifelong interests. In fact, after multiple rejections by various journal editors, he founded his own journal, which became known as *Virchow's Archiv,* earning its pontificating editor the nickname "The Pope." Virchow's contributions to medicine were nonetheless staggering: he was the first to describe (and name) leukemia and understand thrombosis (*see* Virchow's triad). He also was the first to recognize cerebral and pulmonary *embolism* (named that too) and the nature of arterial plugs in malignant endocarditis. He discovered amyloid, myelin, and neuroglia and contributed scores of papers to the understanding of cerebral hemorrhage, meningitis, and various congenital anomalies of the nervous system. By contrast, he had little interest in the emerging germ theory of disease and deeply detested evolution, which he tried to ban from school curricula. Although academically autocratic and reactionary, Virchow was politically very liberal—in fact, almost socialistic. He even helped construct some of the barricades during the 1848 Berlin uprising, a feat that cost him his job. Later, he became an outspoken opponent of Bismarck, who went so far as to challenge him to a duel in 1865 (Virchow agreed but on one condition: that the duel be fought with scalpels). In fact, he never missed a chance to strongly castigate the social injustice and poor hygienic conditions of his time, which he considered

responsible for the frequent and recurrent epidemics. In a report to the government that became almost a political indictment of the industrial revolution, he asked, "Shall the triumph of human genius lead to nothing more than to make the human race miserable?" Still, he didn't limit himself to cursing the darkness, but also lit a few candles—such as securing a good sewerage system and water supply for Berlin. His extracurricular interests included anthropology, medical history, and, above all, archeology. He even accompanied his friend Dr. Heinrich Schliemann to Troy in 1859 (writing an account of his famous discoveries) and concocted the idea of x-raying mummies. When he finally died at 81 from complications of a hip fracture sustained while leaping from a moving tram, it was said that Germany had lost in one single man her leading pathologist, sanitarian, anthropologist, and activist.

36. **What is the best way to palpate a supraclavicular node?**
Have the patient sit up, with head straight forward and arms down (to avoid mistaking a cervical vertebra or neck muscle for a node). Palpate from *behind,* since this allows optimal adaptation of your hand to the patient's anatomy. Conversely, palpate from the *front* in the supine patient, where the lessened gravity may even mobilize the node and thus make it more accessible. End the exam by asking the patient to perform a Valsalva maneuver, or simply to cough. This may "pop" a deeply seated node, thus bringing it within reach of your fingers.

C. UPPER EXTREMITY NODES

37. **What is the best way to search for *axillary* nodes?**
For the left axilla, grasp the patient's left wrist or elbow with your left hand, and lift the arm up and out laterally. Then use the tip of your right fingers to palpate deep into the axillary fossa and roof. Do this first with the patient's arm gently relaxed and passively abducted from the chest wall. Then repeat it with the arm passively and gently adducted. Examine the *right* axilla in a similar fashion, albeit with a reversed hand positioning. This technique allows the patient's arm to remain completely relaxed, thus minimizing any tension in the surrounding tissues that could otherwise mask enlarged lymph nodes. It also is easy to carry out on the *supine* patient, very much as it would be if it were linked with the female breast exam (Fig 18-3).

An alternative technique allows simultaneous examination of both axillae. To do so, ask the patient to lift both arms away from the chest. Then extend the fingers of both your hands and gently direct them toward the apices of the armpits. If you don't want to place your fingers in direct contact with the axilla, you can do this through the patient's gown. Now press your hands toward the patient's body, and move them slowly down the lateral chest wall. This allows you to explore the axillary regions in their entirety.

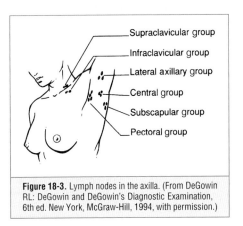

Figure 18-3. Lymph nodes in the axilla. (From DeGowin RL: DeGowin and DeGowin's Diagnostic Examination, 6th ed. New York, McGraw-Hill, 1994, with permission.)

Labels in figure:
Supraclavicular group
Infraclavicular group
Lateral axillary group
Central group
Subscapular group
Pectoral group

38. **What is the clinical significance of axillary adenopathy?**
Very much the same as that of *cervical* adenopathy: *cancer* and *infection* (with a sprinkle of systemic disorders, such as sarcoidosis). Note that axillary nodes should *not* be detectable,

even though at times *small,* mobile, soft, and nontender nodes *can* be felt in normal people. Larger, tender, but still mobile axillary nodes usually reflect *small wounds or infections* of the arm (such as cat-scratch fever, tularemia, sporotrichosis, or staphylococcal and streptococcal infections, but also intravenous drug abuse). Conversely, harder, fixed, or matted axillary nodes indicate spread from malignancies, usually of pulmonary or breast origin (but lymphomas and melanomas, too).

39. **How do you palpate an *epitrochlear* node?**
    By using your right hand to shake hands with the patient's right hand, while at the same time "cupping" the patient's elbow with the fingertips of your left hand. Palpate just above the elbow, along the inside of the upper arm, which is where the epitrochlear nodes reside. Then reverse hands and repeat the maneuver on the contralateral side.

40. **What is the significance of epitrochlear nodes?**
    It depends on whether they are *isolated* or in a *generalized* setting (25% of adenopathies in other regions also will have palpable epitrochlear nodes). Either way, they are rarely benign. In a prospective study of 324 patients, the two most common causes were *infectious mono* and *non-Hodgkin lymphoma/chronic lymphocytic leukemia,* but also sarcoid, HIV, and dermatologic/connective tissue disorders. Historically, the condition has instead been associated with secondary syphilis, lepromatous leprosy, leishmaniasis, and rubella. Finally, an enlarged epitrochlear node also may reflect local inflammation of the hand/forearm. Hence, it is quite common in IV drug abusers.

D. LOWER EXTREMITY NODES

41. **What is the significance of *inguinal* adenopathy?**
    Questionable, since most adults have some degree of it, especially if walking shoeless outdoors. Normally, there are two groups of inguinal nodes: one clustered along the inguinal ligament and the other along the femoral vessels. If benign, these tend to be small, firm, and mobile. Yet inguinal adenopathy also may reflect infection or cancer. Hence, when confronted with nodes, make sure to examine the abdomen (look especially for hepatomegaly/splenomegaly), testes, rectum, breasts, genitals, lungs, and skin (look for melanoma). Most common infections are cellulitis and *venereal diseases* (syphilis, chancroid, genital herpes, and lymphogranuloma venereum). Cancers include instead lymphomas, melanomas, and carcinoma of the penis or vulva. Hence, biopsy of inguinal nodes is usually more informative than that of *femoral* nodes, which often shows only reactive hyperplasia.

42. **What is the node of Rosenmüller-Cloquet?**
    A deep inguinal node just near the femoral canal, which, if pathologically enlarged, may be mistaken for an inguinal hernia. Instead, it is an important "sentinel" for the tumor status of iliac/obturator nodes. First described by the French Jules Cloquet and the German Johann Rosenmüller—an avid speleologist who had a couple of caves named after him.

43. **How significant is a *femoral* lymphadenopathy?**
    Very little. Whereas inguinal nodes are lateral in the groin, femoral nodes are medial and closer to the genital area. They are much less significant clinically. In fact, their enlargement often reflects a simple dermatophytosis of the foot.

44. **What is the significance of popliteal lymphadenopathy?**
    Uncertain. Little data exist in humans, since these nodes are often too deep to palpate, and, if palpable, questionable in significance. Hence, authors like Sapira suggest to not even bother ("the physical examination must *not* be stretched beyond its limits").

E. ABDOMINAL NODES

45. What is Sister Mary Joseph's nodule?

A periumbilical node or hard mass of the navel. It is clinically quite valuable since it represents a direct or lymphonodal metastasis from an intrapelvic/intra-abdominal tumor. The finding was first reported by William J. Mayo in 1928, based on observations by his scrub nurse, Sister Mary Joseph of St. Mary's Hospital, who could predict laparotomy findings by feeling a periumbilical mass while scrubbing the patient's abdomen. This is not surprising since the umbilicus is highly susceptible to intra-abdominal metastases, thanks to its multiple anatomic relations and generous vascular/embryologic connections. In fact, in 20% of cases, umbilical metastasis is the *presenting* manifestation. A total of 407 reports have been published. The usual type is an adenocarcinoma, with the stomach being the most common primary site (23%), followed by ovary (16%), large bowel (10–14%), and pancreas (7–11%). Overall, 52% of cancers are gastrointestinal in origin, and 28% gynecologic; 15% are of unknown primary, and 3% originate instead from the thoracic cavity. In 14–33% of cases, umbilical metastasis is the first (and diagnostic) manifestation of a previously occult neoplasm. In 40%, the nodule is instead an early sign of relapse in a patient with known cancer. Overall, a Sister Mary Joseph's nodule is a bad omen, since survival is less than 1 year (*see* also Chapter 15, The Abdomen, question 7).

46. Who was Sister Mary Joseph?

Sister Mary Joseph was born Julia Dempsey in Salamanca, New York, in 1856. In 1878, she entered the congregation of Our Lady of Lourdes and was assigned to the St. Mary's Hospital in Rochester, Minnesota. There she learned nursing, first working under the guidance of Edith Graham (who subsequently became the wife of Dr. C.H. Mayo) and eventually rising to the position of hospital superintendent, a title she kept until her death in 1939. From 1890–1915, she served as the first surgical assistant to Dr. W.J. Mayo, drawing his attention to the sign that eventually carried her name.

SELECTED BIBLIOGRAPHY

1. Allhiser JN, McKnight TA, Shank JC, et al: Lymphadenopathy in a family practice. J Fam Pract 12:27–32, 1981.
2. Benson JR, Singh S, Thomas JM: Sister Joseph's nodule: A case report and review. Eur J Surg Oncol 23:451–454, 1997.
3. Crook LD, Tempest B: Plague: A clinical review of 27 cases. Arch Intern Med 152:1253–1256, 1992.
4. Dawson PJ, Cooper RA, Rambo ON: Diagnosis of malignant lymphoma: A clinicopathological analysis of 158 different lymph node biopsies. Cancer 17:1405–1413, 1964.
5. De Vriese AS, Philippe J, Van Renterghem, DM, et al: Carbamazepine hypersensitivity syndrome: Report of 4 cases and review of the literature. Medicine (Baltimore) 74:144–151, 1995.
6. Ferrer R: Lymphadenopathy. Am Fam Physician 58:1313–1323, 1998.
7. Fessas P, Pangalis G: Non-malignant lymphadenopathies: Reactive non-specific and reactive specific. In Pangalis GA, Polliack A (eds): Benign and Malignant Lymphadenopathies: Clinical and Laboratory Diagnosis. Chur, Switzerland, Harwood Academic Publishers, 1993, pp 31–45.
8. Fijten GH, Blijham GH: Unexplained lymphadenopathy in family practice. An evaluation of the probability of malignant causes and the effectiveness of physicians' work-up. J Fam Pract 27:373–376, 1988.
9. Habermann TM, Steensma DP. Mayo Clinic Proc 75:723–732, 2000.
10. Hartsock RJ, Halling LW, King FM: Luetic lymphadenitis: A clinical and histologic study of 20 cases. Am J Clin Pathol 53:304–314, 1970.
11. Hartsock RJ: Postvaccinial lymphadenitis: Hyperplasia of lymphoid tissue that simulates malignant lymphomas. Cancer 21:632–649, 1968.
12. Sapira JD: The Art and Science of Bedside Diagnosis, ed 1. Baltimore, Williams and Wilkins, 1990.

CHAPTER 19

THE NEUROLOGIC SYSTEM

Enrica Arnaudo, MD, and Michael D. Kim, DO

"From the brain and the brain only arise our pleasures, joys, laughter and jests, as well as our sorrows, pains, griefs and tears. . . . These things we suffer all come from the brain, when it is not healthy, but becomes abnormally hot, cold, moist or dry."

—Hippocrates, *The Sacred Disease,* Section XVI

"Some seventy years ago a promising young neurologist made a discovery that necessitated the addition of a new word to the English vocabulary. He insisted that this should be knee-jerk, and knee-jerk it has remained in spite of the efforts of patellar reflex to dislodge it. He was my father: Sir William Richard Gowers. So perhaps I have inherited a prejudice in favour of home-made words."

—Sir Ernest Gowers (1880–1966), *Plain Words,* Chapter 5

GENERALITIES

In times of magnetic resonance imaging (MRI) and computed tomography (CT), the neurologic exam may seem almost anachronistic. Yet, as the leading British neurologist McDonald Critchley (1900–1997) once said during one of his U.S. visits, "CT scanning will take away the *shadows* of neurology, but the music will still remain." Indeed, the neurologic exam remains the most sophisticated part of physical diagnosis, still able to pinpoint the location of a lesion ("history tells you *what* it is, but the exam tells you *where* it is"). Of course, good skills, plus mastering of neuroanatomy and neurophysiology are a prerequisite. This chapter will highlight the essentials. But all sections are worthwhile.

1. **What is the purpose of the neurologic exam?**
   To *localize* lesions—that is, to identify the precise site of damage. This is rooted in the *eloquence of the nervous system* (i.e., the unique property that the brain, spinal cord, and peripheral nerves have of "talking to us") insofar as each section performs such a discrete function that any loss can be easily traced back to its level. Hence, neuro *signs* (and symptoms) accurately localize lesions. And this also is why the neuro exam is the bedside tool with the highest sensitivity, specificity, and likelihood ratios. Yet, in contrast to other parts of the exam where inspection or palpation are key, the neurologic exam relies on deductive skills and specific maneuvers. Hence, it is difficult to perform but rewarding. It also is *long*—at least 1 solid hour.

2. **What are the most important components of the neurologic exam?**
   - Mental status
   - Cranial nerves
   - Motor system
   - Sensory system
   - Cerebellum
   - Gait

A. MENTAL STATUS EXAMINATION

3. **What is *dementia*?**
   An *acquired* and *persistent* cognitive impairment that compromises multiple domains of intellectual function (such as memory, language, etc.—basically, *awareness* [i.e., the *content* of consciousness]) while preserving instead perception and *arousal* (i.e., the *level* of consciousness). Hence dementia is *not* coma. Dementia is not *delirium* either, since this is instead an *acute* and often reversible *confusional state* seen in 20% of elderly patients hospitalized for intercurrent illnesses. Dementia is painfully common, affecting 3–11% of adults older than 65, and its prevalence does increase with aging, so that one third of subjects older than 80 (and one half of those older than 90) will eventually suffer from it—something to look forward to. It can be toxic, metabolic, degenerative, inflammatory, infective, or vascular. The earliest signs are often subtle, usually involving short-term memory but otherwise sparing the bulk of the exam. As the disease progresses, *frontal release signs* appear.

4. **What are *frontal release signs*?**
   They are the reemergence of *primitive reflexes* (i.e., signs that are normally present in infants, but resurface in adults only as a result of diffuse frontal lobe disease). Release signs/reflexes include *snouting, rooting, sucking,* and *grasping.* Of these, the most sensitive is *grasping.* To elicit it, place your index and middle fingers in the patient's palm, apply some pressure, and then slowly withdraw them between the patient's thumb and index finger. An abnormal response (involuntary squeezing of the examiner's fingers—with no habituation after three successive strokes) strongly argues for a lesion in the frontal lobes or the deep nuclei and subcortical white matter. Though not too sensitive (13%), it has specificity close to 100%. Contrary to other primitive reflexes (such as *palmomental* or *glabellar*), grasp is never seen in normal subjects.

5. **What are the snouting, rooting, and sucking reflexes?**
   - **Snouting** is the labial pouting/pursing elicited by pressing a tongue blade on the patient's lips.
   - **Rooting** is the shift of the mouth toward a tactile stimulus. It can be elicited by gently stroking the lateral upper lip—or, in newborns, by touching the junction of the lips. This causes head-turning and mouth-opening, as if "rooting" toward the stroke (mom's breast or the bottle).
   - **Sucking** is pouting or sucking following gentle touching of the patient's lip. Normal in infants until weaning, it is absent in adults—except in diffuse frontal lobe injury.

6. **What is the *palmomental* reflex?**
   A brief and involuntary contraction of the ipsilateral *mentalis muscle*, wrinkles and pushes-up the chin boss, while at the same time curving the lower lip *upward* in an inverted "U." This is elicited by stroking the patient's palm (thenar eminence) with a blunt object, from proximal to distal. As a *release sign*, it is often seen in Parkinson's (where it correlates with degree of akinesia), but also in 3–70% of older normal individuals. Note that the muscle is called "mentalis," because its voluntary contraction is often associated with thinking or concentration. Its nerve supply is provided by the *facialis* (CN VII).

7. **What is the *glabellar* reflex?**
   Another primitive (or "release") reflex, very much like the *grasp* and *palmomental.* It involves V and VII, and is elicited by repetitively tapping on the patient's glabella (between the eyebrows). The normal response is a brief contraction of the orbicularis, producing a few blinks after the initial taps that stop after subsequent taps—usually fewer than five. In cases of frontal release, there is instead no *habituation.* Hence, blinking persists as long as tapping continues. This occurs in late extrapyramidal disorders (Parkinson), but also in 3–33% of older normal subjects.

8. **How do you separate "normal" primitive reflexes from the pathologic ones?**
   By judging them like people: by the company they keep. Hence, a "normal" palmomental or glabellar reflex will occur in subjects with otherwise a *normal neurologic exam*. Thus, they will be isolated. In fact, only fewer than 12% of normal individuals have *two* primitive reflexes, and fewer than 2% have *three*. Moreover, *normal* primitive reflexes tend to fade with repetition (i.e., they are *fatigable*). Only 1% of "normal" subjects will continue to exhibit a palmomental reflex after five stimulations. In contrast, patients with real pathology have no habituation.

9. **How long does it take to do a complete *mental status* examination?**
   It can take hours and even days. Yet, for clinical purposes the crucial components can be tested rather quickly. These include (1) level of consciousness, (2) orientation, (3) registration, (4) memory (recall), (5) attention and calculation, (7) intelligence, and (6) language.

10. **What are the most important *levels of consciousness*? How do they deteriorate?**
    There are *four* levels of consciousness. In increasing degree of deterioration they are:
    - **Alertness:** An awake person with normal level of consciousness (alert patient)
    - **Lethargy:** A sleepy patient who needs continuous stimulation to remain awake
    - **Stupor:** An unarousable patient who can still moan, withdraw, or roll around during exam
    - **Coma:** A patient who offers no purposeful response to stimulations of any kind

11. **What is *orientation*? How do you assess it?**
    Orientation is the patients' cognizance of their status in time, place, and person. To assess it, ask them to state the year/date/day/month of interview, their location, and their name (state/county/city/hospital/floor). In organic diseases, the sense of time is the first to be lost, while the sense of person is the last one. Hence, patients who are oriented to time and place but do not know who they are tend to be more psychologic than organic.

12. **What is *memory*? How do you assess it?**
    Memory is the ability to *register* and *recall* prior sensory input. For testing purposes:
    - **Registration:** Ask patients to name three objects and repeat them until fully learned.
    - **Recall:** Distract patients for 3–5 minutes (by doing other parts of the exam, like testing attention and calculation). Then ask them to name the three objects previously learned.

    Most normal subjects can remember three objects after a brief distraction (recent memory). Acute encephalopathies impair *all* aspects of memory (both recent *and* remote). Dementia disrupts instead recent memory and attention span, while preserving remote memory.

13. **How do you assess *attention* and *calculation*?**
    By spelling "world" backward or doing *serial 7's* (i.e., counting backward from 100, in installments of 7, and ending after five subtractions—that is, at 65).

14. **How can one efficiently examine all aspects of mental status?**
    Through a battery of carefully analyzed and validated questions, such as the *Folstein Mini Mental Status Examination (MMSE)*. This consists of 11 items that can be easily administered in 5–10 minutes and are either sensitive for dementia (but not specific), or specific but not sensitive. They evaluate the most important mental status domains (*orientation, registration, attention/calculation, recall,* and *language*), with a final score of 0–30 (<23 being abnormal).

15. **How reliable is the MMSE in assessing cognitive function?**
    Quite reliable. In fact, it has strong likelihood ratios for *identifying* dementia impairments. It is also valuable for *follow-up*, even though only significant for large changes (>4 points).

16. **What is the *clock-drawing* test?**
    Another mental status test. It provides patients with a preprinted circle (4 inches in diameter), asking them to "draw a clock." No further instruction and unlimited time are given. Normal

subjects will draw all 12 numbers, even though not necessarily with proper hands or symmetric spaces between them. Missing one number is still acceptable, but absent figures, irrelevant figures, or unusual arrangements/counterclockwise orientation of figures are *not*. An abnormal clock-drawing test has high specificity for dementia, but low sensitivity (being positive in only 50% of patients).

17. **How do you test for *delirium*?**
By looking for (1) acute and fluctuating change in mental status; (2) difficulty in staying focused or keeping track of what is being said; (3) altered level of consciousness (both in defect and in excess); and (4) disorganized thinking, with flights of ideas, often irrelevant and illogical. Hence, delirious patients exhibit a change in *both* mental status *and* the ability to stay focused. They also may have disorganized thinking or altered level of consciousness.

18. **What is *intelligence*? How do you test it?**
Intelligence is the ability to problem-solve by applying previous knowledge to a new situation and then using *reason*. It can be tested through calculations (serial 7 calculations), vocabulary, fund of knowledge, abstraction (use of proverbs), and judgment (like what to do with a found wallet).

(1) Language

19. **What are the components of *language*? How do you assess them?**
Language involves not only *speech* (verbal language), but also *comprehension* (of what is being spoken to you), *reading,* and *writing*. Hence, the ability to use language is one of the most complex functions of the human brain, whose correct assessment must test *all* of its aspects. Speech impairments include *dysphonia*, *dysarthria,* and *aphasia*.

20. **What is *dysphonia*?**
Dysphonia is *difficulty in phonation*. The voice is usually hoarse, but in the most severe cases, it may be altogether absent (aphonia, mutism). Causes include laryngitis (common cold), hypothyroidism (thickening of the vocal cords from myxedematous deposits), unilateral recurrent laryngeal nerve paralysis, and lesions of the vagus nerve. Reading, writing, and understanding are intact.

21. **What is *dysarthria*?**
From the Greek *dys* (difficulty) and *arthros* (articulation), this is a speech disturbance characterized by difficulty in *articulating* sounds and words. Hence, the quality of speech is impaired and typically slurred, but its content remains intact. Dysarthria is a *motor* impairment with intact cortical/subcortical language capacity. It usually results from paralysis/spasticity of the muscles of phonation (pharyngeal, palatal, lingual, or facial), but also can be observed in cerebellar disease or simple emotional stress. Contrary to most types of aphasia, dysarthria (and mutism) preserves the capacity to read, write, and understand speech.

22. **What is *cerebellar* speech?**
Another disorder of *articulation* of sound, rather than ideation or perception (ataxic speech).

23. **Beside cerebellar speech, what are the two most important types of dysarthria?**
   - **Spastic** dysarthria. This is due to damage of *upper* motor neurons (connecting the cortex to the spine), resulting in excessive and uncontrolled tone.
   - **Flaccid** dysarthria. This is due instead to damage of *lower* motor neurons, compromising all aspects of speech production. Lesions of individual cranial nerve(s) (brain stem stroke or peripheral facial nerve paralysis) also can cause dysarthria. For instance, Bell's palsy may cause difficulty in saying "mo-mo-mo" (*see* Table 19-1).

TABLE 19-1. DYSARTHRIA AND POSSIBLE CRANIAL NERVE INVOLVEMENT		
Syndrome	Sounds	Possible Cranial Nerve Involved
Labial	"mo-mo-mo"	CN VII (facial nerve)
Lingual	"la-la-la-la"	CN XII (hypoglossal nerve)
Pharyngeal	"ka-ka-ka"	CN IX and X (glossopharyngeal nerve and vagus nerve)

24. What is *aphasia*?

From the Greek *aphatos* (speechless), this is an acquired disturbance of language, including its *production* and *comprehension*. Hence, it should not be confused with *mutism* (the inability to produce *sounds*) or *dysarthria* (the weakness/incoordination of speech muscles). In both of these cases, the problem is in the "machinery" of language, not in its ideation or comprehension.

25. What are the most important defects in aphasia?

- Inability to *understand language* (receptive, sensory, posterior aphasia; also called *fluent* or Wernicke's aphasia)
- Inability to *transfer signals* from Wernicke to Broca (conductive aphasia)
- Inability to *properly execute speech* (expressive, motor anterior aphasia; also called *nonfluent* or Broca's aphasia)

Combined Broca's and Wernicke's aphasias constitute *global* aphasia.

26. What are the clinical differences between fluent and nonfluent aphasia?

- **In fluent aphasia (Wernicke's)**, talking is easy, but words are often jumbled and meaningless. There is difficulty in naming objects, repeating sentences, or comprehending. Speech is full of emptiness and gibberish "jargon," even though patients seem unaware of it. In fact, they may even appear confused and almost psychotic. Reading impairment parallels the speech deficit. The responsible lesion is in the temporal or parietal lobe.
- **In nonfluent aphasia (Broca's)**, there is obvious struggling for words and great difficulty with speaking. Language is slow, made up of monosyllabic sentences, and full of latency. In fact, it resembles the labored use of English by tongue-tied foreigners. Although nonfluent aphasics have a hard time naming objects and repeating sentences, their comprehension of *spoken* and *written* material is often quite good. Yet, they may be dyslexic (i.e., making semantic errors and having difficulty in reading highly imaginable words). A writing deficit usually parallels the phonologic deficit. The responsible lesion is in the frontal lobe.

    Pearl. Wernicke's aphasia is fluent, with impaired repetition and impaired comprehension. Broca's aphasia is instead nonfluent, with impaired repetition and intact comprehension.

27. Summarize the common aphasias.

See Table 19-2.

28. Who was Broca?

Pierre P. Broca (1824–1880) was a French surgeon with a prolific career in medicine and neurology. A pioneer in many areas, he described rickets as a nutritional disorder before Virchow, Duchenne's dystrophy before Duchenne, and even the use of hypnotism as a surgical adjuvant. He also was responsible for introducing to France the use of the microscope for cancer diagnosis. An anthropologist with Darwinian sympathies, Broca founded the first Anthropological Society of France and his own anthropological institute. He married the daughter of Dr. Lugol (of Lugol iodine fame) and died at 56 of myocardial infarction.

TABLE 19-2. COMMON APHASIAS

Type of Aphasia	Fluency	Comprehension	Naming	Repetition	Localization
Broca	Nonfluent	Intact	Impaired	Impaired*	Broca area
Wernicke	Fluent	Impaired	Impaired	Impaired†	Wernicke area
Conduction	Fluent	Intact	Impaired	Impaired	Arcuate fasciculus
Global	Nonfluent	Impaired	Impaired	Impaired	Broca and Wernicke areas

*Repetition may be preserved in Broca's aphasia when the lesion is anterior to the Broca area (transcortical motor aphasia).
†Repetition may be preserved in Wernicke's aphasia when the lesion is posterior to the Wernicke area (transcortical sensory aphasia).

29. **Who was Wernicke?**
Karl Wernicke (1848–1905) was a German physician born in what is now Poland. A graduate of Breslau (now the Polish Wroclaw), he described his aphasia in a book written when he was only 26. His interest in localizing lesions was then summarized (sort of) in a three-volume textbook published in 1881, which also contained the description of an encephalopathy caused by alcoholic thiamine deficiency (ataxia, confusion, nystagmus, ophthalmoplegia, and peripheral neuritis). This was later redubbed *Wernicke's encephalopathy* (with Korsakoff describing instead the *psychotic* manifestations of the disease). A cold and aloof man, Wernicke died also at 56, of injuries reported while biking in the Thuringian forest.

30. **What is *perserveration*?**
The difficulty in performing a repeated sequence of actions. Frontal lobe patients, for example, cannot switch easily from one task to the next. Instead, they *perseverate*. For example, when asked to draw a silhouette pattern of alternating triangles and squares, they get stuck on one shape and draw only triangles or squares. A good test of perseveration is Luria's *manual sequencing task,* wherein patients are asked to tap sequentially the table with a fist, then an open palm, and finally the side of the open hand. Frontal lobe patients cannot rapidly repeat the sequence.

31. **What is *cortical* dementia? What is *subcortical* dementia?**
   - **Cortical** dementia is cortical damage resulting in aphasia, dyspraxia, agnosia.
   - **Subcortical** dementia is damage of the basal ganglia, thalamus, rostral brain stem nuclei, and frontal lobe projections. It results in *bradyphrenia,* a unique slowness of thought processes (such as cognition, motivation, and attention) that is *absent* in *cortical* dementia.

32. **What is *dyspraxia*?**
The inability to perform tasks requiring fine motor skills, such as drawing, buttoning, writing, and speaking (verbal dyspraxia). From the Greek *dys* (difficulty in) and *praxis* (doing).

33. **What is *agnosia*?**
The inability to recognize objects by touch alone (*a*, lack of; and *gnosia*, recognition).

B. CRANIAL NERVES EXAMINATION

34. **What is the role of cranial nerve examination?**
An important one, since all cranial nerves have discrete functions that permit accurate localization of lesions based only on exam. Yet detailed testing of *all* cranial nerves is time consuming. Hence, it is unnecessary unless symptoms point toward a specific nerve problem.

35. **How do you test CN I (olfactory nerve)?**
By asking patients to close their eyes, occlude one nostril, and then smell through the open naris a distinctive scent—like cinnamon, cloves, or peppermint. Transient *anosmia* is common, usually resulting from simple colds or intercurrent sinus infection. *Chronic* anosmia (especially if congenital) is instead quite important (*see* Chapter 6, question 33). Note that anosmia can also be seen in frontal/temporal lobectomies or Parkinson's disease.

36. **How do you test CN II (*optic* nerve)?**
By *funduscopy* and *color recognition* (through Ishihara chart or a common and colorful object), but also by two bedside maneuvers, each testing a separate function of the optic nerve:
  - **Visual acuity:**Ask the patient to read an eye chart from a distance of 20 feet. Glasses or contacts are allowed, since the test measures the best corrected vision. A normal person reads at 20 feet letters that others also can read at 20 feet (20/20 vision). A person who reads at 20 feet letters that others can read at *40* is said to have an acuity of 20/40 (*see* Chapter 4, questions 1–15).
  - **Visual fields:** Their assessment can localize damage anywhere from the retina to the occipital lobes, resulting in loss of vision of only a discrete area (or field). The best way to detect *visual cuts* is by confrontation: place yourself head-to-head and eye-to-eye with the patient, while both of you occlude the opposite eye (because while looking into each other's eyes, both you and the patient have the same peripheral vision). To determine whether the patient can see what you see, move objects into his/her peripheral vision, starting from above, then below, then left and right. Patients should be able to see the objects at the same time you do. If they cannot, they probably have a visual cut corresponding to a particular region of peripheral vision (*see* Chapter 4, questions 20–35).

37. **How do you test CN III, IV, and VI?**
Together, since *oculomotor* (III), *trochlear* (IV), and *abducens* (VI) work in concert to produce the various eye movements. To test them, ask patients to hold the head stationary while following your finger as it moves through the main directions of gaze: *left-up, left-middle, left-down,* and *right-up, right-middle, and right-down.* Normal eyes move symmetrically and smoothly. Any restriction or double vision (from inability of the eyes to move together) suggests damage to III, IV, or VI (*see* Chapter 4, questions 84–90).

38. **What abnormal eye movements result from damage to CN III, IV, or VI?**
  - The **oculomotor** supplies medial, superior, and inferior rectus; inferior oblique; and levator palpebrae (which raises the eyelid). It also contains parasympathetic fibers that *constrict* the pupil. Hence, its lesions result in a partially *abducted* eye that is difficult to adduct, raise, or lower. In fact, it is frequently turned *out* (exotropia). There also is a drooping eyelid (ptosis) and a pupil that may be larger (mydriatic) and difficult to constrict. In more subtle cases, there may only be diplopia or blurred vision. A CN III palsy that spares the pupils (i.e., ptosis, and external rotation of the globe, but symmetric and equally reactive pupils) suggests *diabetes*, but also vasculitides and multiple sclerosis.
  - The **trochlear** supplies the superior oblique muscle by extending over a *trochlea*, or pulley. Since this nerve allows us to view the tip of our nose, its lesion will result in an eye that *cannot be depressed when adducted.* Hence, whenever patients pull their eyes *inward* (toward the nose), they will be unable to move them *downward.* This is often subtle. An isolated *right*

superior oblique paralysis results in (1) exotropia to the right (R); (2) double vision that worsens when looking to the left (L); and (3) head tilt to the right (R). The mnemonic is R, L, R (*the marching rule*—conversely, the rule for *left* superior oblique paralysis is L, R, L). This rule and the lack of ptosis and/or mydriasis differentiate the exotropia of CN IV palsy from that of CN III.

- The **abducens** supplies the lateral rectus. Hence, its damage prevents eye *abduction* to the side of the lesion. This results in *double vision on horizontal gaze* only (horizontal homonymous diplopia). It is often injured in patients with increased intracranial pressure.

39. **How do you test CN V (*trigeminal* nerve)?**
   It depends on whether you are testing a *motor* or *sensory* component. The divisions of the trigeminal nerve are shown in Figure 19-1.
   - The **sensory** component is predominant, providing pain, tactile, and thermic sensations to the face. Note that sensation to the tragus, most of the external ear, and angle of the jaw is *not* trigeminal and thus is preserved in diseases of the V (it is supplied instead by cervical sensory roots).
   - The **motor** component is smaller and primarily involved in *chewing*. It travels along the mandibular branch of the V and controls the masseters and lateral pterygoids. If damaged, it causes deviation of the jaw to the paralyzed side when attempting to open the mouth.

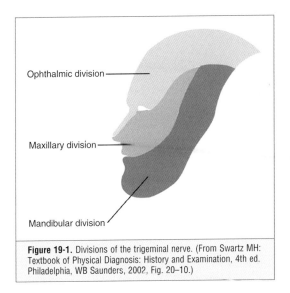

Ophthalmic division

Maxillary division

Mandibular division

Figure 19-1. Divisions of the trigeminal nerve. (From Swartz MH: Textbook of Physical Diagnosis: History and Examination, 4th ed. Philadelphia, WB Saunders, 2002, Fig. 20–10.)

40. **Where are the sensory and motor nuclei of the trigeminal nerve?**
   They are both in the *pons*. Yet the sensory also extends into the *cervical* cord.

41. **How do you test the *sensory* function of CN V?**
   By pinprick or light touch over the areas of distribution of the trigeminal branches: upper (supplied by V1, or *ophthalmic;* forehead), mid (V2, or *maxillary;* cheek), and lower (V3, or *mandibular;* jaw). Sensory function of the ophthalmic branch is also tested by the corneal reflex (*see* question 58).

42. **How do you test the *motor* function of CN V?**
By feeling the masseters during teeth clinching. Contraction must be strong and symmetric.

43. **What are the manifestations of trigeminal motor deficit?**
1. Difficulty clenching the teeth (due to weak *masseters*, at times visibly atrophic)
2. Difficulty deviating the jaw contralaterally (due to weak lateral *pterygoids*)

44. **What is the significance of *unilateral* trigeminal motor deficit?**
It indicates nerve compression (bony metastases) or an ipsilateral pontine lesion. Since trigeminal motor nuclei receive bilateral cortical innervation, hemispheric strokes will *not* affect them. Hence, bilateral masseter weakness suggests *bilateral* hemispheric disease (pseudobulbar palsy).

45. **What is the significance of a sensory deficit of the trigeminal nerve?**
It depends on whether it involves both the face and body, or only the face:
- **Isolated facial anesthesia** suggests disease of the temporal bone or metastatic spread to the ipsilateral mandible and skull base. This presents with numbness to the chin and lower lip ("numb/chin syndrome").
- **Combined facial and body anesthesia** suggests hemispheric and thalamic involvement, typically cerebrovascular. This presents with numbness to the same side of face *and* body (and *contralateral* to the ischemic area), plus hemiparesis and aphasia. Conversely, patients with facial numbness to one side and body numbness to the opposite have a *brain stem* lesion.

46. **What is Hutchinson's sign?**
It is the presence of herpetic vesicles on the nasal tip of patients with *ophthalmic zoster*—an ominous sign, since it suggests higher risk of ocular complications (uveitis and keratitis). This is because the nasal tip, the cornea, and the iris all share the nasociliary branch of the trigeminus. Patients with nasal tip involvement have a 75% chance of ocular involvement (tearing, irritation, photophobia). Still, Hutchinson's is a rather specific (82%), but poorly sensitive (57%), sign.

47. **What is the jaw-jerk reflex?**
A reflex that tests the integrity of *sensory* (afferent) and *motor* (efferent) components of the V. To test for it, place your index finger (or tongue depressor) over the patients' chin, while asking them to keep their mouth slightly open. Then, gently tap the index finger with your reflex hammer. Abnormal responses include jaw deviation or brisk closure. Exaggerated masseteric contraction, often with clonus, suggests upper motor neuron pathology (i.e., above the trigeminal nucleus in the mid-pons). This occurs in 70% of pseudobulbar palsy patients (*see* below, question 65).

48. **How do you test CN VII (*facial* nerve)?**
Through the *muscles of facial expression*. Damage to CN VII causes inability to wrinkle the forehead, tightly close the eye (Fig. 19-2), or smile. It also causes *facial asymmetry* (i.e., ipsilateral widening of the palpebral fissure and sagging of the nasolabial fold).

49. **What determines the difference between *central* and *peripheral* lesions of the VII?**
It's the difference in control of *upper* versus *lower* facial muscles: the upper being supplied by brain stem motor neurons (controlled by *both* sides of the cortex), whereas the *lower* are supplied by brain stem motor neurons (controlled by *only one* side of the cortex).

50. **What are the signs of *central* lesions of the facial nerve?**
Central lesions (i.e., involving either the cortical/upper motor neuron or its pyramidal tracts) result in *contralateral* weakness of only the *lower half of the face*. Thus, patients cannot smile

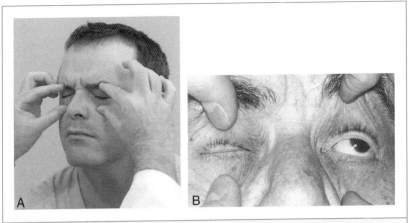

Figure 19-2. *A* and *B*, Testing the strength of eyelid closure. (From Swartz MH: Textbook of Physical Diagnosis: History and Examination, 4th ed. Philadelphia, WB Saunders, 2002, Fig. 20–15.)

(the face draws to the opposite side as they try to do so) or fully open the mouth, but can still wrinkle the forehead and close the eyes. This lower facial weakness only relates to *intentional* movements (i.e., those originating in the *motor* cortex). *Emotional* movements are typically spared, since they originate in the thalamus and frontal lobe.

51. **What are the signs of *peripheral* lesions of the facial nerve?**
   Peripheral lesions (i.e., involving either the brain stem/lower motor neuron or the nerve itself) result instead in *ipsilateral* weakness of the *entire* hemiface. Thus, patients can neither smile, nor open the mouth, nor wrinkle the forehead. Eye closure also is impaired, and the ipsilateral palpebral fissure is wider. Bell's phenomenon is present too. Weakness affects both volitional *and* emotional movements. Separating "central" from "peripheral" facial weakness *is* clinically very important.

52. **Are there any other functions of CN VII that can be affected?**
   Yes. CN VII also controls the anterior two thirds of the tongue, the stapedius muscle, and the lacrimal gland. Hence, its lesions may impair *taste, hearing*, and *tearing*.

53. **What about *ptosis*?**
   This is actually due to lesions of either *CN III* (which controls the levator palpebrae) or the *sympathetic nerves* (which control the Mueller muscle). Do not confuse levator palpebrae with *orbicularis,* which is instead supplied by the VII. Hence, lesions of VII will compromise corneal or glabellar reflexes, but *not* ptosis.

54. **What is *Bell's palsy*?**
   A *peripheral* mononeuropathy of CN VII. Since it involves the nerve directly (i.e., *peripheral* damage), Bell's causes paralysis of both lower *and* upper facial muscles. Hence, there is ipsilateral inability to smile, open the mouth wide, or wrinkle the forehead. Bell's also causes dysfunction in (1) *taste* (reduced in one half of the cases); (2) *hearing* (hyperacusis in 20–30%); and (3) *tearing* (usually increased, due to weakness of the orbicularis, but sometimes reduced as a result of lacrimal gland dysfunction). In 20% of cases, Bell's also may present with facial *hyperesthesia* due to concomitant trigeminal involvement.

55. **What are the causes of Bell's palsy?**
Peripheral paralysis of the VII has been described in infectious mononucleosis, herpes zoster, Guillain-Barré syndrome, parotid neoplasms, sarcoidosis, diabetes, or, occasionally, a cerebellopontine tumor. Yet, by definition Bell's is *idiopathic*, in fact probably viral. This is not an uncommon condition, which even affected heartthrob George Clooney while still in high school.

56. **What is Bell's *phenomenon*?**
It is the upward rotation of the eyeball, triggered by contraction of the ipsilateral *orbicularis*. This is usually *invisible*, since contraction of the orbicularis shuts the eye. Note that Bell's phenomenon is a completely normal event, occurring in anyone as a result of *synkinesis* (from the Greek *syn*, together, and *kinesis*, motion), a fancy term for an involuntary motion that accompanies a voluntary one. Examples of *synkinesis* include the movement of a closed eye that accompanies that of the contralateral open eye or the movement of the arms as a result of leg motion during walking. What makes Bell's phenomenon so unusual is that in patients with *peripheral facial paralysis*, the eyelid on the affected side is unable to close as a result of weakness of the orbicularis. Hence, the physiologic upward rotation of the eyeball becomes suddenly visible.

57. **Who was Bell?**
Sir Charles Bell (1774–1842) was a Scottish neurophysiologist and surgeon. He was *not* the same Dr. Bell who taught medicine in Edinburgh and made a big impression on young Conan Doyle (thus becoming the accidental model for Sherlock Holmes). That was *Joseph* Bell, a mesmerizing teacher who even tried his analytical powers on the mystery of Jack the Ripper, the Whitechapel killer of 1888. *Charles* Bell was instead the soft-spoken son of an Episcopal minister, who after being denied a position in Edinburgh, left for London in 1801. There, he made a name for himself as an artist, thanks to his "Essays on the Anatomy of Painting." He also attended the military hospital of Haslar, where he had plenty of opportunities to treat the casualties of Wellington's peninsular campaign. This triggered a lifelong fascination with *war*, and what it can do to human body and psyche. In 1815, while operating on Waterloo's wounded, he made sketches and drawings that can still be viewed at the Royal College of Surgeons in Edinburgh. He eventually moved back to his native Scotland, but only after founding the Middlesex Hospital and Medical School. He is remembered not only for his palsy *and* phenomenon, but also for *Bell's law*, which states that the anterior spinal roots carry motor fibers, whereas the posterior carry sensory fibers, including proprioception. He also named the "sense of position" as the "sixth sense"—eventually renamed *proprioception* by Sherrington.

58. **What is the corneal reflex?**
A bedside test of CN V and VII. To elicit it, ask patients to look away (so that they cannot see what the examiner is doing), and then use a cotton wisp to *gently* touch the edge of their cornea. The normal response is a protective reflexive blinking, which is *bilateral* (i.e., both eyes blink after stimulation of one) and requires the integrity of both V *and* VII: the ipsilateral V must be intact to receive sensation from the cornea, whereas both facial nerves must be intact to convey the motor response (hence the blinking of *both* eyes). This is a risky reflex since it can cause corneal damage.

59. **What is the significance of an abnormal corneal reflex?**
It depends on the response. If the ipsilateral eye does not blink after corneal stimulation (while the contralateral does), the most likely explanation is *unilateral facial nerve dysfunction*. Conversely, if both eyes fail to blink, the explanation is *unilateral trigeminal nerve dysfunction*, typically in the ipsilateral brain stem. An absent corneal reflex is especially helpful in cases of unilateral sensorineural hearing loss, since it suggests a lesion of the cerebellopontine angle—like an acoustic neurinoma. Yet, an abnormal corneal reflex is poorly sensitive, since it requires a tumor >2 cm. It is not specific either, being absent in 10% of normal elderly subjects.

60. **How do you test CN VIII (*acoustic/vestibular* nerve)?**
    It depends on the function you want to test, vestibular or auditory:
    - **Vestibular function** should be assessed by the Romberg, positional vertigo, and caloric irrigation tests only in cases of vertigo and dizziness.
    - **Auditory function** may instead be compromised in very subtle ways. Hence, the need for routine testing. This can be simply done by asking patients if they can hear whispered words, the soft noise of a ticking watch, or fingers rubbing against each other near the ear. *Conductive* and *sensorineural* hearing loss can be separated by Rinne and Weber tests (*see* Chapter 5, questions 59–65).

61. **How do we maintain balance?**
    Through a complex circuitry that requires intact *positional sense input* (vision, vestibular, and proprioceptive receptors/pathways), intact *sensorimotor integration* (cerebellum), and intact *motor output* (basal ganglia/corticospinal/pyramidal tract). If there is vestibular or proprioceptive damage, the patient will be able to compensate by relying on vision. Yet, darkness (or closed eyes) will remove this compensatory input and thus cause the patient to sway and possibly fall. Conversely, if there is intrinsic cerebellar disease, the patient will be unable to compensate *even with open eyes*. Hence, Romberg is *not* a cerebellar test since patients with *cerebellar ataxia* will not maintain balance *even when they can see*. It is instead a test for proprioceptive receptors and pathways. Thus, it will be positive in conditions of *sensory ataxia* (i.e., affecting [1] the *sensory nerves* (peripheral neuropathy) and/or [?] the *dorsal columns of the spinal cord [tabes dorsalis]*).

62. **How do you perform the Romberg test?**
    Ask patients to first stand up with the heels together, eyes open, and arms by the side. Note any swaying. Then ask them to close their eyes. *Observe for a full minute*. Normal patients may sway a little more with the eyes closed, but will not fall. Vestibular patients will sway a lot more with the eyes closed but will *not* fall. Sensory ataxia patients will instead sway *and* fall with the eyes closed.

63. **Who was Romberg?**
    Moritz Heinrich Romberg (1795–1873) was a well-respected Jewish physician who studied and practiced in Berlin, where he distinguished himself as "officer to the indigent" during the cholera epidemics of 1831 and 1837. A popular and beloved teacher, Romberg translated into German the works of Sir Charles Bell, and then wrote a three-volume textbook of neurologic diseases centered on the relation between altered structure and symptoms and signs. He reported his homonymous maneuver in an 1846 description of tabes dorsalis:

    > . . . the feet feel numbed in standing, walking or lying down . . . as if they were covered in fur . . . the gait begins to be insecure . . . [the patient] puts down his feet with greater force . . . keeps his eyes on his feet to prevent his movements from becoming still more unsteady. If he is ordered to close the eyes while in the erect posture, he at once commences to totter and swing from side to side; the insecurity of his gait also exhibits itself more in the dark.

64. **What is the anatomy of CN IX (*glossopharyngeal*) and CN X (*vagus*)? How do you test them?**
    Axons from several brain stem nuclei mingle together to emerge from the neuraxis through two separate nerves, named by early neuroanatomists as *glossopharyngeal* (IX) and *vagal* (X) (the vagus was so termed since, as a vagabond, it wanders long distances in the body). In reality, the origin of the two nerves is essentially identical. Function also is similar: motor control of the palate and pharynx (plus, for the IX, sensory supply to the pharynx and posterior third of the tongue). Hence, their clinical testing is not entirely separable. Since the brain stem nuclei of these two nerves receive bilateral innervation from the cortex, their dysfunction results from one of three possibilities: (1) bilateral damage to the cortex or pyramidal tracts

(pseudobulbar palsy), (2) brain stem disease (lateral medullary syndrome), or (3) peripheral nerve lesions (jugular foramen syndrome). You can test IX and X by asking patients to say "ahhh" or "ehhh" (*see* Chapter 6, questions 53 and 54) while observing whether the velum of the palate rises symmetrically. Alternatively, you can use the *gag* and *palatal* reflexes. The latter is elicited by touching the patient's palate with a cotton swab, which causes elevation of the soft palate and ipsilateral deviation of the uvula. The gag is instead triggered by touching the posterior wall of the pharynx (or alternatively, the tonsillar area or base of the tongue). It causes tongue retraction and elevation/constriction of the pharyngeal musculature. In unilateral CN IX and X paralysis, these reflexes result in deviation of the uvula toward the normal side. Lesions of the IX also will result in loss of taste in the posterior third of the tongue, and loss of pain and touch sensations in the same area plus the soft palate and pharyngeal walls. Conversely, unilateral paralysis of CN X's recurrent laryngeal nerve will cause hoarseness. *Bilateral* paralysis will cause stridor (requiring tracheostomy).

65. **What is *pseudobulbar palsy*?**
The result of bilateral damage to the pyramidal tracts supplying the nuclei of CN IX and X. This is due to lacunar disease of the internal capsule, and presents with paralysis of both the palate and pharynx (i.e., loss of the gag reflex), but also the tongue, face, and chewing muscles. As a result, patients will be dysarthric, dysphagic, and unable to control facial expression. There also will be spasmodic (and inappropriate) laughing and crying.

66. **How do you rule out the possibility of aspiration in patients with bilateral strokes?**
By testing for *pharyngeal sensation* and *water swallowing* (the latter requires swallowing 50 mL of water in 5-mL aliquots without any choking, gagging, or coughing). Preservation of both functions makes aspiration unlikely; an abnormal water swallow test makes it likely.

67. **And what about the gag reflex?**
It has very little value in predicting the risk of aspiration because swallowing is controlled by different muscles than gagging. Moreover, gag can be absent in many elderly individuals without necessarily increasing the risk of aspiration.

68. **What is the anatomy of CN XI (*spinal accessory* nerve)?**
The accessory nucleus comprises motor neurons from both the brain stem and the upper five or six cervical segments (hence, its name). The spinal axons exit the cord and rise in the neck, where they join axons originating from the brain stem, finally emerging together through the foramen magnum as the *spinal accessory nerve*. This provides motor control to the *trapezius* and *sternocleidomastoids* (SCM). The function of the trapezius is to shrug the shoulders. Its weakness will impair shrugging ipsilaterally. Conversely, the SCM's function is to *thrust* the head forward, *tilt* it toward the same side, and *turn* it toward the *opposite* side.

69. **How do you test CN XI?**
By first looking for asymmetry in the SCMs and trapezii. Then, by asking patients to shrug their shoulders against resistance (which tests the *trapezius*; Fig 19-3) or by having them first turn the head to one side and then attempt to turn it back against your resistance (which tests the *SCM*; Fig. 19-4). To test the right SCM, instruct the patient to turn the head toward the left, hold it there, and to not let you push it back. Then place your hand on the patient's left cheek, and try to force the head toward the midline. When the right SCM is weak, pushing against your resistance will be impaired. Repeat the same for the opposite side. Note that *atrophy* of these muscles reflects a "lower" lesion (peripheral nerve or brain stem/cervical spine). *Weakness*, on the other hand, also may reflect cerebral hemispheric disease. The latter weakens the *contralateral* trapezius and the *ipsilateral* SCM (hence, the patient will be unable to turn the head

toward the hemiparetic side). Disease of the accessory nucleus per se (like syringomyelia) weakens instead (and atrophies) both *ipsilateral* muscles. Hence, the patient will be unable to shrug ipsilaterally or turn the head toward the same side. This also occurs for peripheral nerve lesions.

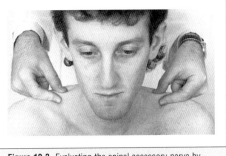

70. **How do you test CN XII (*hypoglossal* nerve)?**
By testing for movements of the tongue. These are controlled by the *genioglossus,* which is supplied by CN XII (running just sublingually in the neck—hence,

Figure 19-3. Evaluating the spinal accessory nerve by testing the trapezius muscle. (From Swartz MH: Textbook of Physical Diagnosis: History and Examination, 4th ed. Philadelphia, WB Saunders, 2002, Fig. 20–19.)

its name). To detect weakness or atrophy, simply ask the patient to stick out the tongue. Hypoglossal weakness will deviate the tongue toward the *weak* side (because the intact genioglossus muscle pushes the tongue contralaterally without meeting any resistance by the weakened muscle). Weakness may result from (1) a contralateral hemispheric cerebral lesion (causing deviation of the tongue toward the hemiparetic side), (2) an ipsilateral brain stem lesion (such as the medial medullary syndrome), or (3) an ipsilateral peripheral nerve lesion. Noncerebral lesions (i.e., lower motor neuron disease) produce also tongue *atrophy* and *fasciculations*.

C. MOTOR SYSTEM EXAMINATION

71. **Which CNS areas participate in the creation/coordination of muscle movement?**
    - **Motor system,** both in its pyramidal and extrapyramidal components (for power)
    - **Cerebellar system** (for rhythmic movement and posture)
    - **Vestibular system** (for balance and coordination of the eye, head, and body movements)
    - **Sensory system** (for afferent input to the spinal axis)

72. **What is the *motor system* made of?**
    - The **pyramidal component** (i.e., the corticospinal level of the motor system). This consists of (1) *upper (cortical) motor neurons* (residing in the posterior regions of the frontal lobes [i.e., the motor cortex]) and (2) the *pyramidal tracts* (i.e., descending corticospinal pathways).
    - The **extrapyramidal component**. This has instead its nuclei of origin in the basal ganglia and their complex connections, creating an elaborate neural organization that works closely with other levels of the motor system to achieve muscular control.

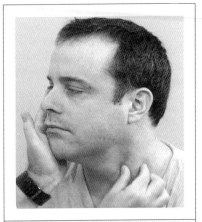

Figure 19-4. Evaluating the spinal accessory nerve by testing the sternocleidomastoid muscle. (From Swartz MH: Textbook of Physical Diagnosis: History and Examination, 4th ed. Philadelphia, WB Saunders, 2002, Fig. 20–18.)

Both pyramidal and extrapyramidal levels converge on the "final common pathway": the *lower motor neurons* of the brain stem (cranial nerves) and spinal cord, whose axons go directly out to skeletal muscles. Cord neurons are clustered in nuclei or longitudinal segments of the anterior gray matter, extending one to four spinal segments (*anterior horn cells*).

73. What is the function of upper motor neurons?
To exert direct or indirect supranuclear control over the *lower* (and more caudal) motor neurons. Upper motor neurons reside mostly in the *motor cortex*, but also in the *brain stem*.

74. What are the manifestations of *upper* motor neuron dysfunction?
Given their function as modulator of lower motor neurons, disease of *upper* motor neurons (or their axons) results in muscles that are initially weak and flaccid, but eventually become spastic, hypertonic, and hyperreflexive. This is associated with pathologic reflexes (such as *Babinski's* and *Hoffmann*) and induced *clonus* of ankle or wrist. Spasticity is especially prominent in the antigravity muscles (flexors of the upper extremities and extensors of the lower), with a *clasp-knife* character due to a variable degree of resistance to passive movements.

75. What are the manifestations of damage to *lower* motor neurons or their axons?
Weakness or paralysis of the involved muscles, with flaccidity, hypotonia, diminished or absent stretch reflexes, and eventually *atrophy*. There also are *fasciculations* (i.e., visible twitches of small groups of muscle fibers), but *no* pathologic reflexes (Babinski).

76. What are the main components of examination of the motor system?
- **Inspection** (for atrophy, hypertrophy, and fasciculations)
- **Palpation** (for cutaneous reflexes, but also for muscle strength and tone)
- **Percussion** (for myotonia and stretch reflexes)

(1) Atrophy, Hypertrophy, and Fasciculations

77. What is muscle atrophy?
From the Greek *a* (lack of) and *trophe* (nourishment), this is the muscular wasting caused by damage to lower motor neurons or their axons. Since these lesions typically interrupt the flow of trophic factors to the muscle, they result in degeneration and wasting of dependent myofibers (and fasciculations too—*see* question 79). Atrophy also may result from congenital muscular diseases or simple disuse, because of either trauma or arthritis. Yet the most common cause is indeed damage to the supplying neuron/nerve. Examples of atrophic muscles include the flat thenar eminence of carpal tunnel syndrome, the prominent metacarpals of polyneuropathy (with loss of interossei), and the atrophic calf of sciatica. To test for it, assess the muscle's three S's: *size*, *symmetry*, and *shape*. Atrophy, hypertrophy, and abnormal bulging/depressions are all important findings in identifying various muscular diseases or abnormalities—especially if asymmetric. Shape may be diagnostic, too, especially when altered by tendinous rupture.

78. What is muscle *hypertrophy*?
The opposite of atrophy. In addition to the Schwarzenegger's type (from overuse and conditioning), hypertrophy may paradoxically reflect a *congenital myopathy*. In this case, it is not associated with strength, but *weakness* (as in the bilateral calf hypertrophy of Duchenne's).

79. What are *fasciculations*?
They are visible, involuntary, and irregular muscle flickerings due to spontaneous contraction of individual motor units. They are typically benign (especially when occurring in the calf). Yet, if widespread, they reflect *denervation*—i.e., problems with *lower motor neurons* or their axons. In fact, interruption of the nerve supply makes the muscle hyperexcitable, thus favoring

the spontaneous contractions of individual fibers. *Tongue* fasciculations are especially ominous, since they occur in one third of patients with amyotrophic lateral sclerosis (ALS).

(2) Muscle Strength and Tone

80. **Which conditions are characterized by reduction in *strength*?**
Paresis and *plegia*, indicating, respectively, a lesser and greater deficit. The prefix "tetra" indicates reduced strength of *all* extremities, whereas "hemi" reflects weakness in just one side of the body, "para" in one station (i.e., either upper or lower extremities), and "mono" in only one limb.

81. **How is muscle strength graded?**
By asking patients to contract a muscle (or group of muscles) as strongly as possible, while at the same time resisting the examiner. Strength is graded on a 6-point scale:
   - 0/5 represents no muscle contraction and no joint movement.
   - 1/5 is visible contraction of a muscle without sufficient strength to move a joint.
   - 2/5 is strength sufficient to move a joint but not to overcome the resistance of gravity.
   - 3/5 is strength sufficient to move against gravity but not to withstand active resistance.
   - 4/5 is strength sufficient to move against gravity *and* to overcome *some* resistance by the examiner.
   - 5/5 is normal strength.
   This system is well accepted and clinically useful but does have flaws.

82. **What are the limitations of muscle strength grading?**
One is the *reference* point, which in unilateral disease is the contralateral (i.e., healthy) limb, whereas in bilateral disease, it is the (arbitrary) standard of the examiner's experience. Still, the real limitation is the 3/5 rating, since only few patients can move against gravity and yet be unable to offer any active resistance. The 4/5 rating also is flawed, since it is too broad for clinical use. Instead use:
   - 4−/5, which offers *little* resistance
   - 4/5, which offers *moderate* resistance
   - 4+/5, which offers *strong* resistance

83. **What muscles should be tested during the neurologic exam?**
The ones the patient reports symptoms on (testing every muscle in the body would be impractical). For a simple screening, it is adequate to test one *extensor* and one *flexor* in each arm and leg, both proximally and distally. Examples include (1) biceps, triceps, wrist extensors, and arm grip for upper extremities; and (2) iliopsoas, hamstrings, anterior tibial, and gastrocnemius for lower extremities. Since simple measurement of strength may *underestimate* the severity of deficit in patients with upper motor neuron disease, special maneuvers may be necessary. These include (1) *upper limb drift* (downdrift and pronation of the affected arm after the patients keeps them both outstretched and with eyes closed); (2) *forearm rolling test* (rapid rotation of forearms around each other, which in patients with hemispheric disease result in the inability to do so with the forearm contralateral to the lesion); and (3) *rapid finger tapping* (rapid sequential tapping of the index finger and thumb together, which is slower in the hand contralateral to the lesion).

84. **What is muscle *tone*?**
It is the permanent state of partial contraction of a muscle, usually assessed through resistance to passive motion, like in passively flexing or extending a joint (for example, arm at the elbow or leg at the knee). To assess muscle tone, instruct patients to "relax," or simply say, "Let me do all the work." Then, support the limb being tested and move it through a full range of motion, one joint region at a time. By doing so (and comparing sides), you can easily identify greater or less resistance.

85. **What are the most common forms of altered tone?**
They are an increase or a decrease in tone (hypertonia or hypotonia). Both reflect motor neuron disease: *upper* (pyramidal or extrapyramidal) for hypertonia, and *lower* for hypotonia.

86. **In addition to lower motor neuron disease, are there any other causes of hypotonia?**
Definitely spinal shock, but also some cerebellar diseases (*see* below, questions 91, 159, and 166).

87. **What are the extreme forms of *hypertonia*?**
   - **Spasticity:** The hypertonia of *pyramidal* tract disease. Resistance is initially low, but gradually increases as the muscle is being progressively stretched by repeat limb extension and flexion. When it reaches considerable tension, there is a protective relaxation and a sudden "clasp-knife" loss of tone, usually toward completion of joint flexion or extension.
   - **Rigidity:** The hypertonia of *extrapyramidal* disease (Parkinson's). It occurs throughout the full range of motion of the joint, with neither *weakness* nor *clasp-knife phenomenon*. It is *constant* (independent of the speed of the examiner's movement) and equal in both extensors and flexors. It may result in a cogwheel (stepwise) or lead-pipe (uniform) resistance to passive movement.
   - **Paratonia:** An increased tone that occurs not at rest, but at the time the limb tested contacts another object. It is a sign of bilateral frontal lobe disease, often associated with dementia.

88. **Name the four commonly used examples of hypertonia.**
   - **Clasp-knife:** Direct proportional increase in resistance, followed by a sudden and giveaway release in tone. It is common in upper motor neuron disease and a feature of *spasticity*.
   - **Lead-pipe:** A steady resistance throughout range of motion. It is a feature of *rigidity*.
   - **Cogwheel:** A ratchet-like resistance during active range of motion. The affected limb gives in intermittently to the pulling by the examiner, as if it were a lever over a ratchet. It is common in extrapyramidal disease, such as Parkinson's, and is a feature of *rigidity*.
   - **Gegenhalten** (German for "against-stop"): A resistance that increases in proportion to how quickly the limb is actively moved, diminishing when movement slows. It is common in frontal lobe diseases, such as Alzheimer's and head trauma, and is a feature of *paratonia*.

89. **What are the clinical features of Parkinson's disease (PD)?**
(1) Rigidity, (2) bradykinesia, and (3) tremor (such as the rolling of pills). A diagnosis of Parkinson's usually requires two of these three findings. False positive rates can be as high as 25%.

90. **What is *bradykinesia*?**
From the Greek *bradus* (slow) and *kinesis* (movement), this is slowness of motion *with* delayed initiation. It is common in early PD, where it can be detected by the blink rate—normally 24 ± 15 times/minute, while typically slower in Parkinson's (12 ± 10/minute, and even 5–6 in most severe cases). Bradykinesia eventually progresses to *akinesia* (i.e., the complete inability to initiate movement).

91. **What is *flaccidity*?**
A *reduced or absent* muscle tone. Hence, an extreme form of hypotonia. In flaccidity, the tested muscle feels unusually floppy. It is a sign of cerebellar disease or damage to lower motor neurons/peripheral nervous system, including the nerves that supply the muscles.

92. **What is *asterixis*?**
An inability to *maintain* muscle tone. It is commonly elicited by having patients close their eyes and then stretch out their arms, with fingers spread and dorsiflexed wrists—as if they were "stopping traffic." This results in rhythmic flexion at the wrist due to sudden loss of tone, causing the hand to *flap* (flapping tremor). It reflects various metabolic encephalopathies (*see* Chapters 20, questions 50–52).

(3) Muscle Percussion

93. **What is the response of a muscle to the stroke of a reflex hammer?**
The normal is *myoedema*. The abnormal is *percussion myotonia*.

94. **What is *percussion myotonia*?**
A prolonged muscular contraction, presenting as a skin "dimple." Typical of myotonic syndromes.

95. **What is *myoedema*?**
The opposite of percussion myotonia: muscle percussion elicits a "lump" and not a dimple.

(4) Reflexes

96. **What are *reflexes*?**
Involuntary muscular contractions elicited by (1) superficial stimuli (*cutaneous* reflexes), (2) muscle stretch (*deep tendon* reflexes), or (3) "release" of primitive reflexes (*see* section on Mental Status previously discussed).

97. **What are the main *superficial* reflexes?**
The corneal, conjunctival, abdominal, cremasteric, anal wink, and plantar (Babinski) reflexes. They all indicate integrity of cutaneous innervation and its corresponding motor outflow.

98. **How do you elicit the *corneal/conjunctival* reflex?**
By gently touching the cornea or conjunctiva with a sterile wisp of cotton. A normal response consists of bilateral winking (*see* questions 58 and 59).

99. **How do you elicit the *abdominal* reflex?**
By drawing a line away from the umbilicus and along the diagonals of the four abdominal quadrants. A normal reflex will draw the umbilicus toward the direction of the line being drawn.

100. **How do you elicit the *cremasteric* reflex?**
By drawing a line along the medial thigh. A normal reflex will elevate the ipsilateral testis.

101. **How do you elicit the *anal wink* reflex?**
By gently stroking the perianal skin with a safety pin. A normal reflex results in puckering of the rectal orifice due to contraction of the corrugator cutis ani muscle.

102. **How do you elicit *muscle stretch* reflexes?**
By briskly tapping the tendon with a reflex hammer. This produces a rapid muscle stretch, which is then sensed by the *muscle spindles*, relayed to the spinal cord, and eventually sent back to the muscle, causing it to contract reflexively.

103. **Is there any evidence that one hammer is better than the others?**
No. Taylor, Queen Square, or Troemner are very much the same. Preference depends on taste.

104. **What are the most important muscle stretch reflexes?**
- For **upper** extremities: (1) brachioradialis (C5–C6), (2) biceps (C5–C6), and (3) triceps (C7–C8)
- For **lower** extremities: (1) quadriceps (patellar—L2–L4) and (2) Achilles (ankle—S1)

105. How are reflexes graded?
On a 5-point scale:
- 0/4 is absence of any reflex (*areflexia*)—despite reinforcement.
- 1/4 is a reduced or weak reflex—usually requiring reinforcement.
- 2/4 is a normal reflex.
- 3/4 is a brisk reflex (*hyperreflexia*).
- 4/4 is extremely brisk hyperreflexia, usually accompanied by *clonus* (from the Greek *klonos*, tumult). This is a self-sustained and rhythmic muscle movement, marked by a rapid sequence of contractions and relaxations, which occurs (and persists) after the clinician has briskly stretched a hyperreflexic muscle and maintained tension on it. Typical of feet, clonus also can be elicited in the quadriceps, jaw, and other muscles.

106. What is the *Jendrassik* maneuver?
A reinforcement technique that can help elicit deep tendon reflexes in apprehensive and tense patients, who, either voluntarily or unconsciously, may be bracing their muscles (Fig. 19-5). During the patellar reflex, have the patient hook together the flexed fingers of the two hands and then pull them apart at the moment the reflex is being elicited. Other re-enforcement maneuvers include having the patient look up at the ceiling, count numbers, read, or cough—all aimed at redirecting the patient's attention, thus relaxing the tested muscles.

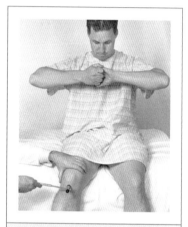

Figure 19-5. Jendrassik's maneuver. (From Swartz MH: Textbook of Physical Diagnosis: History and Examination, 4th ed. Philadelphia, WB Saunders, 2002, Fig. 20–38.)

107. What is the significance of *areflexia* or *hyporeflexia*?
It indicates *lower* motor neuron disease. Hence, it is often associated with other findings of muscle dystrophism, such as fasciculations and atrophy. If localized, it indicates *radiculopathy*.

108. What is the significance of hyperreflexia?
It indicates *upper* motor neuron disease. Hence, it is often associated with other findings of lost corticospinal inhibition, such as spasticity, Babinski, clonus, and exaggerated reflexes, often accompanied by irradiation (such as the jaw-jerk and finger-flexor reflex).

109. What is a finger flexor reflex?
An involuntary contraction of finger flexors in response to sudden stretching. To test for it, tap gently on the palm (or on the distal phalanxes of the index and middle fingers) with your reflex hammer. Alternatively, hold the patient's middle finger between your thumb and index finger, with the other fingers as relaxed as possible. Then, press with your thumbnail on the patient's nail, moving it down until your nail "clicks" over the edge of the patient's nail. This "click" should elicit no response in normal subjects. In patients with upper motor neuron disease, it will cause instead transient flexion of the other fingers (positive *Hoffmann's sign*). In other words, flicking (or nipping) the nail of the second, third, or fourth finger will cause all fingers (and possibly the thumb) to flex. The maneuver is then repeated for the other hand. Hoffmann's is a sign of hyperreflexia. Hence, it indicates *upper motor neuron disease* of the

upper extremities—typically Werdnig-Hoffmann syndrome. Basically, Hoffmann's is to the upper extremities what Babinski is to the lower extremities: a sign of upper motor neuron disease. The sign is linked to the German neurologist Johan Hoffmann (1857–1919), who studied and taught at Heidelberg. Although he discussed the reflex in his teaching (and used it in practice), he never actually wrote it up. This was eventually done by one of his students (Hans Curschmann), who credited his mentor, so that the sign came to be known as Hoffmann's reflex.

110. **Can decreased (or increased) reflexes be normal?**
They can, but in this case they are never associated with other neurologic findings. Hence, judge reflexes the same way you judge people (or murmurs)—by the company they keep.

111. **What are the characteristics of muscle stretch reflexes in *spinal cord disease*?**
They are characteristics of combined upper *and* lower motor neuron disease. Hence, the reflexes will be absent at the level of the spinal lesion (due to lower motor neuron involvement), but heightened *below* the lesion (due to loss of upper motor neuron suppression).

112. **What is a *crossed adduction reflex*?**
A pathologic "irradiation of reflexes" (i.e., the stretching of distant hyperexcitable muscles through spread of the stimulus along the bone—a sign of upper motor neuron disease). To elicit it, strike with a hammer the medial aspect of the patient's thigh tendon. This will contract the *contralateral* adductor, briskly moving medially the contralateral knee in a "scissoring" fashion.

113. **What is the *plantar* reflex?**
A *cutaneous* reflex (i.e., one triggered by skin stimulation) (Fig. 19-6). In normal subjects, a noxious stimulation of the sole leads to a *plantar flexion* of the toes, including the big toe. Conversely, in organic neurologic disease, there will be an *extensor* response (i.e., an upward movement of the great toe). Babinski used this finding to exclude hysterical weakness, which typically lacks "*Babinski*," as this reflex soon came to be known. Note that when stroking the lateral aspect of the sole of the foot, the big toe may display one of the responses shown in Table 19-3 below.

TABLE 19-3. BIG TOE RESPONSES	
Response	**Clinical Significance**
Plantar flexor (toe goes down)	Normal
Plantar extensor (toe goes up)	Common in upper motor lesion (above L5)
Mute (toe doesn't move)	Severe sensory loss or foot paralysis
Withdrawal	Common in metabolic disease

114. **What is the *Babinski sign*?**
It is the original Babinski's: dorsiflexion (or extension) of the big toe in response to stroking of the lateral aspect of the sole (*see* Fig. 19-6). In other words, the big toe goes up. Except for infants (where it is normal), this indicates a lesion of *upper motor neurons or their pyramidal tracts*. It also can occur in metabolic involvement of these tracts, such as meningitis, seizure, overdose, and hepatic/renal encephalopathy. Dorsiflexion of the big toe also may be associated with fanning out of the other toes (as in Babinski's description), yet this is not a requirement

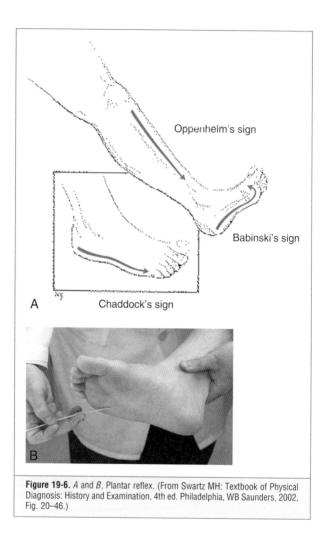

Figure 19-6. *A* and *B*, Plantar reflex. (From Swartz MH: Textbook of Physical Diagnosis: History and Examination, 4th ed. Philadelphia, WB Saunders, 2002, Fig. 20–46.)

for the response to be abnormal. An *extensor plantar response* (or Babinski) is an excellent bedside test: sensitive, specific, and able to pinpoint the lesion.

115. **Are there any false negatives?**
Lack of Babinski can occur in *spinal shock,* or a focal *upper motor neuron disease* that selectively spares the foot muscles. It also can be seen in peroneal paralysis, often as a result of pressure on the head of the fibula—a not infrequent event in bedridden patients.

116. **Name the different techniques to elicit the extensor plantar response**
- **Babinski:** Stimulate the lateral plantar surface of the foot with a blunt point, going from the heel forward, medially crossing the metatarsal pad to the big toe.
- **Chaddock:** Stimulate the lateral aspect of the foot from the heel forward to the small toe.

- **Oppenheim:** Apply pressure with your thumb and index finger to the anterior surface of the tibia downward toward the ankle.
- **Gordon:** Apply deep pressure to the calf muscles.
- **Strumpell:** Apply *strong* pressure on the anterior tibia.
- **Moniz:** Forceful plantar flexion of the ankle
- **Gonda-Allen:** Downward snapping the distal phalanx of the second or fourth toe (Hoffman-like)

The first four are the most used, with decreasing effectiveness from Babinski to Gordon.

117. **Who was Babinski?**
Joseph F. Babinski (1857–1932) was the son of a Polish political refugee. He emigrated to France at age 9, graduated from Paris University with a thesis on multiple sclerosis, and then went on to become one of the foremost neurologists of his time. A tall, handsome, and mustachioed man, Babinski was a committed bachelor, who spent all his life with his much younger brother Henry (a spare time gourmet famous for authoring a popular recipe book under the pseudonym of Ali-Baba), eventually outliving him by 2 years. He was also an unrepentant *bob-vivant*, who once interrupted his ward rounds when the charge nurse informed him that the soufflé was nearly perfect, and who spent many sybaritic evenings at the opera, theater, and ballet. Yet, he was also a clinical giant, who almost single-handedly provided a systematic approach to the neurological exam that has been part of the field ever since. Ironically, his polished skills also allowed him to be the first to recognize on himself the signs of that Parkinson's disease that was to plague him in his final years. Babinski described his eponymous sign (the *"phenomène des orteils"*) at age 39, in a 26-line presentation to the *Société de Biologie*. In that he reported that, while the normal plantar reflex consists of flexion of the toes, a dorsal extension of the big toe identifies pyramidal tract injury. After 7 years, he described the fanning of the other toes. Of interest, the pathological extension of the big toe had actually been reported by Ernst Julius Remak (1849–1911) 3 years before Babinski. In fact, Félix Alfred Vulpian (neuropathologist at the Salpêtrière) also had described it—half a century *earlier*. But it was Babinski who first realized its diagnostic value.

118. **What are movement disorders?**
They are manifestations of *extrapyramidal disease,* impairing the basal ganglia and their complex connections, including the motor integration centers of the brain stem and cerebral cortex. Movement disorders are disturbances of tone, movement, and/or posture. They are either "too much" (hyperkinetic) or "too little" (hypokinetic). A hyperkinetic example is the *intention tremor* of cerebellar disease. A hypokinetic one is the *bradykinesia* of Parkinson's.

119. **How do you examine patients with "abnormal movements"?**
By *observing* and *describing* the abnormal (or absent) movement. Does it occur at rest or during action? During sustained posture or while performing a specific task? Does it involve a specific body region (such as hand or oral-buccal area), or is it diffuse?

120. **What are the most important abnormal involuntary movements?**
They are tremors, fibrillations, fasciculations, chorea, athetosis, hemiballismus, myoclonus, dystonias, tics, asterixis, and seizures.
- **Tremors:** Rhythmic muscular oscillations around a joint, to-and-fro or up-and-down
- **Fibrillations:** Not visible to the naked eye except possibly those in the tongue
- **Chorea:** One of many writhing and twisting motions, which also include *athetosis* and *hemiballismus*
- **Myoclonus:** A sudden and brief (<0.25 second) muscle jerk, shock-like, with twitching of a joint; often asymmetric; isolated or in association with hypoxic encephalopathy/epilepsy
- **Dystonia:** A persistent, fixed contraction of a muscle—such as torticollis or wry neck
- **Seizures:** May result in automatisms of the face or limbs, repeated eye blinks, or tonic-clonic activity

121. **Name the three types of *tremors* and how to elicit them.**
    - **Resting tremor:** Best observed when patients are distracted (i.e., counting numbers with eyes closed) and their hands are lying on the lap. Resting tremor of 4–6 Hz is typical of Parkinson's. Amplitude and frequency of the tremor increase during stress and improve with voluntary movements. The rest tremor of the hand is often described as "pill-rolling."
    - **Postural tremor:** Postural tremor of 6–11 Hz is best elicited by having the arms or legs maintain a particular posture against gravity (i.e., *benign essential tremor of aging*). There also may be titubation of head or jaw and tremulous speech, like in the late Katherine Hepburn.
    - **Action tremor:** Best elicited by having the patient perform common tasks, like drinking from a cup or writing. Most prominent in goal-directed movements (e.g., finger-to-nose testing) and usually associated with cerebellar lesions.

122. **What is *chorea*?**
    From the Greek *khoreia* (choral dance), this is a sudden, rapid, unpredictable, and involuntary movement of the arms, legs, and often the face. It is characterized by purposeless, continuous, and irregular jerks, which may be unilateral or bilateral, at rest or during volitional acts. Eventually, they disappear with sleep. It affects multiple joints (usually distal) and is typical of *Huntington's disease*—an autosomal dominant disorder due to mutation in chromosome 4. This is the degenerative disease that killed Woody Guthrie.

123. **What is *athetosis*? How does it differ from chorea?**
    From the Greek *athetos* (without position or place), this is a constant succession of slow, writhing, sinuous, and involuntary spasms, which can present as flexions, extensions, pronations, and supinations of the fingers and hands. Usually along the long axis of the limbs or the body itself, sometimes involving the toes and feet, too, but *always affecting the proximal limbs*. As a result, the patient may assume different and often peculiar postures. In contrast, chorea is characterized by irregular, arrhythmic, brief, jerky, and spasmodic movements. Still, the distinction between the two is difficult. In fact, chorea and athetosis represent a spectrum of similar abnormal movements of the extremities and face. Hence, the term *choreoathetosis*. Conditions presenting like this include Huntington's disease, Sydenham's chorea, and the chorea of pregnancy.

124. **What is *hemiballismus*?**
    It is a violent flinging movement of half of the body due to lesions of the subthalamic nucleus.

125. **What is *myoclonus*?**
    A *spontaneous*, irregular, and rapid muscle contraction across a joint. It can be (1) *essential* (or idiopathic) and (2) *secondary*. The latter can result from many causes, including trauma, in-born metabolic errors, neurodegenerative disease, medications/toxins, and hypoxic injury. Myoclonus also can be *induced* by external stimuli, such as auditory or verbal.

126. **What is *dystonia*? How can be detected on physical exam?**
    Dystonia is a *sustained muscle contraction*, more prolonged than myoclonus and eventually resulting in *spasms* (i.e., twisting movements or abnormal [and often painful] postures). It is classified according to body region. *Focal* dystonia includes spasmodic torticollis (most common), blepharospasm, and writer's cramp. In *spasmodic torticollis*, the neck muscles (like sternocleidomastoids) are episodically engaged in cramp-like contractions that result in abnormal head posture. Palpation (or electromyogram [EMG]) can isolate the involved muscles. Oromandibular dystonia (a focal dystonia characterized by forceful contractions of the jaw and tongue, causing difficulty in opening and closing the mouth and often impairing chewing and speech) and spasmodic dysphonia (a neurologic voice disorder that involves involuntary "spasms" of the vocal cords, causing interruptions of speech and disrupted voice quality) are other examples of dystonia.

127. **What is a *tic*?**

From the French for "habitual spasmodic movement or contraction," this is an involuntary, repetitive, often complex, rapid, and stereotyped contraction of a single muscle or group of muscles, usually in the face. Forced eye closure, blinking, and sniffing are typical examples. Verbal tics include grunts and throat-clearing. *Echolalia* (parroting speech), *palilalia* (repetition of phrases), *coprolalia* (compulsory uttering of dirty words and obscenities), and *echopraxia* (imitation of movement) may occur, too. Motor/verbal *tics* are diagnostic features of Tourette's.

128. **What is Tourette's syndrome?**

A severe neurologic disorder of childhood/adolescence (but often persisting into adulthood), characterized by facial and body tics, incoherent grunts and barks (probably representing suppressed obscenities), echolalia, palilalia, coprolalia, and a want for touch. First described by Gilles de la Tourette in 1884, it was rumored to have affected very famous people, including Dr. Samuel Johnson and Wolfgang Amadeus Mozart (which would explain his penchant for foul language and nonsensical words so well depicted in Milos Forman's *Amadeus*).

129. **Who was Tourette?**

Georges Albert Édouard Brutus Gilles de la Tourette (1857–1904) was a son of physicians, who studied under Charcot and eventually worked at the Salpêtrière in Paris. Described by his colleagues as "ugly as a Papuan idol with bundles of hair stuck on it," Tourette was an energetic and charismatic teacher who achieved notoriety through his innovative use of hypnotherapy in the management of hysteria. This impressed not only a famous young man like Sigmund Freud, but also a very deranged and paranoid woman, who in 1896 became convinced that Tourette had taken her sanity away. For that she shot him in the head. Tourette managed to survive both this ordeal and the near concomitant deaths of his young son and old mentor, but never recovered. He fluctuated between depression and hypomania until finally losing his job—and mind. He was admitted to a mental institution and died there in 1904.

D. SENSORY SYSTEM EXAMINATION

130. **What are the two components of the sensory system?**

The *noncortical* and the *cortical* sensory systems. The first comprises peripheral nerves and their central pathways to the thalamus; the second one adds to these fibers the thalamic-cortical projections and the somatosensory cortex.

131. **What are the simple sensations conveyed by the *noncortical* sensory system?**

They are *pain, temperature, touch,* and *vibration*. Except for the latter, all originate in skin receptors. And, except for touch, all have well-defined pathways: either nociceptive or proprioceptive.

132. **How are *nociceptive* sensations carried by the nervous system?**

By slow and unmyelinated fibers. Nociceptive input (which includes pain, but also temperature and rough touch) synapses in the posterolateral columns of the spinal cord, crosses anteriorly to the opposite side of the cord, ascends in the spinothalamic tract, synapses in the thalamus, and finally reaches the sensory cortex. Loss of one nociceptive mode (such as temperature) is associated with loss of all other modalities conducted by the same tract (pain and rough touch).

133. **How are *proprioceptive* sensations carried by the nervous system?**

By fast and myelinated fibers. Proprioceptive input (which includes vibration, but also fine touch and joint position) travels in the posterior columns of the spinal cord, synapses in the gracile and cuneate nuclei of the upper cord, crosses to the opposite side in the medial lemniscus, synapses in the thalamus, and finally ends in the sensory cortex (part of the input also goes to the cerebellum). Loss of one proprioceptive modality (like joint position) is associated with loss of all other modalities conducted by the same tract (vibration and fine touch).

134. How do you describe *excess* of, or *lack* of, sensation?

As *hyperesthesia* (excessive, often unpleasant sensation) and *anesthesia* (lack of sensation), the latter being originally limited to touch, but now encompassing all simple sensations. *Hypalgesia* and *analgesia* describe reduction or absence of *pain*. Conversely, *hyperpathia* and *allodynia* describe, respectively, hypersensitivity to painful and tactile stimuli.

135. What is a *dermatome*?

It is a *skin cutting* in Greek; hence, the cutaneous area supplied by fibers from a single dorsal root. Damage to a nerve root (radiculopathy) typically causes sensory loss in just a dermatome. Still, only a few dermatomes are worth remembering, since their anesthesia can identify the damaged spinal segment—a useful finding for localizing the "level" of a cord lesion (i.e., the most caudal cord section that is still functioning):

- C6 (thumb)
- T4 (nipple line)
- T10 (umbilicus)
- L5 (top of foot)
- S1 (bottom of foot)
- S2–S4 (perineum)

136. Which dermatomeric rules should be kept in mind during the exam?

Three:

- **Contiguous dermatomes overlap.** Yet each has a unique "signature zone" (i.e., an area with no overlap that can be used to identify the spinal site of lesion).
- **Tactile dermatomes are larger than pain dermatomes.** Hence, pain testing is more sensitive than *touch* testing.
- **Sensory level in spinal cord lesions can be several segments below the actual lesion.** This is caused by the vascular supply (which may be injured at one level, but cause ischemia at another and more distant section) or the anatomic organization of nociceptive pathways (which carry lower body sensations more laterally than others, thus making themselves more exposed to injury). This does not occur with motor fibers. Hence, whenever there is discrepancy between *motor* and *sensory level*, always trust the motor level.

137. Which sensations should be tested during the neurologic exam?

- A **comprehensive** exam should test (1) *pain* (pinprick), (2) *touch,* (3) *vibration,* and (4) *position*.
- A **screening** exam should test only touch (on all extremities).
- If examining patients presenting with sensory complaints to one extremity, test both touch *and* pain, even though pain testing is usually more sensitive than *touch* testing. If concerned about spinal cord disease (i.e., extensive sensory deficits, involving, for example, trunk or large parts of an extremity), test instead *all* sensations. This may reveal *sensory* dissociation (i.e., loss of one perception, but not of others).

138. How do you assess *pain*?

By using an open safety pin. Assess the patient's ability to differentiate the pin's sharp point from its blunt end. An abnormal response may include increased pain sensation (*hyperesthesia*), diminished pain sensation (*hypesthesia*), or absent pain sensation (*anesthesia*, or numbness). Remember to discard the safety pin after completion of the test.

139. How do you assess *light touch*?

By gently stroking the skin with a wisp of cotton or tissue (for diabetics use instead the Semmes-Weinstein monofilament). Patients should perceive touch as light and symmetric.

140. How do you assess *temperature*?

By touching the patient's skin with two test tubes, one filled with warm water and the other with cold water. Alternatively, ask patients to discriminate between the cold handle of a tuning fork and the warm feel of the examiner's finger. Compare sides to each other and also to a benchmark, like the patient's own forehead (assuming sensation there is normal).

141. What is the clinical significance of *nociceptive loss*?

Loss of pain, touch, or temperature (i.e., nociception) points to a *sensory syndrome*, that is, one caused by damage of any components of the sensory pathways: peripheral nerve (peripheral neuropathy), dorsal root (radiculopathy), spinal segment (spinal cord lesion), ascending pathway (lateral medullary infarction), thalamus, or cortex (cerebral hemispheric syndrome).

142. What are the causes of *hyperpathia* and *allodynia*?

Increased sensitivity to painful (*hyperpathia*) or tactile stimuli (*allodynia*) occurs in peripheral neuropathy, brain stem infarction, and thalamic strokes. It provides no help with localization.

143. How do you assess *vibration*?

By using a 128-Hz tuning fork (Fig. 19-7). To do so:
1. First set it in motion by striking it against your palm from a distance of 20cm.
2. Apply its handle to a bony prominence of the patient's hand or foot.
3. Ask the patient whether he or she can feel the vibration.
4. Compare findings on both sides.
   A normal 40-year-old should perceive vibrations for at least 11 seconds when the tuning fork is applied to the malleolus, and for 15 seconds when it is applied to the ulnar styloid. Aging shortens these times, with an average loss of 2 seconds per decade. Note that applying the tuning fork to a bony prominence is only aimed at improving *transmission* of the input. Applying it directly to the soft tissue would still assess vibration.

144. Which vibration frequencies are well perceived by humans?

Those between 200–300 Hz. Frequencies <100 Hz are instead poorly felt.

145. What is the difference between a nociceptive and a proprioceptive loss?

In contrast to nociception, vibration (i.e., proprioception) can be selectively impaired in spinal cord/peripheral nerves' diseases while remaining instead preserved in cerebral lesions.

146. What is the role of an intact *sense of position*?

It allows us to "sense" joint and limb position, even though our eyes might be closed—like a Global Positioning System (GPS).

147. How do you test for *position sensation*?

First of all, ask patients to shut their eyes. Then, use your thumb and forefinger to grasp the lateral aspect of their great toe (or index finger) (Fig. 19-8). Move it up or down, while inquiring about direction of movement. Patients with intact proprioception should detect joint *movements* of as little as 1–2 degrees, even though 10% of the time they might be wrong in describing *direction*, since motion is more easily perceived than direction.

Alternatively, touch the index finger of the patients' outstretched arms; then ask them to close their eyes, let the arm drop by the side, and find again its previous target with the eyes closed. Since proprioception provides a sense of position that is independent of vision, its loss will cause imbalance—*especially* when vision cannot help (because of closed eyes or darkness).

148. **Which conditions are associated with proprioceptive loss?**
Those that damage (1) the *afferent pathways* (diabetic polyneuropathy), (2) the *dorsal columns of the spinal cord* (tabes dorsalis, B$_{12}$ deficiency, or multiple sclerosis), or (3) the *hemisphere*. Conversely, all of these conditions spare pain and temperature.

149. **How does the *sense of joint position* differ from other sensory modalities?**
Touch, pain, temperature, and vibration are *primary* sensory modalities. Hence, they can occur despite cortical damage. Conversely, upward or downward motions of the patient's limb require cortical integration of both *recognition* and *direction* of movement. Hence, they demand a more complex and *discriminative* cortical sensory function (i.e., an intact contralateral cerebral cortex). In return, this provides a GPS-like perception of joint motion and limb position, *even when the eyes are closed*. Patients with hemispheric cerebral disease may lose this discriminative sensory function *even though they may still maintain* the simple sensations of touch, pain, temperature, and vibration.

150. **How do you assess the discriminative sensory function?**
Through tests that assess the *cortical sensory system* (i.e., the somatosensory cortex and its central connections). These structures allow for higher integration and processing, such as: (1) detection of position and movement of extremities in space (*kinesthetic* sensation); (2) recognition of size and shape of objects (*stereognosis*); (3) tactile sensations of written patterns on the skin (*graphesthesia*); and (4) tactile localization and tactile discrimination on the same side or both sides of the

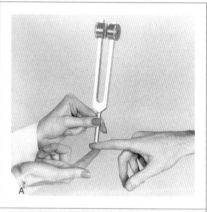

Figure 19-7. Vibration testing. (From Swartz MH: Textbook of Physical Diagnosis: History and Examination, 4th ed. Philadelphia, WB Saunders, 2002, Fig. 20–51.)

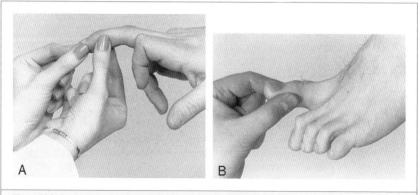

Figure 19-8. Testing of proprioception. *A*, With fingers. *B*, With toes. (From Swartz MH: Textbook of Physical Diagnosis: History and Examination, 4th ed. Philadelphia, WB Saunders, 2002, Fig. 20–52.)

body (two-point discrimination, touch localization and testing for *bilateral simultaneous tactile stimulation*). All these maneuvers require *closed eyes* and *intact simple sensations* (especially touch); otherwise, input to the cortex will be lacking. Abnormal response to any of these tests points to a lesion of either the *contralateral* sensory cortex (i.e., the *posterior* parietal lobe) or the thalamoparietal projections. These compromise proprioception, vibration, and fine touch in the distal extremities, but *not* over the face and trunk. Simple sensations are preserved. Conversely, lesions of the *anterior* parietal lobe (or deeper white matter) impair simple sensations of the contralateral hemisoma (trunk, limbs, and face). Since this dense sensory loss resembles that of thalamic lesions, it is referred to as *pseudothalamic* syndrome.

151. **What is *two-point discrimination (2PD)*? How do you assess it?**
2PD is the ability to distinguish two discrete and simultaneous stimuli of the skin. It is tested with the two needles of either a compass or caliper. By varying needles' distances, one can determine a two-point discrimination *threshold*. In normal subjects, 2PD is 4–7 cm on the body surface, 8–15 mm on the palm, and 3–6 mm on the fingertips.

152. **What is *touch localization*?**
It is the ability to point out with one finger where a touch stimulus was applied. Accuracy in touch localization requires the integrity of the sensory cortex *and* thalamoparietal projections.

153. **What is *stereognosis*? How do you assess it?**
From the Greek *stereo* (solid) and *gnosis* (recognition), *stereognosis* is the ability to identify an object by palpation. *Astereognosis* is the *inability* to recognize shape, form, and size of the perceived object, despite normal primary sensation (i.e., touch, pain, temperature, and vibration). To test for it, place some familiar item (coin, key, safety pin) in the patients' hands while their eyes are closed, and then ask them to identify the object. Lesions of the contralateral sensory cortex (or thalamoparietal pathways) will make this difficult.

154. **What is *graphesthesia*? How do you assess it?**
From the Greek *graphe* (writing) and *esteshia* (sensing), *graphesthesia* is the ability to recognize letters or figures drawn on the palm of the hand. This requires intact *primary sensory modalities* and *discriminative* (i.e., cortical) *function*. Hence, its impairment (*agraphesthesia*) reflects lesions of the right parietal region. To test it, ask patients to identify a number (or letter) you have written on their palm with either your finger or a blunt object (key or back of a pen). The letter/number should be larger than 6 cm, even though fingertips can recognize symbols that are only 1 cm in height. Always repeat the evaluation on the other hand, by drawing a different letter or number.

155. **What is *bilateral simultaneous tactile stimulation*?**
The ability to recognize that two sides of your body are being simultaneously touched.

156. **What is *extinction*? How do you test for it?**
Extinction is the inability to recognize being touched on one side of the body. To test for it, have patients sit on the edge of the table with their closed eyes. Touch them in one particular place of the trunk or legs, and then ask them to open their eyes and point to where they have been touched. Repeat this by touching them in *two* places on opposite sides of the body, simultaneously. Then ask them to point to the areas where they have been touched. Normal subjects will point to both areas, whereas patients with extinction will not do so. Instead, they will point to one area only.

157. **What is the clinical significance of a sensory loss?**
It depends on the area and the extent of the deficit. Sensory loss to only a portion of a limb suggests damage to either a peripheral nerve, or a plexus, or a spinal root. Conversely, sensory

loss to a larger part of a limb (or even the trunk) carries a wider differential diagnosis. A *unilateral* deficit suggests brain stem, thalamic, or cortical lesions, whereas a *bilateral* one suggests polyneuropathy or spinal disease. Also, pay attention to whether the deficit is associated with (1) *a sensory level* (which suggests a complete spinal cord lesion—typically presenting with infra-level weakness, urinary retention, and loss of all simple sensations); (2) *a sensory dissociation* (which suggests an *incomplete* spinal cord lesion); or (3) a *sensory loss on the face* (suggesting a supraspinal lesion, involving either the brain stem, thalamus, or cerebral hemisphere).

E. CEREBELLUM

158. **What are the functions of the cerebellar system?**
To coordinate proprioceptive input and to work with eyes and ears (i.e., vestibularis system) to provide a sense of position in space.

159. **Which clinical findings suggest damage to the cerebellum and its tracts?**
(1) Ataxia, (2) atonia (or hypotonia), (3) asthenia, (4) nystagmus, and (5) dysarthria. Except for atonia and asthenia (which can occur in other lesions of the nervous system), all other manifestations are very typical, since cerebellar diseases interfere with smooth and coordinated movements of arms and legs (*ataxia*), eyes (*nystagmus*), speech (*dysarthria*), and stance/gait. Hence, the tremulous, jerky, and clumsy motions of these patients. For example:
- **Abnormal posture or gait** (truncal ataxia): Due to median cerebellar lesions
- **Intention tremor:** A tremor that worsens at end-of-movement, while approaching the target
- **Dyssynergia** (incoordination): Lack in smoothness of execution of various motor activities
- **Dysmetria:** Inability to control range of movement, resulting in overshooting or undershooting of a target
- **Dysrhythmia:** Inability to tap and keep a rhythm; for example, while tapping the table with a hand or the floor with a foot
- **Dysdiadochokinesia:** Difficulty in performing rapidly alternating movements
- **Dysarthria:** A breakdown of melody and prosody of speech, with poor modulation

160. **Are cerebellar manifestations ipsilateral or contralateral to the site of lesion?**
Ipsilateral.

161. **What is *ataxia*?**
The inability to coordinate voluntary movements into smooth and appropriately directed actions (from the Greek word for *anarchy*).

162. **How do you test for ataxia?**
By observing the patient's gait and by carrying out the following maneuvers, the first two for the upper extremities and the third for the lower. Note, that nondominant hands or upper motor neuron weakness may impair response to these tests, *without implying cerebellar dysfunction*.
- **Diadochokinesia:** From the Greek *diadocha* (in succession) and *kinesis* (movements). This is the ability to rapidly perform alternating movements. To test for it, instruct the patient to pat the knee with the dorsum and palm of one hand, pronating and supinating back and forth. Since this is difficult to perform in cerebellar disease, the test is quite sensitive for ataxia. Observe speed, rhythm, accuracy, and smoothness of movements. Anything that is slow, irregular, clumsy, and inaccurate is abnormal, and suggestive of either *dysdiadochokinesia* (from the Greek *dys*, impaired) or *adiadochokinesia* ("*a*," lack of; complete inability to perform these movements). Another way to test for *diadochokinesia* consists of having the patient touch the tip of each finger with the tip of the thumb, in rapid

sequence, back and forth. Speed, coordination, force, and direction of movement are all affected.

- **Finger-to-finger:** Hold a finger in front of the patient and ask him or her to use the index finger to touch first your finger and then the tip of his/her nose—back and forth several times. Inability to hit the mark in a coordinated fashion indicates cerebellar disease/dysfunction (*dysmetria*). *Intention tremor* and *dyssynergia* may occur, too. Test each hand separately, and keep arms fully extended during testing, since this may precipitate tremors and incoordination.

- **Heel-to-shin-to-knee:** Ask a supine patient to place one heel on the opposite knee, and then slide it smoothly down the shin, over the dorsum of the foot, and back up to the knee. Look for wobbling or unsteadiness. Overshooting (hypermetria) or undershooting (hypometria) represents abnormal responses (i.e., dysmetria).

163. **What is *intention tremor*?**
An oscillating tremor that accelerates in pace on approaching the target during intentional movements—for example, in a finger-to-nose maneuver. Also referred to as "kinetic tremor."

164. **How do patients with *cerebellar deficits* walk? How do they stand?**
They walk with an *ataxic gait*: legs spread wide apart, as in a staggering and "drunk" fashion. Especially difficult is *tandem walking* (i.e., with one foot directly in front of the other [heel-to-toe]), as if on an imaginary tight rope (hence, its use for alcohol intoxication testing). Patients with cerebellar deficits have problems with *stance*, too, which is unbalanced, incoordinated, and with tendency to sway or fall to one side—especially when unassisted by vision (Romberg, *see* also Chapter 1, questions 90–94).

165. **How common is *ataxic gait* in cerebellar disease?**
Very common. In fact, the most common of all cerebellar manifestations.

166. **How is the *muscle tone* of cebellar patients?**
Profoundly reduced. This results in wide swings of the limbs when first raised and then allowed to spontaneously fall. It also results in *pendular knee jerks*, defined as three or more swings produced by a single blow to the patellar tendon.

167. **What is *nystagmus*?**
An involuntary to-and-fro oscillation of the eyes (from the Greek *nystagmos*, nodding). Although usually detected while testing the cranial nerves responsible for eye movements (i.e., III, IV, and VI), nystagmus is *not* actually produced by nerve lesions *per se*, but rather by damage to the brain/brain stem mechanisms responsible for *coordinating* eye movements. Hence, it is a sign of *internuclear ophthalmoplegia*, cerebellar lesions, or vestibular disease.

168. **Is the direction of nystagmus diagnostically helpful?**
Yes and no. In cerebellar diseases, 75% of nystagmus is *horizontal* (i.e., back-and-forth shaking, elicited by lateral gaze); 15% is *rotatory* (clockwise/counterclockwise twisting or rotating); and 10% is *vertical* (up-and-down bouncing of the eye). Yet horizontal nystagmus also can occur in peripheral vestibular disease. Hence, it is not specific.

169. **What is *optokinetic* nystagmus?**
The one elicited by looking at moving visual stimuli. A physiologic response in train passengers who try to fixate objects that are moving rapidly across their field of vision (*railroad nystagmus*).

170. **How is the *speech* of cerebellar disease?**
Dysarthric. In other words: slow, irregular, slurred, and with sudden changes in tempo, volume, and pitch (*scanning* or *staccato speech*), and yet still capable of conveying meaningful

and intelligible words. This is due to discoordination of the muscles of phonation. In contrast to aphasics, patients with cerebellar deficits have no problems understanding or making themselves understood (*see* also questions 19–27).

171. **How common is *dysarthria* in cerebellar disease?**
It is the least common of all manifestations, usually requiring *left*-sided cerebellar disease.

F. GAIT

172. **What is the control of walking? How is gait assessed?**
Walking is a highly complex action that requires integration of motor, cerebellar, vestibular, sensory, visual, and other systems. Hence, almost any abnormality in the nervous system will affect a patient's gait. To evaluate it, ask the patient to first walk normally, then on heels and toes, and finally to perform tandem walking. This simple test will allow you to detect many neurologic deficits, including weakness, incoordination, and dizziness (*see* also Chapter 1, question 71).

G. APPLICATION OF THE NEUROLOGIC EXAMINATION

173. **How do you best evaluate patients with neurologic symptoms?**
By first *localizing* the lesion. Identification of the *cause* comes only *after* accurate determination of the lesion site, since anatomic definition narrows the differential diagnosis.

174. **How can neuroanatomy be applied clinically, given the great complexity of the CNS?**
By thinking in terms of "regions." For clinical purpose, the most important aspects of neuroanatomy comprise only a few regions, with finer detail left to the specialist. From distal to proximal, regions to localize lesions in are (1) muscle, (2) neuromuscular junction, (3) peripheral nerve, (4) root, (5) spinal cord, (6) brain stem, (7) cerebellum, and (8) cerebral hemisphere.

175. **What is the *peripheral nervous system* (PNS) made of?**
(1) The *anterior horn cells* (in the spinal cord and brain stem); (2) *the nerve roots*; (3) the *peripheral nerves*; (4) the *neuromuscular junctions;* and (5) the *muscles*. Damage to any of these structures (*or* to the upper motor neuron) will cause *neuromuscular weakness*. Depending on which structure is affected, there also may be other symptoms.

176. **What are the causes of neuromuscular weakness/paralysis?**
Central or *peripheral* lesions. These include diseases of the (1) upper motor neuron, (2) lower motor neuron, (3) neuromuscular junction, and (4) muscle. The first two are the most common.

177. **What are the manifestations of *upper* motor neuron disease?**
Weakness and loss of dexterity, plus *increased muscle tone* (spasticity), *brisk reflexes* (hyperreflexia), *pathologic reflexes* (Babinski) and, occasionally, *clonus*. In *central* weakness/paralysis, there is neither atrophy nor fasciculations, but possible sensory changes. Note that distribution of weakness always points to the *side* of central lesions, whereas associated neurologic findings indicate the lesion *level*. For example, hemiparesis points to a contralateral central lesion, whereas the associated findings would identify its level: left cerebral hemisphere in patients with aphasia, left brain stem in patients with left sixth nerve palsy.

178. **What is *dexterity*?**
The ability to gracefully coordinate movements. More specifically, the skillful use of hands. In this context, dexterity is a *motor* skill.

179. **How do you separate upper from *lower* motor neuron disease?**
Both cause a weakness that is typically confined to the more peripheral (i.e., distal) muscles and that can be either symmetric or asymmetric. Thus, except for *hemiparesis* (which is a feature of upper motor neuron disease), localization of weakness will *not* separate upper from lower disease. Associated findings, on the other hand, will do so, especially muscle tone, reflexes, fasciculations, and atrophy. In this regard, lower motor neuron disease weakens or paralyzes *muscles,* whereas upper motor neuron disease impairs *movements*.

180. **What are the manifestations of *lower* motor neuron disease?**
Muscle weakness with decreased tone (*hypotonia or flaccidity*), reduced or absent reflexes (*hypoflexia or areflexia*), and frequent sensory changes (typically following the distribution of spinal segments or peripheral nerves). In time, the weak muscles of patients with *peripheral* weakness/paralysis undergo atrophy, and fasciculations appear.

181. **Describe ways to localize peripheral weakness/paralysis**
In lower motor neuron disease, the weakness is always *ipsilateral* to the lesion. Hence, the challenge is not to localize the damage, but to determine its *level*—for example, whether the weakness is due to a lesion of the nerve (*peripheral neuropathy*), spinal segment (*radiculopathy*), or combination thereof (*plexopathy*). For clinical examples, *see* Table 19-4.

TABLE 19-4. CLINICAL EXAMPLES	
PNS Localization	**Clinical Correlate**
Anterior horn cells	Muscle weakness + fasciculations, atrophy, hypotonia
Nerve roots	All of the above + pain and sensory loss in single root or segmental
Peripheral nerves	All of the above in multifocal or length-dependent distribution
Neuromuscular junctions	Muscle fatigability with fluctuations during the day
Muscles	Proximal > distal symmetric muscle weakness with absent sensory loss

182. **What about combined upper *and* lower motor neuron disease?**
A combined peripheral *and* central weakness/paralysis points to a spinal cord lesion, and thus narrows diagnosis to only two entities: *myelopathy* and *amyotrophic lateral sclerosis (ALS)*.

183. **What is *myelopathy*? What are its manifestations?**
Myelopathy is a spinal cord lesion produced by trauma, tumor, or disc disease. It can affect any section of the spinal cord (cervical, thoracic, or lumbosacral myelopathy) and is typically characterized by a *discrete level*, with motor, sensory, and reflex abnormalities both *at* and *below* it. Weakness, for example, is *peripheral* at the level of the lesion (i.e., flaccid, with atrophy and fasciculations), but *central* just below it (i.e., spastic and hyperreflexic). Myelopathy patients also have concomitant sensory findings, which are never present in *ALS*.

184. **What is ALS?**
A degenerative disease of pyramidal tracts *and* anterior horn cells. Hence, its presentation includes both the *hyperreflexia* of upper motor neuron disease (plus Babinski in 50% of cases)

and the *atrophy* and *fasciculations* of peripheral paralysis. Sensation is typically intact (a distinguishing feature from myelopathy). In decreasing order of frequency, onset of symptoms involves the arms (44%), legs (37%), and bulbar muscles (19%). The latter include tongue fasciculations and difficulty with swallowing and phonating.

185. **What are the symptoms of *muscle disease*?**
The most common is *symmetric proximal weakness,* present in more than 90% of myopathic patients. Sensory loss is typically absent, although there may be muscle pain, dysphagia, and weakness of neck muscles. Hence, always ask the following questions:
- Can you arise from a chair, get out of a car seat, get off the toilet, or go up stairs without using your hands? This question checks for *proximal leg weakness.*
- Can you lift or carry objects, such as briefcases, schoolbooks, children, grocery bags, or garbage bags? This question checks for *proximal arm weakness.*
- Is your weakness *symmetric*? Since most generalized processes are slightly asymmetric, there may be some minor differences. Yet, weakness confined to either one limb or one side of the body is very unlikely in pure myopathy.
- Is there any associated numbness or sensory loss? Pain, cramping, and uncomfortable sensations may occur in some myopathic patients, but sensory loss should be *absent.*

186. **After eliciting myopathic symptoms, which findings can you expect on exam?**
Proximal symmetric weakness without sensory loss. *Tone* is normal or mildly decreased, *reflexes* also are normal or mildly decreased, and *atrophy* is seldom significant unless the process is advanced. Similarly, there are no *fasciculations,* although there may be *myotonia*.

187. **What are the symptoms of *neuromuscular junction (NMJ) disease*?**
- Symptoms similar to those of myopathy: proximal and symmetric weakness with intact sensory. Yet, NMJ disease has a unique hallmark: *fatigability* (i.e., the worsening of weakness with use, and its recovery after rest). Since resting improves strength, fatigability does not present as a steady progressive decline during the day, but as *variability* (or *fluctuation*) in strength, as the muscle first fatigues, then recovers, and then fatigues again.
- NMJ symptoms also are very *proximal.* Hence, they affect the facial muscles, resulting in drooping of the eyelids (ptosis), double vision (diplopia), difficulty with chewing and swallowing, slurred speech, and facial weakness.

188. **After eliciting NMJ symptoms, which findings can you expect on exam?**
Proximal symmetric weakness without sensory loss. With repetitive testing, muscles weaken, but after a minute of rest they regain strength. Similarly, sustained muscular activity (such as upward gaze) leads to fatigability and progressive weakness (ptosis). Tone, reflexes, and muscle bulk are normal. There also is neither atrophy nor fasciculations nor sensory changes. There may be, however, ptosis or diplopia.

189. **What are the symptoms of *peripheral neuropathy*?**
The typical is distal and often asymmetric weakness, associated with sensory changes. Atrophy and fasciculations also may appear. Hence, ask the following:
1. *Do you wear out the toes of shoes, or catch the toes and trip?* This checks distal weakness in the legs. Symptoms are typical of patients with a foot drop.
2. *Do you have trouble with grip? Do you frequently drop things?* This checks distal strength in the hands.
3. *Is the process asymmetric?* Some neuropathies are distal, symmetric, stocking-and-glove in distribution, but most are asymmetric.
4. *Have you noticed shrinking or wasting of your muscles (atrophy)? How about quivering and twitching muscles (fasciculations)?*
5. *Do you experience numbness or tingling?*

190. After eliciting neuropathic symptoms, which findings can you expect on exam?
Distal, often asymmetric weakness with atrophy, fasciculations, and sensory loss, such as decreased pinprick, vibration, and occasionally position sense. Tone is normal or decreased, and reflexes diminished. There also may be trophic changes, like loss of hair and nails and smooth, shiny skin.

191. What are the symptoms of root diseases (radiculopathies)?
In addition to pain (the hallmark), radiculopathies have features similar to peripheral neuropathies (i.e., *denervation* [weakness, atrophy, and fasciculations] with *sensory loss*). Weakness may be *proximal* (the most common radiculopathies in the *arms* involve C5–C6 muscles, which are indeed proximal) or *distal* (the most common radiculopathies in the *legs* involve L5–S1 muscles, which are indeed distal). Only pain is unique to root disease and absent in peripheral neuropathy. Pain is severe, often sharp, hot or electric, and commonly radiating down an arm or leg.

192. After eliciting radiculopathic symptoms, which findings can you expect on exam?
Weakness in one group of muscles, such as C5–C6 in the arm or L5–S1 in the legs—sometimes with atrophy and fasciculations. Tone is normal or decreased, and muscular reflexes diminished or absent. Sensory loss has dermatomal distribution. There may be exquisite pain after maneuvers that stretch the root, such as straight-leg raising.

193. What is the presentation of spinal cord disease (SCD)?
The classic one is a triad: (1) *sensory level* (occurring as a band of sensory change around the chest or abdomen or as a sharp level below which all sensation is lost [sensory level is the hallmark of SCD]); (2) *distal, usually symmetric, weakness;* and (3) *bowel and bladder changes.* Hence, questions about SCD should always focus on the following symptoms and signs:

- *Is there a sensory level?* Some patients describe it as a belt, a band, or "tight swimming trunks" around waist or chest.
- *Do you drag the toe or trip because of distal leg weakness?* Lesions of the upper motor neuron or pyramidal tract cause weakness that is usually greatest distally. Hence, they may mimic a peripheral neuropathy.
- *Are your legs stiff?* Pyramidal tract weakness causes spasticity. Hence, patients report their legs as being "stiff" and their knees as unable to bend properly during walking.
- *Is there either retention or incontinence of bowel and bladder?* Note that the bladder is usually much more sensitive to spinal cord injury than the bowel.

194. After eliciting SCD symptoms, which findings can you expect on exam?
Distal weakness, usually worse in the legs than in the arms, and usually worse in the *extensors* (i.e., dorsiflexors of the feet and extensors of the wrists and fingers) than in the flexors. Tone is increased, reflexes are brisk, and the extensor plantar reflex (i.e., Babinski) is usually present. A sensory level is typically found, below which all sensory modalities are diminished.

195. What are the symptoms of *brain stem disease*?
Since the brain stem is basically a spinal cord with cranial nerves stuck in it, brain stem disease is uniquely characterized by *cranial nerve abnormalities*. Symptoms will therefore consist of a combination of *long-tract findings* (such as weakness due to pyramidal tract lesions, and numbness due to spinothalamic tract compromise) plus *cranial nerve findings*. Because the long tracts have crossed (decussated), weakness and numbness will *not* be in the distribution of a level, but rather present as hemiparesis or hemianesthesia. In addition, damage to one side of the brain stem will cause ipsilateral manifestations for the cranial nerves, and

contralateral manifestations for the long tracts. These crossed symptoms are another hallmark of brain stem disease—for example, weakness of one side of the *face* and the opposite side of the *body*. Note that CN lesions commonly cause the big D's: *diplopia* (III, IV, or VI), *decreased sensation in the face* (V), *decreased strength in the face* (VII), *dizziness* and *deafness* (VIII), and *dysarthria* and *dysphagia* (IX, X, and XII). Hence, history should focus on:

- Do you have double vision, facial weakness or numbness, dizziness, or difficulty in hearing, swallowing, or speaking?
- Do you have loss of sensation or weakness on one side of the body? In other words, are long-tract findings present, such as hemiparesis or hemianesthesia?
- Are the findings crossed or bilateral?

196. **After eliciting brain stem symptoms, which findings can you expect on exam?**
A combination of cranial nerve and long-tract abnormalities.
- For **cranial nerves**, there may be ptosis, extraocular movements abnormalities, diplopia, nystagmus, decreased corneal reflexes, facial weakness or numbness, decreased hearing, dysarthria, paralysis of the palate, decreased gag reflex, or tongue deviation.
- For **long-tract abnormalities**, there may be hemiparesis (with a pyramidal pattern of distal weakness), hyperreflexia, hypertonia, and positive Babinski. Hemisensory loss may include decreased sensation to all modalities.

197. **What are the symptoms of *cerebellar disease*?**
Mostly clumsiness and lack of coordination. Since the cerebellum is responsible for smoothing voluntary movements, any impairment will produce abnormalities in the rate and rhythm of motion. Hence, focus on incoordination in the legs and arms, such as:
- Is there a staggering, drunken walk? Alcohol impairs the cerebellum, especially the rostral vermis, which is responsible for the characteristic wide-based gait of intoxication.
- Is there difficulty putting a key in a lock, lighting a cigarette, or carrying out other target-directed movements? Cerebellar tremor is typically worsened by voluntary and intentional movements, especially when the hand approaches the target. Hence, fine/coordinated motions (like extending a key and inserting it into the narrow slot of a lock) are impossible.

198. **After eliciting cerebellar symptoms, which findings can you expect on exam?**
A staggering gait and difficulty with tandem walking. Also, when sliding a heel down a shin, patients may waver it unsteadily. Arms may show tremor and hesitation when the patient tries to touch his or her own nose, the examiner's finger, or another target. Finally, there may be difficulty performing rapidly alternating movements in the limbs, resulting in irregular rate and rhythm.

199. **What are the symptoms of *cerebral hemispheric disease* (CHD)?**
Disease of the brain itself may cause a variety of symptoms: (1) mental status changes and high-function disturbances such as aphasia, (2) hemiparesis, (3) hemianesthesia, (4) visual field defects, (5) involuntary movements, and (6) seizures. Questions to ask include:
- Does the patient have aphasia or altered mental status?
- Do weakness and numbness affect the face, arm, and leg on the same side of the body?
- Is there a visual field defect? Visual fibers run subcortically (in the optic tract, lateral geniculate, and optic radiations) and terminate in the occipital cortex.
- Is there a movement disorder, such as chorea, dystonia, or hemiballismus?
- Any history of seizures? This indicates the paroxysmal discharge of neurons, usually cortical.

200. **After eliciting CHD symptoms, which findings can you expect on exam?**
Aphasia or other mental status changes, plus hemiparesis, hemianesthesia, or visual field cuts.

201. What is *apraxia*? How can you test for it?

Apraxia is the inability to perform upon command simple or complex motor tasks, despite intact motor, sensory, and language functions. It is tested by asking the patient to "stick out the tongue" or "show how to use a comb or a toothbrush." Apraxic patients may be unable to perform these tasks.

202. What is the cause of apraxia?

A disruption of the pathways responsible for skilled motor tasks. These begin in Wernicke's, connect to the prefrontal area via the arcuate fibers, then go to the *left* motor cortex (right side of the body), and finally cross the corpus callosum into the *right* motor cortex (left side of the body). Any interruption eliminates the "how-to" information for simple or complex motor tasks.

H. SPECIAL PROBLEMS—MENINGEAL SIGNS

203. What are meningeal signs?

They are signs of meningeal irritation (i.e., *meningismus*), produced by hemorrhage, tumor, or inflammation. They are primarily three: (1) nuchal rigidity, (2) Kernig's sign, and (3) Brudzinski's sign.

204. What is their mechanism?

A reflex, and thus involuntary, attempt by the patient to prevent stretching of nerves that pass through inflamed meninges. Hence, they represent a defensive mechanism.

205. What is nuchal rigidity (or stiffness)?

It is the involuntary resistance offered by a patient in response to the physician's attempt to flex the neck. It indicates diffuse irritation of the cervical roots from meningeal inflammation. To test for it, place your hand under the patient's head and gently try to flex the neck. In the awake patient, this can often be elicited by simply asking the patient to touch his/her chest with the chin (which triggers pain). Sometimes, nuchal rigidity can be so pronounced as to result in marked extension of the patient's entire body, to the point of resting supine on neck and heels ("opisthotonus," from the Greek *opisthen*, toward the back, and *tonos*, tension).

206. What is *Kernig's sign*?

The involuntary resistance offered by patients to passive extension of the knee from a position in which hips and knees are flexed. Very much like the *straight-leg raising* of sciatica. To test for it, flex the hip and knee on one side while the patient is supine. Then extend the knee with the hip still flexed. Hamstring spasm results in pain in the posterior thigh muscle and difficulty with knee extension. In severe meningeal inflammation, the opposite knee may flex during testing.

207. What is *Brudzinski's sign*?

The reflex flexion of the hips and knees toward the chest in patients whose necks are being flexed. As a result, the patient assumes a *fetal position*.

208. How clinically useful are these signs in the detection of meningitis?

It depends on the underlying process:

- In **acute bacterial meningitis**, the most common sign is *nuchal rigidity* (84% sensitive), followed by Kernig's or Brudzinski's (61% sensitive). Other findings (such as change in mental status, focal neurologic findings, and fever) are more frequent in the elderly. Note that no meningeal sign is specific for meningitis. In fact, neck stiffness can be seen in one third of elderly hospitalized patients *without* meningitis, and Kernig's is often positive in sciatica.

- In **subarachnoid hemorrhage**, the most common finding also is *nuchal rigidity* (sensitivity 21–86%), accompanied by the sudden onset of severe headache (present in 80% of the cases) in an otherwise nonfocal neurologic exam. In fact, nonfocality and nuchal rigidity argue strongly for subarachnoid hemorrhage in patients with an acute neurologic presentation. Stroke or intracranial hemorrhage is much less likely.

ACKNOWLEDGMENT

The author gratefully acknowledges the contributions of Loren A. Rolak, MD, and Cameron Quanbeck, MD, to this chapter in the first edition of *Physical Diagnosis Secrets*.

SELECTED BIBLIOGRAPHY

1. Greenberg DA: Clinical Neurology. New York, McGraw-Hill, 2002.
2. Haerer AF: DeJong's The Neurologic Examination, 5th ed Philadelphia, JB Lippincott, Mosby; 1992.
3. Jankovic J, Marsden CD, et al: Parkinson's Disease & Movement Disorders. Philadelphia, Lippincott, 2002.
4. McGee S: Evidence-Based Physical Diagnosis. Philadelphia, WB Saunders, 2001.
5. Medical Research Council: Aids to the Examination of the Peripheral Nervous System. London, Her Majesty's Stationery Office, 1986.
6. Olson, WH: Handbook of Symptom-Oriented Neurology. Mosby, St. Louis, Mosby; 1994.
7. Patten J: Neurological Differential Diagnosis, 2nd ed London, Springer, 1996.
8. Strub RL, Black FW, et al: The Mental Status Examination in Neurology. Philadelphia, FA Davis, 1977.

CHAPTER 20

THE BEDSIDE DIAGNOSIS OF COMA

Salvatore Mangione, MD

"I live first among the dead and the dying. That is the best world for a physician, but when it lasts too long it becomes overwhelming."
—René Theophyle Yacinthe Laennec, 1810; letter to his cousin Cristophe

"Ignore death up to the last moment; then, when it can't be ignored any longer, have yourself squirted full of morphia and shuffle off in a coma."
—Aldous Huxley, *Time Must Have a Stop*

"His was a great sin who first invented consciousness. Let us lose it for a few hours."
—John, in *The Diamond as Big as the Ritz,* by F. Scott Fitzgerald—uttered before falling asleep

GENERALITIES

1. **How important is the bedside evaluation of coma?**
   —Important, since bedside exam can be used not only to localize the responsible lesion but also to provide *diagnosis* and *prognosis*. Hence, most maneuvers are valuable (in fact, *essential*) for all practicing physicians.

2. **What is coma?**
   From the Greek word for *deep sleep,* coma is a disturbance of *consciousness* characterized by inability of the central nervous system (CNS) to receive, integrate, and willfully respond to environmental signals. Knowledge of anatomic pathways is thus key for a competent evaluation, but this must be combined with an understanding of the many (and often multifactorial) conditions that may disrupt consciousness.

3. **What is consciousness?**
   Our most integrative function and one that provides the essential human characteristics. It is a state of awareness of self and the environment that is determined by two separate functions: (1) *awareness* per se (*content* of consciousness) and (2) *wakefulness* or *arousal* (*level* of consciousness). Each relies on different physioanatomic systems.!

4. **What is the content of consciousness?**
   It is the sum of cognitive and affective mental functions (*awareness*) (i.e., the knowledge of one's existence and the recognition of both internal and external worlds). It depends on the integrity of the *limbic system* (basal forebrain, amygdala, hippocampus, hypothalamus, and cingulum) *and* the *cortex*. Hence, it is a high-level function.

5. **What is stupor? Obtundation?**
   They are gradations of *awareness*. Yet, since both terms lack precision, coma should be assessed by more objective measurements such as the *Glasgow Coma Scale.*

6. **What is arousal? What does it depend on?**
   Arousal is a series of behavioral changes that occur whenever a person awakens from sleep or transits to a state of alertness—the most discernible being opening of the eyes. Arousal

depends on the *ascending reticular activating system* being intact and properly *connected with the diencephalus*. Hence, it is a *subcortical* phenomenon that depends on a functioning brain stem.

7. **Are the patient's eyes open or closed in coma?**
   Closed, since coma is a sleep-like state. Yet they can be open in *metabolic* comas (hepatic or uremic) or in chronic posttraumatic encephalopathies. For example, eyes are open in the late stage of hypoxic encephalopathy, in fact roving around so much as to convince friends, family, and Washington legislators that the patient has finally emerged from coma, when, in reality, the patient has entered *vigil coma (persistent vegetative state—PVS).*

8. **So why are comatose patients unconscious?**
   Because they lack both arousal (*brain stem*) *and* content of consciousness (*cortex/limbic system*). Conversely, PVS patients have arousal (hence, wakefulness), but still lack content of consciousness. Hence, they have awareness/arousal dissociation. In fact, Kinney has defined PVS as a "locked-out syndrome," insofar as "the cortex is disconnected from the external world, and all awareness of it is lost." This is usually due to three causes: (1) widespread and bilateral cortical lesions (hypoxic or ischemic), (2) diffuse damage of intracortical/subcortical connections in the white matter of the cerebral hemispheres (due to trauma or hypoxia-ischemia), and (3) bilateral necrosis of the thalamus.

9. **Why can thalamic lesions cause coma?**
   Because they interrupt the cortex-activating fibers that pass through them. Bilateral *hypothalamic* lesions can cause coma, too, and also present with sleep phenomena, such as yawning, stretching, and sighing.

10. **What is the neurologic basis of coma?**
    It is a *diffuse* and *bilateral* cortical dysfunction. This is either *primary* or *secondary* to a brain stem injury that compromises the ability of the ascending reticularis activating system to arouse the cortex.

11. **What is the ascending reticular activating system (RAS)?**
    A core of gray matter that runs dorsally through the four layers of the brain stem. It connects caudally with the reticular intermediate grey lamina of the spinal cord and rostrally with the diencephalus (subthalamus, hypothalamus, and thalamic nuclei). Its main function is to "power" the cortex (i.e., to provide *arousal*).

12. **So what is the mechanism of coma?**
    By analogy with a computer, we could describe it as a state in which either the *chips* (cortex) or the *generating power* (reticular activating system) are dysfunctional. If the power (brain stem) is off, the computer will not work even though the chips (cortex) might be intact. Neurologically, this will manifest as lack of *arousal*.

13. **Does a unilateral hemispheric lesion cause coma?**
    No, unless there is a preexistent contralateral process or a new secondary brain stem compression (due, for example, to herniation). The latter compromises the RAS, thus causing coma. In all other cases, coma requires extensive damage of *both* hemispheres.

14. **Do all brain stem lesions cause coma?**
    No. The capacity of a brain stem lesion to induce coma depends on its speed of onset, site, and size. Hence, brain stem infarctions or hemorrhages are a common cause of coma, whereas slower lesions (like those of multiple sclerosis or tumor) rarely do so. Note that lesions *below the pons* do not normally result in coma. Finally, drugs and various dysmetabolic states produce coma by depressing both the cortex *and* the RAS.

15. **So what are the causes of coma?**
    - Diffuse or extensive processes affecting the *whole brain* (but primarily the *cortex*)
    - *Brain stem lesions*—including not only primary disorders of the brain stem (such as hemorrhages, infarction, and cancer), but also compression from mass lesions of the posterior fossa (such as cerebellar hemorrhage/infarction)
    - *Supratentorial mass lesions causing transtentorial herniation* with brain stem compression (these are often associated with other neurologic signs, such as third nerve palsy and crossed hemiparesis) (*see* Fig. 20-1)
    - In a large study of "medical comas," 50% of all cases were cerebrovascular in nature, 20% due to hypoxic/ischemic injury, and the rest is a miscellanea of metabolic/infective encephalopathies.

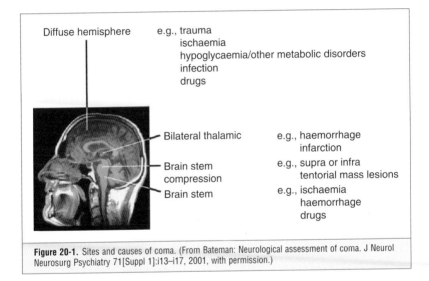

Diffuse hemisphere — e.g., trauma
ischaemia
hypoglycaemia/other metabolic disorders
infection
drugs

Bilateral thalamic — e.g., haemorrhage
infarction

Brain stem compression — e.g., supra or infra tentorial mass lesions

Brain stem — e.g., ischaemia
haemorrhage
drugs

Figure 20-1. Sites and causes of coma. (From Bateman: Neurological assessment of coma. J Neurol Neurosurg Psychiatry 71[Suppl 1]:i13–i17, 2001, with permission.)

16. **What is the function of the neurologic exam in comatose patients?**
    To *localize* the responsible lesion and, possibly, *describe its nature*. In this regard, the exam of comatose patients should categorize them as:
    - **Coma without focal signs or meningism:** The most common; due to dysmetabolic states of the entire CNS: anoxic/ischemic, toxic, drug-induced, infectious, postictal.
    - **Coma without focal signs but with meningism:** Due to subarachnoid hemorrhage, meningitis, and meningoencephalitis
    - **Coma with focal signs:** Due to intracranial hemorrhage, infarction, tumor, or abscess

17. **What is the neurologic exam of a comatose patient?**
    A simple one. Since the cortex of coma is, by definition, dysfunctional, exam is only aimed at assessing *brain stem* function. This is carried out in a rostral-caudal and level-by-level fashion. If all four layers of the brain stem are working properly, then the coma is *cortical* (i.e., one in which the cortex is *primarily* dysfunctional). If one or more brain stem layer is damaged, then the coma is a *brain stem coma* (i.e., one in which the cortex is *secondarily* dysfunctional as a result of direct brain stem damage) (*see* Table 20-1).

TABLE 20-1. CLINICAL ASSESSMENT OF COMA

General Examination

- Skin (e.g., rash, anemia, cyanosis, jaundice)
- Temperature (fever-infection, hypothermia-drugs, circulatory failure)
- Blood pressure (e.g., septicemia, Addison's disease)
- Breath (e.g., fetor hepaticus)
- Cardiovascular (e.g., arrhythmias)
- Abdomen (e.g., organomegaly)

Neurologic Examination

- Head, neck, and eardrum (trauma)
- Meningism (subarachnoid hemorrhage, meningitis)
- Funduscopy

Level of Consciousness

- Glasgow Coma Scale (verbal response, eye opening, motor response)

Brain Stem Function

- Pupillary responses
- Spontaneous eye movements
- Oculocephalic responses
- Caloric responses
- Corneal responses

Motor Function

- Motor response
- Deep tendon reflexes
- Muscle tone
- Plantars

Respiratory Pattern

- Cheyne-Stokes: hemisphere
- Central neurogenic hyperventilation: rapid/midbrain
- Apneustic: rapid with pauses/lower pontine

(Adapted from Bateman DE. Neurological assessment of coma. J Neurol Neurosurg Psychiatry 71[Suppl 1]: i13–i17, 2001.)

18. **What is a level-by-level exam of the brain stem?**

An exam that tests each brain stem layer with at least one neurologic reflex. If the reflex is abnormal, the corresponding brain stem level is considered damaged or dysfunctional. Thus, the neurologic exam of coma relies on four reflexes, one for each of the brain stem layers.

19. **What is the first step in evaluating coma?**

To assess whether there is any response to verbal stimuli. This can be done by asking patients to open their eyes and look up, down, and from side to side. "Locked-in" patients (*see* question 54) will open their eyes on command, and even look up and down, but will be unable to make any other purposeful response. Once this is done, the next step in the evaluation of coma is to test the first and uppermost brain stem level: the thalamus.

20. **Which reflex tests thalamic function?**

The response to pain. Since the thalamus is an integrating center for *all* sensory inputs (with the exception of proprioceptive signals, which travel instead to the cerebellum), thalamic testing requires administration of *painful stimuli*, like compression of the supraorbital nerve. This will induce a facial grimace, which in cases of afferent peripheral lesions of the pain pathways will occur without limb response. Limb response also can be assessed by pressing down on the patient's nail bed with a reflex hammer. Look for presence, symmetry, and nature of the response, since these can localize the lesion.

21. **What are the proper/improper responses of a comatose patient to painful stimuli?**

It depends. The proper response of a conscious, lethargic, or obtunded patient is to withdraw or push away the offending source. Thus, a proper response to compression of the ungual bed with a pencil would be to pull back or push away the examiner's hand. An improper response would be to assume a particular posture—for example, *decorticate* or *decerebrate*.

22. **What are these postures?**

Valuable findings for localization. A *decorticate* posture is a sign of subcortical/thalamic dysfunction. It consists of upper extremities' flexion, with extension and internal rotation of *lower* extremities A *decerebrate* posture consists instead of extension and internal rotation of both upper *and* lower extremities. This is a sign of upper brain stem dysfunction, usually the consequence of midbrain or upper pontine lesions. Finally, lower brain stem damage (low pontine and medullary) will cause no response to painful stimuli, or just extension of the upper extremities with simple bending of the knees (a spinal reflex). Unilateral decerebrate or decorticate responses also may occur, usually indicating unilateral lesions. Overall, it is easy to separate decortication from decerebration by remembering that in de-*cor*-tication the hand points toward the heart (*cor*), whereas in decerebration the hand points away from the heart (*see* Fig. 20-2).

23. **What about other involuntary movements?**

Patients with coma may exhibit various movement disorders (such as myoclonic jerks and tonicoclonic seizures). These are especially common in toxic-metabolic disorders (anoxic encephalopathy) and carry a worse prognosis.

24. **What is the second layer in the brain stem?**

The midbrain.

25. **Which reflex tests the function of the midbrain?**

The *pupillary reflex*. This is elicited by shining a penlight into the patient's eye and then looking for a direct and consensual response (i.e., constriction of both the ipsilateral and contralateral eye). Assessment of pupillary response is very important for localizing the site of lesion in coma

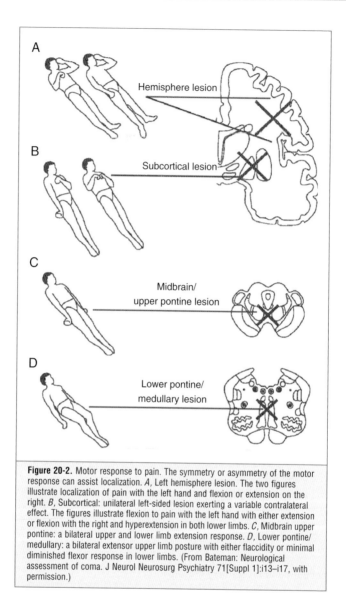

Figure 20-2. Motor response to pain. The symmetry or asymmetry of the motor response can assist localization. *A,* Left hemisphere lesion. The two figures illustrate localization of pain with the left hand and flexion or extension on the right. *B,* Subcortical: unilateral left-sided lesion exerting a variable contralateral effect. The figures illustrate flexion to pain with the left hand with either extension or flexion with the right and hyperextension in both lower limbs. *C,* Midbrain upper pontine: a bilateral upper and lower limb extension response. *D,* Lower pontine/ medullary: a bilateral extensor upper limb posture with either flaccidity or minimal diminished flexor response in lower limbs. (From Bateman: Neurological assessment of coma. J Neurol Neurosurg Psychiatry 71[Suppl 1]:i13–i17, with permission.)

and for separating *structural* from *toxic/metabolic* causes, since pupillary responses are usually preserved in toxic-metabolic states.

26. **What is the significance of pupillary abnormalities?**
Paralysis of the pupil (i.e., inability to constrict in response to light) indicates an ipsilateral dysfunction of the midbrain (*midbrain pupils* = midposition or slightly widened and fixed pupils unreactive to light). *Pontine pupils* are instead bilateral small pupils that still react to light, even though this may only be visible under a magnifying glass. They reflect anatomic lesions in the

tegmentum. *Pinpoint pupils* are both small and constricted but reactive; they often occur in metabolic encephalopathy and may be due to opiates. *Bilaterally dilated pupils* are instead encountered in patients with atropine and scopolamine toxicity (*see* Fig. 20-3). Note the following: (1) drugs that are frequently used in resuscitation from cardiac arrest (such as atropine or dopamine) may have misleading effects on pupillary reactions, (2) *lesions above the thalamus* and *below the pons* usually preserve pupillary reactions, and (3) finally, a third nerve lesion can be differentiated from a contralateral Horner's by the position of the eye and the degree of ptosis.

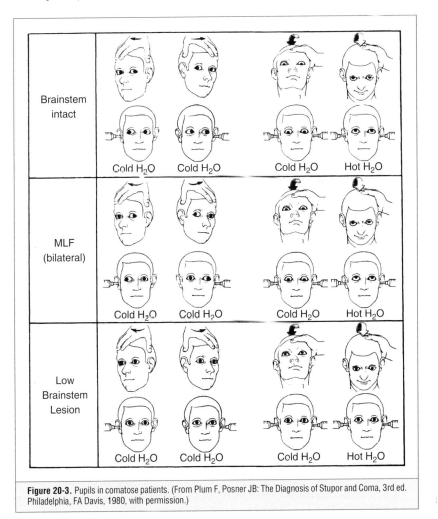

Figure 20-3. Pupils in comatose patients. (From Plum F, Posner JB: The Diagnosis of Stupor and Coma, 3rd ed. Philadelphia, FA Davis, 1980, with permission.)

27. **What is anisocoria?**
    From the Greek *aniso*, unequal, and *kore*, pupil, this is a pupillary asymmetry that is often congenital and physiologic. It is common, being present in up to 20% of the population.

28. **How can one distinguish physiologic from pathologic anisocoria?**
The pupils of physiologic anisocoria have different size (often by <1 mm) but are still reactive to light. Presence of anisocoria may depend on ambient light or time of exam

29. **What is the third level in the brain stem?**
The pons.

30. **Which reflex tests the function of the pons?**
The doll's eye reflex.

31. **What is the doll's eye reflex?**
A very confusing term, first introduced in the heyday of physical diagnosis, when Victorian dolls were more popular, and everyone knew how their eyes behaved. Still, the neurologic description (*oculocephalic reflex*) is preferable, since it conveys an anatomic sense of the pathway. To test this reflex, observe the patient's eyes during passive rotation of the skull. Yet, if you suspect cervical trauma *do not* rotate the patient's head. Instead, do *cold water caloric testing* (*oculovestibular reflex*), a safer way to test the integrity of vestibular and oculomotor systems. To do so, examine the tympanic membrane (to ensure that there is no perforation or impacted cerumen); then, with the patient's head 30 degrees higher than the horizontal line, irrigate the auditory canal with up to 120 mL of ice cold water. In the unconscious patient with intact brain stem function, this will cause the eyes to slowly and tonically deviate toward the irrigated ear.

32. **What is the pathway of the oculocephalic reflex?**
- The *stimulus* is either mechanical (rotation of the patient's head along the horizontal plane) or thermic (injection of a syringe full of liquid in the external ear canal).
- The *receptors* are in the inner ear (semicircular canals and utriculus).
- Once these receptors are activated, the *afferent signal* is carried to the central nervous system via the eighth cranial nerve. This enters the brain stem at the cerebellar–pontine angle.
- The impulse is then taken to the ocular muscles by the *efferent pathway* (third and sixth cranial nerves), eliciting eye movement across the horizontal plane. Since the third nerve resides in the midbrain and the sixth in the upper pons, the electrical impulse will need a "connecting wire" to travel from the lower pons to the upper pons and midbrain. This wire is the *medial longitudinal fasciculus (MLF)*.

Hence, when testing the integrity of the oculocephalic reflex, *we test the integrity of the MLF*. This is important not for the MLF per se, but because the MLF is totally imbedded in the *reticular activating system* (RAS), a crucial structure for *arousal*. Hence, the MLF acts like the canary that was used to identify gas leakage in coal mines. Dysfunction of the MLF indicates dysfunction of the surrounding RAS. Hence, loss of the oculocephalic reflex indicates a lesion in the pontine RAS, thus suggesting a *brain stem coma*.

33. **What is a normal oculocephalic response?**
It depends on whether the patient is awake or comatose and whether the coma is due to a primary (cortical) dysfunction or one secondary to pontine insults. In comatose patients with preserved brain stem function, passive rotation of the head will generate a conjugated movement of the eyes toward the *opposite* side. That is, the eyes do not stay fixed in the midline (as if they were painted), but they *move*. In cases of brain stem damage (with lost reflex), the eyes do *not* move. Instead, they remain in their initial position—fixed like in a cadaver. In *awake* patients, the cortex responds to head rotation by suppressing eye movement, thus inhibiting the oculocephalic reflex (it does so to allow the eyes to see where the head is pointing).

34. **Does any other reflex test the function of the pons?**
The corneal reflex. This elicits blinking of both eyes in response to a corneal sensory stimulus (like touching it with a cotton whisk). This triggers sensory input across the

trigeminal (fifth) nerve, which enters the brain stem at multiple levels, including the pons and medulla. The efferent pathway is then carried out to the orbicularis muscle, along the seventh nerve, eventually eliciting a blinking of the eye. Hence, the corneal reflex consists of a long loop that relies on several connecting wires, such as the MLF, all imbedded in the RAS. Like the oculocephalic, the corneal reflex assesses the function and integrity of the RAS.

35. What is the fourth and lowermost layer of the brain stem?
The medulla.

36. Which reflex tests medullary function?
The one testing the integrity of the most primitive of all function—the cardiorespiratory. Since the medulla houses the major cardiac and respiratory centers, dysfunction of these structures will manifest with cardiorespiratory instability, such as major irregularities of heart rate and rhythm, unstable blood pressure, and *apnea.*

37. What is an apnea test?
It is the inability of the patient to take a spontaneous breath after maximal carbon dioxide stimulation (60 mmHg). It indicates major medullary dysfunction. To carry it out, you need to disconnect the patient from the ventilator, while administering 100% O_2 via cannula. Measure arterial PO_2, PCO_2, and pH after approximately 8 minutes, and reconnect the ventilator. The test is positive if respiratory movements are absent and arterial PCO_2 is 60 mmHg (or 20 mmHg increased over a baseline normal PCO_2).

38. What is the implication of a global absence of brain stem function?
It indicates *death* (*see* question 53). Given its implications, a repeat neurologic exam is usually required at a 12-hour interval. Also, toxic-metabolic states need to be excluded.

39. What is a toxic-metabolic coma?
A wastebasket term indicating a global CNS dysfunction that is possibly reversible, since it is due to exogenous or endogenous toxins. Although toxins can impair *both* the cortex and brain stem, they usually affect the cortex more, since this is less resilient. Hence, coma patients with an intact brain stem should be considered toxic-metabolic until proven otherwise.

40. Can a localized process cause coma?
Only if affecting the brain stem (directly or indirectly [i.e., herniation]). Otherwise, a localized *cortical* process (like a stroke) causes lethargy or stupor, but *not* coma.

41. What are the causes of a toxic-metabolic coma?
They are exogenous or endogenous toxins, affecting the cortex bilaterally and diffusely.
- **Exogenous toxins** are poisons. Hence, a toxic screen should always be carried out.
- **Endogenous toxins** are also poisons that accumulate when there is dysfunction of major detoxifying parenchyma (hepatic, renal, or hypercapnic encephalopathy).
- **Endocrinopathies:** These include hypothyroidism (myxedema coma) and global dysfunction of the hypophysis (panhypopituitarism) or adrenals (Addisonian crisis). In addition, *defects in glucose metabolism,* either in excess (diabetic ketoacidosis or hyperosmolar nonketotic coma) or in deficiency (hypoglycemic encephalopathy), also may cause coma. Finally, *electrolyte disturbances* (hyponatremia and hypernatremia, hypercalcemia, and hypermagnesemia), can do it, too.
- **Subarachnoid toxins:** Direct, generalized poisoning of the cerebral cortex by toxins spreading along the subarachnoid space is another cause of toxic-metabolic coma. The most common culprit is *blood* (subarachnoid hemorrhage) or *pus* (purulent meningitis). Both can be

detected by lumbar puncture. Hence, this should be part of the standard work-up of *all* comatose patients, especially those with meningeal signs.

- **A generalized electrical disturbance** (such as a seizure) also may lead to coma. This can occur during or *after* the crisis (postictal coma). Since subclinical seizures may lack classic tonicoclonic contractions (i.e., patients can be immobile or just exhibit a fine fluttering of the eyelids), all coma patients should undergo electroencephalographic (EEG) testing.
- Finally, a common cause of metabolic coma is **hypoxic encephalopathy (HE)**, a term that is probably incorrect, since the bilateral cortical dysfunction of these patients might be due more to reperfusion injury than true hypoxia. HE affects primarily the cortex, while the brain stem remains mostly intact. Thus, after going through the initial state of coma (i.e., sleep-like), HE patients eventually emerge into *persistent vegetative state,* insofar as their brain stem sends impulses to the cortex (arousal) but the cortex is unable to process them. Hence, the original term of "apallic syndrome" (i.e., one characterized by destruction of the *pallium,* the telencephalon-covering gray matter).

42. **How common is coma due to cardiac arrest?**

Very common. Cardiovascular disease is the leading killer in the United States, accounting for one half of *all* yearly deaths. Of these, a quarter million will not even make it to the hospital (which is the equivalent of all World War II U.S. deaths in just 1 year); 500,000 will instead suffer arrest (and attempted resuscitation) during hospitalization. Survival rates for both groups are dismal: 2–33% for prehospital arrests and 0–29% for inpatient; 80% of all survivors are comatose after resuscitation, making cardiac arrest the third most common cause of coma after trauma and overdose. Rates of meaningful neurologic recovery also are poor, ranging from 10–30%. Given this premise, physical examination provides a universal and valuable tool to gather prognostic information in these patients. It is easy to perform, always available, and quite accurate.

43. **In addition to cardiac arrest, what are the other causes of PSV?**

The Multi-Society Task Force on PVS has classified its causes in three main groups: (1) *acute injuries* (most common being indeed hypoxic-ischemic or traumatic); (2) *degenerative and metabolic disorders,* including dementia; and (3) *developmental malformations* (with the most important being anencephaly). Still, the most common cause of PVS remains hypoxic-ischemic encephalopathy and head trauma.

44. **What is the Glasgow Coma Scale (GCS)?**

It is an important tool for evaluating coma, first introduced by Teasdale and Jennett in 1974. Prior to it, coma assessment was exclusively based on presence/absence of various brain stem reflexes (previously discussed). The GCS has instead provided a standardized way of classifying the condition, and as such has become an international standard. It consists of an ordinal scale calculated from the sum of three components: *motor response, verbal response,* and *eye opening.* Scores range from 3–15 (Table 20-2). Although originally described for traumatic coma, the GCS is equally applicable to *nontraumatic* coma. Still, even though it *does* predict poor neurologic outcome, it is not as predictive as the individual motor and brain stem reflex components (*see* questions 45 and 46). Moreover, assessing motor response requires that you apply *central* pain because peripheral stimulation may cause misleading spinal reflexes that do *not* represent a true motor response. Hence, to give a proper painful stimulus you need to pinch the skin of the supraorbital region or the sternum (using, for example, your knuckles to apply a firm twisting pressure).

45. **What are the crucial maneuvers in the evaluation of hypoxic coma?**

In addition to calculating the GCS, various brain stem reflexes may provide diagnostic and prognostic information. These include the very same ones reviewed before: *the pupillary reflex*

TABLE 20-2. GLASGOW COMA SCALE

Score	Motor	Verbal	Eye Opening
6	Obeys commands	—	—
5	Localizes stimulus	Oriented	—
4	Withdraws from stimulus	Confused	Spontaneously
3	Flexes arm	Words/phrases	To voice
2	Extends arm	Makes sounds	To pain
1	No response	No response	Eyes remain closed

(which involves cranial nerves II and III), and *the corneal reflex* (which involves cranial nerves V and VII); but also *the gag and cough reflexes* (which test cranial nerves IX and X). To elicit a gag reflex, apply a tongue depressor to the posterior pharynx: the normal response is a symmetric rise in the soft palate. If the patient is intubated, you can assess instead the *cough (or carinal) reflex.* This is elicited by applying deep suction through the endotracheal tube to the carina. The normal response is a gasp followed by several rapid coughs. *Vestibular signs* also are quite important, and include the aforementioned oculocephalic (or "doll's eye") reflex.

46. **What signs best predict lack of recovery after cardiac arrest?**
In a meta-analysis of almost 2000 patients, Booth et al. found that the signs with the highest likelihood ratios (LRs) at 24 hours were *absent corneal reflexes* (LR, 12.9), *absent pupillary reflexes* (LR, 10.2), *absent motor response* (LR, 4.9), and *absent withdrawal to pain* (LR, 4.7). At 72 hours, absent motor response predicted death or poor neurologic outcome (LR, 9.2). No sign had likelihood ratios that strongly predicted *good* neurologic outcome. Hence, *lack of pupillary and corneal reflexes at 24 hours and no motor response at 72 strongly argue against recovery.*

47. **Do seizures or myoclonus have significance in coma after cardiac arrest?**
Yes, and both are ominous. Overall, 25–50% of comatose survivors of arrest exhibit either *seizures* or *myoclonus,* usually early in the postresuscitation stage. Seizures may be focal or generalized. Myoclonus refers instead to isolated and sudden muscular contractions, which may also be focal or generalized (the latter involving axial and limb musculature). Remember to discontinue medications that may interfere with the neurologic exam, such as paralyzing agents or sedatives—so ubiquitous in today's intensive care units.

48. **How precise is the clinical exam of coma?**
Quite precise. Five studies have assessed its precision in evaluating comatose patients. Interobserver agreement was good, with little significant change between experienced nurses, residents, and practicing physicians. Overall, the precision of the examination (including GCS and brain stem reflexes) was moderate to substantial.

49. **What is the bottom line for the neurologic exam of coma?**
It is a valuable tool, with moderate to substantial precision and good prognostic value.

50. **What is asterixis?**
From the Greek *a* (lack of) and *sterixis* (fixed position), this is the bilateral flapping tremor of metabolic encephalopathy, particularly impending hepatic coma (*see* Chapter 15, question 79). It was first described in 1949 by Foley and Adams. Foley, a notorious wit, coined the term while

drinking at a Greek bar across from Boston City Hospital. He then used it semiseriously in a paper, not expecting much of it. To his amazement, the word became the official academic term for flapping tremor due to the inability of maintaining a *voluntary* muscular contraction (asterixis requires patient cooperation and thus cannot be elicited in stupor or coma). It consists of involuntary jerking movements, in a typical sequence of flexions and extensions. Since it reflects a lapse of posture, it involves antigravitary muscles, such as those of wrist, metacarpophalangeal, and hip joints, but also toes, eyelids, and even tongue. Still, it is typically assessed in the hands.

51. How can you elicit asterixis?

By asking patients to extend the arms, dorsiflex the wrists, and spread the fingers—as if they were stopping traffic. This usually elicits "flapping" at the wrist. If this is inadequate, ask patients to keep the arms straight while you gently hyperextend their wrists.

52. What is the clinical significance of asterixis?

The most important is hepatic ("liver flap") or renal encephalopathy. But it also may occur in other metabolic encephalopathies, like hypercapnia or electrolyte imbalance (hypokalemia, hypomagnesemia, and hypoglycemia). It may even be elicited (albeit more rarely) in severe congestive heart failure or sepsis. Poisoning (barbiturates, alcohol, and phenytoin [i.e., "phenytoin flap"]) can do it, too, and so can malabsorption. The exact mechanism is unknown, although leading theories include abnormal joint proprioception and disrupted posture pathway in the rostral reticular formation. Thus, the asterixis patient has an inability to maintain posture through muscle tone. Sudden loss of tone at the wrist results in a rhythmic flexion of the hand— hence, the flapping. Asterixis also is a sign of severity, so that hepatic failure *with* it has mortality twice as high as that *without*.

53. What is the definition of death?

An elusive but important one. Prior to intensive care units and ventilatory support, the definition of death was easy: patients were dead whenever their cardiac, respiratory, and neurologic systems ceased to function. Things got more complicated with the development of cardiorespiratory support, since this has almost entirely preempted any rapid and dignified demise once crucial functions have failed. Now it is possible to provide full respiratory and circulatory support, even when there is no detectable neurologic function. This has increased the availability of transplantable organs (still being perfused by a beating heart), but also has made the definition of death more fuzzy. It also has created lots of pain and suffering. To better define death, Ronald Reagan appointed in 1981 a presidential commission that eventually articulated the *Uniform Determination of Death Act,* stating that "an individual who has sustained either (1) irreversible cessation of circulatory and respiratory functions, *or* (2) irreversible cessation of all functions of the entire brain, including the brainstem, is dead." Hence, our current definition of death is a *brain stem death* (or, alternatively, a lack of brain perfusion). This requires *full and global dysfunction of the brain stem,* at each of its levels, with no real need to obtain an EEG. In fact, death is a diagnosis that requires only the exclusion of a toxic-metabolic cause, and two consistent but separate neurologic examinations—12 hours apart. Even though this has become the accepted standard for defining death (and suitability for organ donation) both in the United States and much of the Western world, it still leaves much to be desired. For example, what reasons do we have to believe that the constellation of clinical findings that constitutes brain death actually represents the *true* death of the individual? Although the concept that we are dead when our brains are dead is almost intuitive, it also raises some very difficult questions. For one, many patients currently diagnosed as brain-dead do not actually have (as required by the *Uniform Determination of Death Act*) "irreversible cessation of *all* functions of the *entire* brain." Many, for example, still retain function of the posterior pituitary and other brain parts. Supporters of the definition of brain death have argued that the concept of *whole-brain death* is only "an approximation," and that these residual functions should be ignored because they are *not significant*. This brings us to the inevitable question of what physiologic responses are indeed "significant." Why should the light and corneal reflexes be more important than the neurologic regulation of salt and water? To address this criticism, it has been suggested that these patients are so seriously ill that they will face an inevitable cardiac arrest within a short period (usually 1–2 weeks). Yet this only implies that they are *dying*, not that they are dead. Also, the fact that they have become permanently unconscious does not necessarily make them dead. Although there are no documented instances of patients who, having met criteria for brain death, ever regained any degree of consciousness, persistent vegetative patients are also permanently unconscious, and yet not dead. So, permanent unconsciousness is not enough to define brain death. In short, the most compelling reason for assuming that brain-dead patients are dead is the idea that death is the loss of functioning of the organism "as a whole" and that the brain is such a pivotal component of our overall function, that whenever it can no longer provide the necessary organizational influence, it leaves the body with the inevitable (an unenviable) task of self-disintegration.

54. **What conditions may look like coma but are not coma?**
    - **Locked-in state:** Due to a discrete brain stem lesion, usually involving the junction between the upper and lower two thirds of the pons. Given its high location, there is enough pontine reticularis to preserve consciousness, even though all functions below the lesion are lost. Thus, locked-in patients can only control the high cranial nerves (III and VI), which means that they can move their eyes (and keep them open) but not their extremities. They also can see and hear the examiner but sense neither touch nor pain. Whereas in true coma ("sleep-like" state) the eyes arc closed, in the locked-in state they are *open*—in fact, often *tracking* the examiner (when this happens, instruct the patient, "If you hear me, blink your eyes"). A locked-in state is usually fatal, bringing a merciful death in a matter of days. Yet there have been a few unfortunate souls who have lived trapped in their bodies for months and even years. A famous case involved Jean-Dominique Bauby, a 43-year-old French editor, who became locked-in as a result of a massive stroke. He eventually learned to communicate by blinking his eyes in front of an alphabet chart and even wrote a book about his experience (*The Diving Bell and the Butterfly*), published 2 months after his death.
    - **Hysteric coma:** This is a coma-like state that results from major psychopathology. According to medical lore, it may be identified by raising the patient's hand above his or her face and letting it drop. In contrast to real comatose patients, hysterics will not allow the hand to strike them, but will instead allow it to slowly fall down on the side. Similarly, they might resist the examiner's attempt to open their eyelids.
    - **Catatonic coma** (from the Greek *katatonas*, depressed): Patients often have a history of preexisting depression and develop catatonia after a major intercurrent illness. The eyes are open, and patients are awake, but immobile. Catatonia can resolve with benzodiazepines or short-acting barbiturates (like amytal).

55. **What is uncal herniation?**
    It is a rostral-caudal herniation of the uncus of the temporal lobe, with secondary compression of the brain stem. This causes patients to lose function layer by layer: first the thalamus, then the midbrain and pons, and finally the medulla. Neurologically, there is initial ipsilateral cerebral posturing (decortication and then decerebration), followed by lack of response to painful stimuli, ipsilateral pupillary paralysis, and loss of oculocephalic reflex. Finally, medullary compression and respiratory arrest occur (*see* Fig. 20-4).

56. **What are the most common causes of uncal herniation?**
    Intracranial space-occupying processes, such as ischemic or hemorrhagic strokes, brain abscesses, or tumors. Since brain edema peaks at 48–72 hours following an acute injury, patients who suffer a stroke may become stuporous over time, then comatose, and finally exhibit progressive signs of uncal herniation—just prior to respiratory arrest.

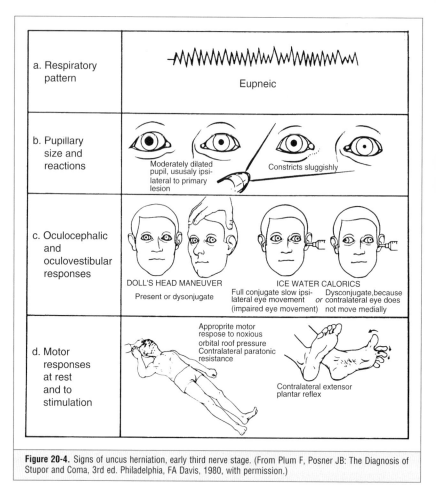

a. Respiratory pattern	Eupneic
b. Pupillary size and reactions	Moderately dilated pupil, ususaly ipsi-lateral to primary lesion / Constricts sluggishly
c. Oculocephalic and oculovestibular responses	DOLL'S HEAD MANEUVER Present or dysonjugate / ICE WATER CALORICS Full conjugate slow ipsi-lateral eye movement (impaired eye movement) or Dysconjugate,because contralateral eye does not move medially
d. Motor responses at rest and to stimulation	Approprite motor respose to noxious orbital roof pressure Contralateral paratonic resistance / Contralateral extensor plantar reflex

Figure 20-4. Signs of uncus herniation, early third nerve stage. (From Plum F, Posner JB: The Diagnosis of Stupor and Coma, 3rd ed. Philadelphia, FA Davis, 1980, with permission.)

57. Is the pattern of breathing helpful in identifying the site of a brain stem lesion?
Yes and no. Some patterns *do* help identify the lesion site. Others are instead less helpful and preferentially triggered by drugs or metabolic states (*see* Chapter 13, questions 23–29).

SELECTED BIBLIOGRAPHY

1. Andrews K: Recovery of patients after four months or more in the persistent vegetative state. BMJ 306:1597–1600, 1993.

2. Bassetti C, Bomio F, Mathis J, Hess CW: Early prognosis in coma after cardiac arrest: A prospective clinical, electrophysiological, and biochemical study of 60 patients. J Neurol Neurosurg Psychiatry 61:610–615, 1996.

3. Bateman DE: Neurological assessment of coma. J Neurol Neurosurg Psychiatry 71(Suppl 1):i3–i7, 2001.

4. Becker LR, Ostrander MP, Barrett J, Kondos GT: Outcome of CPR in a large metropolitan area. Ann Emerg Med 20:355–361, 1991.

5. Booth CM, Boone RH, Tomlinson G, Detsky AS: Is this patient dead, vegetative, or severely neurologically impaired? Assessing outcome for comatose survivors of cardiac arrest. JAMA 291:870–879, 2004.

6. Dougherty JH Jr, Rawlinson DG, Levy DE, Plum F: Hypoxic-ischemic brain injury and the vegetative state: Clinical and neuropathologic correlation. Neurology 31:991–997, 1981.

7. Edgren E, Hedstrand U, Kelsey S, et al: Assessment of neurological prognosis in comatose survivors of cardiac arrest. Lancet 343:1055–1059, 1994.

8. Hawkes CH: Diagnosis of functional neurological disease. Br J Hosp Med 57:373–377, 1997.

9. Krumholz A, Stern BJ, Weiss HD: Outcome from coma after cardiopulmonary resuscitation: Relation to seizures and myoclonus. Neurology 38:401–405, 1988.

10. Plum F, Posner JB: The Diagnosis of Stupor and Coma, 2nd ed. Philadelphia, FA Davis, 1972.

11. Sacco RL, VanGool R, Mohr JP, Hauser WA: Nontraumatic coma: Glasgow Coma Score and coma etiology as predictors of 2-week outcome. Arch Neurol 47:1181–1184, 1990.

12. Snyder BD, Gumnit RJ, Leppik IE, et al: Neurologic prognosis after cardiopulmonary arrest, IV: Brainstem reflexes. Neurology 31:1092–1097, 1981.

13. Snyder BD, Hauser A, Loewenson RB, et al: Neurologic prognosis after cardiopulmonary arrest, III: Seizure activity. Neurology 30:1292–1297, 1980.

14. Snyder BD, Loewenson RB, Gumnit RJ, et al: Neurologic prognosis after cardiopulmonary arrest, II: Level of consciousness. Neurology 30:52–58, 1980.

15. Snyder BD, Ramirez-Lassepas M, Lippert DM: Neurologic status and prognosis after cardiopulmonary arrest. I: A retrospective study. Neurology 27:807–811, 1977.

16. Steen-Hansen JE, Hansen NN, Vaagenes P, Schreiner B: Pupil size and light reactivity during cardiopulmonary resuscitation: A clinical study. Crit Care Med 16:69–70, 1988.

17. Truog RD, Robinson WM: Role of brain death and the dead-donor rule in the ethics of organ transplantation. Crit Care Med 31:2391–2396, 2003.

CHAPTER 21

THE MUSCULOSKELETAL SYSTEM

Salvatore Mangione, MD

"As to my health, thanks be to God, as long as I sit still I am without any pain, but if I do but walk a little I have pains in my legs, but that is, I suppose, caused by former colds and because my legs have carried my body for so long."
                    –Anton Van Leeuwenhoek (1632–1723), in a letter to J. Chamberlayne, 1707

GENERALITIES

This is a difficult area of physical exam, but one necessary in ambulatory medicine and often rewarding. One of 10 patients presenting to a primary care office will do so because of musculoskeletal complaints. Most of these can be diagnosed through a thorough exam, specific maneuvers (Table 21-1), and a proper knowledge of joints' anatomy and physiology.

1. **What are the cardinal signs of joint inflammation?**
    The same as for inflammation in general: *tumor, dolor, calor, rubor*—all originally described by the Roman encyclopedist Celsus in the first century A.D. One hundred years later, the Greek Galen (personal physician to Marcus Aurelius) added *functio laesa* (i.e., the dysfunction of the organ involved). Virchow reiterated this concept in 1858. Note that these signs of inflammation can apply not only to the joint per se but also to the tendons, ligaments, bursa, or muscles *controlling* the joint.

2. **What are *tendons*? What is tendinitis?**
    Tendons attach muscle to bone, thus transmitting muscular force across joints. They are often covered in *tenosynovium*, a sheath of connective tissue and synovium. *Tendinitis* is the general term for disorders of the tendon, including inflammation of the tenosynovium (*tenosynovitis*) and tears of either bone attachment (*enthesis*) or the tendon's body.

3. **How are disorders of tendons differentiated from joint problems?**
    By paying attention to the *pain*. Tendinous disorders cause pain only on (1) passive stretch of the tendon at its extreme range of motion and (2) active joint motion (i.e., requiring muscle contraction). Conversely, *passive joint motion* produces no pain.

4. **What are *ligaments*? What are the findings of a ligament injury?**
    Ligaments attach bone to bone. Injuries present in different ways, based on their degree. Tenderness over the ligament, and pain upon ligament stretching, are the most common manifestations. Abnormal joint motion and gapping with stretching require instead a significant disruption of the ligament. Finally, *ecchymoses* over the site usually indicate severe injury.

5. **What are *bursae*? How do you identify bursitis?**
    Bursae are fluid-filled synovial sacs that facilitate the movement of articulating structures. They can be found over bony prominences and between adjoining muscles with different directions of contraction. Their inflammation (*bursitis*) presents with tenderness and/or fluctuance in the periarticular area, but *not* in the joint per se.

TABLE 21-1. JOINT DISEASES—SPECIFIC MANEUVERS

Joint	Problem	Maneuver
Shoulder	General	Painful arc sign
	Acromioclavicular (AC) arthritis	Cross-body and cross-arm maneuvers
	Bicipital tendinitis	Yergason's and Speed's tests
	Rotator cuff pathology	Gerber's lift-off test, drop arm test, empty can test
	Impingement	Neer (impingement) and Hawkins-Kennedy tests
	Anterior shoulder instability	Apprehension and Jobe's relocation tests
	Inferior shoulder instability	Sulcus sign
	Glenoid labral tears	O'Brien's and anterior slide tests
Elbow	Cubital tunnel syndrome	Elbow flexion test
Wrist	Carpal tunnel syndrome	Tinel's sign, Phalen's sign, flick sign
	Rheumatoid arthritis	Piano key sign
	De Quervain's tendinitis	Finkelstein test (positive)
	Intersection syndrome	Finkelstein test (negative)
Hand	Interosseous tightness versus capsular contraction	Bunnel-Littler test
Hip	General	FABER maneuver
Knee	Patellofemoral syndrome	Patellofemoral grinding test
	Effusion	Bulge sign, patellar ballottement, fluid wave test
	Anterior cruciate ligament	Lachman's test, anterior drawer test, lateral pivot shift test
	Posterior cruciate ligament	Posterior drawer test, tibial sag test
	Meniscal tears	Medial-lateral grind test, McMurray's test, Apley's grind and distraction test
Ankle	Anterior talofibular tear	Anterior drawer test
	Anterior talofibular/calcaneofibular tear	"Talar tilt" test
	Tibiofibular syndesmosis	"Squeeze" test
	Tarsal tunnel syndrome	Submalleolar tap

6. **Describe joint swelling *(tumor)*.**

Swelling is any increase from normal in the joint volume as a result of (1) *bony enlargement* (often due to osteophytes), (2) *synovial proliferation* (i.e., synovitis), or (3) intra-articular *fluid*. Palpation usually allows the examiner to separate these three conditions, insofar as bony enlargement is firm and synovial proliferation is also firm (although palpatory findings may range from indistinct joint margins to sponginess), whereas intra-articular fluid is instead fluctuant.

7. **What is the significance of joint tenderness *(dolor)*?**
   It is another sign of joint pathology. Normal joints can be palpated with significant force without eliciting any pain. Hence, tenderness (ranging from mild discomfort to severe pain) is always abnormal. This also can limit joint *motility*, thus forming the basis of Galen's "functio laesa."

8. **What is the significance of articular warmth and erythema *(calor* and *rubor)*?**
   They indicate pathology, too. Normal joints should be cooler than the surroundings and not red.

9. **What is *crepitus*?**
   It is *palpable crunching* throughout the range of motion of either a joint or a tendon. This may originate from irregularities in the cartilage, bone-on-bone articulation, or tendon per se.

10. **What is the significance of joint *cracking* or *popping*?**
    No significance, unless accompanied by *pain*. Sensation of passive joint *cracking* is common, probably due to tendon or ligament slippage over a bony prominence. This is different from the audible "pop" that can be induced by *actively* "cracking a joint," which is instead due to sudden release of nitrogen gas from the synovial fluid under the negative pressure of joint distraction.

11. **What are the main patterns of joint involvement?**
    - Monoarticular (1 joint)
    - Pauciarticular (2–4 joints)
    - Polyarticular (>4 joints)
    Note that polyarticular involvement can be *symmetric* (with one side of the body mirroring the other [i.e., same joints, or rows of joints, on both extremities]) or *asymmetric* (involving different joints in different extremities).

12. **How do you measure range of motion (ROM)?**
    With a goniometer—always comparing one side to the other.

13. **What are the findings of joint hypermobility?**
    - Ability to oppose the thumb passively to the forearm
    - Hyperextension of fingers
    - >10 degrees of hyperextension of the elbows and knees
    - Ability to touch the palms to the floor with flexion at the waist
    Note that joint hypermobility can be benign or associated with Ehlers-Danlos.

A. THE SHOULDER

14. **What is the anatomy of the shoulder?**
    It results from the confluence of three *bones* (*humerus, clavicle,* and *scapula*) and four *joints* (*glenohumeral, acromioclavicular, sternoclavicular,* and *scapulothoracic*). Everything is kept in place by various static and dynamic stabilizers: the "static" being *labrum,* capsule, and three ligaments (acromioclavicular, coracoclavicular, and coracoacromial); the "dynamic" being the scapular stabilizers (trapezius, rhomboid, and teres major) plus two muscles: rotator cuff and deltoid.

15. **Describe the muscles and tendons of the shoulder.**
    - The **rotator cuff** consists of four muscles: supraspinatus, infraspinatus, teres minor, and subscapularis (mnemonic, *SITS*). Their tendons converge on the humerus, thus allowing for most of the joint movements (abduction of the arm and rotation of the shoulder, both internal and external). They also hold the humeral head in the glenoid cavity, thus stabilizing the joint.
    - The **deltoid** is the largest and strongest muscle, responsible for the later part of abduction and flexion once the arm has been lifted by the supraspinatus. It is visible but rarely injured.

- The **biceps** has two *proximal* heads (hence, the name), which insert into the shoulder: (1) the long head tendon and (2) the short head of the biceps. The *long head tendon* lies in the bicipital groove of the humerus, between the greater and lesser tuberosities and under the *transverse humeral ligament*. This arrangement prevents the humeral head from sliding too far during abduction and external rotation. At the upper end of the groove, the long head of the biceps angles 90 degrees inward, crossing the humeral head and eventually inserting itself into the upper edge of the glenoid labrum and supraglenoid tubercle. The *short head* of the biceps connects instead on the coracoid process. Distally, the two heads of the biceps merge to form the body of the *biceps brachii muscle,* which inserts itself into the radius through its common *distal head*. The biceps is a powerful flexor and supinator of the forearm (i.e., it rotates forearm and hand so that the palm faces upward).

16. **What are the shoulder's movements? How do you test its ROM?**
    The shoulder can actively *abduct, adduct, externally* and *internally rotate, flex,* and *extend*. It has the largest ROM of any joint, since it provides mobility not only to the girdle but also to the hand. ROM is tested as follows:
    - **Abduction:** Ask patients to raise the arms laterally and away from the body: first, to the level of the shoulder and with palms *facing down* (90 degrees of glenohumeral motion), and then above the head and with palms *facing each other* (another 90 degrees, of which 60 degrees are scapulothoracic motion and 30 degrees are combined glenohumeral and scapulothoracic). Normal individuals should complete a smooth 180-degree arc. Average, however, is a little less (150 degrees).
    - **Abduction and external rotation:** Ask patients to place the hand behind the head, trying to reach as far down into the spine as possible. Normal individuals should reach C7. Average range of external rotation with the arm in abduction is 70–90 degrees.
    - **Adduction and internal rotation:** Ask patients to place the hand behind the back, trying to reach with the thumb as far up into the scapula and spine as possible (*Apley's scratch test*). Normal *adduction* is 45 degrees; normal range of *internal* rotation is above T8 (i.e., the lower border of the scapula and the T7 level).
    - **Forward flexion:** Ask patients to trace an arc forward while keeping the elbow straight, ultimately raising the hands above the head as in the "Heil Hitler" sign. Normal range is 0–180 degrees.
    - **Extension:** Ask patients to trace an arc *backwards,* with the elbow straight, arms at the side, and palms facing each other. Normal subjects should place the hand behind their back to 40–50 degrees.
    If active ROM elicits pain, evaluate the same movements through *passive* ROM. To provide your patient with adequate support (and thus ensure maximal relaxation), gently rest one hand on his/her shoulder while using your other hand to move the humerus through the same ROM as previously discussed. Look for pain and crepitus. *Pain* and limitation on active, but not passive, ROM indicate muscular or tendinous problems. *Crepitus* suggests instead degenerative joint disease.

17. **What areas of the shoulder girdle should be palpated?**
    - **Acromioclavicular joint** (top of shoulder, radiating toward the neck)
    - **Long head of the biceps tendon** (anterior shoulder, in the bicipital groove)
    - **Coracoid process** (anterior shoulder)
    - **Rotator cuff** (lateral aspect of shoulder, radiating toward the deltoid insertion)
    - **Glenohumeral joint**
    As a mnemonic for structures to palpate, use *R*eally *G*reat and *B*eautiful *AC*tresses (*R*otator cuff, *G*lenohumeral joint, *B*icipital tendon, *A*cromio*c*lavicular joint).

18. **Can history identify the cause of a shoulder ailment?**
    Yes. For instance, recurrent subluxation in young individuals usually indicates *multidirectional instability*; constant shoulder pain and decreased ROM in diabetics classically reflect *adhesive capsulitis*; pain and weakness in workers whose jobs require recurrent overhead action

suggest *rotator cuff pathology*; shoulder pain after a fall on an outstretched arm argues for *acromioclavicular (AC) lesions*.

19. **What is the general approach to the shoulder exam?**
Always expose *both* shoulders (and *watch* while the patient removes the shirt). Then carry out a systematic exam: inspect, palpate, assess ROM, measure strength, evaluate neurologically, and perform special shoulder tests. Also, examine the cervical spine and upper extremity.
1. **Inspect** for scars, color, edema, deformities, muscle atrophy, asymmetry, and guarding.
2. **Palpate** for pain or point tenderness (the presence of either narrows the exam):
   - Bony and soft-tissue structures, such as coracoid process, acromioclavicular joint, greater tubercle
   - Subdeltoid and subacromial bursae
   - Supraspinatus muscle and its insertion (anteriorly, with arm externally rotated and flexed)
   - Infraspinatus muscle (with arm hyperextended)
   - Major muscle groups and biceps tendon
   - Sternum and sternoclavicular joint
3. **Assess active and passive ROM,** especially in regard to elicited pain and reduced movement.
4. **Determine muscle strength.** This is an essential part of the exam, and comparing side to side may help you locate the area of concern. Always carry it out with *and* without resistance. To isolate the various muscles, use the following maneuvers:
   - *Supraspinatus:* arm forward 90 degrees in the scapular plane and forearm pronated (thumbs *down*, "empty can" maneuver). Drooping of this position suggests full-thickness rotator cuff tears.
   - *Subscapularis* is tested by internal rotation. Arm is rotated internally with the dorsum against the buttock. Actively lift the hand from the buttocks against resistance.
   - *External rotators, teres minor, and infraspinatus* are primarily tested by external rotation (arm on the side and in 90 degrees of abduction).
   - *Deltoids* are primarily assessed by abduction.
   - *Biceps* is primarily tested by elbow flexion and supination.

20. **What is the shoulder pad sign?**
A sign of *bilateral shoulder effusions*. Very typical of amyloidosis.

21. **What are the most common musculoskeletal causes of shoulder pain?**
   - *B*ursitis
   - *I*mpingement (with its complications of *t*endinitis and *r*otator cuff tears)
   - *F*rozen shoulder and *f*racture
   - *D*islocated or unstable shoulder
   - *O*steoarthritis
   Hence the mnemonic, "*B*asically *I* *T*est *R*eligiously *F*or *D*amaged *O*bjects."

22. **What are the origins of *referred* shoulder pain?**
Various. Shoulder (or scapular) pain can originate from many internal organs, including the *myocardium* (angina and infarction), *hepatobiliary system* (cholecystitis), and *diaphragm* (subphrenic abscess). It also may originate from cervical spine and neurovascular entrapment. For example, burning and tingling in the deltoid area may result from irritation of nerve roots, especially C5 and C6. Hence, any patients with shoulder pain who also have C-spine symptoms should have a brief neck exam (with and without resistance) to exclude referred disease.

23. **In addition to history, how else do you identify referred shoulder pain?**
By its being typically nondescript, poorly localized, and not reproducible on shoulder exam.

24. **What is shoulder synovitis? How do you diagnose it?**
Shoulder synovitis is inflammation of the joint. Diagnosis is made by detecting "fullness" just below the clavicle, medial to the deltoid, and clearly visible when compared to the other side. On palpation, there is "bogginess" over the anterior surface of the joint, coinciding with the fullness.

25. **What is acromioclavicular (AC) arthritis? How do you diagnose it?**
It is arthritis of the AC joint, a structure that is minimally mobile but still prone to inflammation. This, in turn, may lead to rotator cuff irritation through the downward protrusion of bony spurs into the tendon. Pain of AC arthritis is initially *vague*, localized to the joint, and possibly radiated to the shoulder, anterior chest, and neck. With time, it may become associated with crepitus and swelling. Pain can be elicited by direct compression of the joint, or by stress maneuvers. These involve (1) cross-body adduction of the arm *behind the back* (which produces pain in the AC joint at the end of adduction); (2) movement of the arm *across* the chest (so that the hand touches the opposite shoulder); and (3) *cross-arm maneuver* (the arm is forward flexed and then adducted across the body). These tests are positive when they elicit pain in the AC joint.

26. **What is AC separation?**
A disruption of the AC joint, usually traumatic. When compared to the unaffected side, the area is swollen, deformed, and painful upon compression or stress maneuvers (such as moving the arm across the chest). In fact, the patient usually keeps the arm very still.

27. **What is bicipital (or biceps) tendinitis?**
Inflammation of the long head tendon. This can be *sudden* (from a direct injury) or gradual. The latter is usually the result of shoulder *overuse* and thus typical of "overhead" athletes: baseball pitchers, racquet players, swimmers, and rowers/kayakers. As the arm is passed into excessive abduction and external rotation, the long head tendon suffers repetitive injury and eventual wear-and-tear. Most commonly, though, the tendon becomes inflamed because of other shoulder problems, such as rotator cuff disease, impingement, instability, or labral tears.

28. **What are the symptoms/findings of bicipital tendinitis?**
Achy anterior shoulder pain, worsened by overhead activity, lifting of heavy objects, and elevated pushing/pulling. Rest is usually beneficial, whereas flexion of the elbow against resistance is detrimental. Pain is vague, though at times it may become localized to the anterior humerus. On exam, there is point tenderness over the bicipital groove, which is the area where the long tendon is anatomically exposed. This lies 3 inches below the anterior acromion and may be best localized by holding the arm in 10 degrees of external rotation. Pain also can be elicited by passive abduction of the arm in a *painful arc maneuver* (*see* question 41), which is typical of impingement syndrome, although at times it also may be positive in patients with isolated biceps tendinitis.

29. **Which specific maneuvers can reproduce the pain of bicipital tendinitis?**
Maneuvers that resist the normal function of the biceps—supination and flexion of the forearm:
- **Yergason's test:** The hand is pronated, the elbow flexed to 90 degrees, and the shoulder in adduction (i.e., arm against the body). With the patient attempting *supination of the forearm* (i.e., palm up), you resist with one hand while with the other you press on the bicipital tendon. The test is positive when it elicits pain and tenderness over the bicipital groove.
- **Speed's test:** Dr. Speed actually never described this maneuver. It was first reported by Crenshaw and Kilgore in 1966, quoting "personal communication" as their source. It is performed by having the patient attempt to flex the affected arm against resistance, after positioning it with elbow extended and forearm in supination (i.e., palm up). Once again, you resist with one hand while you press with the other on the bicipital tendon. The test is positive when it elicits pain over the bicipital groove. As validated by arthroscopy, it has a 14% specificity, 90% sensitivity, 23% positive predictive value, and 83% negative predictive value.

30. **What is the "Popeye" sign?**

    A sign of rupture of the long head of the biceps tendon. The patient reports a sudden, painful, and audible snap, associated with (1) retraction of the biceps belly toward the elbow and (2) bulging over the anterior upper arm—as in the cartoon character "Popeye." In the elderly, this may occasionally result from trauma. Otherwise, it is usually due to long-standing tendinitis. Hence, it is preceded by a long history of shoulder pain, quickly resolving with a painful snap.

31. **What is *shoulder impingement*?**

    A concept first introduced by Neer in 1972 to describe mechanical impingement of the rotator cuff tendon. This runs above the humeral head and glenoid, and below the acromial process, coracoacromial ligament, and acromioclavicular joint. Recurrent friction causes bursitis, tendinitis, and ultimately, tendon degeneration and tearing.

32. **What is the cause of shoulder impingement?**

    Mechanical wear and tear. True tear of the cuff is actually a problem of older subjects, whereas rotator cuff *disease* and impingement tend to affect primarily laborers (whose job requires repetitive and protracted overhead activity) or young athletes (whose sport also involves repetitive overhead motions, such as throwing, swimming, volleyball, and tennis and other racquet-playing activities). Raising the arm over the shoulder forces the humerus against the edge of the acromion. Usually, there is enough room between the acromion and rotator cuff to allow the tendons to slide easily underneath the bone while the arm is being elevated. Recurrent arm-raising, however, eventually creates *impingement* (i.e., friction on the subacromial bursa and the distal part of the tendon). With time, this causes irritation and swelling of the bursa (*bursitis*), further narrowing the space between the acromion and rotator cuff. As a result, impingement on the tendon becomes more severe, which is risky since its blood supply is limited. Hence, the resulting tendinitis and, ultimately, the degenerative damage. *Bony spurs* of the AC joint (which sits directly above bursa and rotator cuff tendons) may further narrow the subacromial space, and so can abnormal acromial morphology (such as a hooked acromion).

33. **How do you diagnose rotator cuff tendinitis?**

    By carefully examining the shoulder and by knowing the *function* of the four rotator cuff muscles (i.e., abduction, external rotation, and internal rotation).

    - The **supraspinatus** is the most important and most commonly damaged of the four. It links the top of the scapula to the humerus, inserting into its greater tuberosity. It is partially responsible for arm abduction (the initial 15–30 degrees are actually produced by the deltoid, the next 60 degrees by the supraspinatus, and the final 90 degrees by the deltoid again). Hence, inflammation of the supraspinatus tendon leads to pain at 30–90 degrees of abduction, as the humerus impinges the tendon against the acromion. It can be easily tested through the *empty can test*.
    - The **infraspinatus** produces external rotation of the humerus, a function assisted by the **teres minor**. The two also cooperate to maintain glenohumeral stability. To test *external rotators* (infraspinatus and teres minor): (1) have the patient abduct both shoulders to 20–30 degrees, while keeping the elbows flexed at 90 degrees; (2) instruct the patient to push the arms outward (externally rotate) against resistance. *External* rotation elicits pain in tendinitis and weakness in tears.
    - The **subscapularis** is the only of the four rotator muscles to originate from the anterior surface of the scapula (the others arise instead in the back). It connects the scapula to the humerus, serving as *humeral head depressor* and, in certain shoulder positions (adduction), as *internal rotator*. Function is evaluated through the "Gerber's lift-off test": (1) have patients place the hand behind the back, with palm facing out, and (2) instruct them to lift the hand away from the back and against resistance. *Internal* rotation elicits pain in tendinitis and weakness in tears.

    Note that given the anatomic closeness of the long head tendon of the biceps (which passes down the bicipital groove in a fibrous sheath between the subscapularis and supraspinatus tendons), patients with rotator cuff disease also may have *biceps tendinitis* (*see* questions 27 and 28).

34. What is the "drop arm" test?

A good way to identify rotator cuff pathology. Ask patient to raise the extended arms to a complete overhead abduction. Those with rotator cuff *tear* will be unable to smoothly bring the arms down to the sides from their abducted position. In fact, they may even display a cogwheel effect.

35. What are the symptoms of shoulder impingement?

The initial one is *pain*—aching and gradual (*acute* and *tearing* suggest instead a rotator cuff *tear*), centered around the anterior-superior-lateral aspect of the shoulder, and occasionally referred to the deltoid region. Pain interferes with sleep (especially when the patient rolls onto the affected shoulder) and is exacerbated by lateral or anterior raising of the arm and by forward flexion and internal rotation of the humerus (as if trying to reach into a back pocket). Pain worsens with time, and the joint may become stiff, causing "catching" sensations upon lowering of the arm. Weakness and inability to raise the arm suggest instead a rotator cuff tear.

36. How do you examine for shoulder impingement?

(1) *By palpating the subacromial space* (which elicits pain in patients with bursitis/tendinitis), and (2) *by assessing the shoulder girdle muscles*, especially during external/internal rotation and abduction. Supraspinatus problems can be identified by *the empty can test*, also described by Jobe, and so named because the patient's position is similar to that assumed when emptying a can. To carry this out, have the patients (1) abduct the shoulder to 90 degrees and forward flex it at 30 degrees and (2) fully rotate the upper extremity (so that the thumbs are pointing toward the floor). While they do so, instruct them to forward flex the shoulder while you are applying resistance from behind. Patients with supraspinatus tendinitis or partial injury to the tendon will experience *pain*. Those with a partial- or full-thickness tear will be instead unable to achieve any forward flexion.

37. Are there any special maneuvers that can be used for testing impingement?

The *Neer (impingement) test* and the *Hawkins-Kennedy test*. Both cause the supraspinatus tendons to rub against the acromion, thus eliciting pain in cases of impingement. Still, beware that it is usually very difficult to clinically identify the location of the problem, that is, to separate bursitis from tendinitis or even partial rotator cuff tears (which is why God created magnetic resonance imaging [MRI]). One possible exception is the *diagnostic subacromial bursa injection*: local anesthetic and steroids injected into the bursa will relieve bursitis but *not* tendinitis nor partial rotator cuff tear.

38. How do you perform the *Neer* (impingement) test?

The patient's forearm is internally rotated, so that the thumb points downward. While standing behind the patient, place one hand on the patient's scapula and with the other hand grasp the forearm and forward flex it, eventually positioning the patient's hand over the head. Forced elevation and internal rotation of the arm cause the greater tuberosity of the humerus to compress the subacromial bursa. This, in turn, squeezes the supraspinatus tendon against the acromion, causing pain in cases of impingement. The test also can differentiate AC arthritis from subacromial bursitis (Fig. 21-1).

39. How do you perform the *Hawkins-Kennedy* test?

Hold up the patient's arm to 90 degrees of forward flexion (i.e., to the shoulder level) and 90 degrees of elbow flexion. Then, forcefully internally rotate the arm to 90 degrees (i.e., thumb pointed down). This causes the greater tuberosity of the humerus to compress the subacromial bursa, and the supraspinatus tendon to impinge against the coracoacromial ligament—thus eliciting pain ("impingement sign"). Hawkins is more sensitive than Neer in detecting subtle degrees of impingement.

40. How else can one elicit pain in supraspinatus tendinitis?

Have the patient hold the elbow against the side and force it into external rotation against resistance.

41. What is the "painful arc" sign?

A *painful arc of motion,* a useful test for evaluating a painful shoulder. Arms are down at the patient's side, and then abducted to 180 degrees above the head (rotating hands as necessary to complete the arc). The maneuver should be smooth and painless. *Impingement disease* (such as supraspinatus tendinitis or partial rotator cuff tear) will produce pain with elevation of the arm above the shoulder level (i.e., in an arc between 40 and 120 degrees). There will be no pain before 40 degrees and no pain after 120 degrees. *Glenohumeral arthritis* instead produces pain *throughout* the arc.

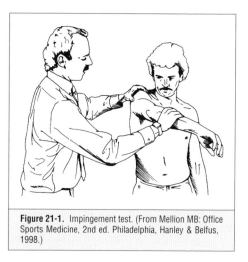

Figure 21-1. Impingement test. (From Mellion MB: Office Sports Medicine, 2nd ed. Philadelphia, Hanley & Belfus, 1998.)

42. What are rotator cuff injuries?

They are a spectrum of diseases (ranging from acute reversible tendinitis to massive tears of the supraspinatus, infraspinatus, and subscapularis) that are common causes of shoulder pain. Although seen in all ages, they usually present after the fourth decade, with peak at 55–85.

43. What are the causes of rotator cuff tear?

Most are the end-result of chronic tendineal degeneration, usually from repetitive friction against the overlying *coracoacromial arch*. This may be due to recurrent overhand motions (as in baseball pitching), but also to more lowly and routine daily activities, such as cleaning windows, washing and waxing cars, or painting. Once the tendons are weakened, excessive force will tear them. This may occur when trying to catch a heavy falling object, trying to lift a big load with the arm extended, or simply falling directly onto the shoulder.

44. What are the *symptoms* of rotator cuff tear?

The most common is *pain,* anterolateral and superior, usually referred to the deltoid insertion, and worsened by holding the arm in an overhead or forward flexed position. The next most common is *weakness* and *decreased range of motion.* In cases of complete tear, there also is inability to raise the arm. Finally, there may be articular clicking, catching, or crepitus.

45. What are the *findings* of a complete rotator cuff tear?

The patient cannot *actively* abduct the arm from 0 degrees. If the arm is *passively* abducted above 90 degrees, there will be inability to hold it up and further abduct to 180 degrees. If the arm is passively lowered below 90 degrees, it will fall to the side (*drop arm test*). Finally, with the elbow against the side, there will be inability to externally rotate the arm.

46. What is glenohumeral (shoulder) dislocation?

A problem as old as mankind (Egyptian tomb murals from 3000 B.C. depict reduction techniques, while Hippocrates fully described them) because the shoulder, being the most mobile joint in the body, is also the one more likely to dislocate. *Anterior* dislocations are the most frequent (95%), followed by posterior (4%) and inferior (0.5%).

47. **What are the causes of dislocation?**
The most common is a traumatic force that overcomes the stability of the joint. *Anterior shoulder dislocations* usually result from abduction, extension, and external rotation (typical, for example, of the preparation for a volleyball spike). Falls on an outstretched hand also are common, especially in older subjects, and so are seizures. Whatever the cause, the resulting blow overcomes the resistance provided by the glenohumeral capsule, the labrum, and the rotator cuff muscles, forcing the humeral head out of the glenohumeral joint and rupturing or detaching the anterior capsule. The *labrum* itself also may tear.

48. **What is the presentation of dislocation?**
The typical is posttraumatic shoulder pain and decreased range of motion. In an *anterior* dislocation, the arm is held in slight abduction and external rotation, the shoulder is "squared off" with loss of deltoid contour, and the humeral head is anteriorly palpable (just beneath the clavicle, in the subcoracoid region). There also will be inability to touch the opposite shoulder, plus resistance to abduction and internal rotation. Given the risk of impingement of the neurovascular bundle, one should always check (and compare) radial pulses and also evaluate the axillary nerve. This can be done by testing pinprick sensation in the "regimental badge" area of the deltoid and through palpable contraction of the same muscle during attempted abduction.

49. **How do you test for glenohumeral instability?**
It depends on the type of instability: anterior versus inferior.

50. **How do you test for *anterior* shoulder instability?**
Through the *apprehension* and *Jobe's relocation tests*. Start with "apprehension" (Fig. 21-2). To perform it, ask patients to lie supine, with the affected shoulder just off the examining table. Grasp the elbow with one hand, and gently bring the arm to 90-degree *abduction* and 90-degree *external rotation*. Then push with your other hand on the posterior aspect of the humeral head, from back to front. Anterior shoulder instability will give a feeling that the arm is about to pop out of the joint. At the same time, patients will experience pain, *apprehension*, and guarding. In the original series of Rowe and Zarins, all 60 cases of anterior shoulder instability had a positive apprehension test. If the patient experiences pain and/or apprehension, move on to the second part of the maneuver: the *Jobe's relocation test*. This is performed in the same position, but this time by pushing on the *anterior* aspect of the humeral head, from front to back, as if relocating a glenohumeral joint that had been partially dislocated by the apprehension test. Patients with primary impingement will have no change in pain, whereas those with anterior instability

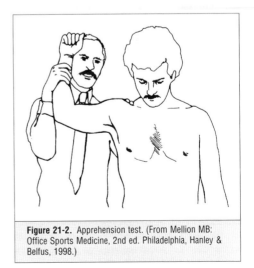

Figure 21-2. Apprehension test. (From Mellion MB: Office Sports Medicine, 2nd ed. Philadelphia, Hanley & Belfus, 1998.)

(subluxation) and secondary impingement will have relief of pain and/or apprehension. When relying primarily on relief of apprehension, the relocation test has sensitivity for anterior instability of 68%; specificity, 100%; positive predictive value, 100%; negative predictive value, 78%; and accuracy, 85%.

51. **How do you test for *inferior* shoulder instability?**
Through the *sulcus sign*. Allow the arms to rest on the patient's side, then pull them down. Compare shoulders. Any *asymmetric* anterior dimpling suggests inferior shoulder instability.

52. **How do you diagnose *multidirectional* instability?**
By the presence of *both* inferior instability (positive sulcus sign) *and* anterior instability (positive apprehension and Jobe's relocation tests).

53. **How do you test for glenoid labral tears?**
Through the O'Brien and anterior slide tests.

54. **How do you perform the *O'Brien test*?**
The patient stands, with arm flexed to 90 degrees and elbow in full extension. Then (s)he adducts the arm to 10–15 degrees medial to the sagittal plane of the body, and internally rotates it, so that the thumb points *down*. The examiner stands behind the patient applying a downward force to the arm. With the arm in the same position, patient is then asked to supinate the palm (thumb pointing *up*), and the maneuver is repeated (i.e., the examiner again applies a downward force to the arm). The test is positive if it elicits pain with the thumb pointed *down* and relieves it with the thumb pointing *up*.

55. **How do you perform the *anterior slide test*?**
The patient is standing or sitting, with hands on hips, and thumbs pointing posteriorly. The examiner stands behind the patient and places one hand on the elbow and the other on the posterior aspect of the top of the shoulder, with the index finger extending over the anterior aspect of the acromion at the glenohumeral joint. Then the examiner applies a force to the elbow and upper arm that is directed forward and slightly superiorly. The patient is asked to push back against this force. The test is positive if it elicits pain and/or pops and clicks in the shoulder. It has sensitivity of 78.4% and specificity of 91.5%. Hence, it is useful but not sufficient.

56. **What is *adhesive capsulitis*?**
A painful shoulder condition often referred to as *frozen shoulder*. This may follow an injury, or more commonly a wrist fracture that caused the arm to remain immobilized for several weeks, possibly triggering an autoimmune process, and eventually leading to severe loss of motion.

57. **What is the mechanism of adhesive capsulitis?**
Inflammation, which "glues" the capsule and surrounding structures into a frozen shoulder.

58. **What are the symptoms of adhesive capsulitis?**
The most common is shoulder pain, causing a reduced range of motion, both on active *and* passive movements. Pain and tightness may occur at night and often interfere with activities of daily living, like getting dressed, combing hair, or reaching across a table.

59. **How is the diagnosis made?**
By history and physical exam. A crucial finding that helps differentiate a frozen shoulder from a rotator cuff tear is the limitation of ROM both on active *and* passive movements. Conversely, a rotator cuff tear limits *active*, but not passive movements.

B. THE ELBOW

60. What are the elbow's movements? Range of motion?
The elbow flexes to 150 degrees (allowing us to touch the shoulder with the thumb). It also extends to 0 degrees. Finally, it provides motion to the *forearm*, making it pronate and supinate to 80 degrees.

61. Is the elbow varus or valgus?
Valgus. With the elbow fully extended, the normal angle is indeed in *valgus* (*cubitus valgus*). Fractures, however (especially in children), may cause a *varus* (gunstock) deformity.

62. What do valgus and varus mean?
This is a very confusing terminology. In orthopedics, *valgus* indicates an *outward* angulation of the "distal segment" of a bone or joint, so that it is "twisted away" (i.e., away from the body, or midline of the limb). Conversely, *varus* indicates its *inward* angulation (so that it is now twisted *toward* the body, or midline of the limb). Note that both terms always refer to the direction in which the *distal segment of the joint* (or bone) is pointing. In fact, when referred to as a *bone*, the bone itself is considered to be the distal segment of the joint. Hence, a varus or valgus deformity of the forearm refers to the arm/forearm joint (the elbow) and *not* to the wrist. Having said that, a normal elbow is in valgus, because with the joint fully extended (and the palms facing upward) the distal segment of the forearm will point *away from the body* (or midline of the limb). If you think this is confusing, wait until you see how it applies to the knee exam (*see* question 213).

63. How do you detect swelling of the elbow?
It depends. Mild swelling can be appreciated as a filling in of the groove between the olecranon and lateral epicondyle. Conversely, moderate to severe swelling causes loss of bony margins on palpation.

64. What is the most common finding of an abnormal elbow?
A flexion contracture. This is the first abnormality to develop and one that often becomes permanent. A common sequela of fracture, *elbow flexion contracture* also may occur in subjects who have to keep their elbow flexed for long periods, like long-distance truck drivers.

65. What is "tennis elbow" (*lateral* epicondylitis)?
The most common elbow injury: 10 times more frequent than *medial* epicondylitis (i.e., "golfer's elbow"), and occurring in 50% of tennis players. The mechanism is overuse wear-and-tear of the proximal attachment of the *extensor/supinator* muscles of the forearm, typically affecting a 30- to 50-year-old recreational athlete. It usually responds to rest and conservative measures.

66. Other than tennis, does anything else cause tennis elbow?
Any activity that requires repetitive contraction of the wrist extensors. This includes hammering nails, picking up heavy buckets, or pruning shrubs. The repeated hyperextension required by these movements eventually results in enthesitis of the wrist *extensors* (i.e., inflammation of the enthesis, that is, the site of tendinous attachment to the bone—actually a more degenerative than inflammatory process. Hence an *enthesopathy*). With time, this leads to tendineal microtears, subsequent fibrosis, and, ultimately, tissue failure.

67. What is the presentation of tennis elbow?
The classic one is *lateral elbow pain*, aching, gradual, at times nocturnal, but typically worsened by hyperextension of the wrist. Pain may eventually spread down the forearm, possibly reaching the back of the middle and ring fingers. Forearm muscles also may feel tight and sore. Activities of daily living (like picking up a cup of coffee or a gallon of milk) often precipitate it. Diagnosis is

made by demonstrating point tenderness over the lateral epicondyle, elicited by grasping and worsened by forced hyperextension of the wrist or by supination against resistance. Flexion or pronation is instead normal (*see* Golfer's Elbow). Range of motion is normal too, although there may be a weakened grip on the affected side. A helpful maneuver is the *chair raise* test, where the patient stands behind a chair and attempts to raise it by placing the hands on top of the chair back, and then lifting. This typically elicits pain over the lateral elbow.

68. What is "golfer's elbow" (*medial* epicondylitis)?
An overuse injury to the proximal attachment of the *flexor/pronator* muscles of the forcarm, commonly seen in the dominant elbow of a golfer. Its mechanism is similar to that of *lateral* epicondylitis, but less common since wrist flexors are stronger and less likely overstressed (*see* Fig. 21-3).

69. What is the cause of golfer's elbow?
Overuse tendinopathy (i.e., the same cause of its more lateral counterpart, "tennis elbow"). This results not only from recurrent swinging of a golf club, but also from any racquet sport that requires repeated *flexion* at the wrist and pronation. Hence, *medial epicondylitis* can affect tennis players who hit their forehand with heavy topspin (or serve poorly), bowlers, archers, weight lifters, various throwers, lumberjacks (who chop wood with axes or run chain saws), and any individual who frequently uses screwdrivers or hammers. Repetitive stress at the musculotendinous junction (and at its insertion over the medial epicondyle) eventually leads to acute tendinitis or chronic *tendinosis,* tendineal microtears, fibrosis, and tissue failure. One half of golfer's elbows also develop ulnar compressive neuropathy, in or around the medial epicondylar groove.

70. What is the presentation of golfer's elbow?
Very similar to that of *cubital tunnel syndrome*. Athletes usually complain of aching pain over the medial epicondyle, triggered by the acceleration phase of throwing. Nonathletes report discomfort even while shaking someone's hand. With more advanced disease, there also may be grip weakness. Diagnosis is made by demonstrating point tenderness over the medial epicondyle, worsened by forced flexion of the wrist against resistance. There also may be pain with resisted forearm pronation, and in more protracted cases, with resisted elbow flexion. Yet, ROM of the elbow and wrist is usually normal. Tinel's sign should be tested over the ulnar nerve, just to rule out ulnar neuropathy. In fact, ulnar symptoms can occur in 25–50% of patients, with occasional/constant numbness and/or tingling radiating down into fourth and fifth fingers.

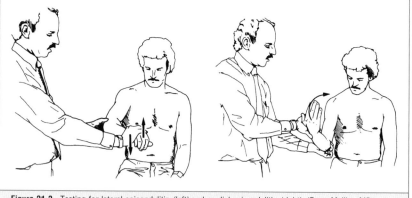

Figure 21-3. Testing for lateral epicondylitis *(left)* and medial epicondylitis *(right)*. (From Mellion MB: Office Sports Medicine, 2nd ed. Philadelphia, Hanley & Belfus, 1998.)

71. **How frequent is ulnar nerve entrapment at the elbow?**
Very frequent. In fact, most ulnar nerve entrapments *do* indeed occur at the elbow (i.e., in the cubital tunnel, which is located on the medial side of it—hence, the term, *cubital tunnel syndrome*). This is the second most common compressive neuropathy after carpal tunnel syndrome, affecting men 3–8 times more often than women.

72. **What are the causes of *cubital tunnel syndrome*?**
Various. Swelling of the elbow joint, bony spurs, constricting fascial bands, or trauma to the ulnar notch have all been implicated. Work also may be a factor, especially when causing repetitive elbow flexion and extension (such as pulling levers, reaching out, or lifting) or protracted direct pressure on the joint (like leaning on the elbow while sitting at a desk, or during a long drive). The ulnar nerve also can be damaged from a direct blow to the cubital tunnel. Still, a clear-cut relationship with occupational activities is not well defined.

73. **What is the presentation of cubital tunnel syndrome?**
Similar to that of *medial epicondylitis* (golfer's elbow), ranging from a vague discomfort at the elbow to frank hypersensitivity, intermittent at first and more constant as time goes by. Exam reveals pain and tenderness in the cubital tunnel, which may radiate proximally or distally. There also may be *sensory changes* in the distribution of the nerve, involving the ulnar side of the forearm and extending into the fourth and fifth fingers. *Paresthesias* also are common, especially after protracted resting upon, or flexion of, the elbow (as when sleeping or talking on the phone). *Tinel's sign* can occur over the medial epicondylar groove, but only in 25% of asymptomatic patients. In later stages, there may be weakness of grip and pinch, plus loss of fine dexterity. Intrinsic muscle atrophy and clawing of the fifth finger (Wartenberg sign) are less common.

74. **How do you diagnose cubital tunnel syndrome?**
Through the *elbow flexion test*. This is carried out by asking the patient to flex the elbow past 90 degrees, supinate the forearm, and extend the wrist. The maneuver is positive if it reproduces discomfort or paresthesia within 60 seconds. Addition of shoulder abduction may further enhance its yield. Differential diagnosis of cubital tunnel syndrome includes other causes of paresthesias and weakness along the C8–T1 distribution, such as cervical disk disease/arthritis, thoracic outlet syndrome, or ulnar nerve impingement at the Guyon canal.

75. **What is olecranon bursitis?**
A common inflammation of the bursa overlying the olecranon. This is located over the posterior tip of the elbow, between the skin and proximal aspect of the ulna.

76. **How does it present?**
Suddenly if due to infection or acute trauma, *gradually* if due to chronic irritation. The hallmark is posterior elbow swelling, quite demarcated, and presenting as a goose egg over the olecranon. Swelling is fluctuant, often recurrent, and usually painless. Yet, it may be associated with point tenderness over the olecranon, worsened by full flexion or pressure, as when the patient leans on the elbow or rubs it against the table while writing. The area may be warm and red, especially with infection (fever). ROM is usually normal, even though pain at the posterior elbow may limit some functional activities (like writing) and prevent the end-range of elbow flexion.

77. **What are the causes of olecranon bursitis?**
Many. Given its superficial location, the most common is acute *trauma* (like falling onto a hard floor) or repetitive *microtrauma* (recurrent rubbing of the olecranon against a desktop during writing). Less common reasons include *infection* (via skin abrasion or hematogenous seeding—septic bursitis), inflammation as part of a *systemic inflammatory* process (rheumatoid arthritis [RA]), and crystal deposition (gout, pseudogout). The last two may present with focal inflammation at other sites.

78. **Which finding differentiates infection from other causes of olecranon bursitis?**
The definitive one, of course, is a positive gram stain or culture of the fluid aspirated from the bursa. Still, if erythema extends *past* the margins of the bursa, infection is the most likely cause.

79. **How do you tell rheumatoid nodules from gouty tophi?**
By palpation: rheumatoid nodules are *rubbery* (whereas tophi are firm) and either subcutaneous, subperiosteal, or intrabursal (whereas tophi are instead subcutaneous or intrabursal, but never subperiosteal). Still, biopsy or aspiration for monosodium urate crystals remains the test of choice. Note that both rheumatoid nodules *and* gouty tophi are quite common at the extensor surface of the elbow, as well as in other sites of chronic and repetitive pressure. Yet, only tophi may occasionally drain to the surface, so that urate can be recovered from an ulcer overlying the nodule.

C. THE WRIST

80. **What is the carpal tunnel?**
A wrist channel, whose floor is formed by the carpal bones and the ceiling by the *transverse carpal ligament*. Through this tunnel flows the *median nerve,* bringing sensory fibers to the palmar surface of the first three fingers and to one half of the fourth finger. It also provides a *motor* branch to the *thenar muscles,* responsible for thumb opposition. Through the tunnel also pass the flexor tendons, providing the hand and fingers with movements that are crucial for grasping. In the tunnel, the median nerve rests on top of the tendons, just below the transverse carpal ligament.

81. **What is *carpal tunnel syndrome* (CTS)?**
An important cause of painful impairment of the hand. It is due to compression of the median nerve at the wrist, resulting in a constellation of typical signs and symptoms. It affects women three times more commonly than men, usually during the third to fifth decades.

82. **What is the cause of CTS?**
Any condition that narrows the carpal tunnel. A major one is *trauma,* especially repetitive microtrauma (such as the one of typing, or operating a jackhammer). Other causes simply swell the tissues delimiting the tunnel, through either inflammation or fluid retention. Among these are rheumatoid arthritis, pregnancy, hypothyroidism, and diabetes (the latter also may cause a direct neuropathy of the median nerve). Smoking, obesity, and caffeine often play a predisposing role.

83. **What are the symptoms of CTS?**
The earliest is *paresthesia* in the median nerve distribution: thumb, forefinger, middle finger, and one half of the ring finger, but typically *not* the small finger. The "asleep" sensation is then followed by *pain*, which may occur during gripping activities, such as sweeping, hammering, or driving. Eventually, pain occurs at rest, and even awakens the patient at night. Hand-shaking (flick sign) can often provide relief. With time, pain and numbness may spread up the arm, into the shoulder, and even to the side of the neck. Eventually, the patient develops *weakness* (and ultimately *atrophy*) of the thenar muscles, making thumb opposition increasingly difficult. This interferes with grasping, including driving, holding a phone, or picking up a newspaper.

84. **What is the physical exam of CTS?**
Once the appropriate history is obtained, two maneuvers are typically carried out: *Tinel's sign* and *Phalen's sign* (first described by the American orthopedist George S. Phalen, 1911–1998) (*see* Fig. 21-4).

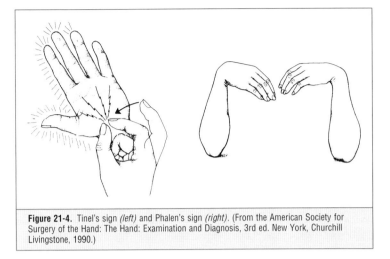

Figure 21-4. Tinel's sign *(left)* and Phalen's sign *(right)*. (From the American Society for Surgery of the Hand: The Hand: Examination and Diagnosis, 3rd ed. New York, Churchill Livingstone, 1990.)

85. How do you elicit *Tinel's sign*?

By asking the patient to hyperextend the wrist while you tap over the median nerve (i.e., over the carpal tunnel) with either a forefinger or the reflex hammer. The test is positive when it reproduces the symptoms (i.e., a tingling sensation along the distribution of the median nerve).

86. How do you elicit *Phalen's sign*?

By having the patient juxtapose the dorsal surfaces of the hands while holding the wrists in hyperflexion for 60 seconds (or less in case symptoms were to occur sooner). This will increase the intratunnel pressure, thus reproducing the tingling. Note that in Phalen's original definition of CTS, diagnosis was established by one or more of three bedside findings: (1) sensory changes of the hand restricted to the median nerve distribution, (2) a positive Tinel's, and (3) a positive Phalen's. Yet, many traditional findings, including *Phalen's, Tinel's,* and the *flick sign* have low sensitivity and limited or no value. Hence, electrodiagnosis has become so crucial that some third-party payers would now not even compensate claims without it. Nerve conduction studies have good sensitivity and superb specificity (49–84% and 95–99%, respectively).

87. How do you elicit the *flick sign*?

By asking patients what they do with their hands and wrists when symptoms occur. The response is positive when the patient demonstrates a flicking motion of hands and wrists—as if shaking down a thermometer. Although initially promising, the flick test also has shown limited utility.

88. How valuable is physical exam in confirming the diagnosis?

Not too valuable. Since the classic signs only occur in one half of the cases, other maneuvers have been suggested, such as: (1) assessing sensory loss in the distribution of the median nerve; (2) looking for atrophy of the *thenar eminence* (which, however, occurs only in long-standing and neglected cases, plus also may result from cervical radiculopathies and polyneuropathies); and (3) testing the strength of the *abductor pollicis brevis* muscle. Findings most helpful in predicting the electrodiagnosis of CTS (which is the gold standard) are: (1) classic or probable Katz hand diagram results (i.e., tingling that primarily involves the thumb and index and long fingers as opposed to the little finger); (2) hypalgesia in the median nerve territory; and (3) thumb abduction weakness.

89. **Who was Tinel?**

    Jules Tinel (1879–1952) was another product of the superb French medicine of the turn of the century. The son of a medical family, Tinel studied with Troisier, Dejerine, Landouzy, and Netter. Convinced by Dejerine to go into neurology, he eventually became chair at the Salpêtrière in Paris. After serving in World War I, he focused on psychosomatic medicine. During WWII, he took a very active role in the French resistance, for which he was imprisoned and even lost his son, Jacques, killed by the Nazis in the death camp of Dora in Neuhausen. After the war, he worked in the Boucicaut Hospital, until his death of heart failure in 1952.

90. **What is the piano key sign?**

    A sign of *rheumatoid arthritis of the wrist*, typically due to a *synovitis* that is stretching ulnar-carpal ligaments and causing dorsal dislocation of the distal prominence of the ulnar head (caput ulnae syndrome). Because of its dorsal subluxation, the ulnar styloid can be pressed volarly on examination, giving the feel of a piano key being pressed down—hence, the name. To elicit it, first stabilize the distal radius with one hand, then grasp the head of the ulna between the thumb and index finger of your other hand. Evaluate freedom of motion, and look for pain or crepitus. Pressing the ulnar head will elicit the piano key sign.

91. **What is a common cause of pain on the *radial* side of the wrist?**

    De Quervain's tendinitis. This is a hand-and-wrist disorder caused by entrapment tenosynovitis of the two thumb muscles' tendons (*abductor pollicis longus* and *extensor pollicis brevis*) as they travel through a retinaculum tunnel near the end of the radius. Thickening of the tendons from either acute or repetitive trauma restrains their gliding through the tendon sheath, thus causing the problem. This sort of friction tendinitis is very frequent in day care workers and new mothers, as a result of awkward hand positions while caring for infants (such as repetitive lifting of babies as they grow heavier). Patients present with aching pain on the thumb side of the wrist and at the base of the thumb, usually noticed when forming a fist, grasping, gripping, or turning the wrist. There also may be swelling over the thumb side of the wrist, point tenderness, and at times crepitation and "triggering" (i.e., catching or snapping when moving the thumb—hence, the term "snapping thumb syndrome"). Because of pain and swelling, there also may be difficulties in moving the wrist and thumb, including opposition. Thus the inability to "pinch." Finally, extrinsic compression of radial branches by the swollen tendon sheath may cause paresthesias on the back of the thumb and index finger. Pain can be elicited by the *Finkelstein test*.

92. **How do you diagnose de Quervain's tendinitis?**

    Through the Finkelstein test, first described by the American surgeon Harry Finkelstein (1865–1939). This is performed by placing the thumb into the palm, closing the fingers around it, and moving the hand in ulnar deviation. Stretching of the involved tendon(s) will reproduce the pain.

93. **Who was de Quervain?**

    Fritz de Quervain (1868–1940) was a Huguenot Swiss, who studied in Bern, trained with Kocher and Langhans, and later on became chair of surgery, dean, and rector at the University of Bern. He retired on the eve of WWII and eventually died of acute pancreatitis in 1940. A prolific writer with a keen interest in thyroid diseases, de Quervain was responsible for introducing iodized table salt in the treatment of goiter, a common problem in mountainous Switzerland. He also was a strong proponent of a general approach to the patient rather than an artificial division into specialties. Finally, he was one of the first clinicians to understand that many cases of postoperative pneumonia were in reality pulmonary infarcts. He reported his tendinitis in 1895, as case series of five patients with tender and thickened first dorsal compartments at the wrist.

94. **What is the "intersection" syndrome?**

A painful wrist condition that can affect individuals who do repeated wrist actions. Patients present with pain on top of their forearm, about 3 inches proximally to the wrist. This also is the site where the two thumb muscles cross over (i.e., *intersect*) the two wrist tendons of the *extensor carpi radialis longus* and *extensor carpi radialis brevis*, both responsible for extending the wrist. Friction tenosynovitis of the wrist tendons eventually interferes with their smooth gliding in the tendon sheath, causing swelling and redness at the intersection point and a pain that can spread either up along the edge of the forearm or down into the thumb. Crepitus may be present.

95. **How do you differentiate de Quervain's tendinitis from an intersection syndrome?**

Both involve inflammation of the wrist tendons, but the pain has different location: in *intersection syndrome,* it is over the *wrist,* at the intersection point , whereas in de Quervain's tenosynovitis is instead over the hand (i.e., in the de Quervain's tunnel [along the edge of the wrist and near the end of the radius]). The Finkelstein's test is positive in de Quervain, but negative in intersection.

96. **What causes the intersection syndrome?**

Overuse of the wrist extensor tendons. This causes the tendons to rub against the thumb muscles, as if they were a violin bow, until, like overused strings, they eventually develop friction tendinitis. Predisposing activities are those that make the wrist curl down (and *in*) toward the thumb. Hence, intersection syndrome is very common in downhill skiers (who have to plant their ski poles deep in powder snow) and also in practitioners of racket sports, weight lifting, canoeing, and rowing. More lowly activities, such as raking leaves against a hard ground or shoveling snow, also can produce stress on the wrist extensor tendons, and thus the syndrome.

97. **What is a wrist ganglion? How is identified?**

Ganglions are benign and often asymptomatic fluid-filled cysts, closely associated with an underlying joint or tendon sheath, and usually connected to it by a stalk. They are the most common soft tissue tumors of the hands and wrists and are not occupationally related. They affect women three times more often than men, usually during the second and fifth decades. They tend to be solitary, rarely exceeding 2 cm in diameter. Although generally asymptomatic, they may present with pain, paresthesias, weakness, and limitation of motion. They can involve almost any joint of the hands and wrists, although their most common forms are: (1) the dorsal wrist ganglions (60–70%), (2) the volar wrist ganglions (20%), and (3) the distal interphalangeal ganglions of the flexor tendon sheath (10–12%). The cysts are smooth walled, translucent, and white. They have a fluctuant swelling that moves with the involved tendon and a mucinous content that is rich in hyaluronic acid, albumin, globulin, and glucosamine.

98. **What is the cause?**

Unknown, although repetitive injuries (like playing tennis or golf) may have a predisposing effect. According to one theory, wrist ganglions are formed whenever wear-and-tear of a joint or tendon sheath allows fluid to escape into a cyst. This also would explain why ganglions have a stalk. Over time, the cyst grows large, since fluid can only enter it but not exit it (one-way valve).

99. **What are the typical wrist findings of rheumatoid arthritis?**

An early finding is swelling of the extensor carpi ulnaris tendon. Later findings include protrusion and instability of the distal ulna, due to laxity of the radial ulnar ligaments. Finally, in more advanced disease the carpal rows sublux toward the dorsal side, causing a bayonet deformity.

100. **What is *Guyon's canal syndrome*?**

It is a compression neuropathy that affects the ulnar nerve as it travels through a wrist tunnel called the Guyon's canal. Note that the ulnar nerve can be compressed either at the wrist (in the Guyon's canal) or at the elbow (in the epicondylar groove). Given its more superficial position at the elbow, the most common site of injury is indeed repetitive *elbow* pressure, such as leaning on it while working or driving. Compression in Guyon's canal requires instead repetitive pressure on the *palm,* often because of excessive wrist and hand twisting. Heavy gripping can do it, too, as in the case of cyclists or weight lifters, but also jackhammer operators and patients on crutches. Finally, fracture of the hamate bone can cause Guyon's canal syndrome in golfers who club the ground instead of the golf ball, or baseball players during batting.

101. **What is the anatomy of the Guyon's canal?**
The floor is formed by two bones (*pisiform* and *hamate*), and the ceiling is provided by the *ligament* between them. Both the ulnar nerve and artery run through the canal. After emerging from under it, the nerve divides into a *sensory* branch (that supplies the fourth and fifth fingers) and a *motor* branch (that supplies instead the interosseous muscles, the adductors pollicis, and the deep head of the flexor pollicis brevis). Note that the hamate bone provides the medial side of Guyon's canal. This includes a small hook-shaped spur (the *hook of hamate*) that serves as attachment for several wrist ligaments. Ulnar compression in the canal is usually caused by either arthritis of the hook or its fracture. Still, this entrapment is much less common than that of CTS. Occasionally, both conditions may coexist.

102. **What are the symptoms of ulnar compression?**
The earliest is *paresthesias,* affecting the fifth finger and the ulnar half of the fourth. As in CTS, symptoms usually occur during the early morning hours, often awakening the patient. There also may be difficulty in opening jars or turning doorknobs, and in opposing the thumb. Later findings include frank pain, followed by atrophy and weakness of the interosseous muscles. Ultimately, there may be clawing of the fourth and fifth fingers with severe intrinsic muscle wasting.

103. **What are the symptoms of *median* nerve compression?**
Pain and numbness along the thumb, index and middle fingers, and radial half of the ring finger.

D. THE HAND

104. **What is the nerve supply of the hand?**
- The **median nerve** supplies sensation to the palmar (or volar) side of fingers one to three, their dorsal and distal aspects, plus the radial half of the fourth finger. It controls motion of the thenar muscles.
- The **ulnar nerve** supplies sensation to both the dorsal and volar side of the fifth and fourth fingers, plus the contiguous portion of the hand. It supplies motor fibers to the interossei.
- The **radial nerve** supplies sensation to the hand's dorsum not reached by median and ulnar. *See* Figure 21-5.

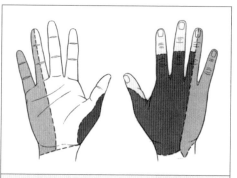

Figure 21-5. Cutaneous innervation from the median nerve *(white area),* ulnar nerve *(light shading),* and radial nerve *(dark shading).* (From Concannon MJ: Common Hand Problems in Primary Care. Philadelphia, Hanley & Belfus, 1999.)

105. **How can you differentiate ostheoarthritis from rheumatoid arthritis (RA)?**
By the pattern of involvement in the small joints of the hand.
- **Rheumatoid arthritis (RA)** is a *symmetric* process, affecting metacarpophalangeal (MCP) and proximal interphalangeal (PIP) joints, but typically sparing the distal interphalangeal (DIP) joints. It is often associated with lateral (ulnar) deviation of the fingers.
- **Osteoarthritis (OA)** is instead *asymmetric*, affecting the DIP and PIP, without involving the MCP.

106. **Describe the typical deformities of rheumatoid arthritis.**
- **Boutonnière deformities** (French for buttonhole): Fixed flexion of PIP, hyperextension of DIP
- **Swan-neck deformities:** Fixed hyperextension of PIP, flexion of DIP
- **Ulnar deviation:** Drift of the phalanges toward the ulnar side at the MCP joints. This is fixed in RA but reversible in Jaccoud's arthropathy (seen in chronic rheumatic fever or systemic lupus erythematosus [SLE]).

107. **What is a *trigger finger*?**
The most common entrapment tendinitis, 20 times more frequent than de Quervain's. It is a painful condition characterized by locking of the affected finger in *flexion* (Fig. 21-6). This is usually due to *tenosynovitis* of the flexor tendon to the digit (hence, its term of *flexor tendinitis*) resulting in palpable swelling of the tendon itself, often nodular. Alternatively, it may be due to inflammation and swelling of the *sheath* surrounding the tendon. Either way, the tendon becomes unable to glide smoothly through the sheath. Hence, whenever the patient forces the finger to bend, there may be a painful snap as the tendon passes through the thickened portion of the sheath into its final flexed position. Then, given its inability to glide back into the sheath, the tendon will *stay flexed*. With more vigorous attempts, either by increased force from the finger extensors or by application of an external force (such as use of the other hand), the

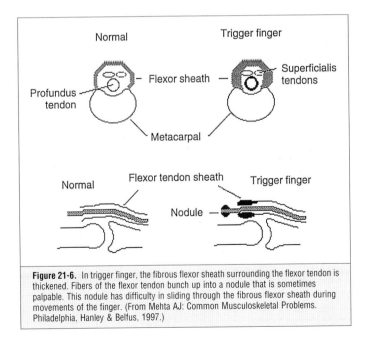

Figure 21-6. In trigger finger, the fibrous flexor sheath surrounding the flexor tendon is thickened. Fibers of the flexor tendon bunch up into a nodule that is sometimes palpable. This nodule has difficulty in sliding through the fibrous flexor sheath during movements of the finger. (From Mehta AJ: Common Musculoskeletal Problems. Philadelphia, Hanley & Belfus, 1997.)

finger will eventually extend, usually with another (and often painful) snap as the tendon passes back through the thickened portion of the sheath—*like a trigger being pulled and released*. Yet, in more severe cases the finger will remain locked. Women are more affected than men, especially musicians, writers, gardeners, and hobbyists, since all these occupations require repetitive gripping actions. Treatment varies, depending on the severity of the condition, ranging from rest, to medications, to surgery.

108. What are the physical findings of a trigger finger?
There is usually tendineal tenderness over the palmar side of the MCP joint. There also may be a palpable nodule and a palpable (and *painful*) click upon the finger's flexion/extension at the MCP.

109. What other typical deformities can be seen in the hand?
- **Mallet finger (or deformity):** This is the inability to fully extend the DIP joint, with some degree of resting flexion. It results from injury to the long *extensor tendon,* causing tendinous lengthening during healing and permanent flexion of the distal phalanx (Fig. 21-7).
- **Heberden's nodes:** Bony enlargement at the DIP joints; typical of osteoarthritis
- **Bouchard's nodes:** Bony enlargement at the PIP joints; typical of osteoarthritis

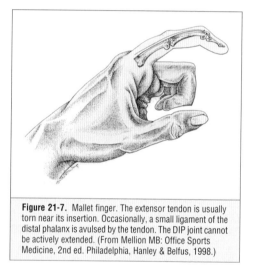

Figure 21-7. Mallet finger. The extensor tendon is usually torn near its insertion. Occasionally, a small ligament of the distal phalanx is avulsed by the tendon. The DIP joint cannot be actively extended. (From Mellion MB: Office Sports Medicine, 2nd ed. Philadelphia, Hanley & Belfus, 1998.)

110. What are Heberden's nodes?
They are painless nodules on the distal interphalangeal joints (Fig. 21-8). These may involve one or more fingers, but typically spare the thumb. The overlying skin is normal, and the nodes are hard, 2–3 mm in diameter, not interfering with fingers' movement, twin in presentation, and typically located on the lateral *and* medial dorsal surface of the DIP (if affecting the PIP, the nodes are instead called Bouchard's). Both reflect localized osteoarthritis. Hence, they are more common in the elderly. Involvement of

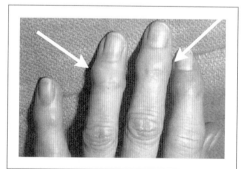

Figure 21-8. Patients with degenerative joint disease of the hands can present with Heberden's nodes *(arrows).* These nodules represent osteophytes at the DIP joint. (From Concannon MJ: Common Hand Problems in Primary Care. Philadelphia, Hanley & Belfus, 1999.)

a single joint is more prevalent in men, whereas multiple involvement is more frequent in women, where the condition is usually postmenopausal and hereditary.

111. **Who were Heberden and Bouchard?**
  - **William Heberden**
    (1710–1801) was an English physician, who studied in Cambridge and practiced in London at the local university. A devout Christian, he was a leading Latin and Hebrew scholar, referred to by Samuel Johnson as "the last of the Romans" ("Dr. Heberden ultimus Romanorum—the last of our learned physicians"). In fact, his reputation as the master clinician of his times eventually gained him a position at the court of King George (the same "mad George" who lost the American colonies) as personal physician to the Queen. He was only 51. His contributions to medicine are indeed staggering, including the aforementioned nodules but also classic descriptions of angina, chickenpox, and night blindness. A lifelong sufferer from gout (which he described masterfully in his "Commentaries on the History and Cure of Diseases"), Dr. Heberden was also able to recognize that his eponymous osteoarthritic nodes ("digitorum nodi") were *not* gouty in origin. In Chapter 28 of the "Commentaries" he wrote:

    > What are those little hard knobs, about the size of a small pea, which are frequently seen upon the fingers, particularly a little below the top, near the joint? They have no connection with the gout, being found in persons who never had it; they continue for life; and being hardly ever attended with pain, or disposed to become sores, are rather unsightly, than inconvenient, though they must be some little hindrance to the free use of the fingers."

    He spent the last 20 years of his life writing his book, commenting that the life of a physician comes in three phases: in the first one you acquire knowledge, in the second one you apply it, and in the third (and last) one you teach it. Words that still ring true today.
  - **Charles J. Bouchard** (1837–1915) was a French pathologist, who studied under Charcot, and then produced the first description of spider nevi in chronic liver disease.

112. **What are Haygarth's nodes?**
  Nodes very different from Heberden's and Bouchard's, since they are *not* degenerative but *inflammatory*. Hence, they present with other signs of inflammation, such as flushing of the overlying skin, increased temperature, thickening of the joint capsule, fluid in the cavity (in part responsible for their fusiform swelling), and limitation of movement. Contrary to Heberden's, Haygarth's nodes can be *painful* and *tender*. They are typical of RA, affecting proximal PIP joints rather than DIP (which RA never involves). Thus, they resemble more Bouchard's than Heberden's. Subcutaneous nodules are very common in RA, having been found on the extensor surfaces of upper extremities (primarily the elbows, but also fingers), knees, ankles, and occiput. Yet, they are not *exclusive* of RA, but can occur in other rheumatic disorders, like lupus, sarcoid, rheumatic fever, syphilis, tuberous xanthomatosis, and granuloma annulare.

113. **Who was Haygarth?**
  John Haygarth (1740–1827) was an English physician from the city of Bath. A Cambridge graduate with a penchant for epidemiology, he eventually set out to study the diseases of the ancient city of Chester, including the value of isolation in infectious diseases and the usefulness of smallpox as a method of immunization. His eponymous work on rheumatism and rheumatic fever was eventually published in 1798, upon his return to Bath.

114. **What are tophi?**
  They are deposits of uric acid (*tophus* is Latin for a calcareous deposit from springs, *tufa*). These can occur over the ears, feet, and hands of gouty patients. In the hands, they are

pathognomonic of the disease (Fig. 21-9), even though they often get confused for rheumatoid nodules.

115. What are Janeway's lesions?
They are small, flat, *nontender*, erythematous, or hemorrhagic macules of palms or soles. Like Osler's nodes (which are instead swollen, *tender*, raised, pea-sized nodules of finger pads, palms, and soles), Janeway lesions are seen in bacterial endocarditis. In fact, before the introduction of antibiotics they occurred in 40–90% of endocarditis patients, but nowadays only 10–23% of cases have them. They also can be seen in SLE, bacteremia without endocarditis, gonococcal sepsis, and marantic endocarditis. They represent either septic emboli or sterile vasculitis, triggered by immune complexes.

116. Who was Janeway?
Edward G. Janeway (1841–1911) was a student of Austin Flint, whom he followed to Bellevue Hospital Medical College in New York, where he established himself as one of the first full-time consultants in American medicine. He had an interest in public service, eventually becoming Health Commissioner for New York and founder of its first Infectious Disease Hospital.

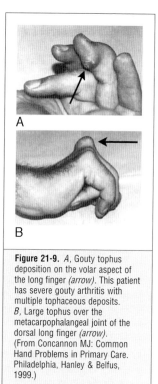

Figure 21-9. *A*, Gouty tophus deposition on the volar aspect of the long finger *(arrow)*. This patient has severe gouty arthritis with multiple tophaceous deposits. *B*, Large tophus over the metacarpophalangeal joint of the dorsal long finger *(arrow)*. (From Concannon MJ: Common Hand Problems in Primary Care. Philadelphia, Hanley & Belfus, 1999.)

117. What is the Pachuco mark?
It is a cross-like tattoo (made with dots rather than lines), which during the 1970s used to be very common over the anatomic snuffbox of intravenous drug abusers (the snuffbox is the hollow space on the radial aspect of the wrist that can be seen when the thumb is fully extended). There it provided a sort of identification card for the drug-dealing world, easily visible upon handshaking. "Pachuco" is actually a Spanish-American term, possibly an alteration of *payuco* (yokel, rustic). The expression has been variously used to identify a Mexican-American youth or teenager, especially one who dresses in flamboyant clothes and belongs to a neighborhood gang.

118. What is the shape of the hand in acromegaly?
Spade-like. Due to enlargement of the distal parts of the body—acromegaly's defining feature.

119. What is arachnodactyly?
It is the spider-like fingers of patients with Marfan's. Described in 1896 by the homonymous Frenchman in a 5-year-old patient, the term arachnodactyly was actually coined 6 years later by Achard. The fingers are thin and long, resembling "the bent legs of a spider." To test for it, use the *Marfan's thumb sign*: ask patients to open their hands and cross their thumbs over their palms as far as possible; then ask them to fold the fingers across the thumb and make a fist. The test is positive if any part of the thumb sticks out beyond the ulnar surface of the fist. The sign is typical of Marfan's, but also can occur in other conditions of joints' hypermobility, like Ehlers-Danlos.

120. Who was Marfan?
Antoine B. Marfan (1858–1942) was a French pediatrician. The son of a provincial medical practitioner, Marfan contributed to several areas of medicine, including the astute observation

that tuberculosis acquired before age 15 seems to provide a unique resilience to patients (which inspired Calmette to develop his bacillus Calmette-Guérin [BCG] vaccine). Very active in public health and service, Dr. Marfan also had a passion for literature and arts, enjoying concert music and trips to Italy, where he was particularly fond of Venetian paintings. Among his many friends was Emile Broca, of whom he wrote a biography. Upon his death, he left most of his fortune to the Society for the Preservation of Infants against Tuberculosis, which he had helped to create.

121. **What is a short fourth metacarpophalangeal bone?**
An unusually short and inwardly dimpled fourth knuckle. This is usually seen in patients with pseudohypoparathyroidism and Turner's syndrome, but even in 10% of normal individuals.

122. **What is the significance of calluses and abrasions on the dorsal aspect of the fingers?**
They are an important clue to bulimia, due to trauma by the teeth during the induction of vomiting.

123. **What is the anatomy of the first carpometacarpal (CMC) joint?**
The first CMC is the *basal* joint of the thumb, the one that articulates its metacarpal bone to the trapezium of the wrist. It is a small joint for man, but a giant one for mankind, since it allowed our ancestors to *oppose* their thumb, which they then used to grasp objects and create "tools," which they then used to whack other fellow hominids, thus taking the first and fundamental step in the evolution of our species—one that eventually gave us the name of *Homo faber* (i.e., the one who creates). Or whacks.

124. **What is CMC squaring?**
It is God's answer to the evolution of the thumb. And since God has a sense of humor, She or He eventually thumbed Her or His nose at us by creating osteoarthritis (degenerative joint disease [DJD]). Carpometacarpal (CMC) squaring is an often-overlooked deformity of the base of the thumb, typical of DJD of the first CMC joint—a common problem, especially among women. The dominant hand is the one most affected, with onset typically after age 40. Initially, the thumb appears unremarkable, but as the disease progresses the CMC subluxes dorsally, starting to protrude proximally to the snuff box (thus creating a *CMC squaring,* or *mushroom deformity*). With time, the CMC becomes even more subluxated and stiff, and as a result the thumb metacarpal joint becomes fixed in *adduction* (i.e., tucked into the palm). As this happens, the only way for patients to lift the thumb off their palms (so that they can grasp) is by hyperextending the MCP joint itself. Eventually, this becomes so painful that the thumb remains frozen into a swan-neck deformity.

125. **What is the presentation of CMC squaring?**
The hallmark is *pain*, first on activity and then even at rest. It is localized at the base of the thumb and usually moderate in intensity, even though at times it may be incapacitating. Tenderness on palpation, crepitus on rotation, and joint limitations in fine motor skills also are typical. Grasp and proximal thumb-index pinching may be limited, and so are activities of daily living that rely on these movements, like using scissors, opening jars, or operating a can opener.

126. **What is a sausage digit?**
It is the inflammation of a whole digit, giving it a diffusely swollen appearance.
A sausage-shaped swelling of a toe or finger (i.e., *dactylitis*, from the Greek *daktulos*, finger) can be quite painful. When unassociated with trauma, it is usually caused by tenosynovitis, and often periostitis as well as arthritis. It is frequently seen in seronegative arthritis, typically

psoriatic, but also sarcoid–related. In psoriasis, it is often associated with pitting of the fingernails (*see* Chapter 3, questions 20–22.

127. **What is a telescoped digit?**
A finger that on exam can be moved in and out like a telescope. A telescoped digit (usually the PIP) reflects extreme joint destruction.

128. **Describe the Bunnell-Littler test.**
It is a test for patients with difficulty flexing the PIP joint, since it can differentiate interosseous tightness from capsular contraction. To carry it out, ask patients to hold the MCP joint in a few degrees of extension, and then flex their PIP joint. If unable to do so, have them place the MCP in flexion, and then reattempt PIP flexion. Those with capsular contraction will not flex the PIP at all, whereas those with interosseous tightness will flex it by using the second maneuver (Fig. 21-10).

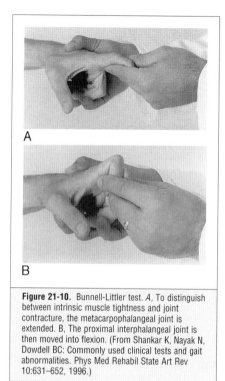

Figure 21-10. Bunnell-Littler test. *A*, To distinguish between intrinsic muscle tightness and joint contracture, the metacarpophalangeal joint is extended. B, The proximal interphalangeal joint is then moved into flexion. (From Shankar K, Nayak N, Dowdell BC: Commonly used clinical tests and gait abnormalities. Phys Med Rehabil State Art Rev 10:631–652, 1996.)

129. **What is a stiff hand syndrome?**
It is thickening of the hands' skin, which becomes waxy and tightened. Also called *diabetic hand syndrome* (or diabetic *cheiroarthropathy*, from the Greek *kheir*, hand), this eventually causes limitation of finger movement, with varying degrees of fixed flexion of the PIP joints. As a result, patients become unable to fully extend fingers or press their palms flat together (prayer sign). It is exclusively seen in protracted type 1 or type 2 diabetes, often paralleling microvascular injury.

130. **What is a paronychia? A felon?**
- A **paronychia** is an infection at the nail margin, accompanied by swelling, erythema, and tenderness of the skin surrounding the nail. As it progresses, the infection points to the finger edge.
- A **felon** is instead a close-space infection of the fingertip *pulp*, usually due to staphylococci and gram-negative organisms. This may start as cellulitis, but eventually evolves into an abscess, with throbbing pain, swelling, and erythema of the finger pad. Although often triggered by wooden splinters or minor cuts (such as lancing for diabetic monitoring), felons have no history of injury in more than one half of the cases. They may represent a paronychial spread.

131. **Can the fingers provide a clue to a patient's sexual orientation?**
Maybe. In a recent *Nature* study, researchers from Berkeley suggested that the length of the index and ring fingers might indeed statistically predict sexual orientation. According to their theory, womb exposure to high levels of androgens would shorten the index fingers of males, causing them to become a little smaller than the ring fingers. Women would have

instead indices that are either longer or, at least, equal to their ring fingers. Researchers carried out their study by going to street fairs in San Francisco and persuading more than 700 fairgoers to have copies of their hands made on portable photocopying machines. They also inquired about family histories and sexual orientations. By doing so, they discovered that gay men have indices even shorter than those of straight men. And, more interestingly, that gay men also have a much greater number of older brothers. And so their theory speculates that womb exposure to even higher levels of androgens (as in cases of many preceding male siblings) would paradoxically induce a gay sexual orientation. This *hypermasculinization* would be the reason why, according to the same researchers, gay men often have longer genitalia and subtle differences in brain structure. It would also explain the finger pattern of gay *women*, which is very similar to that of straight men (i.e., indices shorter than ring fingers), similarly related to high womb exposure to androgens. What is really interesting, though, is that the role of the middle finger hasn't yet been clarified. Maybe in a future study. On a partially related note, Romans-of-old also believed in connections between fertility and fingers—especially the fourth finger of the left hand, which they thought linked to the heart through a unique nerve. That is why they used to "chain" it at time of marriage by putting a ring around it, as a sign of enslavement of both heart and passions. And inside that ring they engraved the words: *"Ubi Tu Gaia, Ego Gaius; Ubi Ego Gaius, Tu Gaia" (When you are happy, I am happy; and when I am happy, you are happy")*. In other words, reciprocal tolerance is key to a successful marriage—good advice for all times.

E. THE HEAD AND NECK

132. How do you assess the cervical spine?
By inspecting for deformities and abnormal posture. Also by palpating for tenderness over the spinous processes, trapezius, scaleni, and sternomastoids.

133. How do you evaluate its ROM?
By asking patients to lift the head back (*extension*), touch chin to chest (*flexion*), chin to each shoulder (*rotation*), and finally touch each ear to the corresponding shoulder, but *without* raising the shoulder (*lateral bending*).

134. How do you diagnose temporomandibular joint (TMJ) arthritis?
By palpating the tragus of the ear and then inserting your index finger in the auditory canal while the patient is opening and closing the mouth. This allows you to assess for *crepitus*, as well as joint swelling and smoothness of articular motion. Finally, watch the mandibular tract *during mouth opening*: normally it is directed *downward*. Any jaw deviation to one side would reflect instead an abnormal TMJ.

135. What is torticollis?
An involuntary rotation of the head to one side. Due to spasm of the cervical musculature.

136. What is occipital neuralgia? What are its findings?
Occipital neuralgia results from impingement of the occipital nerve as it exits the skull at the occipital notch. Its symptom is pain, radiating from the occiput to the vertex of the head. It can be reproduced by pressure over the exit point of the occipital nerve.

137. What is spinal stenosis? How is it classified?
It is a narrowing of the spinal canal, nerve root canals, or intervertebral foramina. Due to degenerative changes of the spine (spondylosis, osteophytes, facet hypertrophy), disks (bulging, herniation), or ligamentum flavum (hypertrophy). It usually affects the cervical or lumbar segments

(rarely the thoracic), eventually causing compression of spinal cord or terminal filaments in the caudal sac (cauda equina). It is common, affecting 5/1000 Americans older than 50.

138. **What are the findings of *cervical* stenosis?**
The most typical are those of cervical *radiculopathy,* with or without myelopathy (i.e., spinal cord dysfunction). This usually involves the *lower cervical spine* (C5–T1), causing radiating arm pain, with numbness and paresthesias in the involved dermatomes. Occasionally, there may be associated weakness in the muscles supplied by the compressed root and changes in reflexes. Fine motor activities (like writing or typing) become difficult, too, and so does the ability to grip and let go of objects. If the *upper* cervical spine is affected, there also may be weakness and wasting of deltoid and shoulder muscles. In contrast to *mechanical neck pain* (which starts in the neck and may spread to the upper back or shoulder, but rarely extends below it), pain from cervical radiculopathy usually spreads farther down the arm. If stenosis is significant, the patient may not only develop finger numbness/tingling, but also signs and symptoms of *myelopathy,* such as clumsiness and difficulty walking (due to a spastic gait with loss of proprioception). In the most severe cases, there may be sphincter dysfunction, with loss of bowel and bladder control. On exam there will be "long-tract signs," such as hyperreflexia and clonus. Knowledge of cervical nerves and their distribution is crucial for examining the hand, elbow, shoulder, and head.

139. **List sensory distribution, reflexes, and motor innervation of cervical spinal roots.**
See Table 21-2.

F. THE THORACIC SPINE

140. **What is the most common type of spinal deformity?**
It is *adolescent idiopathic scoliosis,* a strongly familial condition of unknown etiology.

141. **Describe the difference between *scoliosis* and *kyphosis*.**
- Viewed from the side, a normal spine has an anterior convexity in the neck and lower trunk (*lordosis*), with an interposed anterior concavity in the upper trunk (*kyphosis*). Certain amounts of thoracic **kyphosis** (25–40 degrees) and cervical/lumbar lordosis are indeed normal and in fact necessary for appropriate trunk balance over the pelvis. Excessive misalignment, however,

Root	Sensory Supply/ Area of Pain	Motor Supply/Deficit	Reflex (Loss)
C5	Lateral arm	Deltoid, infraspinatus, supraspinatus	Biceps
C6	Lateral forearm and thumb	Wrist extension, biceps, brachioradialis	Brachioradialis
C7	Middle fingers	Wrist flexors, finger extensors, triceps	Triceps
C8	Medial forearm and little finger	Finger flexors, hand intrinsics	Finger flexors
T1	Medial arm and axilla	Hand intrinsics	None

TABLE 21-2. SENSORY DISTRIBUTION, REFLEXES, AND MOTOR INNERVATION OF CERVICAL SPINAL ROOTS

reflects abnormal kyphosis or lordosis, or more commonly both. Hence, a pathologic kyphosis is one associated with an excessive anterior concavity of the thoracic spine, and a compensatory lordosis of the lumbar segment, often resulting in a protruding belly.

- **Scoliosis** is a side-to-side deviation from the normal frontal axis, with a major curvature pointing toward the right or the left, and a distal compensatory curve pointing contralaterally. Yet, this definition is limited, since the deformity may occur in varying degrees in *all three planes*: back-front, side-to-side, top-to-bottom. The cause is unknown in more than 80% of the cases (especially adolescent girls), but is never the result of unusual sleeping/standing postures or the carrying of heavy weights.

142. **How is scoliosis appreciated?**
By running your finger down the patient's vertebral spine. If scoliosis is present, the finger will follow the spine right and left along its primary and secondary curvatures.

143. **What is Sprengel's deformity?**
A congenital elevation of the shoulder, described in 1891 by the German surgeon Otto Gerhard Karl Sprengel. It results from partial descent of the scapula and produces an asymmetric appearance of the shoulders and upper back. It can be associated with webbing of the neck.

144. **What is the significance of tenderness over the spinous process(es)?**
It suggests pathology of the vertebral body. It is demonstrated by striking your fist at each spinal level, or by firmly palpating over each spinous process. It is highly suggestive of underlying bony disease, such as compression fracture, infection, inflammation (as in seronegative spondyloarthropathy), or tumor.

145. **How do you measure chest expansion?**
Place a tape measure around the chest at the nipple line; ask the patient to first inhale to forced maximal inspiration and then exhale forcefully. The difference in circumference between maximal inspiration and expiration is the *chest expansion,* normally 5 cm (*see* Chapter 13, questions 60, 61, 152, and 153).

146. **What is *winging* of the scapula? How is it demonstrated?**
"Winging" refers to protrusion of the scapula from the chest wall. This can be accentuated by having the patient place both hands on a wall and then push outward.

147. **What are the causes of scapular winging?**
Seven muscles attach the scapula to the chest wall and help maintain its control. Of these, the *serratus anterior* and the *trapezius* are the most important. A winging scapula is usually associated with partial or complete paralysis of the *serratus anterior,* secondary to palsy of the *long thoracic nerve* (strenuous sport/activity, direct trauma, surgical error, and infection). Less common causes include weakness or paralysis of the *trapezius,* and various muscular disorders, such as spinal muscular atrophy and muscular dystrophy.

148. **What are the consequences of scapular winging?**
They are not merely aesthetic, since the compensatory muscular activity required to improve shoulder stability often leads to secondary pain and spasm, plus tendinitis around the shoulder.

G. THE LUMBAR SPINE

149. **What are the normal movements of the lumbar spine?**
It can flex forward and laterally, and it can extend.

150. **What is Schober's test?**

It is a bedside assessment of lumbar spine *flexibility*. It measures the degree of lumbar *forward flexion*, as the patient bends over while attempting to touch the toes (Fig. 21-11). It is carried out as follows: with the patient standing up straight, draw a line at the level of the posterior iliac spine. This corresponds to L5/S1 (i.e., the dimples of Venus, DV). Place a mark on the spine 5 cm below this line and another 10 cm above the line, so that the distance between the two is 15 cm. Then instruct the patient to touch his or her toes (i.e., to maximally flex forward the lumbar spine). If the increase in distance between the marks is <5 cm, the patient has reduced lumbar flexion—an early sign of *ankylosing spondylitis* in young individuals and *degenerative disease* in older ones.

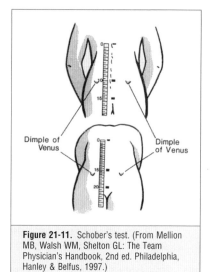

Figure 21-11. Schober's test. (From Mellion MB, Walsh WM, Shelton GL: The Team Physician's Handbook, 2nd ed. Philadelphia, Hanley & Belfus, 1997.)

151. **How valid is Schober's test?**

It correlates with x-ray findings in measuring progressive loss of spinal motion. Hence, it allows for serial evaluation of progressive disease.

152. **How can relative leg length be assessed?**

Stand behind the patient, who, in turn, stands with the feet together and knees extended. Place your hands on the iliac crests. The relative height of each hand provides an assessment of relative leg length. Note, however, that this test is also influenced by scoliosis and relative pelvic tilt.

153. **What are the symptoms of spinal (lumbar) stenosis?**

The classic one is bilateral sciatalgia with *neurogenic claudication* (low back pain radiating down the lateral aspect of the leg, presenting at time with paresthesias).Since this is due to *neurologic* compression rather than arterial insufficiency (which causes instead *true* claudication), the pain will *not* be exacerbated by biking, uphill ambulation, or lumbar flexion. Instead it will be *triggered by walking* (especially downhill) and *relieved by rest*. It also is relieved by sitting, lying supine instead of prone, squatting, lumbar flexion, forward bending, but *not* standing. In fact, standing *exacerbates* it.

154. **How are radicular symptoms reproduced in patients with spinal stenosis?**

By asking the patient to either extend maximally the lumbar spine or flex it laterally.

155. **What are the physical findings of spinal stenosis?**

Very limited. Exam is usually normal and generally unhelpful. The Lasègue test is often negative. The most common findings are wide-based gait, abnormal Romberg, thigh pain following 30 seconds of lumbar extension, and neuromuscular abnormalities.

156. **What is the *stoop test*?**

A maneuver that helps separate neurogenic from vascular claudication. When pain occurs, patients with vascular claudication sit down to rest, whereas those with pseudoclaudication attempt to keep walking, either "stooping" or flexing the spine to relieve the stretch on the sciatic nerve.

157.   What is the *cauda equina syndrome*?
A less common presentation of spinal stenosis. In
addition to bilateral sciatica and lower extremity
weakness, there is perineal/perianal anesthesia in
60–80% of patients, and bowel/bladder dysfunction in
90%. A *cauda equina syndrome* can be a surgical
emergency.

**158.   What is the *Lasègue test*? How is it
performed?**
Lasègue is the straight-leg raising (SLR) test (Fig.
21-12), a maneuver aimed at detecting lumbosacral
nerve root irritation/compression, as in patients with
disk prolapse and sciatica. To carry it out:

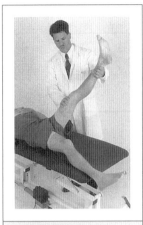

Figure 21-12. Lasègue
(straight-leg raise) test. (From
Shankar K, Nayak N, Dowdell BC:
Commonly used clinical tests
and gait abnormalities. Phys
Med Rehabil State Art Rev
10:631–652, 1996.)

- Ask the patient to lay *supine* and with the legs
straight.
- *Raise one leg with the knee fully extended* (so to
stretch the sciatic nerve) until the
patient experiences radicular pain (i.e., pain referred
down the buttock→ thigh→ calf [L4 irritation→
radiation to medial calf; L5→ lateral calf; S1→ lateral
foot]).
- *The test is positive only if:* (1) pain occurs when the
leg is lifted 30–70 degrees from the horizontal and
(2) pain travels down the leg until below the knee, not solely in the back or the hamstrings.
Note that pain in the low back is *not* a positive test. Posterior thigh pain is not a classic sign
either, but may occur in mild sciatica.
- *Record the angle at which pain occurred.* A normal value is 80–90 degrees. An elevation of
the leg to <70 degrees is clearly abnormal, and yet pain that occurs *before* the leg is raised
to 30 degrees cannot be due to disk prolapse, since this angle is too small to stretch the
nerve root.
- *Perform the sciatic stretch test.* During a standard straight-leg raise, apply dorsiflexion to
the foot (flip test). This maneuver further stretches the nerve and thus increases the pain. A
reverse flip test consists of applying plantar flexion of the foot. This should typically lessen
the pain. If not, it suggests malingering.
- *Flex the knee.* This may relieve the buttock pain, since flexion of the knee causes neither
stretching nor sliding of the nerve root. Conversely, when the leg is raised with the knee fully
extended, up to 1.5 inches of nerve root will slide in and out of the exit foramina of the spine.
- *Sitting straight-leg raising (knee extension) test.* The patient sits on the table edge with both
the hips and knees flexed at 90 degrees and extends the knee slowly. This maneuver
stretches the *lower* nerve roots as much as a moderate degree of supine SLR. If positive, it
will reproduce sciatica symptoms, with pain radiating below the knee.

159.   What is the significance of a positive straight-leg raising test?
It indicates *nerve root impingement*, usually by a herniated disk. It has high sensitivity (91%)
but low specificity (26%), thus limiting its diagnostic accuracy. The "crossed" straight-leg raising
test has instead low sensitivity (29%) but high specificity (88%). Hence, use them together.

160.   What is the "crossed" straight-leg raising test?
The eliciting of pain on the *affected* side as a result of SLR testing on the *unaffected* side.
It reflects severe root irritation. It has higher specificity for disk herniation than the standard
SLR.

161. **How do you perform the "reverse" straight-leg raising test?**
With the patient lying prone, extend the leg at the hip and the knee. Ipsilateral pain in the anterior thigh would indicate *upper* lumbar root disease, a less common site of radiculopathy. The maneuver also is called the prone SLR test, or the *femoral nerve stretch test,* since it does put tension on the femoral nerve and its roots.

162. **What is the "distracted" straight-leg raising test?**
It is an SLR maneuver carried out while the patient is unaware of its being performed. To do so, have the patient sitting rather than recumbent. Then straighten the affected leg at the knee (i.e., do the SLR) while pretending to examine the foot for some unrelated reason—for example, during a Babinski maneuver, or sensory/motor testing, or pulse checking. Patients with organic pain will be positive on both standard and distracted SLR tests. Conversely, patients with nonorganic back pain (malingerers or psychosomatics) will only be positive on standard SLR.

163. **How else can one separate organic from *non*organic back pain?**
By the *Waddell's signs.* In 1980, Waddell et al. reported eight signs (referred to as *behavioral* signs) that in a prospective study of 26 findings in 350 patient evaluations were consistently capable of identifying non-organic back pain (Table 21-3).

164. **Who was Lasègue?**
Ernest-Charles Lasègue was a French internist (1816–1883), who, after contemplating a career in philosophy, got convinced by a mesmerizing lecture of Trousseau to become instead a

TABLE 21-3. WADDELL'S SIGNS	
Sign	**Positive Finding***
Superficial tenderness	Skin discomfort on palpation
Nonanatomic tenderness	Tenderness that crosses multiple somatic boundaries
Axial loading	Report of low back pain
Simulated rotation	Report of back pain
Distracted straight-leg raise	Report of pain in low back or posterior thigh; lessening of pain with continued leg raising; severe pain at 10-degree flexion in patient with no apparent disability
Regional sensory change	"Stocking" or global distribution of numbness
Regional weakness	Sudden, uneven weakness (e.g., "cogwheeling," "dithering") in patient with normal strength on muscle testing
Overreaction to examination	Exaggerated, non-reproducible response to stimulus (grimacing, sighing, guarding, bracing, rubbing)

*The predictive value is greatly improved when three or more positive signs are present.
(Adapted from Waddell G, McCulloch JA, Kummel E, et al: Nonorganic physical signs in low-back pain. Spine 5:117–125, 1980; and from Main CJ, Waddell G: Behavioral responses to examination: A reappraisal of the interpretation of nonorganic signs. Spine 23:2367–2371, 1998.)

physician. After struggling in medical school (he shared a room at the Latin Quarter with Claude Bernard, often wasting rent money on experimental guinea pigs and rabbits), Lasègue became Trousseau's favorite student and close collaborator, eventually delivering in 1867 his eulogy—one of the finest in French language. He himself died at 67 of diabetic complications. A beloved teacher and prolific writer, Lasègue had a special interest in psychiatry, especially psychosomatic diseases. In fact, it was his desire to develop tests and maneuvers that could trap malingerers that eventually led to the discovery of the homonymous sign. As a person, Lasègue was witty, empathetic, and a strong supporter of arts and humanities (in defending a liberal education, he compared the time spent on humanities to the time spent by a soldier polishing his armor). Pierre Astruc relates how Lasègue discovered his homonymous sign.

> ... on one Sunday morning he thinks of the question which he had been asked by Inspector General Dujardin-Baumetz, how to discover the malingerer simulating sciatica. He promised to study the question: it is ever present in his thoughts. While smoking his pipe, he sees Mme. Lasègue seated at the piano while his son-in-law, Cesbron, is tuning his violin. Is not the string stretched over the bridge like the sciatic nerve, which is made taut on the ischium when the lower extremity is elevated? Undoubtedly as he listens to the classical music he has formulated the answer to the Inspector General's question. Tomorrow he will look for the sign in his clinic.

Still, the sign did not appear in Lasègue's *Considération sur la sciatique*. It was only years later that his pupil J.J. Forst put the sign on record.

165. **What is low back pain?**
A problem that afflicts two thirds of all adults at some point in their lives. In fact, it is the second most common complaint in ambulatory medicine, the third most expensive disorder in health care costs (after cancer and heart disease), and the number one cause of work-related disability in the United States. It also is the most common reason for emergency room evaluation. A precise pathoanatomic diagnosis, however, can only be found in one fifth of the cases.

166. **What are the causes of low back pain?**
Other than musculo-ligamentous injuries, the most common cause is age-related degenerative disease of intervertebral disks and facet processes (DJD), resulting in a *nerve root syndrome*. Spinal stenosis, spinal degeneration, and cauda equina syndrome are other possibilities.

167. **What is *a nerve root syndrome*?**
A painful radicular syndrome that can be due to nerve root *impingement,* but also simple *inflammation* or *irritation* (which explains why it may respond to conservative therapies without necessarily requiring surgical decompression). It is common, occurring in 1–10% of the population.

168. **What are the causes of nerve impingement?**
Various degenerative manifestations of the intervertebral disk. From mild to worse, these include *bulging* (where the annular fibers are still intact), *protrusion, extrusion,* and finally *sequestration* (where fragments of disk break off from the nucleus pulposus).

169. **What is the most common site of disk herniation?**
The L5–S1 interspace. Due to thinning of the posterior longitudinal ligament as it extends caudally.

170. **What is sciatica?**
Neuralgia of the sciatic nerve, usually due to lumbar disk disease.

171. **In a nerve root syndrome, can you separate impingement from inflammation/ irritation?**
    - Impingement causes a *sharp and well-localized pain*, typically associated with *paresthesias*; inflammation/irritation causes instead a dull and poorly localized pain with no paresthesias.
    - Impingement also is associated with a *positive straight-leg raising sign*, plus neurologic *deficits* and radiation of the pain below the knee; inflammation/irritation is not.

172. **What are the physical findings of patients with low back pain?**
    They vary from patient to patient. Focus your exam on:
    - **Lumbar range of motion:** Assess this in flexion (Schober's test), extension, lateral bending, and rotation. ROM is usually painful and limited, especially into flexion; however, extension also may be restricted and painful.
    - **Palpation of the lumbar paraspinals:** This may elicit tenderness, as these muscles undergo reactive spasm.
    - **Thorough neurologic evaluation:** This should include pinprick sensation throughout all dermatomes, muscle strength assessment, and muscle stretch reflexes. To separate focal neuropathy from root pathology, the exam also should test two muscles and one reflex for each lumbar root.
    - **Straight-leg raising test:** Carry this out both in supine and seated positions.
    - **Measurements of calf circumferences** (at mid-calf): Differences greater than 2 cm may suggest neurogenic atrophy.
    - **Gait:** To test S1, ask ambulatory patients to walk on their toes. Gait should otherwise be normal.
    - **Rectal examination:** Assess sphincter tone and perineal sensation in any patient with possible cauda equina syndrome.
    - **Pelvic examination:** Only in women complaining of menstrual abnormalities or vaginal discharge.
    - **Functional muscle testing** (Table 21-4).

173. **What are the physical findings of patients with a true herniated disk?**
    There may be no findings at all, except for a positive SLR test. Classic presentation, however, includes numbness in the dermatomes corresponding to the disk involved, with motor weakness and reflex loss. Note that herniated disks have different presentations depending on location:
    - At **L4:** Pain along the front of the leg; weak extension of the leg at the knee; sensory loss about the knee; loss of knee-jerk reflex.
    - At **L5:** Pain along the side of the leg; weak dorsiflexion of the foot; sensory loss in the web of the big toe; no reflexes lost.
    - At **S1:** Pain along the back of the leg; weak plantar flexion of the foot; sensory loss along the back of the calf and the lateral aspect of the foot; loss of ankle jerk.
    - **L5** and **S1:** The two most commonly involved (95% of all disk herniations).

174. **What are musculoskeletal pain syndromes?**
    Syndromes that produce low back pain, like *fibromyalgia* and *myofascial pain*. The former is pain and tenderness on palpation of 11/18 localized areas (*trigger points*, one being in the low

TABLE 21-4. FUNCTIONAL MUSCLE TESTING		
Nerve Root	**Motor Exam**	**Functional Test**
L3	Extend quadriceps	Squat down and rise
L4	Dorsiflex ankle	Walk on heels
L5	Dorsiflex great toe	Walk on heels
S1	Stand on toes	Walk on toes (plantarflex ankle)

back), plus generalized stiffness, fatigue, and muscle ache. *Myofascial pain* is instead loss of ROM in the involved muscle groups plus tenderness over trigger points. Pain radiates along the distribution of a peripheral nerve and is relieved by stretching of the involved muscle group.

175. **What are the other skeletal causes of low back pain?**
   - **Osteomyelitis**
   - **Sacroiliitis:** This results in pain over the sacroiliac joints, radiating to anterior and posterior thighs, and usually worse at night or after prolonged sitting/standing.
   - **Malignancy:** Cancer of the spine can be primary or metastatic. Most primary tumors involve the *posterior* vertebral elements and occur in patients younger than 30. Metastatic tumors occur instead in patients older than 50, usually in the *anterior* aspects of the vertebral body.

176. **What is the Trendelenburg's sign?**
   A sign of weakness of the *gluteus medius*. This originates on the *ilium* (between the anterior and posterior gluteal lines), eventually terminating on the lateral surface of the *greater trochanter*. Its contraction pulls the two insertion sites toward one another, thus elevating the *opposite* side of the pelvis. This typically occurs when the subject stands on one leg: contraction of the gluteus medius of the weight-bearing limb prevents the pelvis from tipping toward the opposite (and unsupported) side, thus keeping it level. When the gluteus medium is weak, the contralateral hemipelvis tips down, the buttock sags, and the unsupported leg hangs lower (positive sign) (Fig. 21-13).

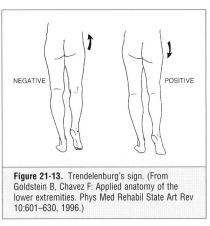

Figure 21-13. Trendelenburg's sign. (From Goldstein B, Chavez F: Applied anatomy of the lower extremities. Phys Med Rehabil State Art Rev 10:601–630, 1996.)

177. **How do you elicit it?**
   Stand behind the patient, and look at the dimples of Venus (i.e., the dimples over the sacroiliac joints). In a patient who is standing upright, with the feet together and weight evenly distributed between the legs, the two DV should be symmetric and at the same level (and so should the two iliac crests and the two buttocks). Then ask the patient to lift one foot off the ground and stand on only one leg, with the other flexed to 90 degrees. Ask him/her to maintain this stance for at least 30 seconds, so as to induce fatigue. In a normal subject, there should be an elevation of the unsupported hemipelvis and buttock (caused by contraction of the contralateral hip abductors, especially the gluteus medius). Sagging of the pelvis indicates a positive Trendelenburg's.

178. **What are the causes of a Trendelenburg's sign?**
   In addition to intrinsic weakness of the muscle (from muscular dystrophy), a positive test suggests congenital dislocation of the hip, poliomyelitis, spinal nerve root lesions (paralyzing the superior gluteal nerve—hence, L5), or greater trochanter fracture (the distal insertion site of the gluteus medius).

179. **What is a Trendelenburg's *gait*?**
   A typical gait of gluteal muscle weakness (*see* Chapter 1, questions 75–80). While stepping from one leg to the other, the glutei are unable to hold up the pelvis, causing it to sag on the unsupported side. As a result, the "swinging" limb may become too low to clear the ground, causing the patient to compensate in one of two ways: (1) *by leaning away from the*

unsupported side, trying to raise the swinging leg in the typical "waddling" fashion of progressive muscular dystrophy (so called because its gait resembles that of a duck), or (2) *by stepping very high on the unsupported side*, so that the swinging leg can clear the ground ("high steppage gait").

180. **What is Hoover's test?**
A bedside assessment of lower extremity strength, based on the principle that whenever a supine patient raises one leg, he or she involuntarily exerts counterpressure with the opposite heel. This response occurs even if that leg is paralyzed. Similarly, if the patient attempts to lift a *paralyzed* leg, he or she will exert counterpressure with the opposite (healthy) heel, regardless of whether any movement at all occurs in the paralyzed limb. This sign is absent in hysteria or malingering, but present in hemiplegia. Hence, it can separate true weakness from poor effort.

181. **How is Hoover's test carried out?**
   - Ask the patient to lie supine with heels off the table. Place your hands below the heels, and then ask the patient to press down on your hands with both feet. If there is hemiplegia, the paralyzed side will exert less pressure.
   - Then place one hand above the nonparalyzed leg, and ask the patient to raise it against your resistance. If the patient produces a good effort, the opposite leg will exert an involuntary downward pressure on the heel, even though it is paralyzed. Failure to do so suggests lack of effort or malingering.
   - Finally, place one hand under the heel of the *healthy* leg, and ask the patient to raise the paralyzed leg. Even in this case, the contralateral (healthy) heel will exert pressure against the examiner's hand. This, however, will be greater than that exerted by the paralyzed leg.

182. **List sensory distribution, reflexes, and motor innervation of lumbar spinal roots syndromes.**
See Table 21-5.

TABLE 21-5. SENSORY DISTRIBUTION, REFLEXES, AND MOTOR INNERVATION OF LUMBAR SPINAL ROOTS

Disk	Root	Motor Deficit	Reflex Loss	Sensory Loss	Area of Pain
L1–L2	L2	Hip flexion	None	Often none (upper thigh)	Across thigh
L2–L3	L3	Knee flexion	Adductor/patellar	Lateral thigh and medial femoral condyle	Across thigh
L3–L4	L4	Inversion of the foot	Patellar	Medial leg and medial ankle (across knee to medial malleolus)	Down to medial malleolus
L4–L5	L5	Dorsiflexion of toes and foot (with L4)	Medial hamstring	Lateral leg and dorsum of foot	Back of thigh, calf, dorsum of foot
L5–S1	S1	Plantar flexion and eversion of the foot	Achilles	Sole of foot and lateral ankle	Back of thigh, calf, lateral foot

H. THE SACROILIAC JOINT

183. **Where is the sacroiliac joint (SIJ)? What is its clinical importance?**
The SIJ is located in the pelvis, between the sacrum and ilium, and is a common but frequently overlooked source of low back pain, both for the *young* (ankylosing spondylitis) and the *old* (DJD). This is not specific to any occupation or sport, but since its symptoms and findings can occur in other low-back pain situations (like herniated disks), diagnosing it is often difficult.

184. **How do I locate the SIJ?**
Sit behind a standing patient and place your fingers over the iliac crests. Your thumbs will naturally fall over the sacroiliac joints, where pressure can then be applied for SIJ tenderness.

185. **What are the presenting symptoms of patients with SIJ disease?**
The main one is a sharp or aching pain in the lower back, usually toward one side. Pain is frequently felt in the groin, often extending down the back of the thigh and occasionally even below the knee, eventually crossing anteriorly. Sacroiliac pain is alleviated by standing or walking, and worsened by sitting down for long drives or plane rides. Numbness, tingling, or weakness in the leg, knee, or foot is rare. In addition to *sacroiliac pain and tenderness*, there may be *reduced motion in the lumbar spine* (*see Schober's test,* previously discussed).

186. **What is the presentation of sacroiliitis?**
Pain and tenderness over the SIJ joints, but no peripheral neurologic findings.

187. **How do you assess sacroiliac joint tenderness?**
There are several maneuvers that test/stress the SIJ, eliciting pain in patients with disease. The simplest one consists in applying pressure over the lateral pelvis in a patient lying on the side. Pain indicates SIJ tenderness. More dynamic maneuvers include Patrick's, Gaenslen's, and Yeoman's tests. Gaenslen consists of maximally flexing *one* hip, while extending the other. To carry it out, ask the patient to lie supine, with one side of the pelvis off the examination table, and the contralateral leg flexed at hip and knee (held up by the examiner). Then extend the hip whose leg is lying below the edge of the table. This will stress both sacroiliac joints simultaneously, eliciting pain on the side being extended.

I. THE HIP

188. **How many muscles control the hip?**
Four groups of muscles: (1) the posterior (represented by the *gluteus maximus* and *the hamstring,* both responsible for moving back the thigh along the sagittal plane [i.e., extension]). Their counterparts are (2) the *iliopsoas* (an anterior muscle) and the *rectus femoris* (one of the quadriceps muscle, the largest anterior muscle). Both are responsible for lifting the thigh up (i.e., flexion). (3) The *adductor muscles* are instead located medially and are responsible for moving the thigh inward (i.e., adduction). (4) Finally, the *abductor muscles* are lateral and made up by the *gluteus medius* and *minimus.* They move the thigh *outward* (i.e., abduction).

189. **What is the normal range of motion of the hip?**
   - **Hip flexion:** Patient supine, knee bent up to the chest and pulled firmly against the abdomen. ROM, 110–120 degrees.
   - **Hip extension:** Patient prone and thigh extended posteriorly. ROM, 10–15 degrees.
   - **Hip abduction:** Patient supine, leg extended and moved laterally. ROM, 30–50 degrees.
   - **Hip adduction:** Patient supine, leg extended and moved medially. ROM, 30 degrees.

- **Hip lateral (external) rotation:** Patient supine, both leg and knee flexed to 90 degrees. Hold the thigh with one hand, and grasp the ankle with the other pushing it laterally. ROM, 40–60 degrees.
- **Hip medial (internal) rotation:** Patient supine, both leg and knee flexed to 90 degrees. Hold the thigh with one hand and grasp the ankle with the other pushing it medially. ROM, 30–40 degrees.

190. **How many bursae does the hip have? Why are they important?**
Three. All are important to know (and examine) since hip pain may be due to *bursitis* and not arthritis.
- The **iliopsoas** (also called iliopectineal): *Anterior on the thigh*, located between the iliopsoas muscle and the hip
- The **trochanteric:** *Lateral on the thigh*, located between the trochanteric process per se and the gluteus medius/iliotibial tract
- The **ischial:** *Inferoposterior on the thigh*, located over the ischium of the pelvis, at the insertion of the hamstring muscles (also known as weaver's butt)

191. **What hip structure can cause *inguinal* swelling?**
The *iliopsoas bursa*. Its inflammation (a rather rare event) can cause anterior hip pain and a fluctuant inguinal mass between the iliopsoas and iliopectineal eminence (or "pelvic brim"). The *snapping hip* maneuver may identify patients with this condition: place your hand on the inguinal crease, while passively flexing, abducting, and externally rotating the hip. Then return the hip to a neutral position. A palpable snap during the last phase of the test suggests iliopsoas bursitis.

192. **Which structures traverse the inguinal fossa?**
From the lateral to the medial: *n*erve, *a*rtery, *v*ein, *e*mptiness, *l*ymph node (all underneath the inguinal ligament). *NAVEL* is the mnemonic.

193. **What are the causes of pain referred to the inguinal area? How do you identify it?**
Pain referred to the inguinal area may originate in a lesion of the *psoas muscle*, such as an abscess or a hematoma. Its psoas origin is confirmed by eliciting pain through hip extension.

194. **What is a trochanteric bursitis?**
It is a painful inflammation of the homonymous bursa. This is a common cause of *lateral* hip pain, especially in older patients. Causes include *acute trauma* (from falls or tackles forcing the subject to land on the lateral hip region) or *repetitive friction* by the iliotibial band (which is an extension of the tensor fascia lata muscle). Runners may be especially at risk.

195. **What are the symptoms of trochanteric bursitis?**
The classic is *lateral hip pain*, even though the joint per se is intact. Pain radiates down the lateral aspect of the thigh (but contrary to sciatica, never all the way into the foot), worsening with internal and external rotation of the hip and pressure during sleep (as when lying in the lateral decubitus position); sometimes the pain even awakens the patient. On exam there is point tenderness over the greater trochanter and bursal swelling, even though this is often difficult to appreciate.

196. **What is "log-rolling" of the hip?**
A test that can separate pain of the hip "joint" from that of other structures. To perform it, roll the leg side to side while keeping it fully extended. Pain so elicited can only originate in the joint.

197. **What is the FABER maneuver?**

A screening maneuver for hip disease. The patient lies supine, while the affected hip is passively *f*lexed, *ab*ducted, and *e*xternally *r*otated. Normally, the lateral leg should be able to lie flat on the examination table with the foot against the opposite knee. A positive test elicits anterior or posterior pain and indicates hip or sacroiliac joint involvement. In an athletic population, a positive FABER test has 88% sensitivity for intra-articular pathology.

198. **How do you detect a flexion contracture of the hip?**

By the *Thomas test*. This consists in asking supine patients to hold their uninvolved leg flexed against the chest (so to flatten the lumbar lordosis) while the examiner moves the symptomatic hip from full flexion to full extension. Inability to lay the affected thigh flat on the examining table (i.e., keeping it instead flexed) indicates a flexion contracture (or deformity). Conversely, a palpable deep click suggests a labral tear.

199. **How should one approach a patient with hip pain?**

By first *localizing* the pain, since anterior, lateral, and posterior pains have different etiologies.

- **Anterior hip pain** is the most common, usually due to *pathology of the joint per se* (osteoarthritis being the most common), with iliopsoas bursitis and involvement of the hip flexor muscle (strain or tendinitis) being other possibilities. *Stress fractures* and *labral tears* are instead less common causes, but not that uncommon in athletes.
- **Lateral hip pain** is usually due to greater trochanteric pain syndrome, iliotibial band syndrome, or meralgia paresthetica. *Greater trochanteric pain syndrome* is a relatively new term that includes trochanteric bursitis and gluteus medius pathology (tear or tendinitis), with the latter being possibly even more common than the former. *Iliotibial band syndrome* is due to repetitive movement of the iliotibial band over the greater trochanter. It is common in athletes. Finally, *meralgia paresthetica* is an entrapment syndrome of the lateral femoral cutaneous nerve. More frequent in middle-aged subjects, it presents with hyperesthesia in the anterolateral thigh, although 23% of patients also complain of lateral hip pain.
- **Posterior hip pain** is the least common presentation and usually suggests a source *outside* the hip joint per se, such as disease of the *lumbar spine* (e.g., degenerative disk disease, facet arthropathy, and spinal stenosis), the *sacroiliac joint,* or hip extensor and external rotator muscles. Or, more rarely, a disruption of the aortoiliac vascular supply.

200. **How should one examine the hip of a patient complaining of pain?**

By first observing the patient's gait, which is going to be *antalgic*. Then by assessing range of motion of the hip (both active and passive), and carefully comparing the affected and normal side. Hip flexion; internal and external rotation; and flexion, abduction, and external rotation (FABER) should be tested, too. The most predictive finding for *osteoarthritis* (DJD) is a decreased range of motion—especially in internal rotation or abduction. For patients with restricted movement in one plane, the sensitivity for DJD is 100% and specificity is 42%; with restricted movement in *three* planes, the sensitivity is 54% and specificity 88%, with a likelihood ratio of 4.4. To ensure that the source of pain is not muscular, muscle strength also should be tested (by doing resisted hip flexion, adduction, abduction, external rotation, and extension). Specialized hip maneuvers should then be carried out. These include not only the Thomas test, FABER, and "snapping hip," but also Ober's test. In this test, the patient lies on the side while the examiner abducts and extends the affected hip before releasing the leg *and* allowing it to drop onto the examination table. Lateral hip pain or considerable tightness may indicate iliotibial band syndrome. Finally, evaluation of hip pain should include palpation of individual structures, like hip flexor muscles, greater trochanter, iliotibial band, and gluteus medius muscle—all maneuvers that can further localize the source of pain. Tenderness over anterior soft tissues would suggest a hip flexor muscle strain (or iliopsoas bursitis), whereas tenderness over the greater trochanter would indicate a trochanteric bursitis.

J. THE KNEE

201. **How common are knee disorders?**
Very common. One of 10 adults reports knee symptoms, with pain accounting for 5% of all physicians' visits, many resulting in diagnostic imaging or subspecialty referrals.

202. **What are the main types of knee disorders?**
(1) Patellofemoral, (2) ligamentous, and (3) meniscal. Basic understanding of knee anatomy and mechanism of injury is crucial for their identification.

203. **Can history identify the site of injury?**
Yes. A careful history (and physical exam) should first of all separate knee problems due to a systemic condition from those that represent instead a *local* musculoskeletal issue. For a local problem, history can then assist the clinician in determining whether this represents a patellofemoral disorder, or a more serious meniscal or ligamentous injury. In this regard, ask the patient to pinpoint the site of pain and assess its duration and impact on activity, the presence of "pops" at the time of injury, and any swelling—especially its timing in relation to trauma. For instance, a large effusion that occurs immediately after trauma would argue in favor of hemarthrosis, most commonly due to a ligamentous lesion (like the *anterior cruciate*). Delayed (or minimal) swelling would instead suggest a meniscal *tear,* especially if associated with *locking.* "Buckling" or "giving way," whether in extension or flexion, would suggest knee instability, often due to ligamentous injury. Finally, pain going up steps, or in the anterior knee while sitting, would indicate patellofemoral dysfunction. Knowledge of the *mechanism* of injury (especially the direction of the force delivered to the knee) also is crucial.

204. **What are the main mechanisms of injury?**
They vary, depending on the type of force applied. A *valgus stress* (i.e., a force that pushes the knee *medially,* but its distal segment [the leg] *laterally*) usually strains the medial collateral ligament; conversely, a *varus stress* (i.e., a force pushing the knee *laterally,* but its distal segment [the leg] *medially*) strains instead the lateral collateral ligament. *Hyperextension* strains the anterior cruciate ligament, whereas *twisting motions* strain both ligaments *and* menisci.

205. **What is the anatomy of the knee?**
The knee is the largest joint in the body (in fact it is composed of *two* joints: the femorotibial and the patellofemoral). It articulates two *femoral condyles* with two *tibial plateaus,* in a modified hinge that relies on patella, ligaments, muscles, and tendons to achieve an extensive ROM.

206. **How many *ligaments* support the knee?**
Four, connecting the femur and tibia and thus providing dynamic stability to the joint. Two of them are external and two internal. The external (or extra-articular) ligaments are the *medial collateral* (MCL) and *lateral collateral* (LCL), which prevent the knee from moving too far from side-to-side. The MCL stretches from the medial femoral condyle to the medial tibia, whereas the LCL stretches from the lateral femoral condyle to the head of the fibula. The intra-articular ligaments are instead: (1) the *posterior cruciate* (PCL) in the front, running from the anterior portion of the femur to the posterior portion of the tibia, whereas in the back is (2) the *anterior cruciate* (ACL). These stabilize front-to-back motions of the tibia and femur, with the ACL preventing the tibia from sliding too far *forward* (hence, *hyperextension* of the knee), and the PCL doing the opposite (hence, preventing *hyperflexion* of the knee). Cruciate ligaments also aid in proprioception.

207. **What are the *menisci*?**
Two semilunar *fibrocartilaginous* ligaments that wedge between the femur and tibia. Their function is (1) to spread the weight of the body over a larger area and (2) to help the ligaments stabilize the joint. If one can imagine the knee as a ball (femur) resting on a flat plate (tibia), the menisci work like a gasket, filling the space between the *femoral condyles* and *tibial plateaus* and thus distributing the weight. Without menisci, the concentration of force onto a small area of the tibial plate would quickly damage the cartilage and lead to arthritis. Thicker on the outside than the inside, they also convert the tibial surface into a shallow socket. And since a round ball in a socket is more stable than a round ball on a flat plate, they enhance the stability of the joint. The *patellar tendon* further stabilizes the joint by connecting anteriorly the quadriceps tendon to tibia and patella. Finally, note that the medial meniscus is attached at its most medial surface to the MCL. Conversely, the lateral meniscus does not have any attachment to the LCL. This is quite important for the knee exam (*see* question 240).

208. **What are the primary *muscles* of the knee?**
The *quadriceps* and the *hamstring,* which are, respectively, the primary *extensor* and *flexor* of the leg. The hamstring lies posteriorly in the thigh, whereas the quadriceps covers instead the anterior, lateral, and medial aspects of the knee. Part of its tendon includes the patella, which sits anteriorly to the two femoral condyles, smoothly gliding over the *patellofemoral groove.*

209. **What is prepatellar bursitis?**
An inflammation of the *prepatellar bursa*—a flat, round, superficial, and fluid-filled structure between the patella, patellar tendon, and skin. Prepatellar bursitis may be due to trauma (like a fall or a direct blow to the knee), although more commonly, it is the result of overuse, like repeated kneeling. Hence, it is frequent in roofers, plumbers, carpet-layers, housemaids, nuns, and overachieving White House interns. It also can be infectious, usually from a skin break, with *Staphylococcus aureus* being the main culprit. Symptoms include knee pain, swelling, redness, and difficulty ambulating. Exam reveals erythema, crepitation, and decreased knee flexion because of pain. There also is fluctuant edema over the lower pole of the patella. Finally, there also is an *infrapatellar bursa* (anserine) just below the knee. As with prepatellar bursa, this, too, can be affected by direct or repetitive trauma.

210. **How do you examine the knee?**
The same way you examine other joints: with a thorough, systematic, and repetitive routine. Always compare side to side, starting with the *unaffected* side. Inspect, palpate, test ROM, assess gait, measure girths, and finally carry out specific maneuvers for integrity of menisci and other knee ligaments.

211. **What do you look for when inspecting the knee?**
In a standing position, look for *misalignments* between the femur, tibia, and patella. In a supine position, look instead for scars, asymmetry, swelling, redness, or chronic deformities. Evaluate the patella, patellar tendon, medial and lateral joint lines, femur, tibia, and tibial tuberositas. Use important landmarks, like *the tibial tuberosities* and the two *condyles* (lateral and medial), both located on the anterior surface of the shin. Since knee problems often limit use of the affected leg, look for wasting of the quadriceps, hamstring, and calf muscles. Finally, watch the patient walk, looking again for misalignments but also for limping or pain.

212. **What is the Q-angle (or "quadriceps angle")?**
It is not a Star Trek member of the "Continuum," but the angle between the tibia and femur—and a great tool for identifying misalignment. To calculate it, draw two lines: (1) one from the tibial tuberositas to the mid-patella and (2) the other from the mid-patella to the anterior superior iliac spine. The normal angle is 15 degrees, although it is wider in women because of their larger pelvis. Wide Q-angles reflect *genu valgus* but also increased patellofemoral contact, thus predisposing to patellofemoral disease.

213. What are the most common types of knee misalignment?

"Genu varum" and "valgum." *Varum* is an angulation of the knees away from each other. *Valgum* is instead an angulation of the knees toward each other. Both can be congenital or acquired. A less-common condition is *windswept knees*, where one knee is varum and the other valgum (*see* Fig. 21-14). If the use of these terms seems to contradict that of question 62, is because of their *etymology*, considering that in Latin *valgum* means "*knock-kneed*," while *varum* means "*bowlegged*." In other words, in a *knock-kneed* person, the femur is deviated *inward* in relation to the *hip* (and thus the term *varum* is correctly applied for the hip, since it refers to the distal segment being angled inward). Yet, in the same knock-kneed person, the opposite situation is found at the *knee*, with its distal segment (i.e., the tibia) now being deviated *outward* (so that the term *valgum* is indeed the one to use for the knee). Hence, it is correct for a knock-kneed deformity to be called both *varum* (at the hip/femur) and *valgum* (at the knee/tibia), although the common terminology is to refer to it as *genu valgum*. Conversely, in a *varum* deformity of the knee, the distal part of the leg below the knee is deviated *inward*, resulting in a *bowlegged* appearance. If this is confusing, just remember that "varum = inward" and "valgum = outward," and that both terms always refer to the direction in which the distal part of the joint points. When the terminology specifies a bone rather than a joint, the bone is taken to be the distal segment of a joint. Thus, a varum deformity of the tibia refers to the femur/tibia joint (the knee) and not to the ankle.

214. Can osteoarthritis cause misalignment of the knee?

Yes. And since it usually affects the *medial* aspect of the joint, it causes primarily *bowing*.

215. How do you demonstrate patellar tracking?

Ask the patient to sit. Then extend the knee, while keeping your finger over the patellar midpoint. During extension, the patella should remain midline in the femoral groove. Any

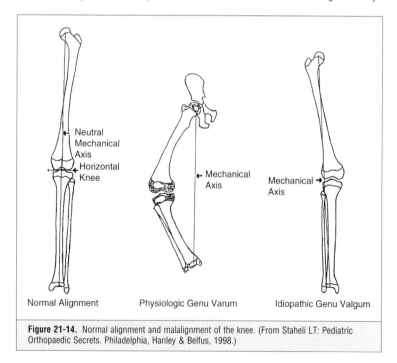

Figure 21-14. Normal alignment and malalignment of the knee. (From Staheli LT: Pediatric Orthopaedic Secrets. Philadelphia, Hanley & Belfus, 1998.)

medial or lateral movement indicates knee misalignment. This, in turn, may predispose to *patellofemoral disease*.

216. **What is patellofemoral syndrome (disease)?**
A constellation of symptoms due to malposition of the knee, resulting in increased/misdirected mechanical forces on the undersurface of the patella. This can be due to unbalanced muscle pull, misalignment between joint surfaces, or excessive knee valgus (i.e., increased Q-angle) with increased lateral forces. All eventually affect the patellofemoral interface and cause the retropatellar cartilage to wear down (*chondromalacia*).

217. **What are the symptoms and findings of patellofemoral disease?**
The most common is knee pain, which is retropatellar and typically triggered by activities requiring knee flexion and forceful contraction of the quadriceps (like squatting or ascending/descending stairs). Pain also is exacerbated by sitting with the knee flexed for a protracted period, such as when driving the car or watching a movie. Hence, the terms "theater sign" and "movie-goer's knee." In fact, these patients often prefer to sit in an aisle seat, where they can keep the knee extended for longer periods. On exam, there may be tenderness along the facets of the patella, the tibial tuberositas, or the patellar tendon. Note that pain elicited *lateral* to the patella usually indicates pathology over the insertion of the iliotibial band; conversely, pain elicited *medial* to the patella (i.e., at the insertion of the medial hamstring) indicates anserine bursal tenderness.

218. **What is *anserine bursitis*?**
A common cause of *anterior knee pain* in athletes or patients. The pes anserine *(goosefoot)* bursa is located with its associated medial hamstring tendons along the proximomedial aspect of the tibia. In case of tight hamstrings, bursitis can ensue, although this also may be due to direct trauma. Pain along the medial aspect of the knee is the presenting complaint. On exam, there is tenderness over the bursa, which is located slightly distal to the tibial tuberositas and two finger breadths medial to it. Management is usually conservative.

219. **How do you test for patellofemoral syndrome?**
With the patient supine, slightly flex the leg to be tested, so that the quadriceps is relaxed. Then, gently push down on the patella with both thumbs, or try to palpate its undersurface. Pain on either of these maneuvers suggests chondromalacia. Now move the patella across the femur: medially, laterally, superiorly, and inferiorly. Crepitus or pain on passive motion also suggests patellofemoral disease. Finally, measure the Q-angle, since wider angles may predispose to it.

220. **What is an *extension lag* of the knee?**
The inability to *actively* extend a knee that can be passively extended by the examiner—another sign of patellofemoral disease. A *flexion contracture* is instead the inability to *passively* extend the knee, a common finding in *intrinsic* knee disease.

221. **What is the *patellar inhibition test* (patellofemoral grinding test)?**
It is patellar pain upon isometric contraction of the quadriceps—an important *apprehension sign* and another clue to patellofemoral disease. To elicit it, have the patient lie supine and with the leg extended. After applying some suprapatellar resistance (i.e., holding the patella in place with one hand), have the patient contract the quadriceps. This will press the inferior surface of the patella onto the femur, thus eliciting pain or crepitus in cases of chondromalacia.

222. **What is the role of palpation?**
Tenderness on palpation reflects different processes based on location:
- If along the joint line, it suggests *meniscal tears*.

- If along the medial side of the knee (and extending above and below the joint line), it suggests *collateral ligament* injury, although this also may be incidental in some morbidly obese subjects. If over the medial femoral condyle, it suggests *osteonecrosis*.
- If over the medial tibial plateau, it suggests *anserine bursitis, stress fractures of the plateau,* or *osteonecrosis*.
- If over the patella, it suggests instead *prepatellar bursitis*—especially if associated with warmth and redness.

223. **How do you palpate the knee?**
Ask patients to sit with the knees slightly flexed, since this prevents other stabilizing elements of the joint from interfering with the exam. Examine the tibial tuberosity, and then move along each side of the tibial plateau, up toward the medial and lateral femoral condyles. Feel the patella.

224. **How do you evaluate the knee's range of motion?**
With a goniometer, and by comparing the affected to the unaffected side.
- **Active ROM:** Have patients bend the knee (flexion); then completely rest it back on the table (extension). Full flexion is 140 degrees; full extension is 0 degrees. A hyperextension of 15 degrees may be normal.
- **Passive ROM:** Grasp the patient's ankle and bend the knee, noting the extent of flexion and extension. If any of these elicits pain, stop and note the point in ROM where it occurred.
- **Crepitus:** Place your hand on the patella, and feel for any crackling sensation during motion. If present, these indicate loss of normal smooth movement between articulating structures, such as the femur, tibia, and patella—an important sign of degenerative joint disease (DJD).

225. **What is osteoarthritis of the knee?**
A common event in large, weight-bearing, and synovial joints. One fourth of people between 55 and 64 show signs in their knees (*gonarthrosis*), while 23% have it in the hip (*coxarthrosis*). Prevalence reaches 39% and 23%, respectively, at ages 65–74, and totality at 75–79.

226. **What is the mechanism of osteoarthritis?**
Trauma, either direct or cumulative. The latter is typical of weight-bearing joints like the knee, and it is due to years of recurrent wear-and-tear. A healthy synovial joint normally allows a significant amount of motion along its extremely smooth articular surface. To do so, it relies on a synovial membrane, an articular (or hyaline) cartilage, an underlying (subchondral) bone, an overlying joint capsule, and plenty of synovial fluid. Osteoarthritis primarily affects the *articular cartilage,* eventually forming tears, first small and then large. With time, these lead to fragmentation into the joint, exposure of the underlying bone, formation of osteophytes, and cystic degeneration of the subchondral bone. Ultimately, the joint undergoes mechanical deformation, resulting in misalignment, instability, and further degeneration.

227. **What are the symptoms of gonarthrosis?**
The classic one is *pain*, insidious, ache-like, and typically worsened by activity/relieved by rest. With time, this becomes persistent and more debilitating. There also may be damage to ligaments or menisci. On exam, the joint may be warm, with crepitus, effusion, and reduced ROM. Gait is often antalgic. Note that gonarthrosis can involve the medial, central, or lateral compartment of the knee—individually or together. Yet, precise location is often difficult to determine on simple exam. Imaging can be much more accurate.

228. **How do you detect knee effusions?**
It depends on the amount. Large effusions can be detected by simple inspection or basic palpation. Inflammatory effusions (like those of infection, gout, or RA) are often associated with *inflammation,* and thus with warmth, redness, and painful movements. Smaller effusions are

instead harder to detect, except for the *bulge sign* (or *milking*), which can identify <15 mL of intra-articular fluid but remain absent in larger effusions. Bulging is demonstrated by a two-step test:

- First stroke upward 2–3 times along the *medial* aspect of the knee. This will "milk" fluid into the suprapatellar pouch (i.e., the superior and lateral aspects of the joint).
- Then push down along the *lateral* side of the knee (from proximal to distal). This will squeeze the fluid back into the medial aspect of the joint, causing the skin to bulge out slightly.

229. **What about intermediate-sized effusions?**
They require either patellar ballottement or the fluid wave test.
- **Ballottement:** With the patient supine, flex slightly the knee and then use the thumb and index finger of one hand to embrace the suprapatellar pouch (located above the patella and communicating with the joint space). Push *down and toward the patella,* forcing any fluid into the central part of the joint. Then, push down on the patella with the thumb of your other hand. In cases of effusion, you will appreciate (1) a palpable click (due to the patellar collision against the femur) and (2) a bouncing back up of the patella itself.
- **Fluid wave (shift) test:** Place one hand around the suprapatellar pouch, and then use the other to squeeze the knee. In cases of effusion, you will appreciate a fluid wave in the suprapatellar area.

230. **What are the mechanisms of ligament injuries?**
- **Cruciate ligaments:** The ACL is typically injured during traumatic *twisting*, wherein the tibia moves forward to the femur, often in association with a valgus stress. Although the foot is usually planted, no direct blow to knee or leg is required. Approximately one half of all patients with ACL injuries also have meniscal tears. PCL injuries are instead 10–20 times less common than ACL injuries, representing less than 7% of all acute knee injuries. They also occur during twisting with a planted foot, but their force of injury is directed instead *posteriorly* against the tibia, while the knee is flexed.
- **Collateral ligaments:** The most common injury results from abduction and external rotation of a knee that is either extended or slightly flexed. An intact MCL helps the ACL in preventing posterior motion of the femur. An injured MCL may instead allow an anterior subluxation of the tibial plateau during flexion, especially in an ACL-deficient patient.
Note that given the forces involved, *ligamentous* tears are often associated with *meniscal* tears. It also is possible to tear more than one ligament at once, with the most common combination being MCL and ACL. Hence, always do a comprehensive exam.

231. **What are the symptoms of ligamentous injuries?**
Usually acute pain, swelling, and often a "pop" (reflecting the tearing of the ligament). After these subside, pain and instability can occur upon movements that require use of the damaged ligament—such as rotation, which now becomes unimpeded.

232. **How does the function of *cruciate* ligaments relate to symptoms?**
- The **ACL** prevents *anterior* motion of the tibia on the femur. Hence, its injury causes an abnormal forward slide of the tibial plateau, giving the feeling that the knee is buckling, or "giving out." Although this may occur with normal walking, it is usually most prominent during pivoting movements, such as quick changes in direction. Injury to the ACL also may cause loss of confidence in the knee's stability, possibly because of its role in proprioception.
- The **PCL** limits the *posterior* displacement of the tibia on the femur. Hence, its injury causes the tibia to slide back. This may occur during knee flexion, or result in hyperextension of the knee, with varus (bowlegged) and valgus (knock-kneed) angulations. There also may be knee buckling, especially during pivoting motions, or when descending stairs.

233. **Which maneuvers test the *anterior cruciate* ligaments?**
(1) Lachman's test, (2) the anterior drawer test, and (3) the lateral pivot shift (or Macintosh) test.

234. **How do you perform the *Lachman maneuver*?**
Have the patient supine, with the knee flexed to 20–30 degrees, and heel on the table toward you. Stand on the patient's side, and hold the femur with your left hand, just above the knee, firmly enough to prevent any movement of the upper leg but gently enough to allow for the hamstrings to relax. Then, use your right hand to pull the proximal tibia *up toward you*, while at the same time stabilizing the femur with your left hand. An intact ACL will limit the amount of distraction by providing a firm end-point. Now reverse your hand position, and repeat the maneuver on the other leg. Compare responses. The test is positive when the end-point is not discrete, or the tibia moves excessively forward (anterior subluxation). Note that Lachman requires a good grasp of the leg; hence, it may be difficult to perform when the patient has large legs or the physician has small hands. In this case, have the patient's leg *hang off* the side of the table.

235. **How do you perform the *anterior drawer test*?**
Have the patient supine, hip flexed to 45 degrees, knee to 90 degrees, and foot/heel resting flat on the table. Stabilize the foot by sitting on its dorsum. Wrap your hands around the knee, with fingers embracing the medial and lateral insertion of the hamstrings and thumbs on the tibial tuberositas, along the medial and lateral joint line. Make sure that the hamstrings are relaxed, then quickly pull and push the proximal part of the leg, testing the degree of distraction of the tibia in relation to the femur. Do these maneuvers in three positions of tibial rotation: neutral, 30 degrees externally rotated, and 30 degrees internally rotated. An intact ACL will provide a *discrete end-point*, abruptly stopping the tibia's forward movement as the ligament reaches its maximum length. No more than 6–8 mm of laxity should be allowed. A positive anterior drawer sign results instead in an unrestrained *forward* motion (i.e., anterior subluxation of the tibia on the femur), indicating a possible tear of the ACL. As always, compare the affected to the unaffected side.

236. **How do you perform the *lateral pivot shift* test?**
By combining a valgus stress (pushing the outside of the knee *medially*) with a twisting force onto a knee that is being flexed. Ask the patient to lay supine, with the affected knee extended and the tibia internally rotated. Place one hand on the lateral aspect of the knee, and push *medially* (thus creating a valgus strain), while at the same time supporting and pulling *laterally* the foot with your other hand. As you slowly flex the knee, keep the foot internally rotated. In a positive test, the tibia "jumps" anteriorly at 10–30 degrees flexion, with an obvious "thud" or "clunk." This indicates the inability of the ACL to prevent anterior subluxation of the tibia onto the femur.

237. **How do you assess the *posterior cruciate* ligaments?**
Through (1) the posterior drawer test and (2) the tibial sag test.

238. **How do you perform the *posterior drawer* test?**
Very much like the anterior drawer test (i.e., with knee flexed at 90 degrees, foot resting flat on the table, and you sitting lightly on it), except that this time instead of pulling the leg *forward*, you should push it *backward*. An intact PCL will give a discrete end-point, whereas a torn PCL will allow unrestrained backward movement of the tibia in relation to the femur.

239. **How do you perform the *tibial sag* test?**
Have the patient flex both knees and hips at 90 degrees; then hold the legs in position by grasping the ankles. Inspect the tibial plateaus for asymmetry. The test is suggestive of PCL tear if one plateau sinks below the patella (i.e., "sagging" in comparison to the other).

240. How do you assess the *collateral* ligaments?

Hold the knee in your hand, freely relaxed and in approximately 15 degrees of flexion (to avoid locking in full extension). Apply first a varus stress (pressure on the *medial* aspect of the joint to test the lateral collateral ligament, LCL), and then a valgus stress (pressure on the *lateral* aspect of the knee, to test the medial collateral ligament, MCL). More specifically, for the MCL, push inward with your left hand along the lateral aspect of the knee, while at the same time applying an opposite force with your right hand. If the MCL is completely torn, the joint will "open up" along the medial aspect. For the LCL, do the opposite: place your right hand along the medial aspect of the knee, place your left hand on the ankle or calf, and push outward with your right hand while applying an opposite force with your left. If the LCL is completely torn, the joint will "open up" along the lateral aspect. An alternative way to test the collateral ligaments consists in cradling the lower leg, and then pressing with your fingers first to the lateral side of the knee (to test the medial collateral ligament) and then to the medial side (to test the lateral collateral ligament). Do this first with the knee flexed at 15 degrees and then at 30 degrees. Any pain or abnormal opening of the joint space indicates instability. When used for the MCL, this maneuver eliminates the medial meniscus from contributing to knee stability and thus tests primarily the MCL.

241. How accurate are these maneuvers?

There is no adequate information for the diagnostic accuracy of maneuvers testing the integrity of *collateral* ligaments. Conversely, the composite exam for tears of *cruciate* ligaments is highly predictive—at least as performed by orthopedic physicians. More specifically:

- **Anterior cruciate ligament:** A *composite* examination for ACL injuries has sensitivity >82% and specificity >94%, with a likelihood ratio (LR) of 25.0 for a positive examination and 0.04 for a negative one. As for individual maneuvers, the anterior drawer test has mean specificity of 67%, with an LR for a positive exam of 3.8 and for a negative exam of 0.30. Lachman is more sensitive than the anterior drawer test, but more difficult to perform. It has a mean sensitivity of 84%, and a specificity that in one study was 100%, LR for a positive test of 42.0, and for a negative test of 0. Finally, the lateral pivot shift test has mean sensitivity of 38% and unknown specificity. Overall, a positive Lachman argues strongly in favor of ACL tear, whereas a negative is fairly good evidence against it. The anterior drawer is the least accurate test.
- **Posterior cruciate ligament:** A *composite* examination for PCL injuries has sensitivity of 91%, specificity of 98%, and LRs of 21.0 (for a positive exam) and 0.05 (for a negative one). The posterior drawer test is the most reliable indicator, with mean sensitivity of 55%.

242. How common are meniscal injuries?

They are the most common knee injury, with more than 1.7 million repairs/resections per year. Many eventually cause joint instability, accelerated DJD, and need for knee replacement.

243. What is their mechanism?

Although at times degenerative, meniscal injuries are more frequently due to *trauma*. Hence, they affect primarily young individuals as a result of either aggressive sports (soccer, football, basketball, and occasionally baseball) or labor activities that predispose to rotational injuries. In sports, most meniscal tears are not due to contact, but to *deceleration*, like landing after a jump, squatting, and twisting. In fact, the most common mechanism is a varus or valgus force onto a flexed knee, with valgus tearing the medial meniscus, and varus tearing the lateral one. Traumatic meniscal injuries also are associated with *collateral ligament tears* (ACL more than PCL). Degenerative meniscal tears occur instead with minimal or no trauma—hence, they are more common in older patients.

244. What is the best way to evaluate a meniscal injury?

Definitely imaging, since all lesions can be visualized by MRI (which is even better than arthroscopy). Yet, meniscal injuries also can be assessed by a series of bedside maneuvers. In fact, in a series of 100 tears confirmed by arthroscopy the clinical diagnosis was correct in 87 cases, correct but incomplete in four, and incorrect in nine.

245. **What are the symptoms of meniscal tear? What are their causes?**
Symptoms are typically due to a torn piece of cartilage interrupting the normal smooth movement of the knee. This can cause acute pain, swelling, and movement limitation, such as joint "locking" or instability (i.e., "giving out"). It also can cause knee *effusion,* usually over hours, but more rapidly in case of hemarthrosis. Finally, denudation of the bone may eventually lead to degenerative arthritis. In the same aforementioned series of 100 cases, repeated popping occurred in 43%, swelling in 51%, and pain localized to the joint line in 63%. Joint effusion has a sensitivity for meniscal tear of 35% and a specificity of 100%.

246. **What are the physical findings of a meniscal tear?**
  - **Antalgic gait.** Limping is very common, since patients may be unable to bear weight and thus exhibit antalgic deviations or compensatory movements.
  - **Effusion** may be evident on knee *inspection* and be subsequently confirmed by ballottement or the fluid wave test.
  - **Atrophy of the quadriceps** may result from long-standing injury and the patient's inability to achieve full extension.
  - **Knee girth** can help identify effusions and atrophy. It should be measured at *the joint line* if looking for effusion, at 5 and 20 cm proximal to the base of the patella if looking for quadriceps' atrophy, and at 15 cm distal to the apex of the patella if looking for calf atrophy.
  - On **palpation,** the most accurate finding is localized tenderness at the joint line. To detect it, ask the patient to slightly flex the knee, then identify the joint line and gently palpate along its medial and lateral margins. Note that (1) the maneuver only assesses the part of the meniscus that is near the joint line (the remainder is not examinable) and (2) location of tenderness is not a fail-proof indication of the type of meniscal lesion.
  - **Locking.** If an anterior tear blocks the motion, there may be difficulty extending the knee. This limits ROM to 20–45 degrees of joint extension, with clicks or snaps after it unlocks arguing strongly for a meniscal lesion (*bounce home test*). Conversely, a posterior tear may render a full flexion painful or just impossible, as in squatting (*Childress test*).
  - **Forced knee flexion** may instead cause medial or lateral pain.
  - Finally, popliteal masses or cysts should be searched for, since a **Baker's cyst** (*see* questions 255 and 256) often coexists with chronic meniscal tears.

247. **In addition to tenderness over the joint line, what other maneuvers can detect meniscal tears?**
(1) Medial-lateral grind test, (2) McMurray test, and (3) Apley's grind and distraction test. Positive results on any of these tests do not necessarily establish the presence of meniscal lesions, but, along with other findings, may help differentiate a tear from other knee injuries.

248. **How do you perform the *medial-lateral grind* test?**
With patients supine, cradle in one hand the calf of the affected leg and place the index finger and thumb of the opposite hand over the joint line. Then apply valgus and varus stresses to the tibia during flexion and extension. The test is positive if you detect a medial-lateral grind over the joint line.

249. **What is the Mc*Murray test*? How do you perform it?**
McMurray is a test of meniscal tears of the middle or posterior horn. For tears of the *medial* meniscus, apply a valgus force and *externally* rotate the foot while extending the knee. For tears of the *lateral* meniscus, apply instead a varus force and *internally* rotate the foot while extending the knee. More specifically: with patients supine and the right knee and hip fully flexed, place your left thumb on the lateral joint margin, while keeping middle, index, and ring fingers aligned along the medial margins. Then use the right hand to passively extend the leg, flex it, and extend it again, but this time with an external rotation of the leg. To do so, first turn the ankle so that the foot points outward (*everted*). Then point the knee outward (*valgus*

stress). In this everted position, first extend and then flex the knee. The test is positive for *medial* meniscal injury when (1) it elicits pain with extension of the knee and external rotation of the leg; (2) it elicits a palpable, audible click or pop over the meniscus; or (3) it elicits locking of the knee. After this is done, flex and extend the knee again, but this time after *internal* rotation. To do so, turn the foot inward (*inversion*), and then direct the knee so that it points inward as well (*varus stress*). Once again, the test is indicative of *lateral* meniscal injury when (1) it elicits pain with extension of the knee and internal rotation of the leg, (2) it elicits a palpable click over the meniscus, or (3) it elicits locking of the knee. Pops, snaps, and clicks are produced as the torn meniscal fragment rides over the femoral condyle during extension. An audible or palpable pop in extreme flexion indicates a posterior horn tear; a click at 90 degrees of flexion indicates a lesion in the midsection of the meniscus.

250. **What is the *Apley's grind and distraction* test? How do you perform it?**
Apley's is a test of meniscal tears in the posterior horn of either the medial or lateral meniscus that also can differentiate meniscal from ligamentous injuries. It consists of rotation *and* compression of the knee. With the patient prone, grab the heel with one hand and flex the knee to 90 degrees. Start with the "grind" part of the test: *compress* the knee (by applying downward pressure on the foot), while at the same time rotating the foot internally and externally. Pain during *this* part of the test indicates a *meniscal* tear. Then *distract* the knee by *rotating* the foot internally and externally, but this time *pull up* on the foot. Since traction on the leg removes pressure on the meniscus, pain during this part of the test indicates instead *ligamentous* involvement.

251. **Who were these folks?**
 - **Thomas Porter McMurray** (1886–1949) was a Belfast-born and educated orthopedist, who taught and practiced in Liverpool for most his life (as first professor of Orthopedics at the local University), until dying suddenly in a railway station at age 63. More than for his writings, he was famous for his lightning-speed skills, which allowed him to remove an entire meniscus in 5 minutes and disarticulate a hip in 10 minutes. He reported his eponymous maneuver in 1938, in an article titled "Observation of Internal Derangement of the Knee" (which borrowed on a term used by Hey in a famous 1803 paper).
 - **Alan Graham Apley** (1914–1996) also was a British orthopedist (plus skier, sportsman, and accomplished self-taught pianist). The youngest son of a Jewish immigrant from Poland who had served in the Tsar's army (and returned home to collect his wife), Apley was born in London and served with the Royal Army Medical Corps in Burma during World War II, where he was wounded. After the war, he became a consultant at the Rowley Bristow Orthopaedic Hospital, where he created a course that, thanks to his showmanship, became legendary.

252. **How accurate are these tests?**
Not as accurate as the maneuvers for evaluation of ligamentous injuries. Using arthroscopy as a reference standard, bedside evaluation has sensitivity of 77% and specificity of 91%, with a positive LR of 2.7 and a negative LR of 0.4. Still, one third of meniscal tears may be missed by clinical screening. Moreover, exam cannot demonstrate location, shape, or length of the tear—something that MRI does instead very well. As for individual findings, joint-line tenderness has a mean sensitivity of 79% and a specificity of 15%, with an LR of 0.9 for a positive test and 1.1 for a negative test. Hence, it is not a super finding, even though its accuracy may be greater for tears of the *lateral* meniscus as compared to those of the medial one. Of the various maneuvers, the medial-lateral grind test is the most accurate, with sensitivity of 69% and specificity of 86%; McMurray is most helpful when positive, with a sensitivity and specificity of 53% and 59%, respectively, and a positive LR of 1.3 and a negative LR of 0.8. Apley has instead a sensitivity so low (about 16%) that many authors even discourage its use. In a series of 100 meniscal tears, at least one of these maneuvers was positive in 79% of the cases. Yet, accuracy may decrease significantly in patients with multiple knee lesions (down to 30%). For example, in cases of acute ACL tear, the sensitivity for associated medial meniscus tear is 45%

and for lateral meniscus tear is 58%. Finally, concomitant presence of a joint effusion lowers the sensitivity for meniscal tear to 35% (specificity, though, is a solid 100%). Overall, exam is more specific than sensitive.

253. **When should x-rays be ordered?**

When the *Ottawa Knee Rules* are met: (1) age 55 or older, (2) tenderness at the head of the fibula, (3) isolated tenderness of the patella, (4) inability to flex the knee to 90 degrees, and (5) inability to take four weight-bearing steps (regardless of limping), both at the time of injury and in the exam room. "Ottawa" does not apply to children. In fact, anyone younger than 12 should have x-rays.

254. **How is *quadriceps atrophy* detected?**

By palpating the quadriceps above the knee and comparing its muscle bulk to the uninvolved side. To quantify atrophy, measure the quadriceps circumference at a point that is 5 *and* 20 cm above the upper pole of the patella. For more subtle atrophies, ask the patient to contract the quadriceps. This will accentuate its anatomy and allow better appreciation of unilateral muscle loss.

255. **What is a Baker's (popliteal) cyst? Where can it be palpated?**

Baker's is a *synovial cyst* (i.e., a collection of fluid that has escaped the joint and collected into a new sac in the popliteal space). First described in 1877 by the English surgeon William Morrant Baker, who reported eight cases, this periarticular cyst represents the most common popliteal mass. It is around 3 cm^3 in size and is often encountered in patients with either inflammatory or degenerative arthritides. To feel it, ask the patient to partially flex the knee, and then palpate the popliteal fossa behind the medial femoral condyle, between the medial head of the gastrocnemius and the semi-membranous bursa. The cyst will present as a fluctuant popliteal swelling. In 10% of patients, it will evolve into a *pseudothrombophlebitis syndrome*.

256. **What is the pseudothrombophlebitis syndrome?**

A syndrome characterized by dissection of a Baker's cyst down the leg and into the calf. This results into swelling and tenderness, often mimicking thrombophlebitis—hence, the term, *pseudothrombophlebitis*. Note that the cyst can also *rupture*. In this case, it presents as an enlarging mass in the calf, with fluid draining down the fascial plane, causing exquisite leg pain, calf swelling, and erythema, plus a crescent-shaped ecchymosis at the medial or lateral malleolus (*crescent sign*). Of interest, the presence of a Baker's cyst per se may predispose to true thrombophlebitis—by compressing the surrounding vein.

K. THE ANKLE AND THE FOOT

257. **What is the function of the ankle?**

The ankle serves as a hinge, which has to support 1.5 times the body weight while walking and up to 8 times while running. Hence, despite being rather sturdy, it is a common site of injury, especially in athletes. A thorough knowledge of the anatomy is key for an accurate diagnosis.

258. **What is the anatomy of the ankle?**

The ankle comprises three bones: distal tibia, distal fibula, and talus. The distal tibia articulates with the talus on its concave plafond, forming the medial malleolus in its inner aspect. The distal fibula articulates with both the talus and distal tibia, forming the lateral malleolus in its outer portion. The malleoli serve as buttresses of the talus, while the talus is the real *hinge*, allowing the foot to *dorsiflex* and *plantarflex*. It comprises a head, neck, and body, with several tubercles arising from the latter. One, the lateral tubercle, arises from the os trigonum. This is a separate ossification center that occasionally may remain unfused, thus causing a painful impingement syndrome. Finally, the talus joins the *calcaneus* on its lower aspect.

259. **How do you approach a patient with ankle injury?**
By determining the *mechanism* of injury, since this can narrow the differential diagnosis. To do so, separate inversion from eversion, plantar flexion, dorsiflexion, or a combination thereof. Also, determine whether the affected joint was previously injured, and what treatment might have been given. Finally, always compare the affected to the unaffected leg (and remove all socks and shoes).

260. **What should one look for in the ankle exam?**
For deformities and swelling, since these may help localizing the affected structure. ROM should then be tested, and compared to the unaffected side.

261. **How do you test ROM?**
By using a goniometer, while the patient sits on the exam table with legs freely hanging down. Test both active and passive dorsiflexion (20 degrees) and plantar flexion (50 degrees).

262. **What ankle structures should be palpated?**
- The **medial aspect of the ankle** comprises the medial malleolus, the deltoid ligament, and the structures just below it. First, palpate the medial malleolus and its posterior border. Then ascend proximally to 6 cm from its distal tip and palpate the deltoid ligament (which runs as a thick structure distally to the medial malleolus). Pain along this course usually suggests injury. Yet, since the deltoid ligament is rarely injured in isolation, any lesion of it should raise suspicion for concomitant pathologies.
- The **lateral aspect of the ankle** consists instead of the lateral malleolus and its three supporting ligaments: (1) the anterior talofibular ligament (near the anterior joint line), (2) the posterior talofibular ligament (from the posterior part of the fibula to a small tubercle on the posterior aspect of the talus), and (3) the calcaneofibular ligament (between the lateral malleolus and a tubercle on the calcaneus). Note that the lateral ankle ligaments are not as thick as the deltoid ligament. Hence, they are more prone to injury. In addition, since the lateral malleolus is longer than the medial malleolus, the talus is more prone to *invert* than evert.
- Finally, examine the **fifth metatarsal,** since this, too, can be injured with the ankle. Tenderness in this area may indicate a fracture/avulsion of the peroneal tendon at its insertion site.

263. **How do you identify an injury of the lateral ligaments?**
By palpation. Since lateral ligaments are thin enough to be very difficult to palpate in isolation, pain on palpation (or even simple swelling) usually indicates injury. Of the three ligaments, the one most prone to injury is the *anterior talofibular*. The *calcaneofibular ligament* is instead torn only after the anterior talofibular ligament, usually resulting in ankle instability. Finally, the *posterior talofibular ligament* is only torn with massive trauma, as in cases of ankle dislocation.

264. **How do you assess the anterior talofibular ligament?**
Through the *anterior drawer test*. To carry this out, have the patient sit on the edge of the bed with the legs freely dangling down. Place one hand on the lower tibia, and wrap the other around the heel. Then pull the heel *forward*, while pushing the tibia backward. The test is positive when the talus moves anteriorly, suggesting a tear of the anterior talofibular ligament. Compare sides.

265. **What is the "talar tilt" test?**
A test of combined anterior talofibular and calcaneofibular tear, an injury severe enough to cause major lateral ankle instability. To carry this out, have the patient sit on the edge of the bed with the legs freely dangling down. Grasp the heel with one hand, and evert the foot while stabilizing the tibia. The test is positive when the talus rocks within the joint.

266. **What is the cause of pain posterior to the fibula?**
Pain behind the fibula and lateral malleolus usually indicates peroneal tendon pathology. This may be confirmed by palpating the posterior fibular groove, while actively resisting dorsiflexion and eversion of the foot.

267. **What is the "squeeze test"?**
A maneuver that identifies injury of the syndesmosis connecting the tibia and fibula. To perform this test, place your hand midway along the lower leg, and gently squeeze tibia and fibula together. Pain along the anterior joint line of the ankle indicates syndesmosis pathology.

268. **When should x-rays be ordered?**
When the Ottawa Ankle Rules are met: (1) inability to take four weight-bearing steps immediately after injury or at the time of the exam and (2) pain with palpation of the lateral or medial malleoli and 6 cm proximally along the tibia and fibula.

269. **What are pes cavus and pes planus?**
The two most common foot deformities (Fig. 21-15). A *pes cavus* has an abnormally high longitudinal arch, whereas a *planus* has lost the arch completely (i.e., flat foot). This loss may be flexible or fixed, insofar as a flexible flat foot has some discernible arch at rest, but loses it with weight-bearing, whereas a fixed flat foot lacks the arch even at rest.

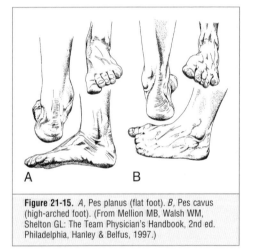

Figure 21-15. *A*, Pes planus (flat foot). *B*, Pes cavus (high-arched foot). (From Mellion MB, Walsh WM, Shelton GL: The Team Physician's Handbook, 2nd ed. Philadelphia, Hanley & Belfus, 1997.)

270. **What ankle deformity is associated with pes planus?**
An *inversion* of the ankle, also called *valgus* or *pronation*. This can be easily appreciated by observing the patient in a standing position. There will be a variable degree of inward rotation of the medial malleolus, and the patient will admit to walking on the inside of the foot.

271. **What are the typical changes of the *rheumatoid* foot?**
Several. RA can in fact cause extensive deformities: (1) pes planus with pronation deformity of the ankle, (2) loss of the anterior arch with widening of the foot, (3) hallux valgus, (4) cock-up deformities of the toes (hammer toes), (5) dropped metatarsal heads, and (6) rheumatoid nodules.

272. **What are hammer toes?**
They are *cock-up* toes, the price the civilized man has paid for the privilege of wearing shoes—usually *short* shoes. Cock-up deformities are caused by ligamentous instability, which in turn leads to subluxation of the *metatarsophalangeal* (MTP) joints and compensatory flexion at the proximal interphalangeal (PIP) joints. Often, the toe no longer touches the floor when the patient stands. As for semantics, a *hammertoe* deformity is characterized by an upward-cocked MTP and a downward-bent PIP. A *claw toe* deformity is one characterized by a cocked-up MTP, but PIP and DIP that are both curled downward—like a claw.

273. **What is hallux valgus? What are bunions?**

Hallux valgus is a common deformity of the big toe, characterized by lateral deviation (i.e., away from the midline—*valgus*) and toward the second toe. Osteophytes may be palpable at the joint line. When the deviation is extreme, there may be a palpable bump (bunion) over the medial border of the first MTP joint, caused by a *varus* (i.e., inward) deviation of the first metatarsal. As a result, the second toe may even override the first toe. This bunion is actually just a fluid-filled bursa, which with time may become inflamed (bursitis). Of interest, hallux valgus and bunion almost never occur in societies that go shoeless. Pointed shoes, such as high heels and cowboy boots, are major culprits in its development. Inelegant but wide shoes, with plenty of room for the toes, reduce the risk of developing the deformity and help reduce the irritation on the bunion if already in place. But they also may get you fewer dates.

274. **Describe the findings with dropped metatarsal heads.**

A dropped metatarsal head is a condition wherein one of the metatarsal bones (usually the second metatarsal) is lower than the rest at the distal end (i.e., subluxated), and can now be palpated along the plantar surface of the foot. Subluxation of the heads is a typical foot deformity of *rheumatoid arthritis*. In this regard, overpronation may play a role, since abnormal weight distributions in an abnormally pronated foot does tend to throw too much weight to the second metatarsal. With more severe degrees of subluxation, the protrusion of the bone is not only palpable, but visible, too. There also may be thickening of the plantar skin (calluses) over the protruding bone. Patients usually complain of pain and the sensation of walking on a stone.

275. **What are corns?**

Areas of skin thickening that develop over toes as a result of chronic mechanical irritation, most commonly from ill-fitting shoes or foot deformities that make shoe-fitting difficult. *Hard corns* develop over interphalangeal joints when a cock-up deformity causes pressure against the shoe. *Soft corns* are instead areas of *interphalangeal* skin thickening, caused by the abnormal pressure as the toes move against each other.

276. **What is Morton's neuroma? How is it demonstrated?**

Morton's is not a true neuroma but rather a perineural fibrosis and nerve degeneration of the common digital nerve (Fig. 21-16). This also is the result of repetitive friction, usually from ill-fitting shoes. It develops most frequently between the third and fourth metatarsal heads (i.e., third web space), but is also found in the second web space. Morton first described it in 1876:

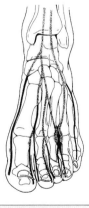

> Patients complain that, as they walk, they are suddenly seized with an agonizing pain at the outer border of their forefoot. They have to stop still and stand on their good foot; they take their shoe off and rub the painful area. After some minutes the pain ceases, but the foot becomes warm and stays so for several hours. When the pain has gone, they are able to walk comfortably. They may experience two attacks in a week then none for a year. Recurrences are variable and tend to become more frequent. Between attacks, there are no symptoms or physical signs.

This Dr. Thomas George Morton (1835–1903) was a Philadelphia born and educated surgeon, who became head physician of many local hospitals (including St. Mary's, Wills Eye,

Figure 21-16.
Morton's neuroma. (From Mellion MB, Walsh WM, Shelton GL: The Team Physician's Handbook, 2nd ed. Philadelphia, Hanley & Belfus, 1997.)

and the Pennsylvania Hospital), until dying of cholera at age 68. Active during the American Civil War, he was for most of his life a hospital administrator, but also a charismatic teacher and an excellent practitioner. In fact, he was one of the first surgeons who were able to remove an appendix after a correct diagnosis, and see the patient survive. His eponymous condition is a rather frequent one, affecting females five times more than males (because of narrower and more pointed shoes?). The most common presentation is sharp and burning pain in the forefoot and toes adjacent to the neuroma. There also may be numbness, often during episodes of pain. In fact, pain is typically intermittent, single or in multiple attacks, with episodes lasting minutes to hours and followed by asymptomatic periods of weeks to months. Patients often describe the sensation of "walking on a marble." Firm squeezing of the metatarsal head with one hand, while applying direct pressure to the dorsal and plantar interspace with the other hand, may reproduce the pain. Conversely, palpation of the actual neuroma is rarely successful.

277. What is the Achilles tendon? What is Achilles tendinitis?

The Achilles tendon is properly named after the "almost" indestructible Achaean warrior, since this is the largest and strongest tendon in the body, but also a weak spot that could lead to demise, like in the case of its namesake. "Achilles tendinitis" is a spectrum of tendon injuries, ranging from inflammation to rupture. Rupture is usually due to overuse, though deconditioning, overtraining, inadequate footwear, use of poor running surfaces, and predisposing intrinsic factors (such as age, pes cavus, and varus deformities) also may play a role. Tendinitis usually develops insidiously, after repetitive stresses during prolonged jumping or running. Patients complain initially of localized burning pain *during or after* activity, such as walking—especially when pushing off on the toes. With time, this progresses to more protracted pain, and, eventually, pain at rest. On exam, there may be tenderness along the tendon. Yet, wear-and-tear degeneration of the tendon (i.e., *tendinosis*) may be entirely asymptomatic.

278. What are the physical findings of Achilles tendinitis?

On palpation, there may be swelling of the tendon sheath (diffuse or at midpoint—i.e., at the Achilles bursa), with nodularity, tenderness, and possibly crepitation. There also may be tenderness where the tendon inserts into the calcaneus (retroachilles bursa). Finally, there may be tendon pain upon passive dorsiflexion of the foot or active plantar flexion (standing on toes).

279. What is Achilles tendon bursitis?

It is an inflammation of the bursae associated with the calcaneal insertion of the Achilles tendon: (1) the *retrocalcaneal* (which is anterior to the tendon, deeply sandwiched between the distal part of the Achilles and the calcaneus) and (2) the *tendocalcaneal* (i.e., Achilles' bursa), which is instead superficial, between the posterior aspect of the tendon and the skin. Both bursae limit the friction of the tendon, and both, if inflamed, may cause posterior heel pain. This may be severe enough to cause limping. The patient also may complain of noticeable redness, warmth, and swelling (often referred to as "pump bump," from the infamous high-heeled shoes—or "pumps").

280. What are the causes of this bursitis?

In addition to bad footwear, rheumatologic conditions also can predispose to bursitis. These include gout, rheumatoid arthritis, and seronegative spondyloarthropathies.

281. What about tendon *tear*?

An Achilles tendon rupture is usually a very dramatic event, often accompanied by an audible *snap* and by the sensation of being violently kicked in the calf. It is typical of older recreational athletes (i.e., "weekend warriors"), whose tendon has undergone degenerative changes that cause it to snap after a sudden eccentric force is applied to a dorsiflexed foot.

282. **What is the presentation of an Achilles tendon tear?**
The patient is unable to run, climb stairs, or plantarflex the ankle or foot (i.e., stand on toes). There is pain, tenderness, ecchymosis, and swelling along the entire gastrocnemius-soleus musculotendinous unit. In patients with *complete rupture,* there is a palpable gap in the Achilles tendon, 2–6 cm above its insertion. To better differentiate complete from incomplete tear, perform a *Thompson test*: with the patient prone and the knee flexed, squeeze the calf proximally to the affected area. The test is negative if it achieves a passive plantar flexion of the foot, suggesting that the Achilles tendon is at least partially intact. If it achieves no ankle motion whatsoever, then the test is positive, and the tendineal rupture is complete. The hyperdorsiflexion sign also may help: with the patient prone and both knees flexed to 90 degrees, maximally dorsiflex both ankles, and compare the injured to the uninjured side.

283. **What is the plantar fascia?**
It is the dense band of tissue that fans out from the anteromedial border of the calcaneus (medial calcaneal tuberosity), providing support for the medial longitudinal arch of the foot. Since the fascia has no elastic properties, repetitive stretching will result in microtears and inflammation. One half of patients also may have spurs. Contrary to popular belief, these do not cause pain per se. In fact, it is the chronic inflammation of the torn fascia that causes the pain. The spurs are more a *result* than a cause of the fasciitis.

284. **What is *plantar fasciitis*? What is its presentation?**
Plantar fasciitis is the most common cause of pain on the bottom of the heel. In fact, pain is on the plantar aspect of the *calcaneus*, dull and similar to that of a toothache. It typically starts upon standing or walking or running. It is usually most prominent with the first morning steps, possibly decreasing as activity progresses, but only to return after a period of rest is followed by resumption of activity. Pain resolves with rest (since this allows contraction of the plantar fascia [i.e., plantar *flexion*]), but restarts as soon as the first *dorsi*flexion step of the day restretches the irritated fascia. Although typically at the heel, pain also may radiate throughout the bottom of the foot and toward the toes. On exam, there is calcaneal tenderness at the midpoint of the plantar surface, but no tenderness with medial-to-lateral heel compression (which would otherwise suggest a stress fracture or osteomyelitis). There also may be heel tenderness with dorsiflexion of the foot or great toe, resolving with plantar flexion of the foot (since this relaxes the fascia). Edema is usually mild. There also may be a radiographic spur at the attachment of the plantar fascia, although this is not the pain's cause (*see* question 283).

285. **What are the causes of plantar fasciitis?**
Repetitive stretching of a tight plantar fascial band, leading to microtears at its calcaneal origin, and chronic inflammation. Hence, it is common in runners and dancers who use repetitive maximal plantar flexion of the ankle and dorsiflexion of the metatarsophalangeal joints. It is especially frequent when activity level is increased, or weight suddenly gained. It is also quite common in situations of prolonged weight-bearing, such as obese patients or policemen ("policeman's heel").

286. **What is *tarsal tunnel syndrome* (TTS)?**
It is to the ankle what carpal tunnel syndrome is to the wrist: an entrapment of the tibial nerve or its associated branches as they pass underneath the flexor retinaculum at the medial malleolus (Fig. 21-17). This leads to numbness, tingling, and pain along the posterior tibial nerve (medial plantar surface of the foot, from first toe to heel). It also may cause motor dysfunction, weakness, and atrophy.

287. What are the symptoms of tarsal tunnel syndrome?
The most common is a vague pain in the sole of the foot. Most patients describe this as burning or tingling. Pain and paresthesias radiate from the medial ankle distally and, occasionally, proximally. Symptoms are typically worsened by activity, especially standing and prolonged walking. They are instead reduced by rest. Findings include (1) *sensory disturbance* (ranging from sharp pain to loss of sensation), (2) *motor disturbance* (with

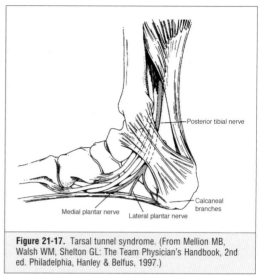

Figure 21-17. Tarsal tunnel syndrome. (From Mellion MB, Walsh WM, Shelton GL: The Team Physician's Handbook, 2nd ed. Philadelphia, Hanley & Belfus, 1997.)

resultant atrophy of intrinsic musculature), and (3) gait abnormality (overpronation, and a limp due to pain with weight-bearing). There also may be pain to palpation along the course of the nerve. If the condition deteriorates, the foot may become numb and weak. Tarsal tunnel syndrome can be demonstrated by tapping beneath the malleolus, which will reproduce (or worsen) the symptoms. In this regard, the *tarsal tunnel tap* is analogous to Tinel's sign in carpal tunnel syndrome.

288. What are the causes of tarsal tunnel syndrome?
They may be extrinsic and intrinsic. In fact, anything that creates pressure in the tarsal tunnel can cause TTS. Extrinsic causes include crush injury, stretch injury, fracture, dislocations of the ankle, and even varicose veins (that may or may not be visible). Intrinsic causes include instead space-occupying masses such as localized tumors or cysts, bony spurs, inflammation of the tendon sheath, nerve ganglions, a venous plexus within the tarsal canal, or simply swelling from a broken or sprained ankle. Note that TTS is more common in athletes, active individuals, or those who stand a lot, since all these people put more stress on the tarsal tunnel area. A *pes planus* (flat foot), also may cause an increase in pressure in the tunnel region, and thus result in nerve compression. The same can occur with excessive pronation or *pes cavus*. Finally, patients with lower back problems (L4, L5, and S1) may have TTS too. In fact, they may have a "Double Crush" issue: one due to the nerve pinch (or entrapment) in the lower back, and the second one in the tunnel area.

ACKNOWLEDGMENT

The author gratefully acknowledges the contributions of Bruce I. Hoffman, MD, to this chapter in the first edition of *Physical Diagnosis Secrets*.

SELECTED BIBLIOGRAPHY

1. Ad Hoc Committee: Guidelines for the initial evaluation of the adult patient with acute musculoskeletal symptoms. Arthritis Rheum 39:1–6, 1996.

2. Anderson AF, Lipscomb AB: Clinical diagnosis of meniscal tears. Description of a new manipulative test. Am J Sports Med 14:291–293, 1986.

3. Castro WHM, Jerosch J, Grossman TW: Examination and Diagnosis of Musculoskeletal Disorders. Clinical Examinations, Imaging Modalities. New York, Thieme, 2001.

4. Chaudhuri R, Salari R: Baker's cyst simulating deep vein thrombosis. Clin Radiol 41:400–404, 1990.

5. Cozen L: Tests for chronic back pain. Contemp Orthop 24:405–410, 1992.

6. D'Arcy CA, McGee S: Does this patient have carpal tunnel syndrome? JAMA 283:3110–3117, 2000.

7. Deville WL, van der Windt DA, Dzaferagic A: The test of Lasegue: Accuracy in herniated discs. Spine 25:1140–1147, 2000.

8. Hawkes CH: Diagnosis of functional neurological disease. Br J Hosp Med 57:373–377, 1997.

9. Jackson JL, O'Malley PG, Kroenke K: Evaluation of acute knee pain in primary care. Ann Intern Med 139:575–588, 2003.

10. Main CJ, Waddell G: Nonorganic signs. Spine 23:2367–2371, 1998.

11. Margo K, Drezner J, Motzkin D: Evaluation and management of hip pain. J Fam Pract 53:420, 2004.

12. Morton TG: Peculiar painful affection of fourth MTP articulation. Am J Med Sci 71:37, 1876.

13. Solomon DH, Simel DL, Bates DW, et al: The rational clinical examination. Does this patient have a torn meniscus or ligament of the knee? Value of the physical examination. JAMA 286:1610–1620, 2001.

14. Sugrue D, McEvoy M, Dempsey J, et al: Diabetic stiff hand syndrome. Ir J Med Sci 152:152–156, 1983.

15. Waddell G, McCulloch JA, Kummel E, et al: Nonorganic physical signs in low-back pain. Spine 5:117–125, 1980.

16. Wipf JE, Deyo RA: Low back pain. Med Clin North Am 79:232–246, 1995.

CHAPTER 22

THE EXTREMITIES AND PERIPHERAL VASCULAR EXAM

Salvatore Mangione, MD

> "In Medicine it is always necessary to start with the observation of the sick and to always return to this as this is the paramount means of verification. Observe methodically and vigorously without neglecting any exploratory procedure, using all that can be provided by physical examination."
>
> —Antoine B.J. Marfan

A. GENERALITIES

1. **What is the role of the extremities' exam?**
    Often examined last, the extremities can still provide important clues to the astute observer. You should focus on the *vascular, musculoskeletal,* and *sensorimotor* components of the limbs. In this chapter, we shall discuss the *vascular* evaluation and address the other two components in the musculoskeletal and neurologic chapters.

2. **Which arteries should be examined in the upper and lower extremities?**
    The major branches of the *brachial* and *femoral arteries* (Figs. 22-1 and 22-2)

3. **Which veins should be examined?**
    - For **lower extremities,** the tributaries of the saphenous system (draining into the femoral vein) (Fig. 22-3)
    - For **upper extremities,** the branches of the brachial veins (deep system) and of the basilic and cephalic veins (superficial system), both draining into the axillary vein (Fig. 22-4)

B. THE PERIPHERAL ARTERIES

(1) Asymmetric Pulses

4. **What causes a weaker and delayed pulse in the left arm as compared to the right?**
    It depends on the patient's age: in younger individuals, it is usually *coarctation,* in the elderly, it is instead an atherosclerotic obstruction or a dissection of the aorta. Depending on the level of obstruction, asymmetry and delay in pulses may only affect the *lower* extremities. Hence, the need to examine *all* peripheral pulses, especially in symptomatic or hypertensive patients.
    A pulse asymmetry can be confirmed by comparing systolic pressure of the two arms or by comparing that of lower extremities to upper extremities.

(2) Raynaud's Phenomenon

5. **What is Raynaud's phenomenon?**
    An exquisite sensitivity of hands and fingers to cold, but also to smoking and emotional stress. Upon exposure to the trigger, fingers exhibit a typical "triple response," which very appropriately for Raynaud follows the colors of the French flag: initial *pallor* and blanching (white), followed by

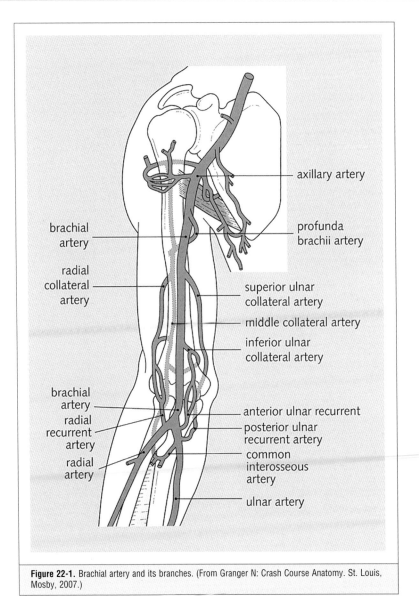

Figure 22-1. Brachial artery and its branches. (From Granger N: Crash Course Anatomy. St. Louis, Mosby, 2007.)

cyanosis (blue), and finally by *rubro* (red). Eventually, the fingers slowly return to their baseline color. Numbness, tingling, or pain accompanies this response. The white-blue-red response may at times be out of sequence, with patients exhibiting a blue-white-red response or even single-color responses (only blue or white).

6. **What causes Raynaud's phenomenon?**
   A spasm of the digital arteries, resulting in ischemia of the fingers, with *pallor* at first and *cyanosis* later (due to increased oxygen extraction from trapped and noncirculating

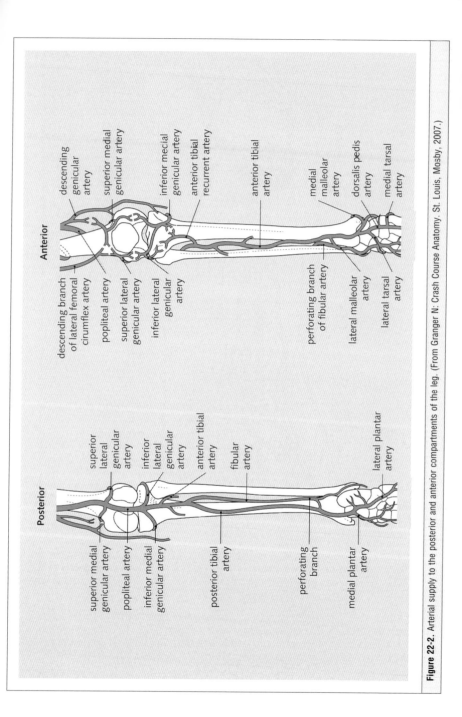

Figure 22-2. Arterial supply to the posterior and anterior compartments of the leg. (From Granger N: Crash Course Anatomy. St. Louis, Mosby, 2007.)

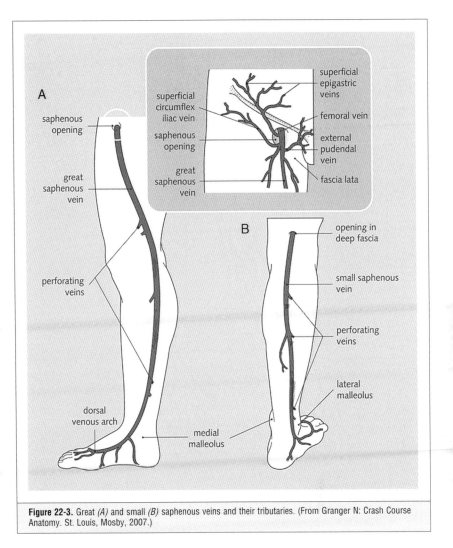

Figure 22-3. Great *(A)* and small *(B)* saphenous veins and their tributaries. (From Granger N: Crash Course Anatomy. St. Louis, Mosby, 2007.)

erythrocytes). The final stage of *redness* coincides with the reperfusion that follows release of the arterial spasm. This also is the phase mostly characterized by numbness or pain (a bit like the numbness and pain experienced in legs that have "fallen asleep"). Severe vasospasm may even lead to infarction and dry gangrene.

7. **How can Raynaud's phenomenon be artificially triggered?**
   By immersing the patient's hand in a bucket of iced water.

8. **What is the clinical significance of Raynaud's phenomenon?**
   It can precede several important disorders, including:
   - **Connective tissue diseases** (systemic lupus erythematosus [SLE], mixed connective tissue disease, rheumatoid arthritis, dermatomyositis, and polymyositis, but especially *progressive systemic sclerosis*, which is present in 17–28% of patients with Raynaud's)

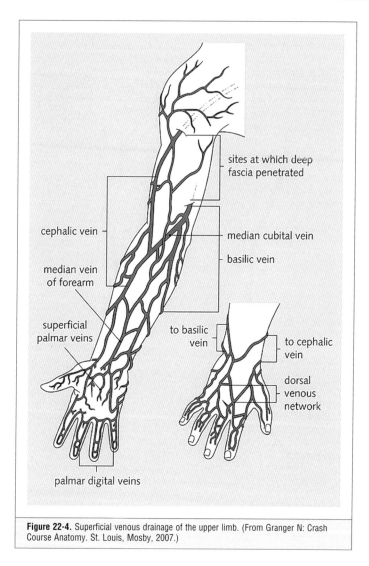

Figure 22-4. Superficial venous drainage of the upper limb. (From Granger N: Crash Course Anatomy. St. Louis, Mosby, 2007.)

- **Hematologic disorders** (cryoglobulinemia, polycythemia, monoclonal gammopathy)
- **Arterial compression syndromes** (thoracic outlet and carpal tunnel syndromes)
- **Vasculitis and atherosclerotic arterial disease**
- **Various drugs and toxins**
- **Recurrent trauma** (use of percussion or vibratory tools)
- **Miscellaneous disorders** (hypothyroidism, reflex sympathetic dystrophy, primary pulmonary hypertension, Prinzmetal angina, acromegaly, Addison's disease). Still, one of five patients with Raynaud's does not seem to have any underlying disorder (i.e., Raynaud's *disease*).

9. **Who was Raynaud?**
   Maurice Raynaud (1834–1881) was one of the great 19th-century French physicians. The son of a university professor, he graduated in Paris at age 28 with a thesis describing his famous

syndrome, which made him an instant celebrity. An excellent clinician and a beloved teacher, he also was passionately interested in literature, history, and the arts. In fact, all his life he sought the chair of Medical History at the University of Paris, but he died before this could come through. His contributions to medical knowledge included the book *Medicine in Molière's Time* and an article on the Greek physician Asclepiades of Bithynia (an opponent of Hippocratic medicine and the unrivaled authority of his times, who treated celebrities like Cicero, Crassus, and Marc Antony). In 1881, Raynaud wrote an address to the International Medical Congress of London titled "Skepticism in Medicine, Past and Present," but died before delivering it.

(3) Allen's Test

10. **What is Allen's test? What does it mean?**
    It is a bedside test for patency of the deep palmar arch and of *radial/ulnar* arteries (Fig. 22-5). Hence, a good way to learn about the risks of radial artery puncture and/or cannulation.
    - Compress the patient's radial artery until blood flow is stopped.
    - Have the patient clench and unclench the hand several times in sequence until there is a visible *blanching of the hand*.
    - When the patient finally relaxes the hand, there will be visible refilling of the capillary bed from the ulnar side, with return of the normal pink color within 5 seconds.
    - *Absence of refilling* (the pallor persists in spite of the hand's relaxation) or *delay in refilling* (return of the color takes longer than 5 seconds) indicates a positive test. This reflects occlusion of either the ulnar artery or the deep palmar arch.
    - Repeat the maneuver on the contralateral hand, comparing size of the refill area and length of refill time.
    - Finally, repeat the entire sequence, but this time compress the *ulnar* arteries, first on the right and then on the left.

11. **Isn't the test conducted by simultaneously compressing the ulnar and radial arteries?**
    Yes, it may be. This is, in fact, a variant of the Allen's test, conducted as follows (*see* Fig. 22–5):
    - Compress both the radial *and* ulnar arteries.
    - Ask the patient to sequentially and vigorously clench/unclench the hand, so as to squeeze all blood out. When the palm finally blanches, ask the patient to relax the hand.
    - Release pressure only on the ulnar artery, and measure the time it takes for the palm to regain its color. This is the refill time *for the ulnar artery*.
    - If refill is *delayed* or *absent* (*see* question 12), do not attempt a radial puncture, but consider instead either a brachial stick or an arterial puncture on the contralateral hand (after similarly checking the arterial supply, of course).
    - Repeat the test, but this time release pressure on the *radial* artery only, thus measuring refill time *for that vessel only*.

12. **How do you report the results of an Allen's test?**
    By indicating (1) the *name* and *side* of the artery compressed (for example, RR for right radial) and (2) refill time expressed in seconds. Thus a RR5/RU3 means that it took 5 seconds to refill the capillary bed of the right palm after releasing the right radial artery, and 3 seconds after releasing the right ulnar artery. Arteries with >15 seconds refill time should not be cannulated. Instead, the contralateral hand should be instrumented.

13. **Who was Allen?**
    Edgar V. Allen (1900–1961) was an American physician. A native of Nebraska and a graduate of that state's university, Dr. Allen eventually moved to the Mayo Clinic, where in 1947, he became professor of medicine. His contributions include the clinical use of coumarin anticoagulants and a landmark textbook of peripheral vascular diseases.

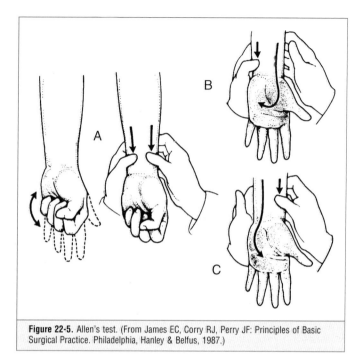

Figure 22-5. Allen's test. (From James EC, Corry RJ, Perry JF: Principles of Basic Surgical Practice. Philadelphia, Hanley & Belfus, 1987.)

(4) Peripheral Vascular Disease

14. **Can peripheral pulses be absent in normal individuals?**
    Yes. *Dorsalis pedis* and *tibialis posterior* are undetectable in 10% of healthy subjects. Congenital loss of one of the arteries usually leads to compensatory increases in the other. Still, only fewer than 2% of healthy subjects lack *both* pedal pulses. Hence, this is usually an important clue to the presence of peripheral vascular disease (*see* question 16).

15. **What is peripheral vascular disease (PVD)?**
    An obstructive condition of the lower extremity arteries, also referred to as *peripheral arterial disease*. Usually caused by atherosclerosis, it affects 8–12 million Americans, with a steadily growing incidence. Although one half of all patients never experience symptoms, the condition represents a risk marker for many other diseases, such as diabetes, hypertension, coronary artery disease, cerebrovascular disease, and aneurysms. Hence, PVD patients have a fourfold to sixfold increase in cardiovascular mortality.

16. **What are the symptoms of PVD?**
    Mostly symptoms of arterial insufficiency, such as exertional limb weakness, resting limb pain (or paresthesia), and poor healing of sores or ulcerations. The classic symptom, however, is *claudication* (from the Latin term for *limping*)—i.e., intermittent limb pain, usually triggered by activity. This affects different parts of the lower extremity, depending on which artery is compromised. Yet, whether obstruction is *high* or *low*, *both* pedal pulses are absent in PVD, an important diagnostic clue (*see* Table 22-1).

17. **What are the physical findings of PVD?**
    (1) *Decreased or absent pulses* (as previously indicated); (2) *atrophic changes in the foot* (such as loss of hair, discoloration of skin, decreased warmth, impaired nail growth, pallor following

TABLE 22-1. SYMPTOMS OF PERIPHERAL VASCULAR DISEASE

Above the Knee

PVD of the *distal aorta* (from below the renal arteries to the common iliacs) will cause claudication of the buttocks, thigh, and calf. It may even compromise erection. Given its high location, all lower extremity pulses will be lost.

Femoropopliteal

PVD will cause *calf* claudication. Femoral pulses are present, but those beyond are absent.

Below the Knee

Peroneotibial PVD will cause either no symptoms or foot claudication. Only pedal pulses are lost. Except for patients with diabetes and thromboangiitis obliterans, this is the least common form of the disease.

elevation, and rubor following dependency); (3) *vascular bruits* (over the involved artery—iliac, femoral, or popliteal); and (4) *increased venous filling time*.

18. **Can these findings predict severity of the disease?**
    No. Vascular bruits and other signs only indicate *presence* of disease; they do not correlate with severity. For severity, the standard assessment is the *ankle-to-arm systolic pressure index* (*see* Chapter 2, questions 117–119). Still, in diabetic patients with significantly abnormal ankle–brachial indexes, the following symptoms/signs predict more severe disease: (1) age greater than 65, (2) history of peripheral vascular disease or claudication in less than one block, (3) diminished foot pulses, and (4) venous filling time longer than 20 seconds.

19. **What is an increased *venous filling time*?**
    It is the abnormally slow (re)filling of foot veins in peripheral vascular disease. To test for it:
    1. Ask the patient to lie supine.
    2. Identify a prominent vein on top of the foot, and then *empty it* by raising the patient's leg to 45 degrees for 1 minute.
    3. Ask the patient to sit up and lower the foot over the edge of the examining table.
    4. Measure how many seconds it takes the vein to become turgid and visible again. Refill time >20 seconds is abnormal.

20. **What is a *capillary refill time* (CRT)?**
    A generally accepted bedside method for assessing peripheral perfusion. To test for it:
    1. Compress the patient's skin for 5 seconds (usually over a digit—in cases of the lower extremity, compress the plantar skin of the distal great toe) and with sufficient pressure to cause blanching.
    2. Release compression, and measure the time in seconds for the compressed area to regain the color of the surrounding skin. More than 2 seconds for the upper extremities (and 5 seconds for the great toe) are considered abnormal.
    Still, these figures have little scientific foundation. In fact, CRT is often longer in women, the elderly, a cold environment, and poor ambient lighting. Hence, a normal CRT indicates good peripheral perfusion, but a *prolonged* one must be interpreted in view of other parameters, such as sex, age, blood pressure, heart rate, cardiac output, and level of consciousness.

21. **What is the Buerger's test?**
   Another bedside maneuver for assessing arterial perfusion to the leg. It consists of examining the color of the patient's leg: first when elevated and then when lowered. Hence, it consists of two stages (Table 22-2). The test is considered positive for PVD when it elicits excessive pallor with *elevation* and intense *rubor with dependency.*

TABLE 22-2. BUERGER'S TEST	
Stage I	**Stage II**
1. Ask the patient to lie supine.	1. Then ask the patient to sit up, and lower the leg over the edge of the examining table—also at an angle of 90 degrees, and also for 2 minutes.
2. Elevate both legs to an angle of 90 degrees, and hold them up for 2 minutes.	2. Gravity aids blood flow, so that color eventually returns to the ischemic leg, although the skin usually turns blue first (as blood is deoxygenated in its passage through the ischemic tissue), and then finally acquires a dusky red flush that spreads proximally from the toes as the post-hypoxic vasodilation takes place.
3. Observe the feet. Pallor indicates ischemia (i.e., the inability of peripheral arterial pressure to overcome gravity).	3. Examine both legs simultaneously because changes are most obvious when one leg has a normal circulation.
4. The poorer the arterial supply, the less the angle to which the legs have to be raised in order to become pale (this was what Buerger originally described as the "angle of circulatory sufficiency").	

22. **How accurate is physical examination for diagnosing PVD?**
   McGee and Boyko compared various findings to the gold standard of *ankle-to-arm systolic pressure index (AASPI)* and found the following signs to be useful and independent predictors of PVD: (1) abnormal pedal pulses, (2) femoral arterial bruit, (3) prolonged venous filling time, and (4) unilateral limb coolness. These also were independent of age, atherosclerosis risk factors, sex, and claudication. Other traditional findings, such as trophic changes of the nails and skin and prolonged capillary refill time, were instead less useful.

23. **Is there any finding that argues against the presence of PVD?**
   Bilateral presence of pedal pulses. Still, beware that as many as one third of PVD patients may have palpable pedal pulses (*see* question 25).

24. **How accurate is physical examination for diagnosing the *distribution* of PVD?**
   Quite accurate. More specifically, findings can predict different levels of obstruction (Table 22-3). Thus, abnormal pedal pulses, a femoral arterial bruit, prolonged venous filling time, and a unilateral cool limb predict the *presence* of vascular disease. Abnormal femoral pulse, iliac bruits, limb bruit, Buerger's test, and warm knees predict instead its *distribution.* Moreover:

TABLE 22-3. PHYSICAL DIAGNOSIS OF THE DISTRIBUTION OF PVD			
Pathology/Obstruction	Finding	Sensitivity	Specificity
Arterial stenosis (of any kind)	Limb bruit	80%	75%
Aortoiliac	Diminished femoral pulse	39%	99%
	Iliac bruits	28%	87%
Distal to adductor canal	Positive Buerger's test	100%	54%
Femoral, at adductor hiatus	Warm knees	73%	75%

- Normal femoral pulses at the level of the inguinal ligament and diminished or absent pulses distally suggest infrainguinal disease alone.
- Loss of femoral pulse just below the inguinal ligament suggests a proximal superficial femoral artery occlusion.
- Loss of popliteal pulse suggests superficial femoral artery occlusion, typically in the adductor canal.
- Loss of pedal pulses is characteristic of disease of the distal popliteal artery or its trifurcation.

25. **What are the limitations of physical exam in evaluating PVD?**
    - 30% of diseased arteries may be palpable. Yet pulses disappear with exercise.
    - Patent arteries may occasionally be nonpalpable. Yet although the dorsalis pedis may be undetectable in 10% of children, the tibialis posterior is absent in only 0.2% of subjects age 0–19. Hence, lack of *both* pedal pulses is a good predictor of PVD.
    - Diabetics may have arteries too stiff to compress, resulting in elevated AASPI.

(5) Diabetic Foot

26. **To what lower extremity complications are diabetics uniquely predisposed?**
    Mostly *infections* and *neuropathic* manifestations (such as ulcers and Charcot arthropathy), both resulting in longer hospitalization and higher mortality. In fact, the "diabetic foot" is the second most common cause (after trauma) for amputation.

27. **What are the predisposing factors?**
    Definitely *atherosclerotic disease*, not only of large and medium-sized arteries (aortoiliac and femoropopliteal), but also of infrapopliteal vessels, to which diabetics are uniquely prone. Still, the most important factor is *peripheral neuropathy*, with loss of muscular coordination and protective sensation, favoring mechanical stress during ambulation.

28. **How common is peripheral neuropathy in diabetics?**
    Very common. Prevalence is 25% after 10 years of disease and 50% after 20 years.

29. **What are the characteristics of this neuropathy?**
    A typical stocking-and-glove distribution, presenting initially with paresthesias (or dysesthesias), and eventually progressing to complete anesthesia. As a result of their inability to sense pressure, every year 2.2–5.9% of diabetics develop a *diabetic foot ulcer*. Especially afflicted are Latinos and Native Americans, among whom the disease is rampant. Hence, the need for early identification of patients at risk, since prompt and meticulous foot care reduces rates of lower extremity amputation by about 50–80%.

30. **What is the best way to recognize peripheral neuropathy in diabetics?**
Nerve conduction studies have long been the gold standard, but they can be time consuming, expensive, and impractical in primary care settings. Conversely, more traditional bedside screenings (loss of vibratory and position sense) are inaccurate, since many diabetics with neuropathy can still sense a cotton wisp, a pinprick, or a tuning fork. Loss of deep tendon reflexes (especially the ankle jerk), foot drop, and muscle atrophy can surely help the diagnostic process, but are often late events. Hence, the bedside standard is the *Semmes-Weinstein (SW) monofilament test,* which provides a simple and inexpensive tool for identifying patients at risk for diabetic ulcers.

31. **What is the Semmes-Weinstein (SW) monofilament test?**
A maneuver designed to test protective sensation in the foot. It measures patients' ability to sense light touch by using a nylon probe (the SW monofilament). This comes in three sizes (4.17, 5.07, and 6.1), which buckle respectively at a constant pressure of 1, 10, and 75-*g* force. Birke and Sims examined all three types in 28 patients with diabetes and 72 with Hansen's disease, and concluded that inability to sense a 10-*g* force pressure (exercised by a 5.07 filament) is a valid and independent predictor for the risk of foot ulceration. Hence, both the International Diabetes Federation and the World Health Organization recommend that 5.07/10-*g* SW monofilament tests are regularly carried out in diabetics.

32. **How is the test conducted?**
By having the patient lie supine with closed eyes, and then pressing the filament against a specific site of the foot, with just enough force to bend the wire for 1 second.

33. **When is the test considered positive for neuropathy?**
When the patient cannot feel the filament at $> 4/10$ sites. Yet there is no real consensus on how to best use the filaments, or even how to interpret the results. In fact, studies have often relied on a different number of testing sites (from 1 to 10) and different criteria for determining protective sensation. Not surprisingly, specificity and sensitivity also have differed. Still, a recent report by Lee et al. used SW monofilament tests on 10 sites, and then evaluated the diagnostic value of each site and their combinations. They found the test to be very sensitive and specific. More importantly, they found that sensitivity and specificity at the third and fifth metatarsal heads were comparable to those of 10 sites taken together. Hence, the inability to sense touch over the plantar aspects of third and fifth metatarsals has equivalent diagnostic value to that of sensing touch in more than four of the 10 traditional test sites (with sensitivity and specificity of 93.1% and 100%, respectively). Thus, a two-site SW monofilament test is as clinically valuable as a 10-site test in screening for diabetic neuropathy. Although limited in its ability to quantify the severity of the disease, this test is simple, cost effective, and practical.

34. **How do you separate an *ischemic* from a *neuropathic* (diabetic) foot ulcer?**
Both occur over toes and trauma sites (especially areas with diminished sensation in diabetics). Yet, neuropathic ulcers usually have a *callous rim*, no pain, and little gangrene. Instead, they have evidence of *neuropathy* (decreased sensation and absent ankle reflex), but not necessarily other signs of peripheral vascular disease.

35. **What about ulcers of chronic venous stasis?**
Their hallmarks are (1) *location* (perimalleolar area of the inner ankle) and (2) *chronic skin changes* (brown hyperpigmentation, stasis dermatitis with skin thickening, and induration). Venous ulcers are also rather painless, warm, and with no gangrene.

36. **What is the role of physical exam in a diabetic ulcer?**
In addition to being comprehensive (diabetes is, after all, a *systemic* disease), the exam should:
- Examine the *ulcer* per se and the general condition of the extremity.

- Assess the possibility of *vascular insufficiency*.
- Assess the possibility of *peripheral neuropathy*.

37. Where is a diabetic foot ulcer located?
It is typically located over one of the following sites:
- **Weight-bearing areas** (75% of all ulcers). These include the plantar surface of the metatarsal heads, tips of most prominent toes (usually the first or second), and tips of hammer toes. Heels and malleoli also may be affected as a result of recurrent trauma.
- **Stress-bearing areas,** such as the dorsal portion of hammer toes

Other findings of the diabetic foot include (1) hypertrophic calluses, especially over pressure points such as the heel, (2) brittle nails, (3) hammer toes, and (4) fissures.

38. What is Charcot's foot?
It is a neuropathic osteoarthropathy resulting from loss of both *sensation* (causing unrecognized microtrauma from ill-fitting shoes) and *motor control* (causing intrinsic muscle weakness and splaying of the foot on weight-bearing areas, thus compounding the trauma). The result is a convex foot with a rocker-bottom appearance, where small fractures remain unnoticed until bone and joint deformities become severe.

39. Which joints are most affected by Charcot's changes?
In addition to tarsometatarsal and metatarsophalangeal joints, Charcot's changes also can affect the *ankle*, causing displacement of the mortise. If neglected, calluses over pressure points will evolve into ulcerations, especially over the medial aspect of the navicular bone, the inferior aspect of the cuboid bone, and the ankle. Sinus tracts from ulcerations may then reach into the deeper planes of the foot and bone, thus leading to osteomyelitis, to which diabetics are also uniquely susceptible. Ulcers deeper than 3 mm and larger than 2 cm^2 are especially predisposed to this complication.

40. Are there any other causes of Charcot's foot?
In addition to *diabetes* (where it affects 2% of the population), a Charcot's foot also can occur in other peripheral neuropathies, including *tertiary syphilis* (which used to be the leading cause of this condition) and *Charcot-Marie-Tooth disease*.

C. THE PERIPHERAL VEINS

(1) Edema

41. What is edema of an extremity?
It is the swelling of a limb caused by accumulation of fluid. This could be *serum* (venous edema), *lymph* (lymphedema), or *fat* (lipedema, *see* Table 22-4).

42. What is "pitting"?
A well-defined depression in soft tissues resulting from application of pressure—something that separates it from the "brawny" edema of hypothyroidism, inflammation, and chronic venous stasis. "Pitting" is due to accumulation of interstitial fluid and thus predominantly localized (but not necessarily so) to dependent areas, like the pre-sacrum of supine patients or the shins of standing/sitting ones. The less viscous and protein-rich the fluid, the more likely the "pitting."

43. How do you elicit pitting edema?
By pressing your thumb for 1–2 seconds over the tibia, dorsum of each foot, and retromalleolar area. Pitting severity is graded from 1 to 4, with 4 being the highest.

44. **How do you grade pitting edema?**
As 1+ (mild pitting, slight indentation); 2+ (moderate pitting, indentation rapidly subsiding); 3+ (deep pitting— longer indentation, leg swollen); 4+ (very deep pitting, leg very swollen).

45. **How does *lymphedema* present? What are its causes?**
Primary lymphedema is bilateral, more common in women, and with onset before 40. *Secondary* lymphedema is instead unilateral, equal in both sexes, and usually occurring after infections (recurrent cellulitis), radiation, surgery, or cancer. These etiologies are all at play in lymphedema of the arm, almost exclusively seen in breast cancer patients as a result of tumor, treatment (surgery/radiation), or a combination thereof.

46. **What is the most common cause of neoplastic lymphedema in the lower extremities?**
Metastatic prostatic cancer in men and lymphoma in women.

47. **How can physical exam help in the diagnosis of edema?**
The most important finding for the interpretation of edema is the patient's venous pressure as assessed through *neck veins examination* (with distention arguing in favor of right ventricular or biventricular failure). Edema *per se* (i.e., without an assessment of central venous pressure) has little correlation with cardiac disease.

48. **How do you separate edema of deep venous thrombosis (DVT) from edema of congestive heart failure?**
DVT causes unilateral edema. Differential diagnosis includes Baker's cyst, cellulitis, and venous insufficiency.

(2) Venous Insufficiency

49. **What is the Trendelenburg's test?**
It is a test of *functionality of leg veins' valves*, first described by Sir Benjamin Brodie in 1846, almost 50 years before Trendelenburg's report (which is why the maneuver is still referred to as the Trendelenburg-Brodie test). To carry it out:
1. Raise the leg of a supine patient above the level of the heart, until the veins are completely empty and collapsed.
2. Apply a tourniquet to the mid-thigh, thereby compressing the greater saphenous vein and preventing it from draining blood.
3. Ask the patient to stand up, and closely observe the leg veins. In normal subjects, the greater saphenous vein will *slowly* refill from below the obstruction. This takes less than 1 minute and is due to unimpeded arterial flow in the face of obstructed venous drainage.
4. Release the tourniquet 60 seconds after standing.
5. Closely observe the leg veins for engorgement.

50. **How do you interpret the test?**
  - If the greater saphenous vein refills rapidly *before* the tourniquet is released, this indicates *backfilling* from incompetent valves of the communicating veins.
  - If the greater saphenous vein refills rapidly *after* the tourniquet is released, this indicates *backfilling* from incompetent valves of the greater saphenous vein itself.
  - Patients with arterial insufficiency may have a false negative test.

51. **Can the saphenous vein serve as a manometer of intra-abdominal pressure?**
Yes. If the saphenous vein has incompetent valves, it may *also* function as an intra-abdominal pressure monitor. Hence, it is to the belly what the internal jugular is to the right atrium. This monitoring function can be carried out by raising the leg at various angles, and then

TABLE 22-4. TYPES OF EDEMA AND THEIR CHARACTERISTICS

	Venous Edema	Low-Protein Edema	Lymphedema	Lipedema	Inflammatory Edema
Pitting	Easy with 1–2 sec pressure Resolves within 2–3 seconds after pressure is released	Easy with 1–2 sec pressure Resolves within 2–3 seconds after pressure is released	Only early in the course. Later on it becomes hard and brawny due to inflammatory and fibrotic changes	No	Only early in the course. Later on it becomes hard and brawny as a result of fibrotic and inflammatory changes
Protein content in edema fluid	Low to normal	Low	High	—	High
Serum albumin	<3.5 g/dL	<3.5 g/dL	>3.5 g/dL	>3.5 g/dL	>3.5 g/dL
Pain	No	No	No	No	Yes
Mechanism	Increased venous pressure (either centrally or locally)	Decreased oncotic pressure	Accumulation of lymph from disruption of lymphatic drainage	Accumulation of fat	Increased vascular permeability
Cause(s)	Biventricular failure Right ventricular failure Venous insufficiency (including side effects of calcium-channel blockers)	Protein-losing enteropathy Malnutrition Cirrhosis Nephrosis	"Primary" (i.e., congenital abnormality of the lymphatic systems) "Secondary" (i.e., damage to lymphatics from infection, radiation, surgery and cancer)	Obesity (especially in women)	Cellulitis

Continued

TABLE 22-4. TYPES OF EDEMA AND THEIR CHARACTERISTICS—CONT'D

	Venous Edema	Low-Protein Edema	Lymphedema	Lipedema	Inflammatory Edema
Gravity-dependent	Yes	Yes, but not necessarily	No	Involves legs but spares feet	No
Diurnal variations	Yes	Yes, but not necessarily	No	No	No
Central venous pressure	Increased	Normal	Normal	Normal	Normal
Neck veins	Distended if mechanism of edema is increased central venous pressure Normal in cases of peripheral venous insufficiency	Normal	Normal	Normal	Normal

studying the level of the column of blood in the saphenous vein both at baseline and after maneuvers that increase abdominal pressure (like coughing or straining).

52. How do you check for presence of *communicating veins*?

By using another maneuver devised by Trendelenburg. This consists of applying a tourniquet on the saphenous vein while the patient is still supine and the varicose veins are engorged. The leg is then raised high above the level of the heart, and varicosities are closely monitored. If they gradually disappear, this indicates that there is a communication between the saphenous and the deep veins, that the valves of these communicating veins are competent, and that the deep venous system is patent. Conversely, if the veins remain engorged, this indicates either occlusion of the deep venous system or absence of the communicating veins.

53. What is the Trendelenburg's *position*?

Originally, it was a supine position on the operating table, with the bed inclined at such an angle that the pelvis was always higher than the head. The Trendelenburg's position is still used during (and after) pelvic operations. It also is used for shock, to redirect blood from legs and abdomen into chest and brain. Since these patients are acutely ill, Trendelenburg's position is often referred to as "the Titanic position."

54. Who was Trendelenburg?

Friedrich Trendelenburg (1844–1924) was the son of a well-known German philosopher. After studying in Glasgow and Edinburgh, he taught vascular surgery in his native Berlin, and then Rostok, Bonn, and, ultimately, Leipzig, where he stayed as surgeon-in-chief until retiring in 1911. An innovator in his field and the founder of the German Surgical Society, Trendelenburg developed the position that still carries his name in order to operate on the pelvis. He experimented, however, in many other areas. For example, he devised a new surgery for varicose veins—hence, the aforementioned Trendelenburg's test(s). He even attempted a pulmonary embolectomy in 1907, yet the first successful embolectomy was not performed until 1924, by one of his former students, Dr. Martin Kirshner (1924 also was the year of Trendelenburg's death, of carcinoma of the mandible). His many interests included a passion for medical history, which prompted him to write a book on ancient Indian surgery, and even an autobiography. Trendelenburg's name is linked not only to the *test(s)* and *position*, but also to the eponymous *sign* and *gait* (*see* Chapter 21, questions 176–179).

55. What is Perthes' test?

Another bedside test of varicose veins, devised by another German surgeon (Georg C. Perthes, the same of Calvé-Legg-Perthes disease fame). It is aimed at determining patency of the deep venous system and competence of the saphenous and communicating veins' valves. It is carried out by placing a tourniquet around the mid-thigh of a standing patient whose leg veins are fully engorged. The patient is then asked to walk for 5 minutes, and the veins are reexamined.

- If the veins below the tourniquet *collapse* as a result of walking, then the deep venous system is patent, and the valves of the communicating veins are competent.
- If the veins below the tourniquet *remain unchanged,* then the valves of *both* the saphenous veins, and the communicating veins are incompetent.
- If the veins below the tourniquet *get more engorged* (and the patient experiences leg pain), then the deep venous system is occluded, and the communicating veins are incompetent.

Perthes' test is based on the "milking" effect that muscle compression exercises on the greater saphenous vein. As a result, walking squeezes blood from the saphenous veins into the communicating system and from there into the deep veins.

56. What is the role of palpation in assessing varicose veins of the saphenous system?

It can provide confirmation of the presence of incompetent valves. To do so, place the fingers of one hand over the engorged saphenous vein (below the knee) while at the same time tapping gently with the other hand the same vein a foot cephalad (above the knee). Valve incompetence results in transmission of the impulse *downward* and *backwards*.

(3) Deep Venous Thrombosis

57. **What is the role of physical exam for diagnosing DVT?**
   It is part of a comprehensive approach, including review of risk factors and symptoms.
   - Commonly reported *symptoms* in suspected DVT include leg pain and swelling.
   - *Risk factors* include instead immobility, paralysis, recent surgery, and/or trauma, malignancy, cancer chemotherapy, advancing age (i.e., >60 years), family history of thromboembolism, pregnancy, and estrogen use. In 50% of DVT patients, a major risk factor is present. Some of these are *major*, whereas others are *minor*. These can then be used to calculate the likelihood of disease (Table 22-5).

58. **What are the traditional physical findings of DVT? How valuable are they?**
   Based on traditional teaching, the physical exam of patients with suspected DVT should include: (1) careful inspection of the leg (looking for pitting edema, warmth, dilated superficial veins, and

---

TABLE 22-5. DIAGNOSIS OF DEEP VENOUS THROMBOSIS (DVT)

Major Criteria

- Active cancer (ongoing treatment, treatment within previous 6 months. or palliative treatment)
- Paralysis, bedridden >3 days, and/or major surgery within 4 weeks
- Localized tenderness along the distribution of the deep venous system in the calf or thigh
- Thigh and calf swelling (should be measured)
- Calf swelling by >3 cm compared with asymptomatic leg (as measured 10 cm below the tibial tuberosity)
- Strong family history of DVT (>2 first-degree relatives with history of DVT)

Minor Criteria

- History of recent trauma (to symptomatic leg within 60 days or less)
- Pitting edema in symptomatic leg only
- Dilated superficial veins (nonvaricose) in symptomatic leg only
- Hospitalization within previous 6 months
- Erythema

Scoring Method

- *High probability:* three or more major criteria with no alternative diagnosis, two or more major and two or more minor criteria with no alternative diagnosis
- *Low probability:* one major criterion and two or more minor criteria with alternative diagnosis; one major criterion and one or more minor criteria with no alternative diagnosis; no major criteria and three or more minor criteria with alternative diagnosis; no major and two or more minor criteria with no alternative diagnosis
- *Moderate probability:* All other combinations

(Adapted from Anand S, Wells P, Hunt D, et al: Does this patient have deep vein thrombosis? JAMA 279:1094–1099, 1998.)

erythema); (2) measurement of leg circumference; (3) appreciation of a palpable cord; and (4) elicitation of Homans' sign (development of calf pain following the forceful and abrupt dorsiflexion of the foot). Yet, all these signs/maneuvers are quite inaccurate. Tenderness, swelling, warmth, and redness of the limb cannot adequately separate patients with or without DVT. In fact, warmth and color of the skin reflect superficial, rather than deep, circulation. A "palpable cord" is also indicative of *superficial* thrombophlebitis—which has no relationship to the deep vein system. Finally, skin changes, pitting edema, and dilated superficial veins may all be caused by other processes, such as venous insufficiency, leg trauma, cellulitis, obstructive lymphadenopathy, superficial venous thrombosis, postphlebitic syndrome, or a Baker (popliteal) cyst—a distended gastrocnemius-semimembranosus bursa that has ruptured into the calf, thus creating a perimalleolar crescent-shaped ecchymosis (*pseudothrombophlebitis*). And as for Homans' sign, it has a low sensitivity and poor specificity.

59. **How accurate is physical exam for DVT?**
    Not much. Given the previously discussed constraints, the sensitivity is only 60–88%, and the specificity 30–72%. In fact, the only important signs of DVT are *tenderness* and *swelling. Calf asymmetry < 2 cm* (when measured 5 cm below the tibial tuberositas) also is abnormal and, if new, argues for DVT until proven otherwise.

60. **What should then be the approach to a patient with suspected DVT?**
    Because of the low sensitivity and specificity of clinical exam, many authors have tried to either combine various signs and symptoms (like the Wells' scoring system for DVT) or have recommended exclusive reliance on noninvasive tests. Still, *five findings* seem to be independently and significantly associated with the presence of proximal DVT: (1) swelling below the knee, (2) swelling above the knee, (3) recent immobility, (4) cancer, and (5) fever. Overall, the sensitivity of a positive clinical examination (associated with the presence of one or more of these independent predictors) is 96%, although the specificity is still low (20%). The absence of any of these findings is associated with a less than 5% chance of proximal DVT. Conversely, the presence of two or more of these clinical findings is associated with a 46% chance of proximal DVT.

61. **In summary, what is the role of bedside examination for the evaluation of DVT?**
    Still an important one. Although individual symptoms and signs are *not,* by themselves, very useful, a careful review of risk factors, symptoms, and signs may nonetheless help determine the *pretest probability of disease*. And thus, it can guide interpretation of noninvasive diagnostic tests. This rekindled value of clinical examination has in recent time led to the hypothesis that when pretest probability of disease and noninvasive tests of lower extremity veins are *concordant*, DVT can be effectively ruled in or ruled out, whereas when pretest probability of disease and noninvasive tests are *discordant*, further evaluation is necessary. This approach has led to the creation of a clinical prediction guide for the management of patients with suspected DVT

62. **Who was Homans?**
    John Homans (1877–1954) was an American surgeon who worked with Harvey Cushing at Hopkins, and eventually became professor of Surgery at Peter Bent Brigham. His interest in peripheral vascular disease led to a monograph on the subject in 1939. He also wrote a very successful surgery textbook based on his Harvard course. Still, he did not name his sign after himself and in fact later in life tried to distance himself from it.

SELECTED BIBLIOGRAPHY

1. Allen EV, Hines EA: Lipedema of the legs: A syndrome characterized by fat legs and orthostatic edema. Proc Mayo Clin 15:184–187, 1940.

2. Anand S, Wells P, Hunt D, et al: Does this patient have deep vein thrombosis? JAMA 279:1094–1099, 1998.

3. Baker WH, String ST, Hayes AC, et al: Diagnosis of peripheral occlusive disease: Comparison of clinical evaluation and noninvasive laboratory. Arch Surg 113:1308–1310, 1978.

4. Birke JA, Sims DS: Plantar sensory threshold in the ulcerative foot. Leprosy Review 57:261–267, 1986.

5. Blankfield RP, Finkelhor RS, Alexander JJ, et al: Etiology and diagnosis of bilateral leg edema in primary care. Ann J Med 105:192–197, 1998.

6. Carter SA: Response of ankle systolic pressure to leg exercise in mild or questionable arterial disease. N Engl J Med 287:578–582, 1972.

7. Carter SA: Arterial auscultation in peripheral vascular disease. JAMA 246:1682–1686, 1981.

8. Christenson JH, Freundlich M, Jacobsen BA, et al: Clinical relevance of pedal pulse palpation in patients suspected of peripheral arterial insufficiency. J Intern Med 226:95–99, 1989.

9. Cranley JJ, Canos AJ, Sull WI: The diagnosis of deep venous thrombosis: Fallibility of clinical signs. Arch Surg 111:34–36, 1976.

10. Criado E, Burnham CB: Predictive value of clinical criteria for the diagnosis of deep vein thrombosis. Surgery 122:578–583, 1997.

11. Criqui MH, Fronek A, Klauber MR, et al: The sensitivity, specificity, and predictive value of traditional clinical evaluation of peripheral arterial disease: Results from noninvasive testing in defined population. Circulation 71:516–522, 1985.

12. DeWeese JA: Pedal pulses disappearing with exercise: A test for intermittent claudication. N Engl J Med 262:1214–1217, 1960.

13. Hall S, Littlejohn GO, Brand C, et al: The painful swollen calf: A comparative evaluation of four investigative techniques. Med J Austr 144:356–358, 1986.

14. Henry JA, Altmann P: Assessment of hypoproteinaemic oedema: A simple physical sign. Br Med J 1:890–891, 1978.

15. Homans J: Exploration and division of the femoral and iliac veins in the treatment of thrombophlebitis of the leg. N Engl J Med 224:179–186, 1941.

16. Insall RL, Davies RJ, Prout WG: Significance of Buerger's test in the assessment of lower limb ischaemia. J R Soc Med 82:729–731, 1989.

17. Katz RS, Zizic TM, Arnold WP, et al: The pseudothrombophlebitis syndrome. Medicine 56:151–164, 1977.

18. Kraag G, Thevathasan EM, Gordon DA, et al: The hemorrhagic crescent sign of acute synovial rupture. Ann Intern Med 85:477–478, 1976.

19. Landefeld CS, McGuire E, Cohen AM: Clinical findings associated with acute proximal deep vein thrombosis: A basis for quantifying clinical judgment. Am J Med 88:382–388, 1990.

20. Lee S, Kim H, Choi S, et al: Clinical usefulness of the two-site Semmes-Weinstein monofilament test for detecting diabetic peripheral neuropathy. J Kor Med Sci 18:103–107, 2003.

21. McGee S, Boyko EL: Physical examination and chronic lower-extremity ischemia: A critical review. Arch Intern Med 158:1357–1364, 1998.

22. McNeely MJ, Boyko EJ, Ahroni JH, et al: The independent contributions of diabetic neuropathy and vasculopathy in foot ulceration. Diabetes Care 18:216–219, 1995.

23. Molloy W, English J, O'Dwyer R, et al: Clinical findings in the diagnosis of proximal deep vein thrombosis. Ir Med 175:119–120, 1982.

24. Mueller MI: Identifying patients with diabetes mellitus who are at risk for lower-extremity complications: Use of Semmes-Weinstein monofilaments. Phys Ther 76:68–71, 1996.

25. Parfrey N, Ryan JF, Shanahan L, et al: Hairless lower limbs and occlusive arterial disease. Lancet 1:276, 1976.

26. Robertson GSM, Ristic CD, Bullen BR: The incidence of congenitally absent foot pulses. Ann R Coll Surg Engl 72:99–100, 1990.

27. Silverman JJ: The incidence of palpable dorsalis pedis and posterior tibial pulsations in soldiers: An analysis of over 1000 infantry soldiers. Am Heart J 32:82–87, 1946.

28. Stein PD, Henry JW, Gopalakrishnan D, et al: Asymmetry of calves in the assessment of patients with suspected acute pulmonary embolism. Chest 107:936–939, 1995.

29. Valk GD, Nauta JJ, Strijers RL, et al: Clinical examination versus neurophysiological examination in the diagnosis of diabetic polyneuropathy. Diab Med 9:716–721, 1992.

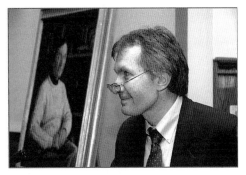

TOP 10+10 "SECRET" REASONS WHY IT IS GOOD TO BE A DOCTOR[1]

1. Because you get to see everyone naked.[2]

2. Because you can park your car on the sidewalk without getting a ticket.

3. Because it is the best excuse for illegible handwriting.

4. Because there is no beat like a heartbeat.

5. Because after working with patients you realize that you are not as neurotic as you thought you might have been.

6. Because you get to meet so many interesting people. For example, lawyers and lawyers and lawyers....

7. Because lots of people are dying to see you.

8. Because you can put your entire family on Valium.

9. Because even if no one sends you a Christmas present, the pharmaceutical companies certainly will.

10. Because the market is always booming. Even if we were eventually to run out of diseases, we could still rely on traffic.

11. Because it is so easy to avoid tedious social obligations. Just say, "I'm on call!"

12. Because you don't need to worry about purchasing a second home, since you'll hardly have time for the first one (same goes for the second significant other).

13. Because you can keep your Italian accent.

14. Because the human body is the same across the planet, although usually a bit thinner.

15. Because you are the first to know whether it will be a boy or a girl.

16. Because Mom and Dad will finally stop wishing for a doctor in the family.

17. Because you don't have to waste your time keeping up-to-date since your patients are dying to lecture you.

18. Because wearing a stethoscope around your neck increases your sex appeal.

19. Because you get to toy around with lots of fancy gadgets.

20. Because God heals and the Doctor collects the fee (B. Franklin).

And, finally, because *Doctor* means teacher, and so you can always fall back on a teaching career. Which sometimes comes with wonderful fringe benefits, like getting a free portrait, giving a Class Day speech, and writing a Physical Diagnosis textbook.

---

[1] By Sal Mangione and Eva Bosma. Written (but not used) for the *2006 Class Day* of Jefferson Medical College.
[2] This is also the number one reason why it's *not* good to be a doctor.

INDEX